LEARNING
CLINICAL REASONING

SECOND EDITION

LEARNING
CLINICAL REASONING

SECOND EDITION

Jerome P. Kassirer, M.D.

Distinguished Professor, Tufts University School of Medicine, Boston, Massachusetts
Visiting Professor, Stanford University, Stanford California
Editor-in-Chief Emeritus, *New England Journal of Medicine*
Physician Emeritus, Tufts Medical Center, Boston, Massachusetts

John B. Wong, M.D.

Professor of Medicine, Tufts University School of Medicine, Boston, Massachusetts
Chief, Clinical Decision-Making Division, Tufts Medical Center, Boston, Massachusetts

Richard I. Kopelman, M.D.

Endicott Professor of Medicine, Tufts University School of Medicine, Boston, Massachusetts
Vice Chairman of Medicine for Education, and Director, Internal Medicine House Staff Training Program
Tufts Medical Center, Boston, Massachusetts

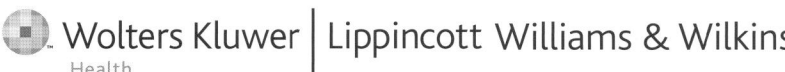
Wolters Kluwer | Lippincott Williams & Wilkins
Health

Philadelphia • Baltimore • New York • London
Buenos Aires • Hong Kong • Sydney • Tokyo

Acquisitions Editor: Susan Rhyner
Managing Editors: Jessica Heise and Jennifer Verbiar
Marketing Manager: Jennifer Kuklinski
Product Manager: Jennifer Verbiar
Senior Designer: Stephen Druding
Compositor: Aptara®, Inc.
Printer: RR Donnelley

351 West Camden Street
Baltimore, MD 21201

530 Walnut St.
Philadelphia, PA 19106

The publisher is not responsible (as a matter of product liability, negligence, or otherwise) for any injury resulting from any material contained herein. This publication contains information relating to general principles of medical care that should not be construed as specific instructions for individual patients. Manufacturers' product information and package inserts should be reviewed for current information, including contraindications, dosages, and precautions.

Printed in China

First Edition, 1991

Library of Congress Cataloging-in-Publication Data

Kassirer, Jerome P., 1932–
    Learning clinical reasoning / Jerome P. Kassirer, John B. Wong, Richard I.
Kopelman. – 2nd ed.
        p. ; cm.
    Includes bibliographical references and index.
    ISBN 978-0-7817-9515-9 (alk. paper)
1. Medical logic. 2. Medical logic–Case studies. 3. Diagnosis. 4. Clinical medicine–Decision making.   I. Wong, John B. II. Kopelman, Richard I. III. Title.
    [DNLM: 1. Diagnosis–Case Reports. 2. Clinical Medicine–Case Reports. 3. Decision Making–Case Reports. WB 141 K178L 2010]
    R723.K38 2010
    610.1–dc22

2009013467

The publishers have made every effort to trace the copyright holders for borrowed material. If they have inadvertently overlooked any, they will be pleased to make the necessary arrangements at the first opportunity.

09 10 11 12
1 2 3 4 5 6 7 8 9 10

To our wives:

Sheridan
Lena
Sheilah

So lying there I knew for the first time the old teacher's frustrations. Just as you cut a little path in their wilderness, you look up—they're gone and you haven't even told them the most important thing. Which assumes of course, that you know it.

Reynolds Price, *The Tongues of Angels, 1990*

FOREWORD

Three quarters of a century ago, T. S. Eliot wrote these prescient lines in his poem "The Rock":

"Where is the wisdom we have lost in knowledge?
Where is the knowledge we have lost in information?"

Perhaps in no time in the history of medicine has information been as prolix and freely available to patients, medical students, house staff, and clinicians as it is now, rapidly accessible with only a finger click on the computer. Information is emphasized in classes, syllabi, journals, and examinations as the bedrock of scientific, evidence-based medicine. However, this information, even if accurate (which it often is not) is evanescent, always tentative: That is the nature of science; information in publications and on the Web is also always general and must be crafted, if it is to be useful, to each individual patient: That is the nature of humanity.

Expert physicians possess and apply vast amounts of information to patient care by using critical, analytic, and efficient clinical reasoning: It is the ability to do this that may be called true knowledge, and it is developed principally by experiential acquisition of the skills both illustrated and illuminated in this invaluable book. Drs. Kassirer, Wong, and Kopelman ask an essential question: Why, with the same information available to all, do physicians of varying skill come to quite different conclusions, with manifestly different implications for patients?

In the past, medical students and residents were exposed to these cognitive techniques applied by their teachers "in vivo" at the bedside and in clinic. They learned by observing these teachers what no textbook could teach: that the application to a patient of information that you do not really know is bad science and, not incidentally, bad art.

Medical students and residents should read this book. Today's medical educational environment—rapid-paced, technologically rich, task-heavy, time-abridged, and algorithmically monitored medicine—has significantly eroded the time students and their teachers spend together with patients or discussing actual cases. Students of medicine have less opportunity to learn by observation and imitation of the way good doctors think. This book can help to fill this gap in their education. Relatively few clinical educators can articulate their reasoning processes as skillfully as the physicians that the authors have persuaded to discuss the cases that make up half of this book. Still fewer have the authors' expertise in the science of decision making, and so their analyses of the case discussions provide insights that simply are not available anywhere except in the pages of this book. The cases and the accompanying discussion and analysis allow the student to slow down the processes of patient care and thoughtfully digest events that whiz by in today's harried, hurried clinical environment.

Clinical teachers should read this book. Thinking quantitatively about clinical information can lead to unexpected conclusions, such as the surprisingly high posttest probability after a negative test in the patient you were sure had the disease the test was designed to detect. Medical schools have tried to teach the principles to guide this form of reasoning for 40 years, but one too seldom hears the words "pretest probability" at the bedside or in the conference room. The main reason is that few clinical teachers feel comfortable enough with the concepts of quantitative reasoning about uncertainty to apply them to a specific patient. This book can help teachers to internalize these concepts, to watch them in action in the case analyses, and to prepare themselves to be better teachers and role models for eager students.

Information and knowledge are fungible. Wisdom lies in knowing how to use information and knowledge, and it is the task of acquiring that wisdom that this volume so ably addresses.

Faith T. Fitzgerald, M.D., M.A.C.P.
Professor, Internal Medicine, and
Associate Dean of Humanities and Bioethics
University of California
Davis School of Medicine, Sacramento, California

Harold C. Sox, Jr., M.D., M.A.C.P.
Editor, *Annals of Internal Medicine*
American College of Physicians, Philadelphia, Pennsylvania
Formerly Joseph M. Huber Professor of Medicine
Dartmouth Medical School, Hanover, New Hampshire

PREFACE TO THE SECOND EDITION

Learning Clinical Reasoning is devoted to clinical cognition, or clinical reasoning; the book is intended both for those who learn it and those who teach it. Clinical cognition comprises the set of reasoning strategies that permit us to combine and synthesize diverse data into one or more diagnostic hypotheses, make the complex tradeoffs between the benefits and risks of tests and treatments, and formulate plans for patient management. Tasks such as generating diagnostic hypotheses, gathering and assessing clinical data, deciding on the appropriateness of diagnostic tests, assessing test results, assembling a coherent working diagnosis, and weighing the value of therapeutic approaches are some of the components. Teaching these cognitive skills is a difficult matter even for outstanding clinician-teachers. No well-accepted comprehensive theory of clinical cognition exists; even the most intelligent and thoughtful clinicians are often unaware of the reasoning processes that lead to their conclusions. As a result, they may explicate these strategies inappropriately or inadequately. Because most books that describe clinical reasoning are based on personal accounts of their authors' cognitive processes, such accounts may be unreliable or incomplete.

Given these limitations, how can clinical cognition be learned and taught? Often, we rely on the "see one, do one, teach one" approach, in which students are expected to learn how to reason about diagnosis and treatment by watching others perform. In this book, we combine a classic approach, namely elaboration of the cognitive principles underlying diagnosis and therapy, with another powerful pedagogic method: learning from carefully chosen examples. Because existing theories of cognition are sufficient to provide only a tentative description of clinical reasoning, we supplement the description of principles by the method that we use to learn medical facts, namely learning by instantiation (that is, from examples). We have long expected students to learn clinical *facts* by example because comprehension of clinical entities is enriched by repeated experience with specific instances of those entities. Students and house officers "work up" one patient after another until they understand the numerous disorders that cause, say, jaundice, the conditions that dispose to early coronary artery disease, and the varied manifestations of acute appendicitis. Here we follow the same pattern, but we do not emphasize medical facts. Instead, we offer specific examples—carefully selected "paradigm cases" of clinical reasoning. These cases were selected not on the basis of their clinical relevance or for their similarity to a "classical case" but because specific aspects of these cases exemplify special aspects of problem solving. We believe that exposure to such examples provides an opportunity to learn much about clinical cognition. In preparing the examples and in explaining the cognitive aspects of each example, we have borrowed liberally from research on cognition in disciplines such as cognitive science, cognitive psychology, computer science, decision science, and organizational behavior. Furthermore, we have used methods of cognitive science to analyze in detail the spontaneous, unstructured problem-solving by expert clinicians. The examples of clinical cognition consist of more than 60 real problem cases discussed by expert clinicians who were asked to "think out loud" as they contemplated unembellished, real clinical material. To guide the learner, we accompany the monologue with detailed comments about the cognitive behavior of the expert.

These examples instantiate many inferences and relevant principles. They illustrate not only optimal reasoning strategies, but also suboptimal reasoning, counterexamples that are helpful in circumscribing a variety of cognitive concepts. We do not claim that this set of examples provides a complete picture of the principles of clinical problem solving, only that alert readers can acquire from them many of the cognitive concepts they need as physicians.

Using examples to learn concepts has special benefits. Learning from books or from direct instruction requires little inference or active participation by the learner, whereas learning by discovery from examples requires considerable inference and active involvement. Learning through inference also generates plausible general concepts that students can incorporate into their reasoning processes. Such learning by discovery through specific examples is more likely to "stick."

This is not a book for learning or teaching interviewing skills or physical diagnosis: We do not offer a formula for taking the history of the present illness, obtaining a review of systems, or carrying out a physical examination. We do not discuss the personal interaction with the patient or provide guidance for obtaining all the relevant data. The reader should not infer that we consider these aspects of a patient encounter unimportant. Nonetheless, except for minor departures, we consider only clinical cognition. For this decision, we make no excuses: The cognitive aspects of diagnosis and therapy are the cardinal functions of the physician, and when they are suboptimal, all other aspects are jeopardized.

Looking back on the first edition, published nearly 2 decades ago, we realize that the fundamental nature of clinical reasoning, namely the diagnostic process and the tradeoffs between the benefits and risks of tests and treatments, has not undergone substantial change. In fact, it is not much different since the time of Hippocrates or that of Maimonides. We gather relevant information from a sick person, draw a tentative conclusion about the nature of the illness, and weigh the value of our available therapies. Nonetheless, in the time since the original publication of *Learning Clinical Reasoning*, profound changes have occurred in the practice of medicine; changes that shape how we approach and use these cognitive tasks.

The pace of medicine has reoriented our approach to diagnosis. Rapid triage in emergency departments and short hospital stays, mandated often by financial considerations, have forced us not only to be much less contemplative and leisurely in our approach to diagnosis, but also to short-circuit the diagnostic process: Thus, we often shave minutes off of the history and physical examination and immediately send the patient for tests. Then we look at the test results, and if a diagnosis is identified, we may not bother to complete the history or physical. "Throughput" sometimes substitutes for thoroughness. Needless to say, this swerve toward efficiency and conservation of resources can sometimes sacrifice accuracy, reduce our opportunity for quiet reflection about what we have learned, and strain the physician–patient relationship.

This is not to say that the venerated approach of taking a full history and carefully mapping out all the positive and negative physical findings is better than the modern "get-a-quick-clue-then-order-a-CT-scan" approach. Given the exigencies of modern medicine and the efficiencies and accuracies of such tests, perhaps the venerated is overrated. Maybe it even makes more sense, in terms of diagnostic accuracy, and perhaps even patient welfare, to short-circuit the diagnostic process by testing even before we have carefully extracted every possible historical fact. Certainly, ordering a quick chest CT scan in a 65-year-old long-time heavy smoker with severe dyspnea and hemoptysis, looking at the blood smear in a 50-year-old woman referred for mental status changes, anemia, and thrombocytopenia, or checking the urine sediment for red cell casts in a 14-year-old boy with hypertension and facial edema cannot be considered bad strategies. We are not advocating short-cutting the diagnostic process, only making the point that its benefits and risks have been inadequately evaluated. We await some creative investigators to set their sights on this issue.

In the meantime, as in the first edition, we focus our attention on the cognitive aspects of diagnosis and therapy. It is important to be explicit about what we mean by clinical cognition and clinical reasoning. We are not so naïve to claim that we know how expert diagnosticians think. In the numerous examples, some saved from the previous edition and updated and many new (all based on actual patients), we show how experts (and some nonexperts) reason out loud as they consider diagnostic and therapeutic dilemmas. What is happening in the circuits of their brains is, quite frankly, unknown. In the years preceding the first edition, a rich body of work in cognitive science and cognitive psychology guided how we applied this work to medicine, and in particular to teaching clinical problem solving. The work of Daniel Kahneman, Amos Tversky, and Arthur Elstein, as well as others, provided a solid framework for analyzing real clinical cases.

Since the publication of the first edition, cognitive scientists have shifted their focus away from analysis of reasoning toward identifying sites in the brain that are activated by various external stimuli. In reviewing the literature, we were struck by how little any of the recent research in medicine or cognitive science brings important insights into the nature of clinical problem solving. Several reformulations of clinical reasoning and how to teach reasoning have appeared but remain similar to ideas we presented decades ago. However, just as the pace of medicine has accelerated, greater appreciation for the use of multiple reasoning strategies, from contemplative analytic problem solving to rapid automatic pattern recognition, has emerged. We have, however, examined relevant information on cognition from the literature published in the intervening years, and where appropriate, added references to such work. In this edition, we have added new citations to both parts of the book.

At the same time, however, medicine's attempts to formalize diagnostic and therapeutic problem solving have proceeded apace. Driven by the high (and increasing) cost of care and by large variations in how medicine is practiced from one town to another, from one state to another, and even from one physician to another, attempts have been made to put the practice of medicine on a firmer scientific basis and to codify or formalize the approach to diagnosis and management. The evidence-based medicine movement seeks to examine available clinical data, organize it, and even put a value judgment on it. A new discussion on evidence-based medicine is now given in the first part of the book, and illustrated cases are given in the second part. The next step beyond assessing evidence is applying it, and we also include in both parts a discussion of clinical practice guidelines and how they are applied. An understanding of guidelines has become increasingly important, in that insurers and the government rely on adherence to guidelines to determine what services they will or will not reimburse.

Learning (and teaching) clinical reasoning is critically dependent on the use of illustrative examples and, in particular, examples of poor as well as excellent instances of clinical reasoning. In our research that preceded publication of the first edition, we published dozens of examples of physicians getting it right or completely missing the mark. We argued then that a salient example of a cognitive error was as valuable a lesson in clinical reasoning as an example of correct reasoning, and we had published a detailed categorization of cognitive errors in the hope that by identifying them and categorizing them, it might be possible to avoid making them. As a consequence of several studies by the Institute of Medicine, errors in medicine have become a matter of public discussion in the years since *Learning Clinical Reasoning* was first published. Although the focus on medical errors has been principally on systemic factors such as recording flaws, communication failures, and equipment mishaps, we believe that personal errors in cognition have not received sufficient attention, and we have added more on such errors to this edition.

Our interest in clinical cognition has been generated, informed, and renewed weekly by our regular participation in morning report in the Department of Medicine at Tufts Medical Center in Boston as well as several other academic institutions in Boston, New Haven, Cleveland, and Palo Alto. The format of these teaching exercises is conducive to identifying instances of excellent and faulty reasoning, to commenting on diagnostic strategies, to discussing the complex tradeoffs between the benefits and risks of test and treatments, and to correcting flawed reasoning in a nonthreatening environment. We have insisted in these conferences to be uninformed about the nature of the case being presented, and thus to share in the uncertainties of the case with all other discussants. By being "in the same boat" as all others (except, of course, the physician who presents the case), we exhibit our own misconceptions, our own lack of knowledge, and our own errors.

The original impetus to publish *Learning Clinical Reasoning* came after we published 78 monthly installments of a series called "Clinical Problem Solving" in the controlled circulation journal *Hospital*

Practice. The series was later adapted for the *New England Journal of Medicine*, in the pages of which it continues.

In some languages, the words "teaching" and "learning" are subsumed by the same word. It is our belief that the best way to teach and learn clinical medicine is by exposure to one case after another, and that the best way to learn how to reason about clinical diagnosis and therapeutics is to be exposed, under the tutelage of a seasoned clinician, to multiple examples of savvy and faulty reasoning. Watching an expert clinician dissect out the important elements of a clinical dilemma, come to a diagnosis, and treat a patient skillfully is an exemplary experience. We hope that this new effort affords glimpses of such beauty.

J.P.K.
J.B.W.
R.I.K.

ACKNOWLEDGMENTS

We acknowledge Samuel Proger, William Schwartz, Sheldon Wolff, Jeffrey Gelfand, and Deeb Salem, all chairs of Medicine at Tufts University; Ralph Horwitz, chair of Medicine at Stanford University; and John Harrington, Nicolaos Madias, and Michael Rosenblatt, successive deans at Tufts University School of Medicine for their encouragement and support. We are grateful to generations of house staff at Tufts Medical Center (formerly New England Medical Center) and Caritas Christi in Boston, Yale School of Medicine in New Haven, Case Western Reserve University School of Medicine in Cleveland, and Stanford Medical Center in Palo Alto for educating the authors and willingly providing material for many of the cases. We thank June Osborn and George Thibault of the Josiah Macy Jr. Foundation for their support. We thank Stephen Pauker, Mark Estes, Joseph Rencic, Michael Barry, William Mackey, Debra Poutsiaka, Lawrence Tierney, David Battinelli, Faith Fitzgerald, and Robert Utiger for the development or review of case material. Cora Ho helped to discover important citations. Peter Szolovits of MIT and G. Anthony Gorry of Rice University provided helpful perspectives on the fields of artificial intelligence and cognitive science. We are grateful to Stuart Mushlin, James Hallenbeck, and Arthur Elstein for helpful suggestions on the penultimate draft of the manuscript. We acknowledge the help of Anita Yu for invaluable administrative assistance and our editors, Jessica Heise and Jennifer Verbiar at Wolters Kluwer, for their patience and forbearance.

A NOTE ABOUT THE BOOK'S FORMAT

Part I consists of a brief overview of clinical reasoning, followed by detailed discussions of its components. All of the principal concepts considered in this part are highlighted in bold at the time of their first use. Definitions of these concepts are provided in the Glossary. Following the subheadings in Part I, extensive cross-references are given to the cases in Part II that elaborate on these problem-solving concepts.

Part II consists of more than 60 real cases organized in chapters that parallel the cognitive processes described in Part I. Each case contains edited transcripts of prospective problem solving by experts, analyses of the clinical reasoning by the authors, and references to the literature. These case discussions and their analyses richly supplement the narrative descriptions of reasoning in Part I. As a guide to the reasoning strategies considered across the segments of the book, the outlines of Parts I and II are identical: Cases are placed in the chapter of Part II most appropriate for the reasoning strategies they illustrate. Abundant references to the literature are found in the analyses of the case discussions in Part II. Case analyses that contain such references are indexed in the headings of the chapters in Part I.

CONTENTS

Foreword by Faith T. Fitzgerald, M.D., M.A.C.P. and Harold C. Sox, Jr., M.D., M.A.C.P.   vii

Preface to the Second Edition   ix

Acknowledgments   xiii

A Note About the Book's Format   xiv

I   The Processes of Clinical Reasoning

1. Overview 3
Introduction   3
Diagnosis is an Inferential Process   5
Problem-Solving Strategies   5
Diagnosis Based on Hypothesis Generation and Testing   5
Alternate Concepts of Diagnostic Strategies   6
Therapeutic Principles   6
Linking Diagnosis and Treatment   7

2. Diagnostic Hypothesis Generation 8
Hypotheses and Cues   8
The Cognitive Basis of Hypothesis Generation   8
Hypotheses as a Context   9
Expertise and Error   9

3. Refinement of Diagnostic Hypotheses 11
Where Refinement Begins and Ends   11
Context and Diagnostic Classification   11
Hypothesis Evolution   12
Sequence of Data Collection   12
Reducing Diagnostic Uncertainty   13
The Differential Diagnosis   14
Relation to Formal Probabilistic Approach   14

4. Use and Interpretation of Diagnostic Tests 15
The Function of Tests   15
Quantifying Testing Decisions   15
Sensitivity and Specificity   16
Bayes' Rule   17
Testing Principles   18

Bayesian Revision for Multiple Results   19
Bayesian Revision for Multiple Diseases With Multiple Attributes   21
Pragmatic Considerations in the Probabilistic Approach   22
Interpreting Results   23
When to Test   23
The Threshold Concept   24
The Therapeutic Threshold   24
Testing Thresholds   25

5. Causal Reasoning 28
Definition   28
Using a Causal Model   29
Where in the Diagnostic Process Does Causal Reasoning Fit?   29
Explaining Relations Between Variables   30

6. Diagnostic Verification 31
Definition   31
Criteria of Validity   31
Premature Closure   31
The Penultimate Result: A Working Diagnosis   32

7. Therapeutic Decision Making 33
Principles   33
Treatment Under Conditions of Uncertainty   33
When the Value of Therapeutic Choices is Close   34
Incommensurate Options   34
Quantitative Therapeutic Decision Making   34

8. Examining Evidence 36
Introduction   36
Evidence-Based Medicine   36
Asking Questions   36
Searching for Evidence   37
Summarizing and Appraising Evidence   37
Applying the Evidence   37
Practice Guidelines   38

9. Cognitive Errors 39
Scope   39
Classification   39
Some Errors may have a Psychological Origin   39
The Nature of Cognitive Errors   39
Cognitive Biases in the Laboratory   40
Consequences of Cognitive Biases   40
Strategies for Avoiding Cognitive Errors   41

10. Some Cognitive Concepts 42
Cognitive Science   42
Studying Mental Processes   42
The Structure of Memory   42

Search Strategies   44
Characteristics of Expertise   46

11. Learning Clinical Problem Solving 48
Facts Versus Process   48
Pedagogic Principles   49
A Specific Example   49
The Goal Should Determine the Format   50
Learning by Instantiation   50
Learning Clinical Problem Solving Versus Problem-Based Learning   51

II   Cognition at the Bedside: A Set of Examples

12. Introduction to the Cases 55

13. Diagnostic Hypothesis Generation 56
Case 1. Generation of Diagnostic Hypotheses   56
Case 2. Hypothesis Triggering by an Expert   60
Case 3. A Diagnostic Coup   63
Case 4. A Quick and Accurate Solution   66
Case 5. Better Late Than Never   69
Case 6. A Hit After a Miss   73
Case 7. The Critical Role of Context in the Diagnostic Process   76
Case 8. A Masked Marauder   81
Case 9. A Serious Lack of Focus   84

14. Refinement of Diagnostic Hypotheses 89
Case 10. What is a Differential Diagnosis?   89
Case 11. An Orderly, Sequential Approach   94
Case 12. Weak Reasoning: Diagnosis by Drug Reaction   96
Case 13. Narrowing Down the Diagnostic Options   100
Case 14. A Picture is Worth a Thousand Words   104
Case 15. Strategies of Information Gathering   108
Case 16. A Fatal Flaw in Sutton's Law   113
Case 17. How to Disregard Red Herrings   118
Case 18. Discrimination: The Problem of Look-Alikes   121
Case 19. Location, Location, Location   125

15. Use and Interpretation of Diagnostic Tests 128
Case 20. Interpreting a Negative Test Result   128
Case 21. Diagnosis and the Risks of the Primrose Path   131
Case 22. Searching for a Pony   134
Case 23. Interpreting Hoofbeats: Can Bayes Help Clear the Haze?   137
Case 24. Short-Circuiting the Diagnostic Process   143
Case 25. The Bypass on the Way to the Bypass   145
Case 26. It is What You Believe That Counts   148
Case 27. Renal Rescue by Reverend Bayes   152
Case 28. A Diagnostic Fluke   155
Case 29. Surprise!   157

Case 30. Tripping Over Technology   161
Case 31. The Probability of a Probability   165

16. Causal Reasoning 169
Case 32. Judging Causality   169
Case 33. Post Hoc, Ergo Propter Hoc   171
Case 34. The Case for Causal Reasoning   175
Case 35. The Tricky Task of Attributing Causation   180
Case 36. The Right Answer for the Wrong Reason   183

17. Diagnostic Verification 186
Case 37. A Point-By-Point Dissection of Clinical Reasoning   186
Case 38. Leaving No Stone Unturned   188
Case 39. Verification   192
Case 40. A Meticulous Approach   196
Case 41. A Diagnostic Quandary   199
Case 42. Diagnosis by Fiat   203
Case 43. Iron Pyrite and Diagnostic Confirmation   207

18. Therapeutic Decision Making 209
Case 44. The Surgeon Opts to Operate: Why?   209
Case 45. Treat or Keep Testing?   211
Case 46. Watch and Wait, or Operate?   216
Case 47. An Apple or an Orange?   218

19. Examining Evidence 223
Case 48. A Difficult Tradeoff   223
Case 49. Making Judgments When the Evidence is Not Definitive   225
Case 50. Using and Citing Published Evidence   227
Case 51. A Little Math Makes the Medicine Go Down   229
Case 52. A Rewarding Pursuit of Certainty   234
Case 53. Treating Before Knowing   239

20. Cognitive Errors 244
Case 54. A Defective Detective   244
Case 55. Remedies for Faulty Hypothesis Generation   248
Case 56. A Disaster Averted   252
Case 57. Derailed by the Availability Heuristic   255
Case 58. Wrong Diagnosis, Wrong Tests, Wrong Treatment   262
Case 59. Reconsidering Failures of Therapy   266
Case 60. The Cheetah and the Snail   267
Case 61. A Collection of Cognitive Diagnostic Errors   271

21. Some Cognitive Concepts 275
Case 62. A Message about Methods   275
Case 63. Memory: How We Overcome its Limitations   279
Case 64. Diagnosis and the Structure of Memory; Disease Polymorphism and
       Mental Models   281
Case 65. Intuitive and Inspirational, or Inductive and Incremental?   286
Case 66. Knowledge and Clinical Expertise   291

22. Learning Clinical Problem Solving 295
Case 67. Learning Clinical Reasoning from Examples   295
Case 68. Making a Silk Purse out of a Sow's Ear   299
Case 69. Optimizing Case Discussions   304

Glossary   308
Bibliography   313
Index   325

The Processes of
Clinical Reasoning

CHAPTER 1   Overview

INTRODUCTION

Clinical reasoning is the essential function of the physician; optimal patient care depends on keen diagnostic acumen and thoughtful analysis of the tradeoffs between the benefits and risks of tests and treatments. As benchmarks for considering these issues, here are several real examples:

A 33-year-old man presents to the emergency room complaining of headache, facial flushing, and urticaria of the trunk, which he had never had before. Based on these limited data, most physicians would fail to make the correct diagnosis in this patient, but a clinician who had access to only this information suspects an unfamiliar disorder, namely scombroid poisoning. Twenty minutes later another man who ate bluefish in the same restaurant as the patient comes to the emergency room with the same complaints. Scombroid poisoning was the correct diagnosis.

A 62-year-old woman treated successfully 13 months earlier for exophthalmic goiter and thyrotoxicosis with propylthiouracil develops an alteration in her voice, regurgitation of fluids through her nose, and progressive weakness in her extremities. For 1 month, several physicians are unable to determine the nature of her problem, but then another physician immediately recognizes that the patient is suffering from a form of myasthenia gravis associated with recovery from hyperthyroidism. He verifies the diagnosis and treats the patient effectively for this disorder.

A 49-year-old man with cholangiocarcinoma develops renal failure and anemia after treatment with five cycles of fluorouracil, adriamycin, and mitomycin over a period of 1 year. A clinician unaware that such a complication is known to be caused by mitomycin nonetheless makes a diagnosis of hemolytic uremic syndrome and correctly attributes it to mitomycin.

A 66-year-old woman with long-standing hypertension and cardiac failure admitted to the hospital with breathlessness is found to have distended neck veins, pulmonary edema, an S_3 gallop, and a rough 5/6 holosystolic murmur radiating to the left axilla. After intubation for hypoxemia, she develops a picture of cardiogenic shock. Treatment with dopamine and then norepinephrine and nitroprusside fails to raise her blood pressure. Several physicians are baffled and expect the patient to succumb, but another physician notices a "spike and dome" configuration on her arterial tracing, a brisk carotid pulse with a bisferiens quality, and augmentation of the arterial pulse in the beat following a ventricular premature contraction. He diagnoses asymmetric septal hypertrophy, stops all drugs, including digoxin, and administers intravenous saline and phenylephrine. The patient recovers promptly from the hypotensive episode.

A gastroenterologist, in reviewing a histologic specimen from a 52-year-old man with acute appendicitis, believes that the diagnosis rendered by more than one pathologist (carcinoma of the appendix) is an incorrect interpretation, and he advises the patient against having the right hemicolectomy that has been recommended. The patient follows his advice and remains well with no evidence of cancer for more than 30 years.

A diagnosis of cirrhosis is made by two physicians in a 37-year-old schoolteacher with ascites, peripheral edema, temporal wasting, and palmar erythema. Liver biopsy is said to confirm the diagnosis. A consultant exhibits skepticism about the diagnosis because liver function tests are virtually normal. He extracts a previously undetected 4-year history of breathlessness and finds distended neck veins and a cardiac murmur, and an echocardiogram demonstrates that the correct diagnosis is silent mitral stenosis.

A 55-year-old man with a history of alcohol and benzodiazepine abuse is brought to the emergency room in a coma and is found to have profound metabolic acidosis. A physician systematically analyzes the patient's electrolytes, anion gap, and osmolar gap, finds oxalate crystals in the patient's urine sediment, diagnoses intoxication with ethylene glycol, and treats the patient promptly. The patient recovers.

These brief vignettes are descriptions of actual occurrences. They display exceptional cognitive proficiency by some physicians when others had exhibited suboptimal performance, and they illustrate graphically the critically important nature of the reasoning processes of the physician,[1] both "intuitive" (rapid pattern recognition) and "analytic" (deliberative and exhaustive) reasoning as examples of the extremes of the "cognitive continuum."[2-7] Few would contest the notion that no matter how competent a physician may be at other tasks, outcomes cannot be optimal if these reasoning skills are deficient. Indeed, the prime function of the physician is clinical reasoning: to suspect the cause of a patient's symptoms and signs, to gather additional relevant information, to select necessary tests, and to recommend therapy. Although no one would doubt that cognitive skills are the basis for these tasks, medicine has developed few methods to enhance the acquisition and development of these problem-solving skills. Instead of discussing how diagnostic hypotheses are initiated and refined and how testing and treatment decisions should be formulated, teachers of clinical medicine have substituted standardized histories and physicals, book chapters that list the myriad causes of individual symptoms, an apprentice system in which the student is expected to imitate others, formal approaches to recording patients' problems, and lock-step algorithmic charts for blind guidance. None of these methods focuses on the essential reasoning processes that are critical to optimal performance. The last several decades have witnessed considerable growth in our understanding of human reasoning and, in particular, clinical reasoning from fields generally not considered part of the fabric of clinical medicine. Research in these disciplines, namely **cognitive science, decision theory**, and computer science (in particular, **artificial intelligence**), provides insights into the critical cognitive processes that form the basis for both teaching and learning the principles that underlie diagnosis and management. These insights into the process of medical reasoning also form the basis for identifying errors in clinical **cognition** and improving the quality of medical care.[6,8,9]

Part I of this book describes many of the insights identified in recent years. It begins with a brief overview of the processes of diagnosis and management decision making and then elaborates on five aspects of the diagnostic process: generation (evocation) of diagnostic hypotheses, refinement of hypotheses, diagnostic testing, causal reasoning, and diagnostic verification. The book continues with a discussion of therapeutic decision making, evidence-based medicine, and cognitive errors in diagnosis. To introduce the reader to unfamiliar concepts derived from disciplines outside of medicine, we also consider some cognitive concepts underlying problem solving, knowledge, and memory. The final discussion offers some views on how to learn and how to teach the processes that are considered.

Throughout Part I, extensive references are given to the cases in Part II. These cases generally are in three parts: real clinical problems selected for their capacity to elicit significant aspects of clinical reasoning, prospective discussion of the problems by **experts**, and detailed analyses of the reasoning used. The analyses, focused around the specific clinical problems, elaborate extensively on the cognitive principles discussed in Part I. As with any new discipline, some of the expressions used in this book may not be familiar, and some have not achieved universal acceptance. For that reason, an extensive glossary is provided.

The book is about reasoning in clinical medicine. Because theories of human problem solving (including clinical problem solving) are incomplete, some of the concepts described here must be considered tentative. Although many of these concepts are new to medicine, they are sufficiently accepted by cognitive scientists to be adapted for use in learning and teaching. The cognitive aspects of diagnosis have been studied quite extensively, but few studies have been carried out on management decision making, that is, the process by which physicians make testing and treatment decisions. This lack of information on physician behavior impedes our ability to assemble a comprehensive description of testing and therapeutic decision making. Nonetheless, we borrow generously from the principles inherent in **prescriptive**, or **normative**, approaches to decision making such as

Bayes' rule and decision analysis.[10,11] These principles have been elaborated in sufficient detail to explain the rationale for many testing and treatment decisions.

DIAGNOSIS IS AN INFERENTIAL PROCESS

In the process of diagnosis, the clinician makes a series of **inferences** about the nature of malfunctions of the body. These inferences are derived not only from existing observations (historical data, physical findings, and "routine" studies), but also from invasive tests and responses to various interventions. Inferential or **inductive reasoning** proceeds until the clinician has identified a "**working diagnosis**," a diagnostic category sufficiently acceptable to establish a prognosis, dictate a therapeutic action, or both. When making diagnostic inferences from clinical data, the clinician uses many strategies to combine, integrate, and interpret the data. Clinicians make extensive use of rules of thumb or short-cuts (designated **heuristics** by cognitive scientists) in the process of gathering and interpreting information. Rather than rely on statistical data on disease **prevalence** to generate **diagnostic hypotheses** from a set of findings, for example, they often assess the likelihood of diseases on the basis of the salience of the findings or familiarity: the resemblance of the findings in a given patient to those of a known disease. By reducing the need to ask an inordinately large number of questions, these rules of thumb make the task of information gathering manageable and efficient. By and large, judgments based on heuristics are accurate and appropriate, although on occasion they can be faulty.

PROBLEM-SOLVING STRATEGIES

Studies of human cognition suggest that problem-solving strategies depend on the nature of the clinical problem being addressed and even more on the expertise of the clinician. Nonexperts tend to use nonselective strategies that, although they are applicable across a wide range of clinical settings, are nonspecific, rather **weak problem-solving methods** and inefficient in generating specific hypotheses. Experts, on the other hand, typically employ **strong diagnostic problem-solving** approaches tailored to a particular problem or situation usually in the domain of their expertise. Rather than casting their nets broadly, experts quickly focus on a problem by recognizing patterns, formulating problems in semantically meaningful "**chunks**," gathering data relevant to a perceived specific solution of the problem, and applying familiar, "prepackaged" actions.

DIAGNOSIS BASED ON HYPOTHESIS GENERATION AND TESTING

At the inception of a diagnostic encounter, the first step is generation, or evocation, of one or more diagnostic hypotheses. The diagnostic process focuses on one or more evolving hypotheses. Typically, the clinician generates initial hypotheses merely from a patient's age, sex, race, appearance, and presenting complaints, but sometimes such hypotheses emerge exclusively from physical findings or from laboratory data. Additional hypotheses are **triggered** as new findings emerge. A diagnostic hypothesis can be either quite general (such as infection) or quite specific (such as acute inferior myocardial infarction). It can take several forms, including a state (inflammatory process), a clinical disorder (acute transplant rejection), a syndrome (nephrotic syndrome), or a specific disease entity (polycythemia vera). The formulation of a preliminary hypothesis on the basis of only a few observations is critically dependent on the cognitive ability to relate a new situation to past experience.

Diagnostic hypotheses serve an essential function: They form a **context** within which further information gathering takes place. This context, a diagnostic category of some kind (e.g., acute bacterial meningitis), provides a model against which a given patient's findings can be assessed. The context is the **framework** for further hypothesis assessment. It specifies both the findings that should be present and those that should be absent if the patient has a given disorder. Diagnostic reasoning proceeds by progressive **hypothesis modification and refinement**. Some hypotheses are made more specific, some previously triggered hypotheses are deleted, and some new ones are added. It is not clear how much of the diagnostic process is driven by hypotheses as described here and how much is driven simply by the availability of data from the patient's history, the physical examination, or the laboratory. Quite likely, elements of cognitive approaches driven by hypotheses and those driven by data are frequently intermingled.

Verifying a diagnostic hypothesis is the penultimate task. It creates a working diagnosis that is used to plan further action. Because the diagnostic process is inferential, all diagnostic hypotheses (even those refined by extensive data gathering and interpretation) necessarily reflect a belief or a conviction by the physician regarding the nature of the condition from which the patient suffers. Verifying a hypothesis is a kind of test of its validity. It involves assessing a hypothesis for its **coherency** (are all physiologic linkages, predisposing factors, and complications appropriate for the suspected disease in this patient?), its **adequacy** (does the suspected disease encompass all the patient's findings—normal and abnormal?), and its **parsimonious** nature (is the suspected disease a simple explanation of all the patient's findings?), often referred to as **Ockham's razor** or the law of parsimony, from the fourteenth-century philosopher William of Ockham, who advocated "entia non sunt multiplicanda praeter necessitatem," which can be interpreted as recommending that the simplest solution (i.e., the one with the fewest assumptions and factors) may be the best. Verifying a hypothesis also requires eliminating competing hypotheses (can any other disease[s] explain the patient's findings better than the current hypothesis?). This process produces one or more working diagnoses that form the basis for the next step in patient management—arriving at a certain forecast about the patient's subsequent clinical course, taking no further action, ordering additional tests, or treating the patient. As noted later, such choices are a function not only of the probability that a patient is suffering from one or more given diseases, but also of the benefits to be derived from further testing, the risks of further testing, and the benefits and risks that accrue from treatment.

ALTERNATE CONCEPTS OF DIAGNOSTIC STRATEGIES

How much physicians use a general problem-solving approach such as the one just described is open to question. Quite likely, nonexperts rely on it considerably more than experts. The **hypothesis generation**/testing concept came into question because diagnostic accuracy seemed dependent more on a mastery of content (knowledge of disease and patterns of diseases) than on any specific strategy.[4,12] Researchers in the field have subsequently tried to identify the nature of such knowledge structures and the mechanisms of their retrieval. Some suggest that diagnosis proceeds by matching the characteristics of a new case to a previously encountered specific instance or to a general resemblance of cases previously seen.[4,12] Others propose that clinicians develop mental models, abstractions, or prototypes and use a kind of pattern matching approach to diagnosis. Still others have hypothesized the existence of "illness scripts"—cognitive structures somewhat analogous to the **frame** structure of some artificial intelligence computer programs.[13,14] Finally, some workers in the field have opined that a variety of methods (including all of the aforementioned) are used flexibly to solve diagnostic problems.[8,12,15] What this means is not certain, but what does seem to be clear is that in the absence of an extensive knowledge base for a disease or complaint, novice and experienced physicians alike are more likely to resort to the hypothesis **generation and testing strategy** discussed earlier.[12,16,17] Experts who have a finely honed knowledge of disease probably use this strategy principally when dealing with a particularly difficult diagnostic dilemma.[12]

THERAPEUTIC PRINCIPLES

The principles of diagnosis and therapy are inextricably intertwined. Because a diagnosis is an inference about a patient's illness, we can never be absolutely certain that the disease label we assign to a patient's illness is correct. For this reason, we will inevitably treat some patients who do not have the disease and inevitably fail to treat some who do. Both circumstances deprive some individuals of appropriate therapy. To the extent that the treatment is effective but also produces harmful side effects, patients who have the disease for which the treatment is designated will derive the benefit of therapy, offset to some extent by the risk of therapy. Treated patients who do not have the disease, however, derive no therapeutic benefit but nonetheless are subjected to the risk.

LINKING DIAGNOSIS AND TREATMENT

The interplay between diagnostic hypotheses and the benefits and risks of tests and treatments can be envisioned effectively in terms of decision thresholds, a concept derived from decision science. A **threshold** is the probability of a disease at the point at which two choices (e.g., treating vs. not treating; treating vs. further testing) have equivalent value. The threshold is thus a benchmark for action: At disease probabilities lower than the threshold, one action is appropriate, whereas at disease probabilities greater than the threshold, a different action is appropriate. A threshold can be calculated using the methods of decision analysis from data on the benefits and risks of diagnostic/tests and treatments, or it can be estimated.

Thresholds define diagnostic and therapeutic interactions. When deciding whether or not to administer a treatment for a suspected disease, the efficacy and risks of the treatment for the disease determine how confident a physician must be in the diagnosis to make treating the patient a better choice than not treating. For treatments with a high ratio of benefits to risks, the **therapeutic threshold** is quite low, and treatment can be given even when the probability of disease is relatively low (e.g., penicillin for suspected streptococcal throat infections). For treatments with a low ratio of benefits to risks, on the other hand, the therapeutic threshold is quite high, and the physician must be quite certain that the patient has a given disease before administering therapy (e.g., thrombolytic therapy for suspected myocardial infarction). Of course, low efficacy of treatment, high risk, or both can contribute to such a low ratio of benefits to risks.

CHAPTER 2 — Diagnostic Hypothesis Generation

HYPOTHESES AND CUES

(Cases 1–4, 16)

In our daily life, we are constantly generating hypotheses about our environment—about our visual images, how the physical world operates, our expectations of events, and our perceptions of people. These hypotheses provide a framework for interpreting all of our unstructured experiences. **Diagnosis**, a special case of unstructured problem solving, is initiated when a physician evokes, formulates, or triggers one or more hypotheses from a set of cues that emanate from an encounter with a patient.[18–22] The cues that initiate hypothesis generation are varied. Sometimes a single symptom, such as dysuria, or a single physical finding, such as prominent facial bones, triggers a diagnostic possibility. At other times, even a single laboratory result, such as an elevated serum calcium concentration, does the same. Most often, however, the cues are multiple: The patient's age, sex, race, appearance, and presenting complaints constitute a familiar set. We formulate hypotheses at first contact, and we continue to evoke new hypotheses as long as we fail to satisfy ourselves that we have the "right answer." Although hypothesis generation usually is the first step in diagnosis, it continues as we refine our existing diagnostic hypotheses and eliminate those hypotheses that are no longer tenable.

Diagnostic hypotheses take on many forms and lie on a spectrum from quite general to highly specific. Forms include disease entities, syndromes, involvement of an organ system, or even such notions such as "healthy," "sick," or "desperately ill." Along the scale of specificity, hypotheses might range from a vague notion such as infection, to more specific entities such as gram-negative sepsis, to highly specific disorders such as meningococcal meningitis.

THE COGNITIVE BASIS OF HYPOTHESIS GENERATION

(Cases 1, 3, 6, 23, 57, 63)

The process of hypothesis generation is best understood in the framework of modern cognitive science, which holds that the brain is an information processor that manipulates semantically meaningful "chunks" or packets of information. Such information chunks are represented in memory, but theories conflict about the nature of their storage. No matter how the information is represented, access to it evokes or generates a hypothesis about the state of a patient. Hypotheses are generated rapidly—probably tentatively at first as candidates for acceptable hypotheses, and then, if they are consistent with existing data, they are accepted as plausible explanations for a finding or a set of findings. Quite likely, only a small number of hypotheses remain active at any given time. Given the limited ability of **short-term memory** to manipulate only 5 to 10 items at a given time, one can presume that this memory restriction also pertains to diagnostic hypotheses.[23,24] If so, many hypotheses must be quite evanescent as others take their place, even though discarded hypotheses can and do re-emerge at a later stage in the process.

Some of the factors known to be important in the generation of diagnostic hypotheses include disease prevalence, heuristics (rules of thumb), and the gravity or seriousness of a patient's condition. Triggering hypotheses according to a disease's (or condition's) prevalence presumably is an optimal approach, but it is uneconomical as a cognitive function because it requires considerable memory storage and processing, including checking for consistency against available clinical data.[25,26] Instead of this cumbersome approach, we often rely on heuristics to evoke hypotheses.[27] One commonly used short-cut is designated the

representativeness heuristic, an approach that relies on the resemblance of a set of findings to those of some well-defined clinical entity. The findings of simultaneous cough, dyspnea, and travel to California might trigger the hypothesis "coccidioidomycosis," for example, even though the prevalence of other diseases that cause both symptoms is far greater than that of the fungal infection. Another commonly used short-cut is the **availability heuristic**.[27,28] This approach is a function of familiarity with a given clinical entity, usually because a certain pattern of findings evokes a readily recallable, particularly striking clinical entity.[29] The triggering of the hypothesis "pheochromocytoma" in response to the finding of a sudden, severe increase in blood pressure is such an example. As with the representative heuristic, however, there is no guarantee that a hypothesis evoked by the availability heuristic accurately reflects disease prevalence.

Still another short-cut used in hypothesis generation is related to the physician's ever-present vigilance for life-threatening manifestations or complications of a disease. Repeatedly, physicians engaged in the diagnostic process change from generating hypotheses based on any of the mechanisms described earlier and instead evoke hypotheses for these diagnostic imperatives when early diagnosis and treatment is critically important for a patient's well-being. In the midst of the process of generating hypotheses based on prevalence, representativeness, or availability, physicians often evoke hypotheses that identify life-threatening manifestations or complications. Such hypotheses (sepsis, shock, pulmonary edema, acute myocardial infarction, hyperkalemia) may be generated without regard to prevalence, but they focus on the value of alertness to serious events while the "routine" part of the diagnostic process is underway. This type of medical rule of thumb may be merely a special case of known heuristic mechanisms such as availability.

or constrain, a patient's problem and provide a context (or **problem space**) for further diagnostic reasoning and exploration.[30,31] Each diagnostic hypothesis evokes a template of possible clinical findings against which a given patient's findings can be compared. The diagnostic hypothesis "nephrotic syndrome," for example, mandates the presence of heavy proteinuria, typically includes hypoalbuminemia, edema, and hyperlipidemia, and encompasses an exceptionally large array of syndrome characteristics that include predisposing factors (diabetes mellitus, amyloidosis, systemic lupus erythematosus), short-term complications (venous thrombosis), long-term complications (accelerated atherosclerosis), pathophysiologic associations (sodium intake and edema formation), and histopathologic correlations ("spikes" on silver stain in one of the cases— membranous nephropathy). Thus, when the nephrotic syndrome becomes a hypothesis, its many characteristics become a framework against which a patient's findings are assessed. Within this framework, or context, new data are gathered and assessed and hypotheses are preserved, rejected, or refined.

The value of the context lies in its capacity to guide the subsequent diagnostic process.[32] The context helps the physician to formulate appropriate questions as he or she takes a history of the present illness, directs certain specific aspects of the physical examination, and identifies tests that might provide additional relevant clinical data. Evidence suggests that physicians do not simply gather data without regard to diagnostic hypotheses, and that they do not simply accumulate facts until a diagnosis becomes evident. Rather, they gather relevant data within a defined context. The context serves as a guide for predicting which information might be useful to gather, which tests might be helpful, and which diagnostic procedures deserve further attention.

HYPOTHESES AS A CONTEXT

(Cases 7, 8)

Given that maximum uncertainty characterizes the initial state of a diagnostic encounter, hypotheses form an essential function: They frame,

EXPERTISE AND ERROR

(Cases 3, 9, 54, 58, 66)

Clinical experience and expertise clearly enhance the quality of hypotheses generated. Knowledge of the various clusters of cues that should trigger certain hypotheses and knowledge of the characteristics of diseases and syndromes that become the context for further diagnostic resolution facilitate the process of hypothesis generation.[19] "Book knowledge" is insufficient for optimal hypothesis generation, in part because diseases and syndromes vary far more in their attributes (combinations of clinical findings at onset, clinical course) than those characterized in "classic" textbook descriptions. Indeed, experience with one patient after another with a given disease or syndrome produces the enriched model of a disease or syndrome against which we measure new cases.

The process of hypothesis generation, however, is imperfect. When a patient's disease is common and its manifestations are typical, when a patient's clinical findings are representative of a certain disease, and when one or more striking clinical features point toward a specific diagnostic entity, the correct diagnosis often emerges quickly. Neither disease prevalence nor the heuristic solutions described before guarantee that the correct diagnosis will be generated initially, nor do they guarantee that the correct hypothesis will ever be evoked. Both rare diseases and common diseases with atypical manifestations can be overlooked, and perceptual errors (e.g., failure to recognize that a patient has the classic physical features of acromegaly) can lead to faulty or insufficient hypothesis triggering. No special reasoning skills will suffice to trigger diagnostic hypotheses if the physician does not have sufficient knowledge about disease entities or about the full range of expected manifestations of these entities. A lack of either makes hypothesis generation at best faulty and at worst totally lacking.

CHAPTER 3

Refinement of Diagnostic Hypotheses

WHERE REFINEMENT BEGINS AND ENDS

(Cases 1, 12, 13, 16, 17, 37, 38)

After hypotheses are evoked, the process of **hypothesis refinement**, also known as "**case building**," ensues. Hypothesis refinement is an evolving, sequential process of data gathering and interpretation. Repeated inferences yield a series of provisional approximations (intermediate diagnostic hypotheses) that are revised continually in an iterative process until one or more diagnostic hypotheses satisfactorily explain all available clinical data. The process begins with a small number of hypotheses generated from a set of clinical findings. It proceeds by elaborating questions that elicit further data and by interpreting the data obtained. Initial hypotheses are revised, refined, and often made more specific. Some hypotheses are added and some are deleted. The process of hypothesis refinement uses a variety of reasoning strategies (probabilistic, causal, and deterministic) and often involves the use of diagnostic tests to discriminate among existing hypotheses. After relevant data are accumulated, diagnostic refinement merges into **diagnostic verification**—the process in which one or more hypotheses are accepted as sufficiently valid to permit further decision making (testing, therapeutic, or prognostic). This chapter considers details of the refinement process. Subsequent chapters describe the probabilistic approach to combining clinical data and the use of causal (physiologic) reasoning in the process. Causal reasoning, which depends on the cause-and-effect relations between clinical variables, is discussed later because it functions chiefly in the later phases of the diagnostic process as we attempt to verify our hypothesis.

CONTEXT AND DIAGNOSTIC CLASSIFICATION

(Cases 7, 9, 63, 64)

The context within which problem solving occurs is a function of the cognitive representation of the problem in memory. As noted in Chapter 2, this context can be as general as "infection" or as specific as "unexplained hypoglycemia." The context frames the problem, constrains the number of possible explanations, sets a limit on the number of operations to be applied to the problem, and serves as a basis for expectations.[30–32] These expectations are the predictable, anticipated findings and are based on some mental model of the disease. When an attempt is being made to classify a given patient within a diagnostic hypothesis, the varied characteristics of the clinical disorder become the basis for such expectations. Given a hypothesis of acute appendicitis, for example, features expected in appendicitis (right-lower-quadrant tenderness, leukocytosis) are sought as more clinical data are obtained. In addition, features not expected in appendicitis (disorientation, cough, normal white cell count) can be evaluated and explained. Thus, the representation of disease entities in memory is a critical factor.[8,12,13]

A central question is how new instances (a patient with certain clinical manifestations) are compared to existing entities in memory and indexed or classified. Clearly, the characteristics of the context critically determine the efficiency and accuracy of diagnostic refinement. If a clinical entity (appendicitis again as the example) is defined narrowly according to its textbook description or according to its typical or classical descriptions, features that occur in its variants (such as diarrhea when the appendix is in a retrocecal location) might be considered to exclude the diagnosis. Repeated experience with variations of disease entities fills out the expectations, that is, the normal and abnormal findings that are associated with a given entity.

How is such experience stored and accessed? For many years, it has been assumed that information about a new case is compared to some case prototype, or abstract model, stored in memory.[6,33] It has been further assumed that the abstract description is sufficiently detailed to contain all variations of the disease, as well as rules about how the disease relates to other diseases or conditions. This theory argues that memory consists of abstract descriptions that evolve by compiling and compressing information into a single model, or prototype, as we encounter more and more patients with a certain disease. To the extent that a single abstract model could exist, a new case would be assessed by comparison to this abstract description.

Another theory, based on studies in the domain of **case-based reasoning**, supposes that knowledge is stored in a symbolic structure known as a **script**.[6,13,34] In medicine a disease script would comprise patient-specific scenarios containing personal features, predisposing factors, causative agents, and clinical manifestations tied together both by causal links and chronological relations. A script might consist of a description of an illness, the natural course of the illness, the possible interventions, the sequences of events, and the outcomes. Scripts could vary from representing clinical data in a highly physiologic format on one hand (i.e., containing a detailed causal model or physiologic or anatomic model) to a smaller, more efficient, highly compiled format on the other (i.e., containing only relations between findings in the form of diagnostic labels, e.g., radiologic, pathologic, or dermatologic findings). One recently developed concept holds that much of the indexing or classification by physicians of new instances is carried out not against a single prototype of the disease but against multiple stored prototypes or even actual recalled cases (**instance scripts** or **exemplars**) of the disease seen by a physician in the past. Given the range of manifestations seen in a set of patients with a single disease entity (i.e., the **polymorphism** of that disease), the notion that multiple cases are stored in memory for later comparison with new cases is attractive. A more detailed discussion of the structure of memory is given in Chapter 10, section The Structure of Memory.

HYPOTHESIS EVOLUTION

(Cases 1, 10, 12, 16, 33)

Although initial diagnostic hypotheses provide the framework for data gathering, they may or may not survive. When new data are consistent with an existing mental model (however it is constructed), the hypothesis remains active and may become even more specific. A hypothesis of "infection" may evolve into "urinary tract infection," then into "pyelonephritis," and finally into "left-sided *Escherichia coli* pyelonephritis." Alter-natively, hypotheses deemed interesting initially may be dropped quickly when further data fail to support them. The process should not be viewed as an orderly one in which hypotheses that initially are quite vague always are progressively specified. Although this pattern does occur, others are observed as well. An initial hypothesis may be highly specific (e.g., Cushing syndrome), and it may not change as more information is obtained. Usually, diagnostic hypotheses become more or less credible with each new clinical datum, but hypotheses may disappear only to reappear later. A given hypothesis may be considered highly probable when only a few cues are available; later it may be nearly dismissed only to become prominent again when all available data are obtained. A diagnostic hypothesis may have to be abandoned when data appear that are inconsistent with it. In such instances, replacement hypotheses must be generated to account for the data. It seems quite likely that clinicians do not simply continue to collect hypotheses indefinitely during a diagnostic encounter, only to narrow down to one or two after all information has been gathered. Rather, evidence is strong that the cognitive limitation of **working memory** to a small number of items constrains the number of hypotheses in active memory.[27,30] This constraint probably pertains to the concept of differential diagnosis, as discussed later.

SEQUENCE OF DATA COLLECTION

(Cases 14, 24, 45)

Clinical data need not be accumulated according to a fixed pattern. Although data are typically sought first from the history, then from the physical examination, and then from the laboratory, this pattern of data gathering is more a matter of historical precedent than of cognitive necessity. In fact, data may first emerge from a patient's physical appearance (gait, tremor, or facial features), from the laboratory (an unexpected low hematocrit or a high serum calcium), or from a test (a blood pressure measurement made in a shopping mall). Hypothesis refinement demands no special sequence of data collection, although some optimal sequence probably does exist. Initially, expert clinicians do focus heavily on data from the patient's history and previous records (a particularly rich data source), but they readily switch to an aspect of the physical examination or a diagnostic test in the interest of gathering a pertinent piece of data whenever appropriate. On the other hand, conceding that it is appropriate to gather data out of sequence does not invalidate either the traditional questions asked as part of a "review of systems" or the "routine" physical examination. Such approaches have valid goals, including gathering of baseline data, avoidance of errors in drug administration, identification of risk factors, case finding for diseases that are uncommon but important to identify, and disclosure of critical psychological and social issues.

The sequence of data accumulation has increased in importance, given the foreshortened pace of medical diagnosis, especially in emergency departments, where the rapid triage of patients often begins with a brief acquisition of a patient's presenting complaint and is followed immediately by the ordering of one or more diagnostic tests. Whether it is more efficient, and just as accurate, to "short-circuit" the diagnostic process in this manner has never been evaluated. Until we learn more about the benefits and risks of this approach, we continue to recommend the process described previously.

REDUCING DIAGNOSTIC UNCERTAINTY

(Cases 9, 12, 15, 18, 38)

Early in the process of **hypothesis revision** when only a small set of cues is available, the number of possible disorders that could explain this set of cues often is quite large. At this stage, **diagnostic uncertainty** is at its highest (i.e., differentiation among the various diagnostic hypotheses is at its nadir) and the number of questions that a physician might ask to elicit the data needed to narrow the number of hypotheses is at its peak. The process that the physician uses to gather data follows no preordained pattern and in this framework can be characterized as unstructured problem solving, yet diagnostic hypotheses do lend some structure to the process. Most of the time a lock-step or algorithmic method cannot substitute for this unstructured approach simply because of the large problem space (i.e., the constrained environment that guides the possible operations and solutions to a problem) in which the problem must be solved. Questioning

is guided by hypotheses, which may be related to probabilistic relations between clinical variables. Diagnostic efficiency requires that the questions that are asked are the ones most likely to reduce diagnostic uncertainty. To do so requires that the data obtained from such a question, whether positive or negative, should produce the largest change in disease probability. Several strategies for eliciting information are used.[35-38] One is a **confirmation strategy**, in which information is sought that might be expected to enhance a highly likely hypothesis.[19] Another is a disconfirming or **elimination strategy**, in which information is sought to reduce the likelihood of an unlikely hypothesis. Of course, when either of these strategies alters the likelihood of any hypothesis, the likelihood of one or more remaining hypotheses also must change. A reduction in the likelihood of a leading hypothesis, for example, forces remaining hypotheses to be more prominent.

When only a few possibilities remain, a **discrimination strategy** can be invoked to seek specific information to discriminate among these remaining hypotheses.[19] Frequently these few diseases bear close resemblance to each other in their clinical manifestations (e.g., constrictive pericarditis and severe biventricular failure; or polyarteritis nodosa and systemic atheroembolism) and are often mistaken for one another. In such instances, differences in the prevalence of the disorders, subtle differences in the clinical characteristics of each, and the results of specific laboratory tests may be required to discriminate among completing diagnostic entities. In some instances, the response to therapy becomes a final discriminator.

The process of hypothesis refinement can be carried out mathematically, but expert clinicians rarely rely on formal **probabilistic models** as they engage in diagnostic reasoning. Instead, they use a variety of rules of thumb or heuristics previously described. These simplifications are useful shortcuts, and although they are not precise reflectors of prevalence or other probabilistic associations between clinical variables, they are convenient and frequently correct. As uncertainty increases, physicians rely even more on their clinical intuition.[39]

The goals of questioning and data accumulation are several: to identify highly likely diagnostic hypotheses, to disprove unlikely hypotheses, to forge causal links between clinical phenomena, to differentiate among existing hypotheses, and, as noted before, to find hypotheses that are particularly critical to preserving a patient's well-being (diagnostic imperatives).[40]

THE DIFFERENTIAL DIAGNOSIS

(Cases 10, 18, 38)

As attempts are made to refine hypotheses, clinicians often assemble a list of surviving, competing hypotheses commonly known as a **differential diagnosis**. However, no single definition of a differential diagnosis is universally accepted. Such lists are assembled early in the process from single or multiple cues, and they may or may not be ordered according to some hierarchy (such as physiologic categories or disease probabilities). Some clinicians define a differential diagnosis as a small final set of remaining hypotheses for which the discrimination strategy described previously is used.[41,42] We prefer to consider the entire process of hypothesis refinement as one that differentiates among diagnostic possibilities. According to this definition, a differential diagnosis comprises the entire evolving, sequential, and iterative diagnostic process from generation of hypotheses to establishment of the working diagnosis.

RELATION TO FORMAL PROBABILISTIC APPROACH

(Cases 23, 27, 42)

It is useful to set this evolving process against an explicit process of diagnostic revision that is based on probability theory and that uses Bayes' rule for recalculating the likelihood of various diseases. This comparison is of particular value because of the close parallelism between the implicit reasoning processes that physicians use to revise and refine diagnostic hypotheses with new information and the formal, prescriptive process that calculates these revisions.[12]

Bayesian analysis requires that a physician assembles a complete set of diagnostic hypotheses that could explain a given set of clinical findings. For each hypothesis, a set of relevant attributes is identified (historical findings, physical findings, complications, predisposing factors, laboratory results) that might help discriminate among the diagnoses. The **pretest** or **prior probability** of each diagnostic hypothesis is specified numerically, as is the probability that each attribute is found in each disease entity (the **conditional probability**). Then, a calculation is made of the likelihood of each disease entity, given the disease prevalence and the probability of each clinical attribute. The resulting revised probabilities (the **posterior probability**) represent the likelihood of various disease entities, given the prevalence and the presence of the specified attributes. This process requires that all possible diseases be specified prospectively because omitting even rare possibilities may eliminate the correct diagnosis. As long as a complete set of diagnostic hypotheses is assembled at the onset of an analysis, Bayes' rule can be applied sequentially as information is gathered. Thus, Bayesian analysis is best applied after considerable data are already available. Bayesian analysis seeks to combine information as a clinician would, but according to formal mathematical rules. A detailed example of how Bayesian analysis is used in diagnostic hypothesis revision when multiple diseases and multiple attributes of these diseases are under consideration is given in Chapter 4, section Bayesian Revision for Multiple Diseases with Multiple Attributes.

Use and Interpretation of Diagnostic Tests

THE FUNCTION OF TESTS

Diagnostic testing is an information-gathering task that differs from the processes discussed in the previous chapter only in respect to the risks and costs that tests incur. Testing is used in the process of hypothesis refinement to help formulate a working diagnostic hypothesis, defined previously as one that is sufficiently unambiguous to set the stage for making decisions about further invasive testing, treatment, or judgments about prognosis. Because diagnostic tests elicit new information, they usually reduce diagnostic uncertainty and are often used selectively to distinguish among competing hypotheses. Tests virtually devoid of risk (e.g., those obtained by collection of blood and urine) and those low in cost are not different in their information-processing function from the direct questions asked the patient or from the findings gleaned from the physical examination.

QUANTIFYING TESTING DECISIONS

(Cases 20, 23, 26, 27, 29–31)

Physicians order diagnostic tests and process the data from these tests implicitly, but we have little data on the cognitive basis of the decisions to carry out the tests and their interpretations of the results. We do have extensive experience, however, with the prescriptive, quantitative approaches alluded to in the preceding section. Elaboration of these quantitative approaches yields valuable principles of diagnostic testing. In fact, because many test results are expressed numerically, such data are particularly amenable to quantitative interpretation. However, data from tests are not the only information that can readily be expressed in probabilistic terms. The frequency of clinical symptoms, findings, complications of tests, favorable and morbid outcomes, and the efficacy and risks of therapies all can be expressed in probabilistic terms.

Before describing techniques for combining probabilistic information, some attention must be paid to the concept of probability as it applies to medical diagnosis. A probability is an expression of likelihood—an opinion of the relative frequency with which an event is likely to occur. In medical practice, a probability is a belief about some aspect of a patient's state of health; it can never be known with certainty and can only be estimated. The basis of the belief could ideally be objective from large collections of such data, but usually such collections of data are unavailable or not readily at hand, so the usual source of these estimates becomes subjective opinion on the basis of personal experience with like cases.

Because probabilities have their basis in different data sources, not all probabilities are alike. Some probability assessments can be accepted with considerable confidence and some with little confidence. Our confidence in a probability assessment is couched in terms of **ambiguity**: The greater our uncertainty about the validity of a given probability assessment, the greater is the ambiguity. Ambiguity in probability assessments increases when available information is scanty, when data are unreliable, and when the **test results**, facts, or opinions of putative experts are conflicting. The least ambiguous probability assessments are those solidly grounded in large bodies of data. Unfortunately, such data are not always available, and in some instances, the physician must accept considerable ambiguity in his or her probability assessments.

Probabilistic interpretation of the results of diagnostic tests is invaluable in the process of discriminating among diagnostic hypotheses because the approach combines both the physician's diagnostic hypothesis before testing and the test result itself. These concepts are effectively understood in terms of certain kinds of probabilities. A prior probability is a belief about the likelihood of a diagnostic hypothesis—for example, the prevalence of a disease such as acute myocardial infarction among patients presenting with chest pain. This pretest probability may be modified by all information collected up to that point, including symptoms and signs. A posterior probability represents the revised belief in the likelihood of the diagnosis (myocardial infarction) after interpreting the test result (e.g., one or more creatine kinase or troponin levels). Test characteristics are defined as conditional probabilities, that is, as probabilities specific to certain (disease) conditions. Conditional probabilities describe the frequency with which a given result (e.g., an elevated creatine kinase [CK],) occurs in a given disease and in all other diagnoses of potential interest. In a patient suspected of having an acute myocardial infarction, for example, alternative possible hypotheses of potential interest might include angina pectoris, acute pericarditis, esophageal spasm, and anxiety. Conditional probabilities for an elevated CK would describe the frequency of high CK values in each of these alternate hypotheses. Combining the prior probabilities of acute myocardial infarction and its diagnostic competitors with the conditional probabilities of the CK results in each of the diagnostic hypotheses yields posterior probabilities (revised probabilities after testing) of all diagnostic possibilities under consideration. These probabilistic data can be combined implicitly without formal calculations, but experience shows that many physicians fail to combine such data accurately when interpretation is carried out in an implicit fashion. For this reason, carrying out an actual calculation of posterior probabilities has special advantages.

SENSITIVITY AND SPECIFICITY

(Cases 20, 23, 26)

When considering only the presence or absence of one disease, the conditional probabilities of test results can be described as the **sensitivity** and **specificity** of a test (Fig. 4.1). The sensitivity of a test applies to patients known by some independent criterion to have a given disease. It is defined as the **true-positive rate** or equivalently the probability of a positive test result in patients known to have the disease (a mnemonic is PID for "positive in disease"). Unfortunately, few tests are exclusively positive in patients with a given disease (**pathognomonic**) and exclusively negative in those who do not have the disease (sine qua non). Overlaps are virtually the rule. Negative test results in patients known to have the disease are described as false negatives. The specificity of a test applies to patients known by some independent criterion to be free of the disease (a mnemonic is NIH for "negative in health"). It is therefore the **true-negative rate** or equivalently the probability of a negative test result in patients known not to have the disease. Positive test results in patients who do not have the disease are considered to be false positives. Given the nearly universal overlap between test results in patients who have and who do not have the disease, it is necessary to define a positivity criteria or cutoff point above which the test is considered

TEST RESULT:

		POSITIVE	NEGATIVE	
DISEASE:	PRESENT	TRUE POSITIVE	FALSE NEGATIVE	TOTAL WITH DISEASE
	ABSENT	FALSE POSITIVE	TRUE NEGATIVE	TOTAL WITH NO DISEASE
		TOTAL POSITIVE TESTS	TOTAL NEGATIVE TESTS	

Figure 4.1 • Outcomes of a test with a binary result (either positive or negative) in a population of patients who either have or do not have a given disease. As shown, patients with the disease may have a positive test (true positive) or a negative test (false negative); patients who do not have the disease may have a negative test (true negative) or a positive test (false positive). The probability of a true-positive result in patients with the disease is the sensitivity of the test, and the probability of a negative result in patients who do not have the disease is the specificity of the test.

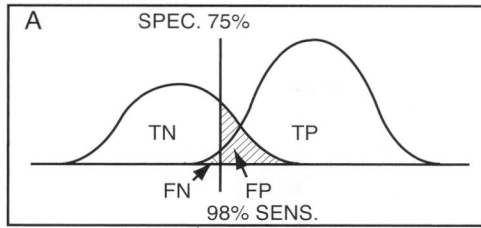

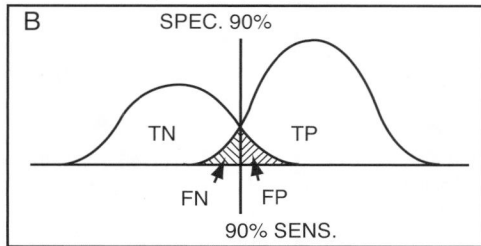

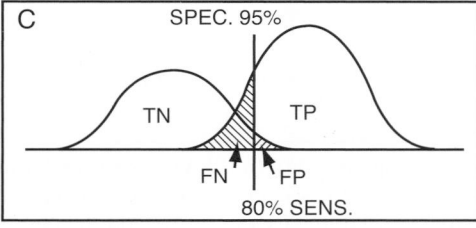

Figure 4.2 • Interpretation of a test, the results of which are in the form of a continuous function. Individuals who do not have the disease have low test values and are distributed under the shorter curve on the left. Patients with the disease have high test values and are distributed under the taller curve on the right. However, test values in normal and in diseased individuals overlap. The vertical lines represent different cutoff points or positivity criteria: for each of the three segments of the figure, any value of the test to the right of the cutoff point is defined as a positive test and any value to the left of the cutoff point is defined as a negative test. Segment B, in the middle of the figure, defines a cutoff point with equal sensitivity and specificity. With this criterion as the cutoff, the true positives (90% of those with the disease) are to the right of the cutoff, and the true negatives (90% of those who do not have the disease) are to the left of the cutoff. As the criterion for a positive test is made stricter (segment C, bottom), the specificity increases but the sensitivity is reduced. As the criterion for a positive test is made more lax (segment A, top), the sensitivity increases, but the specificity falls. FN, false-negative result; FP, false-positive result; SENS., sensitivity; SPEC., specificity; TN, true-negative result; TP, true-positive result.

positive and below which it is considered negative. If the cutoff point is made stricter (i.e., raised), then the number of **false-negative results** increases (or, equivalently, sensitivity decreases); however, the number of **false-positive results** decreases (or, equivalently, specificity increases); and vice versa (Fig. 4.2).

BAYES' RULE

(Cases 20, 23, 30, 51)

We present a specific example of calculations with Bayes' rule when both sensitivity and specificity are known. Although this "prostate cancer screening test" example is simplistic, it illustrates the relevant principles. Surveillance Epidemiology and End Results (SEER) data suggest that the prevalence of prostate cancer is 108 of 1,000 men aged 60 to 64 years. Of note, if prior screening with a highly sensitive test had been performed previously, the incidence of disease since the prior screening test should replace the prevalence estimate as the pretest likelihood of disease. In this case, assuming a screening test 1 year ago, the annual incidence of prostate cancer would be between 2 and 9 of 1,000, depending on race. Based on a published study,[43] 71% of patients known to have prostate cancer have a positive test (sensitivity) and 51% of patients known to be free of cancer (benign prostatic hyperplasia [BPH]) have a negative test (specificity) (the data are summarized in Table 4.1). In the population described, what is the significance of a positive test? How likely is it that a person with a positive test has cancer? Calculations are shown in the accompanying figures.

TABLE 4.1	
Data for the Prostate Cancer Screening Test: Prostate-Specific Antigen (PSA)	
Prior Probability (equivalent here to disease prevalence)	**0.108**
True-positive rate (sensitivity)	0.71
False-negative rate (1 − sensitivity)	0.29
True-negative rate (specificity)	0.51
False-positive rate (1 − specificity)	0.49

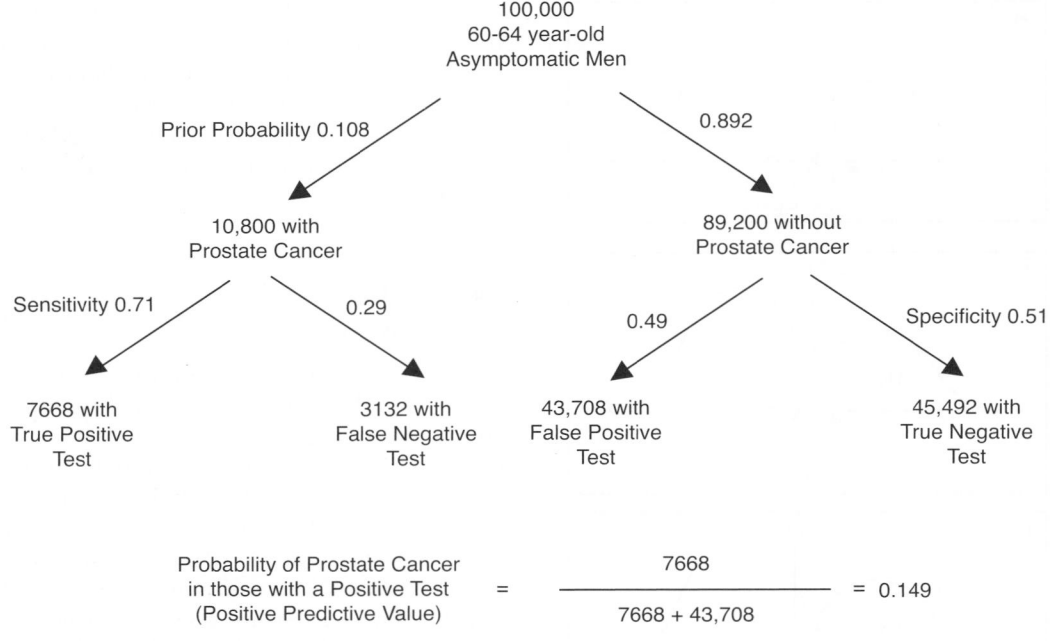

Figure 4.3 • A "tree" or flow diagram approach to the prostate-specific antigen (PSA) "cancer test" using Bayes' rule. This illustrates one solution to the PSA prostate cancer test described in the text. Starting with a population of 100,000 individuals, of whom 108 of 1,000 are expected to have cancer, we add the positive tests in those with cancer (true positives) to those who do not have cancer (false positives) and determine the fraction of patients with a positive test who actually have the disease (true positives divided by the sum of true positives and false positives). The origin of the data in the figure is shown in Table 4.1. With the relatively low specificity of the test at 0.51, more than 85% of positive tests are found in patients who do not have cancer. The low prevalence and the high false-positive rate of the test (0.49) account for this result.

Three different approaches to the calculations are illustrated: a "tree" or flow diagram approach (Fig. 4.3), a tabular approach (Fig. 4.4), and the use of Bayes' formula (Fig. 4.5). More detailed examples of the actual use of Bayes' rule, or Bayesian analysis, are given in Part II (see Cases 23 and 30).

TESTING PRINCIPLES

(Cases 20, 22, 23, 29)

Bayes' rule combines data on sensitivity and specificity of tests with prior probabilities, yielding a probabilistic view of various diagnoses that incorporates the test results. The application of Bayes' rule to diagnostic testing yields important testing principles: The specificity of a test is critical for case finding, especially when screening asymptomatic patients, because the higher the specificity, the lower is the false-positive rate. In populations in which disease prevalence is low, most positive tests will be false positives unless a test is exceptionally specific so that almost all patients without disease have a negative test. Indeed, if the disease prevalence is extremely low, a test (if it is the only one available) should not be done unless it is nearly perfectly specific. Thus, when a test is highly specific, a positive test result helps "rule in" a disease (a mnemonic is Positive SpIn for "positive test with high specificity rules in the disease"). Tests that are not highly specific are most useful for screening if they are applied in populations with a high disease prevalence. When other confirmatory tests are available, a test with only a moderately high specificity may be worth using (assuming no cost and no risk) as an initial screening test if it has high sensitivity. For example, screening for HIV typically involves enzyme immunoassay (EIA) followed by Western blot testing, a very sensitive test followed by a more specific test if the first test is positive

	Prior Probability	Conditional Probability	Product	Fraction with Positive Test	Posterior Probability
Prostate Cancer	0.108	0.71	0.07668	$\dfrac{0.07668}{0.51376}$	0.149
No Cancer	0.892	0.49	0.43708	$\dfrac{0.43708}{0.51376}$	0.851

Sum of positive tests = 0.51376

Figure 4.4 • A tabular solution to the prostate-specific antigen (PSA) "cancer test" using Bayes' rule. The prior probability of each condition (cancer or no cancer) is multiplied by the conditional probability (in this case the probability of a positive test, given each condition). The products are summed, and the fraction of positive tests in each condition is calculated. Note the similarity between this calculation and that shown in Figure 4.3. For interpretation, see legend for Figure 4.3.

for a disease in which accurate diagnosis has a high **expected utility** or benefit. Thus, when a test is highly sensitive, a negative test result helps "rule out" a disease (a mnemonic is Negative SnOut for "negative test with a high sensitivity rules out disease").

BAYESIAN REVISION FOR MULTIPLE RESULTS

The previous example of prostate-specific antigen (PSA) screening involved the simplest model of **Bayesian revision** (disease either present or absent;

USE OF BAYES' FORMULA

$$P(D+|T+) = \frac{P(D+) \times P(T+|D+)}{P(D+) \times P(T+|D+) + P(D-) \times P(T+|D-)}$$

Where

$P(D+)$	=	disease positive (prostate cancer)
$P(D-)$	=	disease negative (no cancer)
$P(T+|D+)$	=	true-positive rate (sensitivity)
$P(T+|D-)$	=	false-positive rate (1 − specificity)
$P(D+|T+)$	=	probability of cancer among those with a positive test

For this particular patient:

$$P(\text{prostate cancer}) = \frac{0.108 \times 0.71}{0.108 \times 0.71 + 0.892 \times 0.49} = 0.149$$

Figure 4.5 • Solution to the prostate-specific antigen (PSA) "cancer test" using Bayes' formula. Note that the calculation is identical to that shown in Figures 4.3 and 4.4.

TABLE 4.2

Data for the Prostate Cancer Screening Test: Prostate Specific Antigen (PSA)

PSA Level (ng/mL)	Prostate Cancer	No Cancer (Benign Prostatic Hypertrophy)
0–3.9	0.29	0.51
4.0–5.9	0.21	0.21
6.0–9.9	0.23	0.18
≥10	0.27	0.10

test either positive or negative). A more refined estimate of prostate cancer can be based on knowing the actual PSA result, or "how positive it was." To do so, results that are reported as continuous

variables or patterns (e.g., serum enzymes, serum electrolytes, electrocardiographic stress tests, or in this case PSA results) usually must be broken into discrete intervals or discrete categories so that they can be used in calculations. Instead of simply positive or negative, test results describe several levels of positivity. Table 4.2 summarizes the likelihood of different PSA levels for prostate cancer and for BPH.[43] Figure 4.6 illustrates the likelihood of prostate cancer if the PSA is 12 (10 or above). Figure 4.7 illustrates the results for a PSA of 7.0 (falling in the 6.0–9.9 range). In these cases, the interpretation of a test result no longer depends on the result simply being positive by falling above a cutoff value. Thus, the previous sensitivity and false-positive rate (1 – specificity) conditional probabilities cannot be applied. Rather, conditional

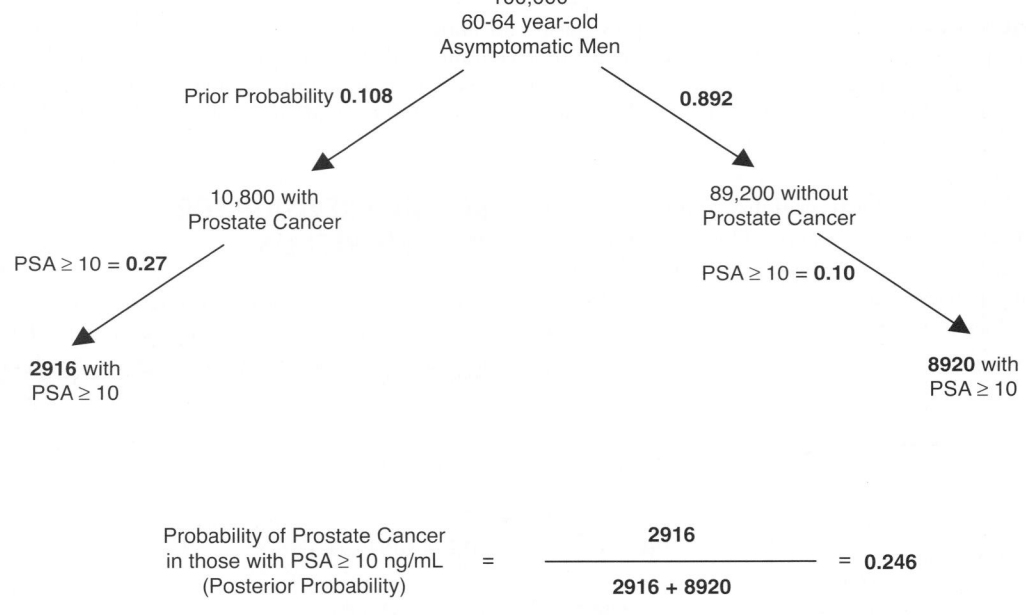

Figure 4.6 • Solution to the prostate-specific antigen (PSA) "cancer test" for a specific test range. This figure demonstrates the benefit of knowing the exact PSA result (Table 4.2). Sensitivity and specificity are typically defined as test values falling above or below a "cutoff" value or positivity criterion. However, in a given patient, the positive or negative results may be close to or far from this cutoff. For a test result of 12 (exceeding 10), which is far from the 4.0 positivity criterion, the likelihood of cancer is higher at 0.246 than the 0.149 for a positive test in Figures 4.3 to 4.5. With regard to simply an entire group of patients with positive test results, some have results close to 4 and others have values that are much higher, greater than 10. Patients with benign prostatic hyperplasia, however, are much less likely to have results exceeding 10, so the likelihood of cancer is this subset with high PSA (greater than 10) is consequently higher because false positives drop. Note that if 10 were used as a positivity criterion cutoff, many patients with cancer would have negative tests and be missed, so choosing a cutoff is a tradeoff between false-positive and false-negative results, balancing the benefit of treating true positives against the harm of treating false positives.

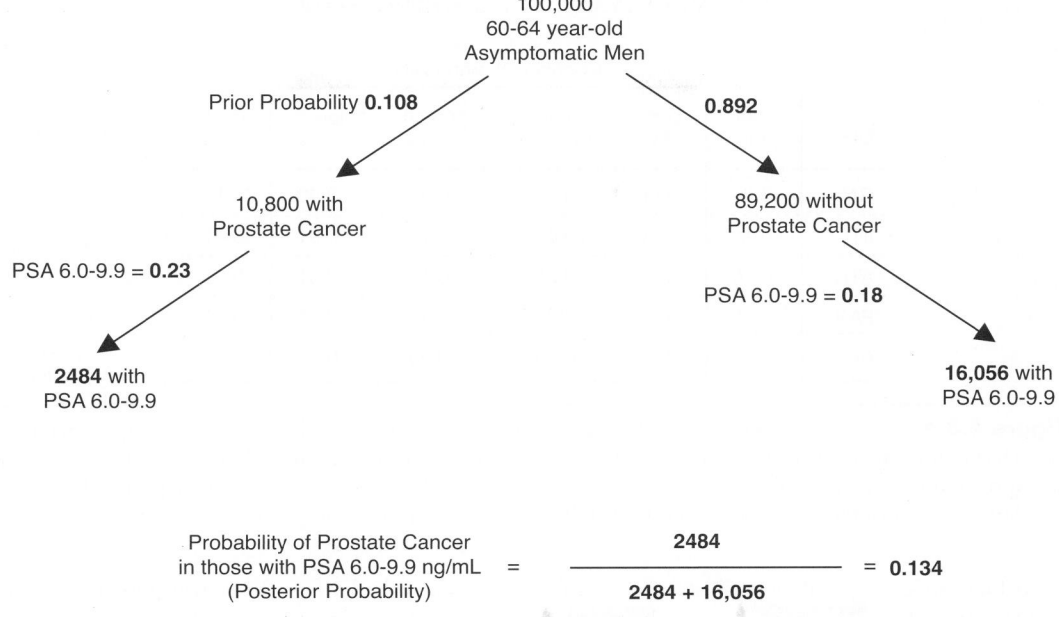

100,000
60-64 year-old
Asymptomatic Men

Prior Probability **0.108**   **0.892**

10,800 with   89,200 without
Prostate Cancer   Prostate Cancer

PSA 6.0-9.9 = **0.23**

PSA 6.0-9.9 = **0.18**

2484 with   **16,056** with
PSA 6.0-9.9   PSA 6.0-9.9

$$\text{Probability of Prostate Cancer in those with PSA 6.0-9.9 ng/mL (Posterior Probability)} = \frac{2484}{2484 + 16,056} = 0.134$$

Figure 4.7 • Solution to the prostate-specific antigen (PSA) "cancer test" for a specific test range. As in Figure 4.6, this figure demonstrates the effect of knowing the exact PSA result. For a test result of 7.0 (between 6.0 and 9.9), which falls closer to the 4.0 positivity criterion cutoff, the likelihood of cancer is a bit lower at 0.134 than the 0.149 for a positive test in Figures 4.3 to 4.5 and the 0.246 for a test result of 12 in Figure 4.6.

probabilities become the likelihood of a result of 10 or greater or the likelihood of a PSA falling between 6.0 and 9.9 among patients with and without prostate cancer.

BAYESIAN REVISION FOR MULTIPLE DISEASES WITH MULTIPLE ATTRIBUTES

(Cases 23, 27)

Having expanded the simplest model of Bayesian revision (disease either present or absent; test either positive or negative) to include ranges of test results, we can consider an even more complex model in which several diseases are under consideration, each of which has two or more attributes. Indeed, the physician often considers several diseases during the process of differential diagnosis and needs to interpret how his or her suspicion of each of these diseases changes in the light of new information.

For a specific example, let us consider how the differential diagnosis can be carried out using Bayesian analysis. Suppose we have a 70-year-old man who had a cardiac catheterization 8 days ago

and since then noticed a reduction in urine output. He gives a history of vomiting and has been taking a nonsteroidal anti-inflammatory drug for arthralgias that appeared in the last week. He now has acute renal insufficiency. His examination and a variety of laboratory studies have narrowed the diagnostic possibilities to five conditions: glomerulonephritis (GN), interstitial nephritis (IN), acute tubular necrosis (ATN), functional acute renal failure from dehydration (FARF), and atheromatous embolism (AE). We will assess the diagnostic significance of two of his physical findings—hypertension and livedo reticularis; and two laboratory results—a urine sediment containing few abnormalities and a low hemolytic complement level (Fig. 4.8). Let us assume that the prior probabilities of these five diseases are those given in the figure, and that the approximate conditional probabilities shown for each of the clinical attributes (hypertension, livedo reticularis, sparse sediment, and low complement) have been obtained from a survey of the literature on acute renal failure. The figure shows the prior probabilities, the conditional probabilities, and the calculated posterior

BAYESIAN ANALYSIS FOR ACUTE RENAL FAILURE

DIS.	Prior prob.	Conditional probabilities				Post. prob.
		B.P. 190/120	livedo reticularis	sparse sediment	low CH50	
GN	0.29	0.60	0.05	0.01	0.40	0.019
IN	0.10	0.10	0.05	0.15	0.01	<0.01
ATN	0.40	0.05	0.05	0.15	0.01	<0.01
FARF	0.25	0.01	0.20	0.95	0.01	<0.01
AE	0.01	0.80	0.60	0.95	0.40	0.977

Figure 4.8 • Use of Bayes' rule in the differential diagnosis of multiple conditions when multiple attributes of each condition are being considered. AE, atheromatous embolism; ATN, acute tubular necrosis; B.P., blood pressure in mm Hg; DIS., disorder, FARF, functional acute renal failure; GN, glomerulonephritis; IN, acute interstitial nephritis; Post. prob., posterior probability; Prior prob., prior probability.

probabilities. This calculation illustrates several features: first, that a "diagnosis" is in truth a **probability distribution** for a set of diagnostic possibilities (in this case, the various types of acute renal failure), and second, that the estimate of the prior probability of any given disorder and the relation between the conditional probabilities have major effects on the outcome of the analysis. In this example, glomerulonephritis was a likely diagnosis initially, and two features (hypertension and hypocomplementemia) argue in favor of this diagnosis, yet because a sparse sediment and livedo reticularis are rare in this disorder, the posterior probability is quite low. More important, atheromatous embolism was quite unlikely initially, but because the likelihood of most of the attributes was higher in atheroembolism than in the other disorders, the diagnosis of atheroembolism after considering these findings is highly likely. This example illustrates how clinical features other than test results can be used in formal, quantitative decision making using Bayes' rule. The analogy of this mathematical approach to the implicit process of hypothesis refinement described before should be quite evident.

PRAGMATIC CONSIDERATIONS IN THE PROBABILISTIC APPROACH

(Cases 23, 31, 42, 43)

An unambiguous definition of all disease entities under consideration is an essential element of

Bayesian calculations. Whenever possible, definitions of disease entities should be based on some "**gold standard**," that is, some relatively irrefutable standard that constitutes recognized and accepted evidence that a certain disease exists. Histologic evidence is the most frequently accepted criterion, although biochemical markers (enzyme analyses) and genetic markers (gene probes) already have substituted in many instances. When the questions regarding clinical attributes of a given disease are being formulated, all possible variations in these manifestations must be considered. Disease attributes vary according to factors such as the stage of the disease and the age of the patient in whom the disease occurs. In addition, a disease may not be stable: Because it may be evolving even as the diagnostic process is underway, the probability of certain attributes may change over time.

The formal application of Bayes' rule has many advantages. When objective data are used for sensitivity, specificity, and disease prevalence, calculated posterior probabilities represent statistically valid approaches to combining the data. To the extent that some of the data are not solidly rooted in experimental studies, the interpretation of an analysis can be tested by altering the particular variable (e.g., the prior probability) and repeating the calculations. This process—**sensitivity analysis**—also is used in decision analysis.

As the acute renal failure example illustrates, Bayes' rule need not be confined to use with clinical data in the form of sensitivity and specificity. These quantitative techniques also can be applied to clinical radiologic or pathologic findings. All that is needed is to specify the probability of any given finding in various competing diseases. As illustrated in the acute renal failure example and in Case 23, multiple findings (e.g., results of several biochemical studies) can be considered simultaneously. Multiple findings also can be considered serially with Bayes' rule. When such findings are considered serially, the posterior probability after one finding is used as the prior probability for assessing another finding.

When using Bayes' rule, several caveats should be heeded: (1) Making a calculation with Bayes' rule does not require that every possible disease under consideration be listed separately. Diseases can be combined and even a "**catchall hypothesis**" residual diagnostic category can be included if necessary (such as "other etiologies of acute renal failure"). Of course, all possible relevant diagnoses must be included in the list, or else the actual diagnosis might never surface. (2) To avoid counting the same information more than once, each disease must be mutually exclusive of all other diseases under consideration and each conditional probability used in a calculation must be independent of the others. (3) Certain diseases cannot be appropriately considered simply as either present or absent. Because stages of diseases often have different manifestations, any quantitative analysis must recognize the clinical manifestations and test results in various stages of the disease. Because of these caveats, especially when simultaneously considering many findings or diseases, mathematical predictive modeling methods such as logistic regression or neural networks have become preferred.

Although the formal application of these quantitative techniques is an invaluable benchmark for all considerations of diagnostic testing, frequently no formal quantitative approach is needed when interpreting the results of tests. Nonetheless, because our descriptions of diagnoses often comprise rather nonspecific terms such as "compatible with," "suggestive of," "likely," "highly likely," and "virtually certain," and because physicians often falter when they combine probabilistic concepts intuitively, reverting to a quantitative approach in some circumstances has merit.

INTERPRETING RESULTS

(Cases 20, 23, 26, 29)

When we are not certain how to interpret some clinical data or are confronted with surprising, conflicting, or counterintuitive results, Bayes' rule is worth invoking. Surprising results do occur from time to time, and the principles of Bayesian analysis help with their interpretation. Given a low prior probability, the characteristics of a test result critically determine how a positive test result is interpreted. A slightly positive test increases the posterior probability of disease only slightly, whereas a dramatically positive test result increases the posterior probability substantially. The latter is true because highly positive test results (e.g., a serum sodium concentration of 160 mEq/L or a 3-cm round, solid mass in the kidney on a renal ultrasound) virtually never occur in normal people.

WHEN TO TEST

(Cases 23, 25, 28–30, 45)

The foregoing discussion centers on the interpretation of tests, but decisions to carry out tests are equally important. Clearly, testing is superfluous when the test result can be expected to have no effect on subsequent decision making. When a disease is highly unlikely, further tests to disprove the diagnosis often are not needed. When a disease is highly likely, confirmatory tests are also often unnecessary. Increasing the diagnostic likelihood of a disease to near certainty or decreasing the likelihood of a disease to virtually zero by successive testing is in itself not a rational use of tests. Testing is most useful when the result, either positive or negative, can be expected to alter the posterior probability sufficiently to influence some subsequent decision (usually another decision to test or a decision to treat). Decisions to use tests should not be made on the basis of test accuracy alone; the risk of performing the tests as well as the efficacy and risks of available therapies should be included into the decision to use the test. Bayesian analysis only calculates probabilities; other methods are needed to deal with these everyday complex tradeoffs.

THE THRESHOLD CONCEPT

(Cases 24, 29, 30, 45, 51, 52)

The threshold concept explicitly considers both the likelihood of disease and the tradeoffs between the risks and benefits of tests and treatments; it uses simple principles to identify when to test and when to treat. When a treatment for a suspected disease is extremely effective and low in risk and the probability of disease is quite high, it may be appropriate to avoid using a risky test and give the treatment without complete confidence that the disease is present. With a less effective treatment or a risky treatment, the physician's confidence in the diagnosis must be quite high to avoid giving the risky treatment to patients who do not have the disease. When assessing a treatment, multiple factors must be considered, including the cure rate, the extension in life expectancy, and the alleviation of suffering. In addition, any measure of the value of a treatment must represent the net effect of both the efficacy and the risk of that therapy. The cost of a test is, of course, another factor. When a test is expensive but virtually risk-free and the disease sought has a large potential in terms of a patient's well-being (e.g., an abdominal ultrasound for abdominal aortic aneurysm or CT scan for hemangioma of the liver), then the use of the test often is warranted even if the condition being sought is uncommon.

As discussed briefly, the threshold concept combines these issues explicitly. It incorporates factors such as test accuracy, therapeutic efficacy, and the risks of the tests and treatments and offers guidance in decisions to use diagnostic tests. Of course, some of these issues (the likelihood of a diagnosis, the efficacy and risks of therapy) also influence decisions to use a treatment. Thus, because testing and treatment thresholds are closely related, both will be discussed here instead of discussing testing here and treatment later. To explain how the interrelations among the sensitivity and specificity of tests, the risks of testing, and the risks and benefits of treatment are merged in the threshold concept, we will consider a simplified clinical situation in which a hypothetical patient either has or does not have a single disease, in this case pulmonary embolism: That is, pulmonary embolism is either present or not. To describe the therapeutic threshold, we will first make the as-

sumption that we have all of the patient's clinical data and the results of a D-dimer test, but that the most definitive tests—spiral computed tomography scan or pulmonary arteriography—are not available. We also will make the assumption that the only treatment being considered is the use of heparin. Our decision, then, is to treat with heparin or to withhold treatment. The factors that influence this choice are imbedded in the threshold concept.

THE THERAPEUTIC THRESHOLD

(Cases 22, 45, 51)

At the extremes of diagnostic certainty, the relations between the confidence in a diagnosis and a therapeutic intervention are readily apparent. If one is confident on clinical grounds that a patient has had a pulmonary embolus, one should be willing to give heparin as long as the benefits of treatment outweigh the risks (e.g., gastrointestinal hemorrhage). At the other extreme, if one is confident on clinical grounds that the patient has not had a pulmonary embolus, one should not, of course, give heparin. At likelihoods of pulmonary embolism between definitely present and definitely absent, the decision to treat is a function of how likely one considers the probability of an embolus, the magnitude of the benefits of anticoagulation, and the magnitude of the risks of therapy. Indeed, some probability of pulmonary embolism exists between 0 and 1 at which the value of giving or withholding treatment are equivalent. This "break-even" probability is known as the threshold probability, or specifically the therapeutic threshold (Fig. 4.9). At disease probabilities greater than the threshold, treatment should be given, whereas at disease probabilities lower than the threshold, treatment should be withheld. As shown in Figure 4.10, the higher the ratio between benefits and risks of treatment, the lower the likelihood of disease required to give treatment. The lower the ratio (i.e., the lower the efficacy of treatment and/or the higher the risk), the more certain one must be of the diagnosis before administering the treatment. If the suspicion of pulmonary embolism is only moderately high and there is no increased risk from heparin, heparin should be given, whereas even if the suspicion of pulmonary embolism is moderate,

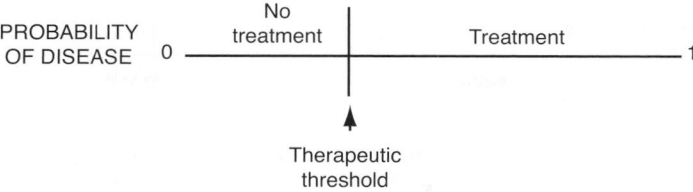

Figure 4.9 • The therapeutic threshold. The probability of disease is represented from 0 to 1 on the horizontal line. The therapeutic threshold is calculated from data on the likelihood of a given disease and the benefits and risks of available therapy. The threshold is a benchmark for action: At disease probabilities less than the threshold, treatment is withheld, and at disease probabilities greater than the threshold, treatment is given. The assumption is made that no additional tests are available to further assess the probability of disease. When no such tests are available, the thresholds in this are applicable.

heparin should be avoided when the risk of treatment (serious bleeding) also is high.

TESTING THRESHOLDS

(Cases 25, 29, 30, 51)

A test that can help differentiate whether a disease is present reduces uncertainty: A positive result increases the probability of the disease and a negative test reduces its likelihood. Depending on the characteristics of a given treatment, the test result may make the **posttest probability** of disease sufficiently high or low to alter the decision in favor of administering treatment or withholding it, respectively. These principles are embodied in the concept of **testing thresholds**, which are benchmarks for the use of diagnostic tests. If, as noted in the preceding section, the two therapeutic choices for a patient

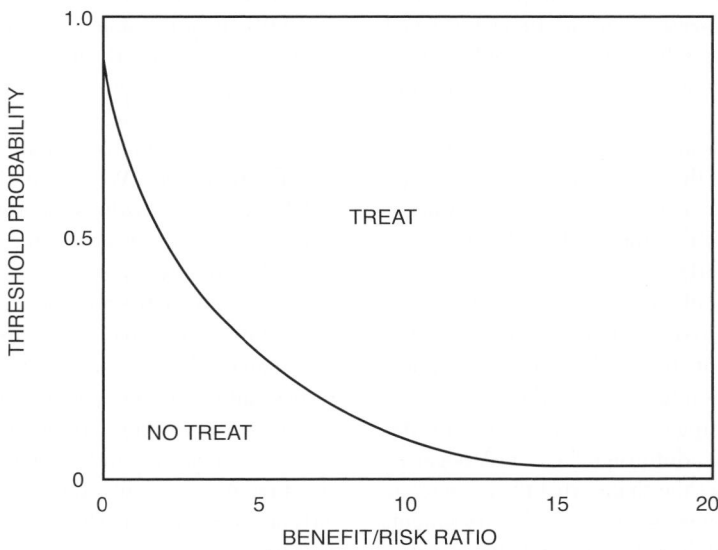

Figure 4.10 • Relation between the benefits and cost (risk) of a treatment and the threshold probability. For a given benefit/cost ratio, treatment is preferred (TREAT) when the probability of disease in an individual patient exceeds the threshold value. The lower the ratio between benefits and costs, the more certain must the physician be of the diagnosis before prescribing therapy. As in Figure 4.9, the threshold is calculated from data on the likelihood of a given disease and the benefits and risks of available therapy. (Modified from Pauker SG, Kassirer JP. Therapeutic decision making: a cost–benefit analysis. *N Engl J Med.* 1975;293:229–234; with permission.)

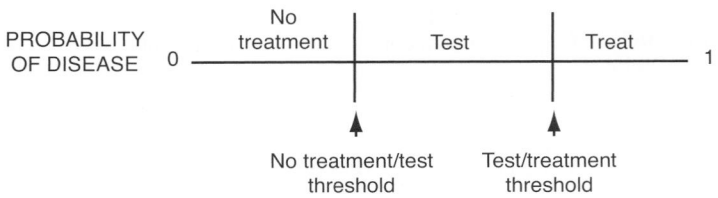

Figure 4.11 • Testing thresholds. The probability of disease is represented from 0 to 1 on the horizontal line. The two thresholds are calculated from data on the likelihood of a given disease, the benefits and risks of available therapy, the sensitivity and specificity, and the risks of a given diagnostic test. As in Figure 4.9, the thresholds are benchmarks for action: At disease probabilities less than the no-treatment/test threshold, treatment is withheld and the test is not used. At disease probabilities greater than the test/treatment threshold, treatment is given, also without testing. At disease probabilities between the two thresholds, the test is carried out, and the result of the test dictates the action taken (withholding vs. giving the treatment).

suspected of having a given disease are withholding treatment or giving the treatment, and if treatment should be withheld when the disease is absent and given when the disease is present, then the "break-even" probability at which the value of giving the treatment and not giving the treatment is the same as the therapeutic threshold. If, however, a diagnostic test is available that has the potential of altering the likelihood that the patient is suffering from the disease, then the clinician is faced not with two choices, but three: withholding therapy, ordering the test, and treating without testing (Fig. 4.11).

The decisions at the very lower end and the very upper end of the probability scale are not affected by the existence of the test: The clinician will still withhold treatment when the disease is highly unlikely and still give the treatment when the disease is virtually certain. In both of these circumstances, the physician should not carry out the test. At intermediate probabilities of disease, however, the test result might have an influence on the choice of not treating or treating, and the optimal decision then is to administer the test. A negative test result decreases the chance that the patient has the disease and argues against giving the treatment; a positive test result increases the probability of disease and argues in favor of giving the treatment. The probability value at which the choice to give no treatment and the choice to use the test are equal in value is the test threshold for deciding between no treatment and testing, and the probability value at which the choice to administer the test and the choice to give the treatment are equal in value is the

treatment threshold for deciding between testing and empiric treatment.

Testing thresholds are a function not only of factors such as the accuracy of the test (sensitivity and specificity) and the risk of the test but also (in the case of the therapeutic threshold) of the efficacy and risks of treatment. Once the thresholds are calculated from these factors or estimated by the physician, they are interpreted as follows (Fig. 4.11): When the estimated likelihood or probability of disease falls below the no-treatment/test threshold, the optimal choice is not to give the treatment. When the disease probability exceeds the test/treatment threshold, the optimal choice is to give the treatment. When the disease probability falls between the two thresholds, the optimal choice is to carry out the test and to either treat or not treat, depending on the test result.

Returning to the pulmonary embolism example, suppose now that a pulmonary arteriogram is available. Threshold calculations would include values, tailored to the specific patient if necessary, on the sensitivity and specificity of the test, the efficacy of heparin, and the risk of heparin. Derived from this calculation would be two thresholds: a probability at which the value of the two strategies of not treating with heparin and performing the arteriogram are equivalent (the no-treatment/test threshold), and another threshold at which the value of the two strategies of performing the arteriogram and giving heparin are equivalent (the test/treatment threshold). The tripartite choice between no heparin therapy and no arteriogram, performing the arteriogram, and administering heparin without carrying out the arteriogram would be made on the basis of the physician's assessment of whether the patient is suffering from the disease. At low probabilities of pulmonary embolism, no treatment is given and no testing is performed; at high probabilities of pulmonary embolism, heparin is given without arteriography; and at intermediate probabilities of pulmonary embolism, the choice of withholding heparin or giving it is dependent on the result of arteriography.

Whether testing decisions are made on the basis of formal threshold calculations or implicitly, the factors that influence the decision to use a test are evident in this model of diagnostic and therapeutic decision making.

CHAPTER 5

Causal Reasoning

DEFINITION

(Cases 32, 34, 35)

The process of arriving at a working diagnosis requires interpretation of new data in light of existing information and assessment of the relations among all of the clinical findings. In carrying out these tasks, the physician makes repeated attempts to "tie all the findings together." The probabilistic approach, such as that described earlier, represents one of the methods used, and the use of standard, **compiled knowledge rules** or **categorical reasoning** (e.g., if a patient has rheumatoid arthritis, splenomegaly, and leukopenia, consider Felty syndrome) is another. Indeed, much of the reasoning in medicine depends on probabilistic and categorical associations between clinical variables. Still another powerful approach is causal reasoning. **Causal reasoning** is an aspect of the diagnostic process based on the cause-and-effect relations between clinical variables or chains of variables. It is a function of the anatomic, physiologic, and biochemical mechanisms that operate in the normal workings of the human body and the pathophysiologic behavior of these mechanisms in disease. In addition to its basis in the mechanisms of normal and abnormal pathophysiology, causal reasoning relies on commonsense notions of causality, such as the beliefs that an effect is usually generated by a known cause, that cause and effect are related in time and space, and that a cause and its effect are generally similar in intensity and magnitude.[44-46]

Certain kinds of clinical reasoning are better described in terms of a **causal model** than in terms of the probabilistic associations between variables. Take, for example, the interpretation of a normal creatinine level 1 hour after a patient develops acute anuria. A probabilistic model that explains this apparent contradiction (a normal creatinine value in the face of zero kidney function) would strain credibility. Yet the physiological explanation is simple, complete, and revealing: Because creatinine is produced in the muscle at a constant rate even when kidney function is nil, an insufficient amount would accumulate over such a short time following renal shutdown to produce a perceptible rise in the serum level. This example is based on a causal or physiologic model of reality. The capacity to make inferences from the observed clinical findings also depends on the principles embedded in this model. Such models abound in all domains in medicine but are especially common in nephrology, cardiology, pulmonology, and endocrinology because of their strong underlying physiologic knowledge base.

When applying causal reasoning, the physician examines clinical variables and includes them if they help to explain the model. A model is created for each patient, although a single model can be applicable for many patients in many clinical settings. Such a model is a coherent system that is capable of explaining its components, the range of possible variations, and the nature of findings in a particular patient. If the same model is not applicable for the next patient with a problem similar to that for which it was created, additional features of the model might be required and some existing features might have to be deleted.

To explain how a causal model can support a clinician's performance by simulating possible courses of the disease and its modification by treatment and how such a model can serve as a coherency criterion for hypotheses about the patient, an example is presented here from the domain of fluid and electrolyte equilibrium. Assume that a patient with clinical and laboratory findings suggestive of the syndrome of inappropriate secretion of antidiuretic hormone (SIADH) has a high urinary sodium excretion: Does this finding influence the suspected diagnosis? We could assess this finding in a probabilistic framework (e.g., we might say that 85% to 95% of patients with SIADH have a high sodium excretion), or, alternatively, by understanding the pathophysiology of SIADH, we could examine how the finding "fits" with the diagnosis. If our model of SIADH contains (as it should) the concepts that such patients are volume expanded, that volume expansion promotes sodium excretion, and that sodium excretion in SIADH typically matches sodium intake, we would understand readily that a high urine sodium excretion not only is consistent with the diagnosis of SIADH, but also that it adds to the credibility of that diagnosis. We also would be in a position to explain a low urine sodium excretion if that were the finding instead. In this instance, despite the presence of SIADH, urine sodium is low, presumably because the patient is ingesting little salt.

USING A CAUSAL MODEL

(Cases 11, 32, 33, 35, 36)

We often are alerted to the possibility that we should be using a causal model when abnormal findings or events violate normal expectations. This deviation produces the context within which further data gathering and interpreting takes place. To carry out this interpretive process, we generate a causal model, typically a chain of related features consisting of stimuli and their responses.[44,46–48] When invoking a causal hypothesis involving two or more variables, we assess the links between stimuli and responses for their strength. The strength of this link can be assessed by the satisfaction of several criteria. Is the entire causal chain credible? Does a given change in a response correlate closely with the change in the stimulus? Is there substantial congruity of duration and magnitude between response and stimulus? Is there close contiguity in time and space between a response and a stimulus (did one event follow another sufficiently closely to allow us to accept that the first event caused the second)? When these tests are satisfied, one gains confidence that a given stimulus and a suspected response are related.[48–50]

Note that in describing the outcome of causal reasoning we deliberately use the notion of "confidence" in the relationship between cause and effect. We do so because causality virtually never can be proved; the stronger that the elements of causality are, the more likely it is that the effect can be attributed to the cause. Just because a given effect commonly quickly follows, a stimulus is not sufficient justification for attributing the effect to the cause.[51] Common sense does not always lead us to correct conclusions about causality, as evidenced by the mistaken notions that getting chilled causes upper respiratory infections and that stormy weather causes arthritic pain to worsen. Similar considerations lead to caution when attributing a rare complication to a drug that is new to the market.

In medicine, we are always attempting both to validate and to debunk causal relations. Indeed, the final step in assessing a causal hypothesis is

testing it for alternate possible explanations. Simply because a given causal hypothesis appears to explain a set of findings does not necessarily prove that this causal chain is the correct one. Alternative constructions of the causal chain must be sought and their strengths assessed before accepting one model and not another.

WHERE IN THE DIAGNOSTIC PROCESS DOES CAUSAL REASONING FIT?

(Cases 11, 33, 34)

Causal reasoning can be applied in several steps of the diagnostic process. Early in the process, probabilistic reasoning is more likely to be helpful than causal reasoning in generating hypotheses. Because causal models are dependent exclusively on fundamental knowledge about physiologic function and dysfunction and the cause-and-effect relations between clinical events, they are specific to disease entities and independent of the patient population. By contrast, probabilistic models are dependent on the specific population from which the patient is drawn. Because diagnostic hypotheses are so critically dependent on disease prevalence, causal reasoning is a rather weak approach when the required task is triggering such hypotheses, whereas probabilistic reasoning is quite strong. The assertion, for example, that a 60-year-old heavy smoker with hemoptysis is far more likely to have lung cancer than a 20-year-old nonsmoker with the same symptom is based predominantly on disease prevalence rather than on the mechanisms of bleeding. Nonetheless, causal reasoning can be useful early in the diagnostic process when formulating a context: If the possibility of a pathophysiologic state has been triggered by some findings, the state may provide the context for further data gathering. When physical examination in a 37-year-old man admitted for cough, hiccups, and extensive lesions in the lung disclosed that the patient had bilateral gynecomastia, attention immediately shifted to the possibility that metastatic germ cell was the etiology of his pulmonary nodules. Further studies proved the diagnosis to be correct. In addition, once a possible cause has been proposed, causal reasoning allows us to assess whether the cause can explain the observation. The SIADH example given before illustrates the interplay of these reasoning strategies. Once the diagnosis of SIADH was triggered, the causal model made it possible to check the appropriateness of either a high or a low urinary sodium excretion. Causal models also help us to understand when certain findings do not fit within the framework of a given hypothesis. Such a signal then becomes a trigger for generating new hypotheses.

When a complete or nearly complete causal model can be constructed, it can be useful in the process of hypothesis refinement. In one aspect of hypothesis refinement, namely the interpretation of diagnostic tests, causal models can be used to check the validity of probabilistic models constructed to assess the data from diagnostic tests. As described in the preceding chapter, probabilistic models require that each disease under consideration be mutually exclusive of all others and that conditional probabilities under consideration be independent of each other. Causal models, because they encode dependence among the parameters they encompass and because they provide an understanding of the relations between variables, can identify circumstances in which the independence assumptions of a probabilistic model are invalid and can provide valuable guidance for correcting a poorly constructed model.

Causal reasoning may be most valuable when diagnostic hypotheses are undergoing final checking and a "working diagnosis" is being formulated (see later discussion of diagnostic verification). In that phase of the diagnostic process, a diagnosis is assessed for its coherency, namely, whether the physiologic or causal associations are reasonable, appropriate, and complete. This step involves determining whether a patient's findings are consistent with recognized pathophysiologic manifestations of a suspected disease.[19] A causal model is essential to this process: In a patient suspected of having hyperthyroidism based on the combination of clinical findings and a plasma thyroxine concentration that is only slightly elevated, the finding of a suppressed level of thyroid-stimulating hormone is a critical finding to verify the diagnosis. In this instance, suppression of pituitary function by excessive circulating thyroid hormone is the causal link that helps to confirm the hypothesis of hyperthyroidism.

Proper application of the causal approach can yield a rigorous guide to therapy because the treatment can be based on efforts to reverse the string of events that produced the disordered state. If, for example, one understands that chloride depletion is a regular consequence of the enhanced bicarbonate reabsorption that accompanies sustained hypercapnia, it follows clearly that replacement of depleted chloride stores will be necessary during any process in which hypercapnia is rapidly reversed. Any probabilistic approach to this therapeutic problem would be, at best, necessarily complex or opaque and, at worst, grossly inadequate.

EXPLAINING RELATIONS BETWEEN VARIABLES

(Cases 11, 33, 34, 36)

An important strength of causal reasoning is its capacity to provide an explanation for a given finding, especially when the relation is not immediately obvious from either probabilistic associations or from already compiled knowledge or concepts. A causal model also makes it possible to tie various clinical findings together in a common framework: The effect of dietary sodium intake and sodium excretion in patients with SIADH, mentioned earlier, is such an example. A causal approach provides a consistency check among related findings: Two common findings may have a strong probabilistic (or statistical) relationship, yet they may be causally inconsistent. Causal reasoning can help to identify such discrepancies.

DEFINITION

(Cases 37–39, 56)

Before a diagnosis is accepted as a basis for action, namely prognostication or therapy (i.e., a working diagnosis), it must be subjected to a detailed validity assessment. The processes used in this assessment are described here as diagnostic verification. This process makes a final check of a patient's findings against known patterns of the disease or suspected diseases. When a given patient's manifestations are identical to those of a known clinical entity, further search for a diagnosis usually is not required, and action can be taken. When some clinical feature differs from the known pattern of a clinical entity, however, a judgment must be made: Is the feature merely a variation of that entity, or is the finding sufficiently unusual that it raises doubts about the current diagnostic hypothesis? This dilemma is particularly likely when the tentative diagnostic hypothesis is a disorder that the physician encounters infrequently. In such instances, detailed review of disease manifestations in source materials may help to determine whether a particular clinical finding is consistent with the current hypothesis.

CRITERIA OF VALIDITY

(Cases 12, 17, 38–40, 43)

Given the nature of evidence, one must always maintain some element of doubt even with biochemical, histologic, or radiologic confirmation of a diagnosis. Several criteria are useful in helping to decide whether a diagnostic hypothesis qualifies as a working diagnosis. One "test" assesses diagnostic adequacy.[19] A diagnostic hypothesis is considered adequate when it encompasses all surviving hypotheses and when it accounts for all the patient's findings, whether abnormal or normal. Another "test" or criterion is coherency. A diagnosis is coherent when a patient's findings are consistent with the altered pathophysiology of the hypothesized disease state.[19] As noted in the preceding chapter, it is in this phase of the diagnostic process that detailed causal models are most helpful. Parsimony is another criterion, although no specific guidelines for its assessment exist. A parsimonious

diagnosis represents the simplest possible explanation of all the findings.[19] Generally one tries to find a single diagnostic hypothesis that explains all findings, but in some instances several diagnoses must be invoked to explain all of a patient's findings and to achieve confidence that clinical features are physiologically and causally consistent with the hypothesized entity. **Falsification** is also used during **hypothesis verification**. Falsification, an approach commonly used to discredit scientific hypotheses, is the process by which certain features that are unequivocally inconsistent with the tentative hypothesis discredit this hypothesis and thus call for new hypotheses or revision of competing hypotheses. This process consists in a systematic consideration of alternative, feasible hypotheses as a last step before accepting a given disease entity as the working diagnosis.[19] The credibility of a diagnosis is also a function of its likelihood. After all information is collected, a diagnosis with the highest probability is the most credible. Many schemes have been devised to determine when the probability of a diagnosis is sufficiently high to consider the diagnosis verified, but all are arbitrary. Neither a specific probability value (e.g., 0.95) nor a scoring mechanism based on approaches that give credit for findings that are present and subtract credit for findings that are not present have a solid scientific basis as a verification tool. Beyond verification, these schemes do not account for the benefit and risk of appropriate treatment for that diagnosis or the risk of harms for unnecessary treatment.

PREMATURE CLOSURE

(Cases 5, 8, 12, 33, 39, 53, 56)

Accepting a diagnosis before it is fully verified is often known as **"premature closure."**[52,53] Premature closure cannot be avoided simply by avoiding hypothesis generation. Indeed, physicians almost invariably generate hypotheses early in a diagnostic encounter when only a few cues are available. Nonetheless, inappropriate and premature acceptance of a diagnostic hypothesis may be avoided if one insists that all data be considered before accepting a diagnostic hypothesis as verified. The "tests" considered in the previous chapter on causal reasoning, namely adequacy and coherency, are mechanisms that help to avoid making a diagnosis that is incomplete or wrong. Sometimes, an acceptable diagnosis may not emerge even after all available data have been collected and considered. In such circumstances further testing, further patient observation, or both may be necessary. Alternatively, sometimes a detailed re-examination of the patient and a reanalysis of the significance of individual clinical features or findings reveal hypotheses not yet considered. Some observers have hypothesized that seasoned clinicians may be at greater risk of premature closure.[54]

As data emerge, the process of diagnostic refinement requires probabilistic revision, which can be a source for errors.[6] *Overconfidence* bias refers to physicians having a greater belief in the correctness of their diagnosis than necessarily warranted,[55,56] which may lead to premature closure. *Conservatism* reflects the tendency to insufficiently raise or lower the likelihood of a diagnosis as would occur with formal Bayesian probabilistic revision. Other errors include *acquiring redundant evidence* or *confirmatory bias* (confirmation testing at the expense of elimination strategies), *incorrect interpretation* (placing greater weight than warranted on confirmatory data and discounting or ignoring negative findings), *base-rate neglect* (ignoring or not considering appropriately pretest likelihoods, especially those that are very high or very low), and *ordering effect* (the influence of the sequence of the presentation of information).[6,56]

THE PENULTIMATE RESULT: A WORKING DIAGNOSIS

(Cases 9, 39, 41)

Working diagnoses should be highly likely and parsimonious. They should explain all principal clinical findings and should be coherent, in the sense of causal and physiologic relations. They survive the test that no competing diagnostic hypotheses are plausible. Such hypotheses usually produce valid predictions, both of test results and of the patient's future clinical course. After all efforts have been made to identify the most plausible diagnostic hypothesis, considerable uncertainty may still remain. At some point, despite remaining uncertainty, prognostic and/or therapeutic decisions must be made. The basis for making such decisions is discussed in the next chapter.

CHAPTER 7

Therapeutic Decision Making

PRINCIPLES

We make every effort to select a treatment according to scientific principles. We try to avoid anecdotal reports of therapeutic efficacy and risk because factors such as placebo effect and individual variation in reactions to treatment can cloud the interpretation of individual responses. To avert these confounding variables, we rely heavily on randomized, controlled trials of therapeutic approaches. To qualify as an appropriate study, patients must be assigned to treatment randomly; neither the patient nor the physician must know which treatment is being administered; outcomes must be important ones (deaths and disability rather than intermediate test results); outcomes must be measured and defined with precision; and analysis of data must be done using accepted methods. Such trials are laborious, expensive, and subject to flaws, both in design and implementation, yet controlled studies have provided many invaluable therapeutic insights. Often, however, even the best of the randomized, controlled studies provide only an anchor point or a benchmark when it comes to selecting therapy for an individual patient. To the extent that a given patient differs notably from the individuals studied in a randomized trial, that patient's response to the treatment also might well differ. Patients can differ in many ways, including their age, sex, race, genetic makeup, severity of illness, and the stage at which their disease is encountered. In addition, physicians often encounter a clinical problem for which no randomized, controlled trial has been carried out. When the patient fails to match a cohort in a controlled trial or when no such trial is available, the physician's judgment is the fallback position. The elements of therapeutic judgment become critical in such circumstances, forming the basis for the ability to evoke principles in making therapeutic decisions in the face of uncertainty.

TREATMENT UNDER CONDITIONS OF UNCERTAINTY

(Cases 41, 44, 48, 50, 53)

Therapeutic considerations frequently focus on the specific characteristics of one or another treatment, including the efficacy of a drug or of an interventional approach, and the risks of treatment. However, these important influences on choices of one therapeutic approach over another seldom occur in isolation. Treatment decisions often must be made before a diagnosis has been confirmed; furthermore, in some circumstances diagnostic uncertainty is never resolved, yet treatment decisions must be made. The principles described in Chapter 4 guide decision making under conditions of diagnostic uncertainty. Restated briefly, they are as follows: When the efficacy of the available treatment for a given disease is low or if the risk of the treatment is unusually high (or both), the treatment should only be given if the probability of the disease is quite high. On the other hand, if the risk of the treatment is negligible or if the efficacy of therapy is unusually high, the treatment can be given even when the probability of the disease is quite low (see Fig. 4.10).[57,58] Therapeutic implications of test use follow similar rules. When the probability of disease is very high, a negative test result usually will not reduce the suspicion of disease sufficiently to change the original assessment of the need for treatment. If so, the test is unnecessary. When the probability of disease is very low, a positive test result often will not increase the suspicion of disease sufficiently to change the physician's mind about the lack of a need for treatment. If so, the diagnostic test also is superfluous. However, if the test result can be expected to alter the probability of disease sufficiently to influence the decision to give or to withhold a treatment, then the test should be used.[57,59]

WHEN THE VALUE OF THERAPEUTIC CHOICES IS CLOSE

(Cases 25, 26, 46, 50, 51)

Unfortunately, the threshold determinations discussed in detail under diagnostic testing may not provide a definitive answer to the decision on whether to give or withhold a treatment. Just because a disease probability falls above or below a threshold, the differences in value between giving no treatment and giving treatment may be quite small and thus may be clinically insignificant.[60] When comparing the choice of withholding versus giving a treatment or when comparing two treatments, the clinician tries to assess the benefit of one approach over another. In many instances, this benefit is large and the decision is clear. In some instances, however, no clear therapeutic approach dominates. A difference of only a few days in life expectancy between two choices may imply that the decision between the choices is so close that neither choice predominates. When two or more choices are imperceptibly different in their perceived values (or expected utility, in the language of decision theory), the decision is considered a **close call**, or a **toss-up**.[60] In such circumstances, minor differences in patients' preferences may help to decide whether to give one treatment or another. When testing is one of the choices, a desire of the patient to know a test result may be sufficient to move the decision toward further testing. The principal problem in dealing with therapeutic toss-ups lies in judging the clinical relevance of a small marginal benefit. A difference of several years of life expectancy between two treatments seems like quite a lot, whereas when the difference is only several days or weeks, the physician could easily recommend either treatment. However, even a difference of a few weeks could be important to a particular patient. Given these features of therapeutic decision making, patients' preferences must always be taken into consideration. Doing so is especially important when differences in the outcomes of two choices are quite small.

INCOMMENSURATE OPTIONS

(Cases 46, 47)

Therapeutic decision making often involves making complex tradeoffs between choices that are not easily balanced against one another. In some instances, the choice may lie between one approach in which the risk of therapy is immediate and the expected beneficial effect of therapy is long term, and another approach that involves no immediate risk but with which there are important possible long-term unfavorable outcomes (e.g., the morbidity and mortality associated with immediate cholecystectomy for asymptomatic gallstones vs. the later enhanced risks of subsequent surgery for serious complications of gallstones at an older age). In other instances, one must weigh the immediate effects of a particular therapy on morbidity and mortality versus the long-term effects of that therapy on the quality of a patient's life (e.g., the risks in terms of morbidity and mortality of joint replacement for an arthritic hip vs. the long-term benefit of surgery in terms of improved mobility).

QUANTITATIVE THERAPEUTIC DECISION MAKING

(Cases 23, 30, 45, 47, 51)

Many therapeutic decisions must be made before all diagnostic information is available and before we are confident of a diagnosis. In many instances, selection of therapy is simple and straightforward because extensive experience has confirmed the value and safety of a given approach. In such instances, we develop comfortable and familiar categorical **rules of procedure** ("treatments of choice") that guide our decision making. Given the repetitiveness of our day-to-day patient experiences, this practice generally stands us in good stead. Nonetheless, situations often arise in which the patient or clinical setting is in some way atypical—the operative mortality may be higher than usual because of a patient's risk factors and comorbid illnesses, there may be considerable diagnostic uncertainty, or the efficacies of alternative therapies may be in doubt. Sometimes we are confronted with innovative techniques for testing or novel therapies, developments in health technology for which we do not yet have adequate information.[61] When these problems stretch the judgmental capacities of physicians, a quantitative approach to therapeutic decision making known as decision analysis can be used. Decision analysis applies probability and **utility** theory to therapeutic decision making under conditions of uncertainty.[10,11] The process requires structuring the therapeutic dilemma as a **decision tree** that contains all choices and outcomes, specifying the probability and the utility (value) of each outcome, and making a calculation from these data to determine the optimal choice. Given the quantitative nature of the data used in this decision-making process and the ease by which computerized decision trees can be recalculated, the data used in the analysis can be tested for its influence on the decision. The process by which the robustness of a decision is assessed by testing it against reasonable limits of the data is called sensitivity analysis. In sensitivity analysis, the effect of any single probability or sets of probabilities can be tested. The effect of utility values can be assessed in the same manner. One can ask, for example, whether the decision would be different if the probability of a certain therapeutic response were higher or lower, or if the quality of life (i.e., the utility) of a given outcome were higher or lower.

Because computer programs can carry out extensive calculations with combinations of probabilities and utilities, thresholds can be derived not only for the probabilities that affect a decision, but also for critical outcome measures (utilities). If necessary, the effect on the decision of variations in multiple variables can be appraised simultaneously. Even though computer technology has greatly simplified construction and assessment of decision trees, decision analysis for complex clinical problems must be used with considerable caution by inexperienced individuals. Because such analyses are quite sensitive to decision tree structure and the data used in the analysis, it is better to leave such analyses to experts. Even experts use their common sense and clinical judgment in interpreting the results of decision analyses when the outcomes are counterintuitive. In such circumstances, the analysts scour their assumptions, check the structure of their decision models, and return to literature searches before assuming that their analysis is rational.

INTRODUCTION

The preceding chapters considered the processes by which diagnoses are made and described approaches to understanding the tradeoffs between the risks and benefits of tests and treatments. However, process is never sufficient to deal with clinical medicine, even the simplest cases. There is no substitute for marrying effective clinical decision making with hard facts about disease entities and the characteristics of diagnostic tests, therapeutic agents, medical devices, and surgical treatments. In the past, there was a tendency to rely on a physician's recall of facts from his or her intuition or experience and their application to the decision at hand, but in an effort to reduce the remarkable variation in clinical practice between one physician and another and between physicians in different parts of the country, a new standard of factual use has emerged, often called "evidence-based medicine."

Because our goal in this book is to elaborate on the processes underlying diagnosis and clinical management, a detailed exposition on evidence-based medicine is not appropriate, but the student or resident beginning to understand these processes must also have a framework of how the facts and the processes intersect.

EVIDENCE-BASED MEDICINE

(Cases 23, 48–50)

The intention of this discipline is to replace intuition, unsystematic clinical experience, and pathophysiologic rationale with solid, experimental-based evidence for clinical decision making.[62] Evidence-based medicine can be defined as "the conscientious, explicit and judicious use of current best evidence in making decisions about the care of the individual patient. It means integrating individual clinical expertise with the best available external clinical evidence from systematic research."[63] To practice evidence-based medicine involves formulating clinical questions explicitly and searching for evidence that might bear on the decision; summarizing and appraising the evi-

dence; and applying the evidence for the patient's benefit.

ASKING QUESTIONS

The process starts with a patient and his or her clinical problem, leading to the formulation of a critically important question that affects clinical decision making. Questions such as "Should my patient receive long-term anticoagulation for a single episode of pulmonary embolism?" or "Should my patient have back surgery for severe pain thought to be caused by spinal stenosis?" or "Should I recommend that my patient undergo bronchoscopy for a lung lesion?" cannot be answered without detailed information about the risks and benefits of anticoagulation, the outcomes of spinal surgery, and the chance of having cancer and risks of bronchoscopy, respectively.

Evidence-based medicine makes a distinction between foreground and background questions. Background questions involve general knowledge about a condition, such as etiology, manifestations and treatment—for example, who develops hypertension, what are the symptoms of hypertension, and how does hypertension arise? Foreground questions require specific knowledge necessary for the treatment of individual patients; for example, in 60-year-olds with mild hypertension (systolic blood pressure 140 to 179 mm Hg), are angiotensin-converting-enzyme inhibitors more effective than beta-blockers in minimizing cardiovascular events (or adverse effects, e.g., developing diabetes)? If so, how much more effective? The formulation of the question involves four components, often represented by the acronym PICO:

Patient: Describe the patient or population.
Intervention: Describe what you want to do.
Comparison: Describe what are you comparing with the intervention.
Outcome: Describe the effect that you want to examine.

Common categories of clinical questions involve diagnosis, screening, etiology, prognosis, harms (potential risk or adverse effects), and economics.

SEARCHING FOR EVIDENCE

It is often surprising to beginning students that the evidence base for many common clinical problems has many deficiencies. In fact, studies are always underway to fill in the gaps in our knowledge base, as well to keep it current. Nonetheless, the strength of evidence varies considerably from field to field. To standardize the classification of evidence, a scheme has evolved to define the strength of medical evidence supporting a therapy or strategy as hierarchical, a fundamental principle of evidence-based medicine.[64] The highest level of evidence is the so-called "N-of-1 randomized, controlled trial," in which a single unique patient is randomized to placebo or intervention, such as two identically appearing pills for blood pressure.[65] Because randomized, controlled drug trials yield only an average observed effect, some individuals in the study population will have a substantial benefit and others will have no effect. The N-of-1 trial clarifies definitively whether a particular individual with his or her unique genetic makeup and dietary and lifestyle habits will indeed respond, for example, to a particular blood pressure medication. The next highest level of evidence is a systematic review of randomized trials of patients with a single condition, evaluating not only repeatability of the benefits and risks, but generalizability in different patient populations and clinical settings. Next in the hierarchy is a single randomized trial. Subsequent levels of evidence include a systematic review of observational studies, followed by a single observational study. Of course, heed must be taken of the potential biases of observational studies. Physiologic studies and unsystematic clinical observations comprise the lowest levels of evidence.

Search efforts begin by seeking the highest possible level of evidence. In this information age, an abundance of potential sources exist, in particular on the Internet. With regard simply to free public Web sites that provide dedicated medical information, the National Library of Medicine and the National Institutes of Health–sponsored PubMed (http://www.ncbi.nlm.nih.gov/sites/entrez?db=pubmed including), which has more than 17 million citations dating back to the 1950s, and the Agency for Healthcare and Quality Guideline Clearinghouse (http://www.guideline.gov/) deserve mention. Numerous tutorials now exist online and in print to assist with literature searching.[66,67] Increasingly, search engines in the public domain, such as Google and Google Scholar, are valuable sites for starting an evidence-based information search.

SUMMARIZING AND APPRAISING EVIDENCE

Summarizing and appraising the evidence combines clinical expertise with knowledge in epidemiology, statistics, and clinical trial design. Summarizing the study involves determining the study type in the hierarchy of evidence, patient population, inclusion and exclusion criteria, statistical methods, and outcomes. The appraisal criteria typically consist of a series of structured questions specific to the type of study being evaluated. For example, when examining a randomized, controlled trial involving therapy, key questions to assess the validity of the study include the following: (1) Was treatment assignment randomized? (2) Were all patients enrolled in the trial accounted for and their final outcome assigned? (3) Was follow-up sufficiently long and complete? (4) Were investigators blinded to treatment assignment? (5) Were the patient groups similar at the start? and (6) Were groups treated equally except for therapy? Many journal articles and books provide help in appraising the quality of any study.[64,68–71]

APPLYING THE EVIDENCE

The medical literature provides evidence of varying quality, but because of the need for researchers to keep the number of variables to a minimum, the data in an individual study may or may not be representative of any particular patient. Compounding this application of evidence from one group of patients to individual patients is that analysis of subgroups of a study is more likely to yield spurious results in the absence of replication or statistical adjustment for multiple comparisons.[72] Moreover, even when results are considered "statistically significant," the physician must assess whether any difference is clinically significant: Small significant differences between one treatment and another may not matter in decision making (see Chapter 7). Finally, every patient is unique in his or her preferences for risk and the values that he or she places on medical outcomes consequent on any testing and therapeutic decisions under consideration. Thus, another fundamental principle for evidence-based medicine is that "Evidence is never enough for clinical decision making."[64] The ultimate goal for clinical reasoning is to use evidence-based practice and integrate the best research with clinical expertise and patient values for optimum care.

PRACTICE GUIDELINES

Clinical practice guidelines are compiled recommendations issued by professional organizations and are based largely on published data. They are generally intended as an aid to therapeutic decision making once a working diagnosis has been achieved. Because guidelines must be somewhat general, it may be difficult to extract a recommendation for an individual patient, and some extrapolation may be required. Guideline developers attempt to use systematic and explicit methods to encourage their transparency and acceptance. Most guidelines separate the strength of the recommendation regarding benefits versus harms from the certainty of the benefit or precision regarding the quality of the evidence supporting the recommendation.

CHAPTER 9

Cognitive Errors

SCOPE

Unfortunately, errors in diagnosis and treatment selection are common occurrences in medicine, and in 2000, the Institute of Medicine estimated that nearly 100,000 deaths yearly could be attributed to some kind of error.[73] Errors can range from as important an error as removing a normal kidney instead of a diseased one to as minor an error as missing a scheduled dose of a drug by a few minutes. Some of the many causes of medical errors include poor communication among doctors or other members of a medical care team, inadequate staff, equipment failure, misinterpretation of doctors' orders, mistaken patient identity, misuse of drugs and laboratory tests, and wrong diagnosis. Many of these errors are "systemic," that is, they can be attributed to glitches, flaws, and inefficiencies in our "patch quilt" medical care system.[73] These mistakes have been studied extensively, and many methods have been implemented to repair the defects. These systemic issues, however, are not within the scope of this book: Here we consider only the errors in diagnosis and treatment attributable to flaws in reasoning. However, errors of both varieties—systemic and cognitive—can coexist, and often do, as recent studies attest.[52,74]

CLASSIFICATION

(Cases 16, 27, 54, 55, 57, 58)

If diseases can be considered errors in normal structure and function, and if diseases can be classified by type, etiology, pathogenesis, epidemiology, prevention, and treatment, then by analogy diagnostic errors can be considered fallacies in normal clinical reasoning, and such errors can be organized and classified.[52,75–77] The classification of errors parallels the categories of the diagnostic process. Such categories include errors in hypothesis generation, context formulation, hypothesis refinement (information gathering and processing), and verification. An additional category called "no fault" encompasses errors that a physician could not be expected to avoid (Table 9.1). Experience shows that such errors can be identified unambiguously, that

multiple errors of different types may be present in a single diagnostic endeavor, and that many errors can be attributed to inadvertent cognitive biases.[52] Many examples of such errors are described in the cases in Part II.

SOME ERRORS MAY HAVE A PSYCHOLOGICAL ORIGIN

(Case 5)

Errors in diagnosis can also have their source in many factors that are neither "systemic" nor strictly cognitive. A physician may miss a pertinent physical finding, receive a faulty laboratory result, or be misinformed about factual data. Many other errors exist in which a judgment seems to be influenced by psychological factors. Such errors have been attributed to factors such as **ego bias, hindsight bias, physician regret**, reciprocation, and others.[78–80] Another error occurs when physicians exaggerate the probability of a given diagnosis when one possible outcome is perceived as exceedingly unfavorable. This error is a kind of value-induced bias. Here we consider only the errors introduced by faulty information processing.

THE NATURE OF COGNITIVE ERRORS

(Cases 31, 36, 39, 54–58)

Faults in clinical cognition that provoke diagnostic errors presumably are the consequences of inadequate knowledge, defective information processing, or some combination of the two. Although we have little data on the relation between the structure or adequacy of physicians' knowledge and the commission of errors, some information on the interplay between cognitive processes and knowledge is available. In some instances, defective hypothesis generation can be attributed to improper interpretation of clinical cues, to failure of properly identified cues to raise the possibility of a given disease, or to lack of knowledge to invoke a disease. Another error occurs when a correct diagnosis is eliminated even though the clinical findings actually are consistent with this diagnosis. This error can be ascribed to the clinician's overly specific

TABLE 9.1
Classification of Cognitive Errors
Faulty hypothesis generation
Faulty context formulation
Faulty information gathering and processing
Faulty estimation of disease prevalence
Faulty interpretation of a test result
A faulty causal model
Overreliance on a clinical axiom
Faulty verification, including premature closure
"No-fault" errors

expectations for the disease. In such instances, physicians presumably have constructed a faulty model of the disease. On some occasions, physicians fail to recognize that observed findings are at odds with those of the suspected disease (a failure of verification). This error can be attributed to an overestimation of the allowable range of variation for findings in a given disease and is another example of a faulty disease model. Rather than the disease model being too restrictive like the one described before, the model in this instance presumably is too broad.

COGNITIVE BIASES IN THE LABORATORY

(Case 57)

In the everyday process of problem solving, people use short-cuts known as heuristics. These quick, intuitive judgments are often correct and produce the desired result, yet many studies show that people (including physicians) sometimes make errors in information processing when using these heuristics.[81–83] Perhaps some of the common heuristics are best understood in their "pure culture," that is, as they are studied in the psychology laboratory. Investigators have generally used simple problems as their experimental models and nonphysicians as their subjects, and they identify quite clearly the errors that people make when using these heuristics. The representativeness heuristic—a technique used in probability assessments—derives from the practice of assessing the likelihood of an event on the basis of its

close resemblance to other well-defined events. In one classic experiment in the psychology laboratory, this error was revealed by describing the personal attributes of an introverted and meticulous individual and then asking subjects whether they thought the individual was most likely an engineer, a physician, an airline pilot, or a librarian. Indeed, subjects were confident that the individual was a librarian even if the description was scant, unreliable, or outdated and even though librarians are fewer in number than those in the other professions listed. The availability heuristic involves assessing the chance of some event or outcome on the basis of readily recallable similar events or outcomes. The event or outcome may be particularly easy to recall because a given event was quite striking or impressive, because a combination of findings brings it readily to mind, or because the causal connections between events makes a given outcome quite imaginable. In a classic laboratory experiment that revealed this error, subjects were asked to judge how many people on a list were men and how many were women (half were of each sex). Manipulating the list to contain either a disproportionate number of famous men or famous women induced the subjects to guess that the numbers were not evenly split between the sexes. Another heuristic identified in these psychological studies is that of **anchoring**. This approach involves assessing the likelihood of an event or an outcome based on some starting point or some initial value. In another classic experiment, one group of subjects was asked to estimate the product of $8 \times 7 \times 6 \times 5 \times 4 \times 3 \times 2 \times 1$ and another group was asked to estimate the product of $1 \times 2 \times 3 \times 4 \times 5 \times 6 \times 7 \times 8$. The median score of the former group was 2,250 and of the latter group was 512.

CONSEQUENCES OF COGNITIVE BIASES

(Cases 16, 43, 52, 56–58)

Cognitive biases similar to those identified in laboratory experiments do taint everyday clinical reasoning and can influence clinical outcomes. Indeed, physicians make many errors similar to those described by the psychologists. In a study carried out some years ago, physicians presented with a hypothetical test for cancer (which they agreed was similar to tests in their everyday practice) made grossly incorrect interpretations of a positive test because they ignored the base rate of cancer in the population. Among the cases in Part II, we identified errors in the use of both the representativeness heuristic and the availability heuristic (see cases 1, 3, 13, 14, 54, 57). Although we did not identify an error attributable to the **anchoring heuristic**, other studies clearly show that physicians do make such errors.

It should be pointed out that, by and large, people are excellent problem solvers, and questions have been raised about the applicability of these laboratory exercises to real-world problem solving. Indeed, the real world often consists of redundant cues and multiple measures of the same cue, and the context in actual problem solving is likely to be far richer in content than that of the artificial constraints of a laboratory experiment. Nonetheless, many of our cases and those of others illustrate not only the existence of these cognitive biases in day-to-day medical decision making, but also the gravity of such errors.[82,83] Serious emotional consequences and many morbid outcomes can result from such faulty reasoning.

STRATEGIES FOR AVOIDING COGNITIVE ERRORS

This book focuses on examples of excellent and faulty reasoning, assuming that exposure to both kinds of examples sensitizes students to recognizing and avoiding errors. In addition, we have provided descriptions of many of the common cognitive biases. As diagnostic processes become increasingly automated, steps are being built in that reduce reliance on knowledge and memory, and these approaches further reduce many errors. Some have suggested that other educational approaches can reduce errors, such as regularly requiring thorough consideration of alternate diagnostic possibilities, developing strategies based on specific diagnostic categories, organizing clinical information so as to simplify the cognitive task, monitoring one's cognitive processes, and regularly revisiting important diagnostic decisions before acting on them.[79,83] These ideas are interesting, but, like the method of instantiation presented here, they have not been subjected to much evaluation,[84] and some are less optimistic about the benefit of "debiasing" to change how we think.[85–87]

CHAPTER 10

Some Cognitive Concepts

COGNITIVE SCIENCE

(Case 65)

Cognition—the process of perceiving and knowing—underlies all of human problem solving and decision making. In recent years, attempts by scientists in several fields to understand cognitive processes have converged within the discipline of cognitive science. Cognitive science views the mind as an information processor that receives, transforms, retrieves, and transmits information. The discipline seeks to learn how information is stored and how the processes that interpret this information operate. In this chapter, we describe briefly some of the theories about the storage of information, the characteristics of memory, the nature of strategies for searching material stored in memory, the nature of expertise, and the attainment of expertise.

STUDYING MENTAL PROCESSES

(Cases 62, 65)

Scientists and philosophers have struggled for centuries to understand the structure and function of the mind. For many years, theories of cognition were formulated by learned people based on their personal, introspective theories of their own mental processes. In recent years, however, the theories derived from such introspective approaches have come under considerable question because of inconsistencies between them and experimental observations.[88,89] Because introspection is not considered trustworthy, other approaches to understanding the function of the mind have evolved. Prominent among these approaches is the detailed analysis of transcripts of recordings of individuals who were "thinking aloud" as they solved problems, including clinical problems (the process of **protocol analysis**, or **transcript analysis**).[18,19,36,47,61,89,90] Typically a problem is presented to a subject; the subject describes what he or she is doing while solving the problem; the session is recorded and transcribed verbatim; and a **domain expert** then analyzes the transcript. This so-called **descriptive approach** to the study of reasoning assumes that speaking while thinking is not

dissimilar to thinking without speaking. Although investigators who use transcript analysis acknowledge that not all mental strategies are captured by this technique because some mental processes may not be verbalized, such as the short-cut heuristics described earlier,[88,91] they infer that the transcripts provide selective glimpses of intermediate points and illuminate states that people pass through as they solve problems.[90,92–94] They assume that the analysis provides a running series of responses of behavior from which one can infer the sequence of mental states and reasoning processes that operate in solving problems. In many instances, data from transcript studies have been implemented as a working computer program. This implementation provides evidence that the information obtained in such studies is sufficient to perform the task at hand, although few would claim that the computer program directly models the function of the mind.

THE STRUCTURE OF MEMORY

(Cases 63, 64, 66)

The mechanisms by which knowledge is stored are avidly debated. One hypothesis, the **physical symbol system hypothesis**, argues that information is stored in the form of symbols that represent objects, events, and relations between these elements. The form in which symbols might exist is actively debated. One such form is a structure known as **production rules**. A production rule (also known as a **condition–action pair**) is a **compiled** form of **categorical knowledge** in the form of an "**IF-THEN**" statement, with the IF part of the statement representing some semantically meaningful condition (e.g., a symptom cluster such as dyspnea on exertion and orthopnea) and the THEN part of the statement representing some action to be implemented whenever the IF condition is satisfied. In the case of this particular IF example, the THEN part might be "generate the hypothesis left ventricular failure." Another form is a structure called a frame. A frame is a list of declarative (factual) and procedural (processing) aspects for dealing with a given entity. A frame for a disease entity would contain some hierarchical structure into which the entity fits, findings necessary and sufficient to define the entity, factors that cause the disorder, complications of the disorder, approaches to distinguish it from other entities, and some mechanism to score the relative importance of expected findings. Although frames have been implemented as computer-based diagnostic decision support, they have not added much to our understanding of human cognition.

A third symbolic form has been named a script, a complex description of a particular kind of experiential episode, such as a patient encounter. According to this hypothesis, our memory does not contain abstract descriptions or models of diseases but instead comprises individual specific "training cases," and we interpret a new case by recalling a similar specific instance or example (called an exemplar) for comparison.[95–97] A discipline known as case-based reasoning exploits the notion of exemplars as an approach to understanding reasoning.[98–101] Case-based reasoning holds that the storage of specific cases is important in diagnosis. The concept proposes that routine diagnosis is done by reference to knowledge structures that contain case-specific information about the context in which the disease develops, the clinical features, a description of the malfunction, and the disease's consequences.[13,97–102] Such knowledge is thought to be tied together with causal links and organized in a temporal sequence that integrates the events as a cohesive story. This story is thought to be the content of a script. According to this hypothesis, diagnosis involves identifying the information obtained for a patient, searching for an appropriate script by some process of pattern recognition, selecting the script, and verifying the script. Scripts can be prototypes of disease (the most general) or they can be exemplars, that is, descriptions of individual patients (the most specific).

This concept holds that knowledge of clinical medicine may exist at various levels and that this knowledge changes as expertise develops. The first and most elementary level contains extensive pathophysiologic details in some kind of network.[47] After experience with more cases, these causal models become simplified, compressed, and compiled.[47,103] The second level consists of such compiled knowledge constructed into general diagnostic skeletons that describe either a category of disease or a specific disease entity. The third level consists of multiple exemplars, that is, idiosyncratic scripts based on actual experience with a specific patient (instance scripts). This hypothesis supposes that learning proceeds through a series of transitory stages, starting with pathophysiology, proceeding with a compiled version, and ending at the highest level with exemplars.[13,34] The attractiveness of the hypothesis is in the capacity of these multiple stored exemplars not only to represent disease polymorphism, but also to explain expertise. Expert diagnostic performance, according to proponents of this hypothesis, is achieved after accretion of a myriad of exemplars in the form of instance scripts. Presumably experts use pathophysiologic knowledge only when the problem is difficult and other methods fail (i.e., when script knowledge does not apply or is not available).[47,103] This concept is consistent with experiments on expertise in the field of physics: Such studies show that expertise is a function of knowledge structures available in several different forms.[96]

If there are symbolic knowledge structures in memory, scripts are not the only ones. Where no specific script exists (e.g., when an individual encounters a new situation), presumably a set of general rules exists to solve the problem. We suppose that many different knowledge structures could be accessed to solve such a problem. Such structures could include items, goals, themes, and plans.[102] In medicine, certain forms of knowledge that cut across disease entities might be stored in nonscript form, possibly as rules (perhaps the IF-THEN rules described earlier). Forms of knowledge that might be coded in this fashion include prevalence of disease and characteristics of tests and treatments. It is difficult to imagine, for example, that we index the efficacy of computed tomography scans or the complications of various drugs according to specific disease entities or individual exemplars. It seems more likely that we store the characteristics of procedures and therapies in some kind of generalization independent of specific diseases. Furthermore, it seems quite unlikely that only a single script is accessed when searching for a solution to a problem. Given the powerful effect of reminding (i.e., certain concepts remind us of others within the same domain and even in different domains, just as physical objects and events have reminding effects), a given set of circumstances can bring to mind a solution to the problem at hand even if the circumstances and the problem are not related.[102] Reminding is an essential aspect of understanding a new situation as a function of previously processed situations.[102]

Finally, some hold that the brain is a parallel computational device, and that representations of the world are held not as symbolic structures in the form of rules, frames, or scripts but as distributed patterns of activity across a network of neurons. This hypothesis, known as **connectionism** or **parallel distributed processing**, proposes that meaningful patterns are generated when sets of neurons are activated jointly and that knowledge is stored in the interconnections among a large number of processing units, namely neurons. This concept gains credibility from studies in which large, rapid, parallel processing computers ("neural networks") have been programmed to simulate a number of functions such as vision, pattern recognition, and cognitive information processing.[104–106]

Storage and retrieval of information depend on the functioning of memory. **Long-term memory** appears to be infinite in capacity, and although information in it is long lasting, retrieval from it is slow.[107] Working memory, otherwise known as **short-term memory**, contains only information under active manipulation. It is widely accepted that working memory is limited in capacity to some 5 to 10 items, and that its contents rapidly change as attention shifts away from the items.[23,108] Retrieval from working memory, however, is rapid. **Skilled memory** is a special adaptation of long-term memory. It is thought to contain chunks of semantically meaningful material organized into elaborate cognitive structures. In other words, by clumping bits of information into easily remembered salient "chunks," recall of these items from memory is enhanced. When information is organized in this fashion, long-term memory becomes an effective extension of short-term memory.

SEARCH STRATEGIES

The search for a solution to a problem (including a diagnostic problem) involves developing a representation of the problem, making inferences about possible solutions, gathering and interpreting data, wending a path toward a solution, deciding on the "best" solution, and "confirming" the result. In this discussion, we explore the nature of **search strategies** in solving diagnostic problems.

To set the stage for our discussion of search strategies, we pose this simple problem: Suppose you are looking in your file of 300 papers on pulmonary embolism for a specific reprint. Let us assume that there is no other access to the data. You remember seeing the reprint in your file recently, but it is not in the pulmonary embolism folder. No one else has access to the file. How do you find the reprint? You might consider checking each of the 300 reprints or selecting reprints at random, but these strategies are highly inefficient and time consuming. Alternatively, you might speculate that you placed the paper in the wrong folder and look in other folders that are related to pulmonary embolism by some semantically meaningful association: for example, anticoagulation, postoperative complications, phlebothrombosis, or membranous nephropathy. In the latter strategy, you are making an educated guess and then testing it.

How is this example relevant to searches for solutions to medical diagnostic problems? Most medical problems are not as simple as this. First, many do not have a straightforward solution, such as finding the one and only reprint. Second, many medical problems have more than one solution: Two diseases might interact—one might cause the major clinical manifestations and another might cause only a few others. Third, manifestations that initiate a search for a solution are sometimes quite specific and other times quite vague. The search for a solution may be relatively easy when a heavy smoker presents with cough and hemoptysis but far more difficult when a previously healthy person presents with malaise and weakness. In both medical examples, of course, a **systematic search** through all possible causes of the individual clinical manifestations is neither efficient nor effective. The "review of systems" probably will turn up interesting and important clues in both hypothetical medical examples but will not be likely to give the "answer."

"Weak" Problem-Solving Methods

An exhaustive or **random search** is almost never successful except for trivial problems. When such general search strategies are applied to complex problems, the process takes the form of a combinatorial explosion.[109] Nonetheless, a random search strategy is the standard against which all problem-solving methods must be measured. When we do not know precisely how to proceed, we use so-called weak problem-solving methods that are sufficiently general to be applied widely.

Two recognized weak methods are the **generate-and-test strategy** and **means-end analysis**.[110] They are useful mainly for general problems that have clear-cut solutions and occupy a small problem space. The generate-and-test strategy is the least focused and is nearest to the systematic search, as exemplified in the hunt for the missing reprint. In the generate-and-test strategy, one selects almost randomly among all possible actions and then pursues them until some progress is evident.[110,111] Then one reassesses (i.e., tests) the situation. In essence, one keeps trying different approaches until something works. This strategy works best when the set of choices is small and there is a systematic procedure for ensuring that each choice is tried only once.

In means-end analysis, one identifies a difference between a current state (reprint lost) and a goal state (reprint found) and uses various mental operations to reduce or remove the difference.[110,111] Weak methods are broadly applicable but not highly specific. Nevertheless, they impose some order in solving a problem in a domain that a person knows little about, and they are often a vast improvement over exhaustive searches or blind trial-and-error searches.[111]

"Strong" Problem-Solving Methods

In contrast to the poorly directed, general, and domain-independent nature of the weak methods described, strong methods are purposive, highly directed, and narrowly applicable. They are characterized not only by rapid recognition of patterns, but also by efficient formulation of problems in meaningful chunks. Solution of problems by these methods proceeds from available data, hypotheses about the problem's solution, or both. Which aspect of the process (i.e., data or hypothesis) takes precedence is not fully understood. The two principal approaches, namely a **data-driven strategy** and a **goal-directed strategy**, are described, respectively, as "working forward" and "working backward" (a list of terms used by cognitive psychologists is provided in Table 10.1).

The data-driven strategy (working forward) starts with data, works toward hypotheses, and

TABLE 10.1

Strong Problem-Solving Methods: Terminology

Goal Directed	Data Driven
Working backward	Working forward
Top-down reasoning	Bottom-up reasoning
Backward chaining	Forward chaining
Conceptually driven reasoning	
Expectation-driven processing	
Inference-driven processing	

is propagated by available information.[47,112] This approach assesses the possible actions, chooses the one that seems best, observes the action, and iterates in this manner to arrive at the solution. In the data-driven strategy, the solution starts with data and builds up, finding parsimonious structures in which to imbed the data.[107,113] An essential principle of such reasoning is the need to account for all available data. Expert physicians use this approach: They start with data, use highly elaborate representations of a problem, and apply principles to develop further data.[107,113]

Goal-directed reasoning (working backward) starts with hypotheses, motives, or goals; according to expectations derived from these hypotheses, it accumulates data leading to a solution.[18,19,61,107,113] Hypothetico-deductive reasoning is a kind of goal-directed reasoning in which a problem can be broken down into smaller units with smaller subgoals, with the smaller problems solved first.[109] Much human problem solving is thought to involve goal-directed reasoning, including computer programming.[114] Many artificial intelligence programs are based on this strategy.[109,115]

There have been conflicting claims about the kind of reasoning applied in some domains. In medicine, some studies have described diagnostic behavior as goal directed, others have claimed it to be data driven, and some have found it to be both. At least some discrepancies in these conclusions can be attributed to artifacts of experimental design. When little information is given, goal-directed reasoning seems to predominate.[18,19,61] When large quantities of clinical data are provided to subjects (as in our clinical discussion) or when causal explanations predominate, the problem solving appears to be principally data driven.[47,116] Combinations of data-driven and goal-directed reasoning also have been observed.[116]

Trying to unravel how much of our reasoning is goal directed and how much is data driven is analogous to the chicken–egg problem. Although we are not certain which comes first, there is little doubt that the reasoning strategies often are intertwined and that the process of discovering solutions to problems can at any time involve data or hypotheses. In fact, goal-directed processing can be interrupted opportunistically to examine data.[107] This is consistent with our familiar practice of attending single-mindedly to solving a problem while at the same time remaining alert to relevant data as they emerge. Even an approach that at first glance might be thought of as strictly data driven—for example, visual perception—involves substantial conceptual (hypothesis, or expectation-driven) processing.[107,117] Indeed, our expectations have significant effects on perceptual recognition: An object that fits its context is perceived better. In fact, when the context is misperceived, as it is from time to time during ordinary visual perception or diagnostic problem solving, gross errors can occur.[77] Further research is likely to clarify the circumstances in which various reasoning strategies are used.

CHARACTERISTICS OF EXPERTISE

(Cases 2, 3, 11, 66)

The game of chess provides a model in which to explore expert problem solving. Although common sense suggests that expert chess players plan ahead further or consider more moves or think faster, evidence suggests that experts construct a mental representation of board positions relevant to possible moves. They then recognize these perceptual units (chunks) and respond when they see a certain configuration (pattern recognition).[110,118] Consistent with the limitation of working memory to a handful of items (see case 63), chess experts apparently identify six or seven configurations at a time and act on those. Experiments show that experts in physics solve problems in the same fashion: They recognize typical physical situations and

"conditions," which evoke the application of some established physical principle.[119]

A picture of expert problem solving emerges from these experiments. Rather than rely on analytic thinking, experts use previously compiled mental procedures in their domain of expertise. They build a representation of the problem in terms of basic principles and store necessary procedures in working memory for subsequent activation, and their procedures are organized around an efficient strategy.[110,112,120] The expert has a deeper comprehension of the problem, bases his or her diagnostic approach on an elaborate representation of the problem, and reasons forward at a more abstract level than the novice.

In achieving these highly purposive searches, experts rely heavily on their experience with similar cases.[121] They also appear to use various heuristics. Heuristics are rules of thumb, tricks, strategies, simplifications, or devices that drastically limit searches for solutions in large problem areas but do not guarantee a solution.[109] General heuristics are probably useful in solving many problems. When more and more information is required to solve a problem—for example, in chess, physics or medicine—heuristics become narrowly applicable in a given domain or even in subsets of that domain.[111]

Novices use crude and cumbersome search methods; they are tentative and uncertain. Experts recognize patterns and are purposive. The evolution from novice to expert problem solver requires both knowledge and experience. To be most efficient, sophisticated problem solving requires specialized, domain-specific knowledge and experience. Experts who have extensive clinical knowledge typically use compiled mental procedures (perhaps the "chunked" information described before) in their domain to build a representation of the problem in terms of basic principles, store problem-solving procedures, organize these stored procedures around efficient strategies, and use domain-specific heuristics to limit searches. Evidence suggests that experts in medicine also store a great number of "illness scripts" that describe either individual patients or multiple prototypes of an illness in which the clinical data are organized in a highly compiled format.[122,123] By contrast, novices have been noted to build elaborate causal or pathophysiologic scripts because they have a limited library of compiled scripts. Some have argued that novices in medicine develop the more efficient problem-solving strategies characteristic of the expert as they gain experience and store more and more compiled scripts. There is little doubt that repeated purposive exposure to material (i.e., experiences that involve active learning) enhances long-term recall, which in turn would enhance problem solving. Studies suggest that other techniques may enhance learning.[114] Immediate feedback, which provides a signal that an error has been made (without giving away the answer), helps a person to develop an appropriate mental rule or procedure. Learning by discovery is another mechanism that presumably captures semantically meaningful material and compiles it for later use. "How-to-do-it" information generally prevails over "how-it-works information."[110] Nonetheless, with respect to learning skills, formal instruction diminishes in importance, and the value of purposive practice increases. The venerable homily rings true: Practice makes perfect.

CHAPTER 11

Learning Clinical Problem Solving

FACTS VERSUS PROCESS

(Cases 46, 60, 67, 69)

We have centuries of experience in teaching the knowledge basis of medical practice. Lectures, reading assignments, demonstrations, and laboratory experiments are tried and true formats for learning the fundamental principles of medicine (anatomy, physiology, molecular biology, and genetics). Repeated encounters with patients in a kind of apprenticeship, heavily supplemented by independent study, remain the usual educational approach for accumulation of the knowledge of clinical medicine. There is little doubt that learning medical facts is a critical determinant of expert performance. Yet biochemical and physiologic principles and medical facts represent only one aspect of the cognitive burdens on the physician. Beyond the substantial knowledge requirement is the need to apply that knowledge to solve clinical problems. This task has many varied components: extracting reliable information, evoking a set of diagnostic hypotheses, synthesizing a patient's clinical findings coherently, concisely and coherently representing a patient's problem,[8,124,125] comparing such findings with accepted models of disease states, selecting diagnostic tests that help to differentiate among hypotheses, establishing a diagnosis sufficiently acceptable to evoke an action, and making decisions that encompass the tradeoffs between the risks and benefits of tests and treatments.

Ordinarily, little attention is given to teaching clinical problem solving. Students and house officers are expected to learn these concepts by observing others engaged in the process. Most medical textbooks are simply compendia of medical facts, and many medical journal articles report scientific advances, but neither source explains how to incorporate this knowledge into a diagnosis or how to think about the tradeoffs just described. Some have cataloged problem-solving processes, and some have itemized the diverse possible causes of individual symptoms, but because a single symptom (lightheadedness, for example) is a manifestation of so many diseases that vary in severity from a

vasovagal attack to a life-threatening arrhythmia, elaborate lists or even descriptions of the causes of individual symptoms are of little value to the student.

Case presentations and clinicopathologic conferences presented in the traditional style (i.e., a format in which all clinical data are presented and a clinician discusses the case) also have important limitations. Although this format is effective in elaborating on a patient's illness and its management, the presynthesized formulation of the patient's findings virtually precludes discussion about the significance of individual findings, sets of findings, and the rationale for gathering information or selecting diagnostic tests. The rich lode of knowledge to be garnered from the process of reasoning through these intermediate steps about these essential issues is lost in these kinds of teaching exercises. In addition, discussions after the fact (after all information is available) are subject to **retrospective bias**: the appropriate hypotheses, questions, tests, and treatments always seem clearer when the outcome is already known.

How can we improve on the way we teach and learn clinical reasoning? As we gain deeper understanding of general problem solving, including notions of problem framing, inferential reasoning, strategies for searching, the characteristics of memory, and the application of heuristics, we may be able to improve our capacity to teach clinical problem solving. A detailed description of the elements of clinical reasoning, such as that given in Part I of this book, also should enhance how we both teach and learn the cognitive business of medicine because it provides an unambiguous road map of processes involved and a language for contemplating problem-solving methods. Clearly, however, our understanding of general problem solving and clinical problem solving as a specific case remains incomplete. Nonetheless, research in these disciplines does provide some principles that guide the teaching of clinical cognition.

If clinical problem solving is an unstructured iterative process in which inferential reasoning evolves, refines, and verifies diagnostic hypotheses that lead to a working diagnosis, it follows that simulating the process might provide an improved approach to teaching it.[5,8,126] Such an approach is described here and is abundantly illustrated by the cases in Part II. It is applicable to the teaching of problem solving in diverse settings—small groups of house officers or students doing clinical rotations, entire classes of students in introductory courses to clinical medicine, grand rounds, specialty conferences, and even demonstrations to large audiences. It should be emphasized that although this approach is solidly grounded in experimental studies on cognition inside and outside of medicine, there exist no data on whether the approach is a better method of learning clinical problem solving than traditional methods. On the other hand, this limitation does not differ in its lack of a reliable evaluative mechanism from many other teaching approaches.

It should also be noted that flat-footed statements about how knowledge is structured in memory[4,8,13,33,124] should be viewed with great caution, and although such theories may be helpful in thinking about clinical problem solving and teaching it, they are just that—theories—and should not be taken as fact.

PEDAGOGIC PRINCIPLES

(Cases 60, 69)

A few principles guide our approach. First, to simulate a patient's clinical problem realistically, clinical data are presented, analyzed, and discussed in the same chronological sequence in which they were obtained in the course of the encounter between the physician and the patient. Second, instead of providing all available data completely synthesized in one cohesive story, as is the practice in the traditional case presentation, data are provided and considered only a little at a time. This approach is designed to mimic the actual process of data accumulation and interpretation. Third, any cases presented should consist of real, unabridged patient material. Simulated cases or modified actual cases should be avoided because they may fail to reflect the true inconsistencies, false leads, inappropriate clues, and fuzzy data inherent in actual patient material. Finally, the careful selection of examples of problem solving ensures

that a reasonable set of cognitive concepts will be covered.

A SPECIFIC EXAMPLE

(Case 69)

Let us consider the approach as applied at the undergraduate level with one clinician-teacher and a small group of students on a clinical rotation. The student who comes prepared to present the case is the only participant who has any information about the patient and provides all the clinical data. Rather than begin with a complete summary of all of the patient's clinical findings (the traditional case presentation), however, the student supplies only the patient's age, sex, race, and reason for seeking medical attention. This student subsequently provides only specific information as it is requested. Participants ask questions that produce more data, but they must first justify the question—the diagnostic hypotheses they have in mind, the rationale for asking the question, and what they anticipate learning from it.

After the group has concurred on the appropriateness of a question, the student provides the answer. The questioner is then asked to interpret the information elicited by the question and to explain how it influences the earlier diagnostic hypotheses. Did it change or modify the current diagnosis? Did it suggest a need to take some immediate action? Did it make some previously unexplained finding comprehensible? Did it uncover some complication of the patient's illness?

The serial questioning, justification, and interpretation continues until all relevant material has been extracted or until all important diagnostic and management issues have been discussed. In more advanced groups, such as residents or subspecialty trainees, the instructor can dispense with the history and physical rapidly and focus on the rationale for invasive or expensive tests, therapeutic approaches, and the tradeoffs among management options.

The emphasis of this didactic approach is on assessing information as it is encountered in the course of a patient's workup. The student learns how to accumulate and interpret clinical findings as they surface. This ability to develop a fact-finding strategy is what students and house officers must learn: Patients rarely "present their case" to the doctor. The method exposes all of the intermediate details of the diagnostic process. With guidance, an assembled group can assess the validity of a questioner's hypotheses, discuss the reasons for seeking certain information at any particular point, or consider the appropriateness of pursuing more details concerning a certain symptom, sign, or laboratory result. When a faulty hypothesis emerges, the instructor can promptly explain why it is incorrect. If certain questions fail to characterize a symptom adequately when such an elaboration would be expected to yield a great refinement of a diagnostic hypothesis (e.g., chest pain), the instructor can immediately point out this fault. The essence of this format is that any addition to the student's knowledge occurs precisely when information is being digested, not at some later time when the student is trying to assimilate facts out of context. At any time the instructor can explain the pathophysiology of certain disease manifestations, comment on diagnoses being considered, make an observation on the nature of a participant's diagnostic strategy, identify gaps in available data, describe certain diagnostic principles, or show how diagnostic hypotheses can be used to guide the questions asked. The instructor may also reject a request for results from expensive or risky tests until the set of diagnostic hypotheses has been narrowed sufficiently from other data or when testing is grossly inappropriate.

For large groups, some modification of this approach is needed. Rather than use an individual to provide the data, the clinical material can be organized in "chunks," also in the same sequence in which they were obtained. The cases in Part II are presented in this format. Rather than have multiple discussants, a single clinician can describe his or her reasoning processes. A skilled facilitator to guide the discussion is useful.

THE GOAL SHOULD DETERMINE THE FORMAT

The structure of a case presentation should be determined by the goal of the didactic exercise. If the goal is to have participants extract essential elements of the history (as it might be in the case of a patient with unexplained fever after returning from a tropical country), then it would be appropriate to offer only minimal information to begin the session (such as the patient's age, sex, chief complaints, and identity of the country) (see cases 2, 12, 56, and 60). If the goal is to contemplate the significance of a set of laboratory data, then an alternative dataset should be offered initially (see cases 23 and 46). If the goal is to examine which tests or treatments are appropriate, then additional history and physical examination might be presented. (see cases 11, 29, and 50) If the goal is to examine difficult clinical choices, then a complete history, physical examination, laboratory findings, and imaging results should be presented (see cases 44 and 49).

Sufficient material should be presented to establish the appropriate context and properly set up the desired discussion. Providing information such as "A 75-year-old man with fever and a rash" will be too vague and unfocused for detailed discussion of the patient's problem if the actual information is "A 75-year old man with diabetes, psoriasis on treatment with immunosuppressive drugs, fever, and a new rash." Finally, important historical information should not be omitted in an effort to add to the mystery of the case. Omitting a drug from the patient's history, for example, when the drug could be the cause of an adverse event and was known at the time of the patient encounter should be discouraged.

LEARNING BY INSTANTIATION

(Cases 67–69)

The use of carefully selected examples is an important principle in learning clinical reasoning. Learning from examples certainly is not new in medicine. For years, we have taught clinical facts by exposing students to many different examples of the same kind of clinical problem (such as jaundice or acute renal failure) because comprehension of clinical entities is enriched by repeated experience with specific instances of these entities. In the cases provided in Part II we follow a similar pattern, but we emphasize reasoning rather than the medical facts. We offer multiple specific, annotated examples of both optimal and faulty clinical reasoning.

Using examples to learn concepts has special benefits. Learning from books or from direct instruction requires little inference or active participation by the learner, whereas learning by discovery from examples requires considerable inference and active engagement. Because of the active involvement, learning by discovery through specific examples may be more likely to "stick." Learning through inference also generates plausible general concepts that, in turn, become useful in future similar and related contexts.

We have selected the examples for Part II carefully. Although our selection of clinical material does not exhaustively encompass all cognitive concepts, we have tried to choose patient problems that **instantiate** (exemplify) the specific inferences that we wish the reader to make. We describe a sufficient number of broad examples to evoke, by inference, a large array of appropriate and relevant principles. However, we have avoided describing only examples of optimal reasoning because a reader might well overgeneralize an inferred concept from such examples. To avoid such overgeneralization, we also furnish negative examples: In this context, negative examples are instances of faulty clinical reasoning. Such counterexamples are helpful in circumscribing the concepts that we want to teach. Counterexamples that are "near misses," namely, negative examples that just miss being positive by a small number of attributes, may be particularly helpful in elaborating on a reasoning strategy.

Each case covers a small fragment of the broad range of reasoning processes used in clinical medicine. Because knowledge of mental processes is at best incomplete and at worst filled with missteps and blind alleys, we should exercise caution in being too confident that we fully understand these complex processes. Nonetheless, we believe that the issues, principles, and concepts we consider provide a unique framework for both learning and teaching clinical reasoning.

LEARNING CLINICAL PROBLEM SOLVING VERSUS PROBLEM-BASED LEARNING

It is important to explain how the processes of learning diagnostic problem solving and therapeutic decision making that are described here differ from problem-based learning. Problem-based learning relies on the direction and supervision of a facilitator to guide students in solving compiled clinical problems. The goals of problem-based learning are to impart a large number of skills, including careful history taking, efficient literature searching, independent learning, recognizing one's limitations, being able to communicate with others, acquiring methods of problem solving, and critical reasoning. Because problems are presented in their entirety, detailed interpretation and analysis of clinical information as it emerges is not possible without the biasing effect of subsequent clinical facts. Often, no universal set of cognitive guidelines is provided to the students by the facilitators. By contrast, the learning processes described here focus on a narrow domain, namely clinical cognition. Both by a narrative description of the processes underlying diagnosis and therapy and by a large number of carefully selected examples, the cognitive tasks of the clinician are described and elaborated. The singular goal is to learn clinical reasoning.

Cognition at the Bedside: A Set of Examples

CHAPTER 12

Introduction to the Cases

We selected cases in this collection to illustrate one or more features of clinical reasoning. Each chapter in Part II is parallel to the detailed summaries in Part I. All of the clinical data in the cases come from real patients. To preserve important examples of clinical cognition for their didactic value, we updated the clinical material in many of the cases from the first edition with diagnostic tests and treatments in current use. As before, nearly all of the clinical material is organized in "chunks," namely, collections of semantically meaningful information organized to reflect the actual sequence in which data were obtained. To the extent that this sequence mirrors reality, the reader should attempt to confront and solve the same dilemmas as did the physicians originally responsible for the patients' care. Because the reasoning behind the solutions to these quandaries cannot be identified in real time, we presented these chunks of information to a clinician (in most instances an expert and in no instance one of us) and asked him or her to "think out loud" as they solved the problem. We recorded their utterances, transcribed them literally, and edited them lightly to maintain a consistent style. We then analyzed the content of the transcripts and described many of the cognitive aspects in some detail in an accompanying comment. In each case, the analysis focuses on the specific details of each patient and thus places the context of reasoning directly "at the patient's bedside."

It will come as no surprise that the cognitive content of each case is an admixture of various aspects of the diagnostic process and/or a mixture of diagnostic and therapeutic issues. Indeed, the blending of diagnostic problem solving and testing and treatment decision making is a characteristic of a physician's day-to-day experience. The cases have been inserted into the chapter most suited to its discussion and to the principles considered, yet a given case often crosses over into several different chapters. Because many cases were published originally as a self-contained, monthly journal installment, in some instances a given concept is discussed in more than one of the cases. Differences in orientation of these discussions of clinical cognition justify this occasional redundancy.

As in Part I, definitions of unfamiliar terms are found in the Glossary.

Because a complete theory of clinical reasoning has not been elaborated but many important principles of cognition are recognized, the cases in this part provide invaluable specific examples of these principles. Finally, because they were discussed by real clinicians, they provide insights not readily gleaned from a straight declarative description of how doctors are *supposed* to solve problems.

CHAPTER 13

Diagnostic Hypothesis Generation

CASE 1. GENERATION OF DIAGNOSTIC HYPOTHESES

> A 52-year-old man experienced gradually progressive loss of control of his right arm and leg over the last 3 months. His family reported heavy alcohol use, up to 1 pint a day, for more than 20 years. He had no known history of trauma, but he did complain of intermittent occipital headaches. The patient had smoked approximately one pack of cigarettes per day for the last 30 years.

This man had abused his body for many years in two ways—with excessive alcohol consumption and cigarette smoking—both of which increase the likelihood of several major medical problems. With alcohol abuse, the problems of liver disease, pancreatic disease, infectious diseases, and hypertension come immediately to mind. Smoking increases the risk of ischemic heart disease and cancer of the lung and of other organs, particularly the genitourinary tract. This patient is, therefore, at much greater risk for those problems than any 52-year-old man with no history of alcohol abuse and smoking.

This patient's symptoms were gradually progressive, and I think that is the key point, at least in the context of his history. As a nonneurologist, I like to divide central nervous system problems into acute problems—such as strokes or hemorrhage, or ischemic episodes either from thrombosis or embolus—and chronic problems. The chronic problems could range from metabolic disorders to toxic problems to space-occupying lesions and, I am sure, a variety of other things. I would be particularly concerned about space-occupying lesions in this patient. The fact that the symptoms are unilateral suggests that it is not one of the global disorders that affect alcoholics, such as Wernicke encephalopathy or Korsakoff syndrome. He has lost motor control without, at least as far as we are told, any change in mental status. This again suggests that it is not a metabolic problem related to his alcohol abuse or smoking. With the information at hand, I am concerned about the possibility that he has a space-occupying lesion on the left side of his brain in the part of the cerebral cortex that would account for the loss of function of his right arm and leg.

I would want to examine him, and I also would push a little bit more for a history of trauma to evaluate the possibility of a subdural hematoma.

> Physical examination was unremarkable, except for right-sided ataxia with past pointing and impaired rapid alternating movements. Vital signs were normal. No abnormalities were evident on examination of the lungs. He was not jaundiced, and the liver was not palpable. He had no spider angiomas and no evidence of portal hypertension. No head trauma was evident.

It is suggested that there is no evidence of alcoholic liver disease because of the absence of the usual stigmata of alcoholic cirrhosis. He is not jaundiced, he does not have an enlarged liver, and he does not have spider angiomas. There is no evidence of head trauma, and we are back to a primary neurologic problem. Now we are told that he has right-sided ataxia with past pointing and impaired rapid alternating movements, which is more consistent with the history than the earlier information. This does sound like loss of control of his right arm and leg rather than loss of function in the extremities. Nevertheless, I am still interested in a problem on the left side of the brain. This raises the problem of localization, in that the problem may be more cerebellar than cerebral. I do not know the results of his Romberg test and which side he fell to. Given this information, you have to be sure that there is no mass lesion in the head. I would be interested in a chest x-ray, as well as a head scan, because I believe the most common brain tumor is not primary but metastatic, with lung being the most common site of the original disease.

The hemoglobin was 18.1 g/dL, hematocrit 58%, white blood cell count 9,200, and platelet count 181,000.

I suspect I would have been more interested in looking at the chest x-ray first, for the reasons I stated. Now we know that the patient has polycythemia; his hemoglobin and hematocrit are elevated without any change in white blood cell count or platelet count. This is consistent simply with hypoxemia from the long history of smoking. I must say I am impressed by a hematocrit of 58% in somebody who to our knowledge has no respiratory symptoms. That hematocrit level seems a little high for the kind of hypoxemia that one usually sees in a patient who smokes, but that would probably be the most likely situation statistically. A more intriguing possibility is that if this patient turns out to have a space-occupying brain lesion, as I think he will, a potential cause of the increased hematocrit would be a metastatic renal tumor that is also secreting erythropoietin. That is speculative, but whether or not I found an abnormality on chest x-ray, I would need to make sure that there is no lesion in the kidney as well. Renal cell cancer notoriously metastasizes to the lung and can then metastasize to the brain.

All liver function studies were normal, as were kidney function studies and urinalysis. Chest x-ray and arterial blood gases also were normal.

This normal information is helpful. First, it again lowers the likelihood of any problem from alcohol. I should have mentioned earlier that alcoholics with cirrhosis also have an increased incidence of hepatomas, despite normal physical examinations and normal liver function tests. That is unlikely, however, in this patient. The normal kidney function and urinalysis are not very helpful. Most patients with renal cell tumors have a normal urinalysis. The arterial blood-gas determination is quite helpful. I previously observed that polycythemia could be caused by either hypoxemia or some nonhypoxic stimulus to the bone marrow, with tumor-associated production of erythropoietin a good possibility. The normal arterial blood gases mean we have a distinctly unusual cause of polycythemia. A major possibility would be a tumor secreting erythropoietin or an erythropoietin-like substance. It would be interesting if we had a measurement of erythropoietin, but I do not think it would affect my approach to the patient.

A computed tomography (CT) scan of the head showed a cerebellar mass.

This result accords with the physical findings of right-sided ataxia and impaired rapid alternating movements. The question is whether we need to invoke anything other than the cerebellar mass as the cause of his neurologic symptoms and polycythemia. I think this is certainly a sufficient explanation for his neurologic abnormalities, and it could also explain the elevated hematocrit. I do not have a list in my head of all of the tumor-associated causes of polycythemia, but I think some cerebellar tumors have been associated with the release of erythropoietin or some erythropoietin-like substance.

As I stated earlier, brain tumors are still more likely to be metastatic than primary. I would be interested in a CT scan of the abdomen before doing anything to determine what is going on in his head. Whether he would require an arteriogram or whether an MRI (magnetic resonance imaging) scan would be able to make a clearer diagnosis is beyond me. I would need help in deciding that.

At surgery, the patient was found to have a large cerebellar hemangioblastoma.

Analysis

There is little argument that the initial cognitive task in the process of diagnostic problem solving is the generation of one or more hypotheses, a process variously described as evocation, hypothesis generation, hypothesis formulation, and, in the language of artificial intelligence, triggering.[20–22,127–132] Such hypotheses are generated in response to cues (typically a patient's appearance, age, sex, race, and presenting complaints) but sometimes by one or more laboratory or radiologic findings. In fact, we argue that generating hypotheses from laboratory findings alone is an entirely legitimate enterprise, even though conventional teaching warns us to get and interpret the laboratory data only in their proper sequence (see case 14).

TABLE 13.1	

Sequential Hypotheses Proposed in a Patient with Gradually Progressive Neurologic Symptoms

Major medical problems	Alcoholic liver disease
Liver disease	Head trauma
Pancreatic disease	Primary neurologic problem
Infectious diseases	Problem on the left side of the brain
Hypertension	(Mass lesion) more cerebellar than cerebral
Ischemic heart disease	Mass lesion in the head
Cancer of the lung	Primary brain tumor
Cancer of the genitourinary tract	Metastatic tumor
Acute central nervous system (CNS) problems	(Metastatic) lung (tumor)
Strokes	Hypoxemia (from) smoking
Brain hemorrhage	Space-occupying brain lesion
Ischemic CNS episodes	Metastatic renal tumor that is also secreting
(Cerebral) thrombosis	Erythropoietin
(Cerebral) embolus	Problem from alcohol
Chronic CNS problems	Hepatomas
Metabolic disorders	Renal cell tumors
Toxic problems	(Polycythemia related to) hypoxemia or some
Space-occupying lesions	nonhypoxic stimulus
A variety of other space-occupying lesions	Tumor-associated production of
A variety of other things (involving the brain)	erythropoietin
Space-occupying lesion (of the brain)	Unusual cause of polycythemia
Global disorders that affect alcoholics	Tumor secreting erythropoietin
Wernicke encephalopathy	Tumor secreting erythropoietin or an
Korsakoff syndrome	erythropoietin-like substance
Metabolic problem related to alcohol abuse	Anything other than the cerebellar mass
Metabolic problem related to smoking	Tumor-associated causes of polycythemia
Space-occupying lesion, left side of brain	Cerebellar tumors
Subdural hematoma	Brain tumor . . . metastatic
	Primary brain tumors

In several cases, we give specific examples of hypothesis generation for patients with both common and rare diseases (see cases 2 and 17). We also give examples of faulty hypothesis generation, some of which led to unfortunate outcomes (see cases 16 and 27). In this discussion, we pay attention to the initial phase of the diagnostic process, namely hypothesis generation. Fortunately, research on the organization of memory (see cases 63 and 64) and a series of studies on the nature of hypothesis generation make it possible to dissect this initial process and to identify some of its components.

As a prelude to this discussion, we first consider the hypotheses generated in the diagnos-

tic exercise described. A total of 52 hypotheses were mentioned as the discussant reacted to the data provided to him (Table 13.1). The initial cues provided were a rich collection of facts about the patient, which included seven items: the patient's age and sex, the progressive nature of his complaints, the location of the weakness in his right arm and leg, and a history of both alcohol abuse and cigarette smoking. In response to these seven cues, the discussant raised 28 hypotheses, of which the 21st (space-occupying lesion of the brain) eventually was found to be correct. Several aspects of the problem-solving exercise are notable from the standpoint of the hypotheses that were generated. First, the alcohol and cigarette addictions were powerful hypothesis evokers. Approximately 24 of the hypotheses mentioned by the discussant are consequences of use of these agents. Second, a large (possibly even disproportionately large) number of hypotheses—16 in all—were cancer related. Third, the discussant made use of two catchall hypotheses. The significance of these will be covered later.

The reader should be cautioned against assuming that the hypotheses generated in the foregoing transcript are necessarily an accurate reflection of how the discussant usually solves diagnostic problems. First, the case material was discussed as part of a didactic exercise, and it seems likely that some of the discussion was directed at displaying a complete differential diagnosis and possibly even displaying the discussant's knowledge. Second, the clinical material was not gathered by the clinician in the usual fashion (i.e., from the patient, by an interactive process) but rather was provided in chunks on a set of slides. The latter concern seems less important as a factor that interferes with the veridicality of the process (i.e., its reflection of real-life clinical problem solving) because the discussant is quite likely to receive information in the same fashion when he functions as a consultant and has cases presented to him.

What prompts the generation of these hypotheses? Are some clues more important than others? Do people hold off evoking hypotheses until considerable data are available, or do they often generate hypotheses with only flimsy data and then check them by some process when more information becomes available? Do features that increase the plausibility of already held hypotheses have a greater impact on the generation of new hypotheses than features that reduce the plausibility of such hypotheses? Are searches for new hypotheses constant throughout a diagnostic problem-solving session? Are there heuristics in hypothesis generation that reduce the search for plausible diagnostic possibilities? How is the plausibility of a hypothesis assessed?

Research on hypothesis generation has been done chiefly in nonmedical domains. Although it has been confined to the psychology laboratory and has for the most part encompassed hypotheses activated by a single cue, the results of such studies and the theories produced from them provide interesting and relevant insights into the medical diagnostic process. One model of the nature of hypothesis generation that satisfies the experimental findings in humans has the following components:

- Plausible candidates for active hypotheses are retrieved from memory in a recursive (i.e., repetitive), relatively slow search by some as-yet-undefined executive process that initiates, guides, and ends the search.
- These plausible candidate hypotheses often are generated with only minimal and incomplete cues, and thus the candidate hypotheses may not be consistent with all the available data.
- Given that the candidate hypotheses may be inconsistent with all the data, a consistency check is used to determine whether the data are explained by the hypothesis. If they are, the hypothesis becomes active.
- In contrast to the initial search for candidate hypotheses, the check for consistency is a high-speed process, probably because it involves relationships already in active memory.
- Because some of the candidate hypotheses will not explain all the data, some will be rejected.
- Compiling a set of active hypotheses often involves adding a catchall category to the list—that is, a hypothesis that encompasses possibilities that have not yet occurred to the reasoner.
- Hypothesis generation occurs far more frequently when the plausibility of a set of hypotheses is low than when it is high.
- Finally, the model proposes that active hypotheses are linked with a cluster of data rather than only a single item.[25,26,133,134]

Given the limited capacity of working (short-term) memory, the number of hypotheses retrieved from long-term memory would be excessive if hypotheses were generated from a single item.[23] Single items—cough, for example—evoke an enormous number of possibilities, whereas cough, fever, pleuritic chest pain, and blood-streaked green sputum evoke far fewer. This model is supported by experimental studies using college students as subjects, and the reader is referred to these studies for further evaluation.[25,26]

This model answers many of the questions posed earlier. Still unexplained are the factors that elicit hypotheses. Evidence from a variety of sources suggests that heuristics play an important part.[27] The representativeness of a set of cues with respect to a recognizable pattern is known to be a powerful stimulus,[135] and availability—the resemblance to readily recallable items in memory—is another.[27,28] In fact, studies show that when physicians generate diagnostic hypotheses, they do so by recalling those disease processes most prevalent in their institution.[29]

These psychological studies of the process of hypothesis generation confirm the results of earlier studies of clinical problem solving that diagnostic hypotheses are generated in response to only a small number of clinical cues.[18,19] Many of the hypotheses are eliminated as new data become available, but retrieving many hypotheses and retaining only a few appears to maximize diagnostic performance.

The opening discussion discloses some of the features outlined in the model just described. The discussant generated a large number of hypotheses from the initial seven cues provided to him. Some of these hypotheses (stroke, intracerebral hemorrhage, and ischemic heart disease) appear to be quite ephemeral. Those transient hypotheses presumably did not survive a consistency check and were discarded. By contrast, other hypotheses (brain tumor and space-occupying lesion of the brain) survived the checking process, are cited repeatedly, and presumably remain active throughout. The discussant does make use of two catchall hypotheses, presumably to formulate a full set of possible diagnoses. At one time, he considered "a variety of other things," and at another time, he considered "anything other than the cerebellar mass."

Finally, we can speculate on what cues and associations evoked the various hypotheses. The patient's age and sex probably had little relevance, but the gradually progressive weakness in the arm and leg probably were powerful cues. Although the alcohol and tobacco abuse probably were irrelevant in this patient, they were powerful cues that evoked many hypotheses over a broad range of diagnostic possibilities involving multiple organs. The elevated hemoglobin and hematocrit were also important cues that generated several hypotheses, but over a much narrower range. The discussant repeatedly invoked a cancer, a tumor, or a space-

occupying lesion to explain the findings. We can only speculate why, because he offers no clues. Perhaps these diagnoses came to mind simply because of the prevalence of tumors and cancers in the population of patients familiar to the discussant, or perhaps only a single one of the initial cues (gradually progressive) was so representative that it alone pointed to this highly plausible possibility.

The generation of hypotheses is one aspect of diagnostic reasoning that can be studied fruitfully. A valid, relevant, and appropriate set of hypotheses is critical for the next sequential steps in the process, namely gathering and interpreting further information and selecting the appropriate diagnostic tests.

CASE 2. HYPOTHESIS TRIGGERING BY AN EXPERT

> A 24-year-old Chinese man came to the Emergency Department complaining of weakness of his arms and legs for 10 to 12 hours.

There are so many causes of weakness that I find it difficult to be very specific. I take it, however, that we are dealing with real muscle weakness and not simply a general feeling of fatigue. Two features are helpful: The weakness is in all extremities, and it is of recent onset. It would be useful to know whether the patient had had similar episodes in the past and whether the weakness was more pronounced proximally than distally. Proximal weakness suggests a myopathy and distal weakness a neuropathy. It is also possible that the weakness is a manifestation of a metabolic disturbance or some other systemic process.

> A resident came to assess the urgency of the patient's condition. Deciding that the patient could wait until other, more urgent problems were under control, the resident requested that several laboratory tests be performed pending examination. One hour later, the laboratory reported the following results: sodium 143 mEq/L, potassium 2.0 mEq/L, chloride 108 mEq/L, total CO_2 28 mEq/L. Blood urea nitrogen (BUN) 13 mg/dL, creatinine 0.7 mg/dL.

> Hemoglobin 16.7 g/dL, hematocrit 49%. White blood cell count 9,000. Erythrocyte sedimentation rate 1 mm/hr.

The most impressive value is a serum potassium of 2 mEq/L, which is very low. The other electrolytes, in particular the normal bicarbonate, suggest that the hypokalemia is an isolated finding not associated with an acid-base disorder. Renal function is normal. The patient is not anemic. The sedimentation rate is normal, as is the white count. A low serum potassium alone can cause weakness. One possibility that comes to mind in a Chinese patient with muscle weakness and a low serum potassium is hypokalemic periodic paralysis. This disorder occurs either alone in a familial form or, in Chinese patients in particular, in association with thyrotoxicosis. Typically, in hypokalemic periodic paralysis with or without thyrotoxicosis, the weakness comes on over a short period of time, either after a carbohydrate load or after vigorous exercise.

Of course, there are many other causes of hypokalemia. We need to consider disorders that produce excessive loss of potassium from the gastrointestinal tract or kidney. I would like to know if there is a history of diuretic use, and if the patient is hypertensive. Hyperaldosteronism and Cushing syndrome should be considered, although the patient does not appear to be alkalotic. If he is normotensive, Bartter syndrome would be a possibility, but this disorder is extremely rare, especially for his age. Finally, we need further information to evaluate the possibility of thyrotoxicosis.

> Returning to the patient immediately after receiving the laboratory report, the resident learned that the patient had been born in Hong Kong. He had lived in England for the last 18 months, and he had been in the United States for 2 weeks. The patient said he had had similar episodes over the last 2 years, characterized each time by weakness sufficiently severe to prevent him from climbing stairs. He claimed that the current episode was the worst he had experienced.

The history of similar episodes is quite helpful. Also, the fact that the weakness prevented the patient from climbing stairs strongly suggests that he has proximal muscle weakness. If we were to learn

that he had trouble lifting objects over his head or combing his hair, we would be even more convinced that he has proximal muscle weakness. The travel history sometimes can be important. Hyperthyroidism can be unmasked when a person moves from an iodine-deficient area to an iodine-replete area, by providing the thyroid with some substrate. In this case, however, I doubt that this history is relevant because Hong Kong is not a particularly iodine-deficient area, nor is England.

> The current episode of weakness began several hours after the patient had eaten a dinner consisting of rice, pork, and two bottles of beer. Mild weakness that evening was followed the next morning by difficulty arising from bed and inability to walk.

As I mentioned, a high carbohydrate load is a typical precipitating factor for the weakness of hypokalemic periodic paralysis. Typically, the symptoms are progressive and may last up to 24 hours but usually not longer than that. It would be pertinent to ask whether this was an unusual meal for him and whether there were comparable antecedent factors in his previous episodes. Even though at the peak of the weakness he had difficulty even arising from bed, he may have been recovering when he was being evaluated in the emergency room, since the resident found that he was not extremely weak. Under these circumstances, no urgent therapeutic intervention would be necessary.

> The history was negative for vomiting and diarrhea and use of cathartics and diuretics, and the patient had never been hypertensive. He denied having polydipsia or polyuria. The family history was negative for any disease characterized by weakness.

All of these are important negatives that exclude the more common causes of hypokalemia. I think we can be quite secure with the diagnosis of hypokalemic periodic paralysis. There are three forms of familial periodic paralysis, which are distinguished by the serum potassium concentration during the attacks of weakness: hyperkalemic, normokalemic, and hypokalemic. The periodic paralysis in hyperthyroid patients is of the hypokalemic variety and usually is not familial. In this patient, the family history is certainly against the familial form of hypokalemic periodic paralysis. That being the case, one would want to look carefully for signs and symptoms of thyrotoxicosis.

> Review of systems revealed only that the patient was more anxious than usual, that he had lost several pounds over the previous 6 months despite a good appetite, and that he found warm weather difficult to tolerate (he was seen in July). He was constantly warm and perspiring.

At this point, I would say that thyrotoxicosis is a very likely diagnosis. The physical findings will be of obvious interest.

> The patient was thin. His temperature was 36.6°C, blood pressure 142/70 mm Hg, pulse 100 per minute and regular, and respirations 20 per minute. There were no abnormal eye signs. The thyroid gland was palpable and not overtly enlarged and contained no nodules. Cardiac, pulmonary, and abdominal examinations were normal. Muscle strength had improved markedly: Strength in the hands was judged to be normal, and in the arms and legs, it was 4+ on a scale of 5. Deep tendon reflexes were reduced in both the arms and legs. The remainder of the neurologic examination was normal.

His pulse pressure is mildly increased, and assuming he was resting and not anxious, his pulse rate of 100 is high. In a young person with thyrotoxicosis, the resting pulse rate is almost always over 90. The thyroid gland is usually but not always enlarged. He still had mild weakness of his arms and legs. Muscle weakness, particularly proximal, is very common in hyperthyroidism, and it often takes specific questioning or formal muscle testing to elicit it. One would have expected the deep tendon reflexes to be abnormally brisk. They are described as reduced, perhaps because of persistent hypokalemia-induced muscle weakness. There is a distinction in the extent to which the extremities move during the reflexes and in the timing of the movement. It is the timing of the reflexes that is most reliably abnormal in thyrotoxicosis. If the patient is hyperthyroid, Graves disease is the most likely cause, especially in a young person. No abnormal eye signs were found, but they are present in only one third of patients with Graves

disease. The fact that the thyroid gland contained no nodules certainly is compatible with Graves disease.

> Two hours after the initial laboratory results were obtained, serum potassium was 3.4 mEq/L.

The serum potassium returned toward normal without any specific treatment, concomitant with the improvement in muscle strength. This is typical of hypokalemic periodic paralysis. I am satisfied with this diagnosis. The links between hypokalemic periodic paralysis, thyrotoxicosis, and the peculiar ethnic prevalence are not well understood. The cause of the hypokalemia in this disorder is equally obscure. What we know is that the total body potassium is normal, and the hypokalemia seems to reflect a pronounced shift of potassium from the extracellular to the intracellular space. There is some thought that this shift may somehow be linked with abnormal calcium fluxes and that abnormalities of intracellular calcium pools may be responsible for the muscle weakness, but the precise details have not been worked out.

> The following laboratory results were reported the next day: total thyroxine 13.6 μg/dL (N = 4.2 – 12). Thyroid hormone binding ratio 1.92 (N = 0.82 – 1.2). Free thyroxine index 26.1 (N = 5.5 – 11.5). Thyroid-stimulating hormone (TSH) <0.35 μU/mL.

These results confirm the clinical diagnosis. The greatly elevated binding ratio indicates that the serum concentration of thyroxine-binding globulin is abnormally low. This finding is most often familial, but there are some drugs that can give this picture. This illustrates the importance of using the thyroid hormone binding ratio; when people who have low thyroxine-binding globulin levels become hyperthyroid, the total thyroxine level does not accurately reflect the degree of thyrotoxicosis.

Now that the diagnosis has been made, one should treat the thyrotoxicosis because the periodic paralysis disappears when patients are rendered euthyroid. Interestingly, beta blockers have been reported to abort the attacks of weakness in hypokalemia, perhaps because of their effects on potassium distribution. If the attacks were frequent while the patient's thyroid disorder was being brought under control, beta blockers would certainly be indicated as part of the regimen. During the course of treatment of the thyroid disease, the patient should be instructed to avoid vigorous activity and high carbohydrate loads to prevent recurrent attacks.

Analysis

This diagnostic problem-solving session is not an ordinary one, and not many physicians would have approached the problem in the same fashion as the clinician did here. Before we disclose *why* the session is unusual, it is worth describing *how* it is unique. Notice that after the first chunk of data was provided, the clinician jumped to the conclusion that he might be dealing with a metabolic disturbance and that after the second chunk, the first diagnosis he posits is the correct one—hypokalemic periodic paralysis with thyrotoxicosis. Here is a highly specific postulate—a rare condition—yet it is the leading diagnosis for this clinician and the diagnosis on which he focuses throughout the rest of the diagnostic encounter. In fact, he discards many far more common causes of hypokalemia and tenaciously builds a case for the rare disorder. Few students and not many house officers would have been so confident and so narrowly directed.

Two aspects of this direct approach are worth considering. The first is that this clinician happens to be an endocrinologist and as such is intimately familiar with the syndrome. Studies of specialists show this behavior clearly: Solving clinical problems in their field, they ask fewer questions and mention the correct diagnosis sooner than specialists in unrelated areas would in solving the same problem.[19] Second, the initial clues were far more specific to this clinician than they would be to the majority of less experienced or less expert physicians. Weakness alone would have been a rather nonspecific finding, but to the expert, weakness in an Asian male patient conjured up a rare diagnostic possibility.

Lest the uninitiated conclude from this exercise that every patient first should be assumed to have a rare disease before common ones are considered, they should understand the medical cliché that common diseases occur most commonly and

that the kind of highly directed diagnostic problem solving exhibited here requires considerable experience, knowledge, and expertise. The aphorism that "when one hears hoof beats on the street, one shouldn't look for zebras" is a good and solid clinical rule. It is striking, nonetheless, how in this instance a "zebra hunt" paid off.

CASE 3. A DIAGNOSTIC COUP

> A 38-year-old man with a history of a cardiac transplant for dilated cardiomyopathy 5 years earlier and renal failure secondary to cyclosporine toxicity complained of diffuse muscle pain and weakness.

Knowing why the patient had dilated cardiomyopathy might be helpful. If he is an alcoholic, for example, that might affect my interpretation of subsequent events. In my experience with patients with muscle disorders, clinicians frequently do not report patients' actual symptoms. Myalgia means the muscle hurts. It does not necessarily signify that the muscle is weak, and it does not necessarily imply that rhabdomyolysis is present. It is possible to have severe myalgias and still have a normal CK (creatine kinase) level and preserved strength. The same is true for muscle weakness, which is a loss of power. It does not necessarily have any implication for either pain or chemical evidence of rhabdomyolysis. Clearly these symptoms and signs can overlap. We must remember that the patient is immunosuppressed. I would want to know how he looks, and how he responded to viral infections in the past. Statistically I think a viral syndrome would be the most likely cause, given the limited information so far, even in a cardiac transplant recipient.

> For the past 1 to 2 months he had some difficulty arising from a chair, and during the past week he had a 2-day episode of diarrhea with mild nausea and vomiting. Diarrhea resolved, but the nausea and anorexia persisted. For 2 days, the extremity weakness worsened, and he developed diffuse myalgias. He also said that he had mild difficulty swallowing. He had no paresthesias.

The month-long history is very valuable. Difficulty arising from a chair implies a real myopathy or muscle weakness. In myopathies, we often see predominant involvement of the larger muscles, so it is not uncommon to see symptoms related to the pelvic girdle or shoulder. We should also keep in mind that patients who are receiving cyclosporine may also be receiving corticosteroid therapy, and we need to keep steroid myopathy in mind. The 2-day episode of diarrhea, nausea, and vomiting makes me wonder if the patient could be on colchicine. I think there is a slightly higher incidence of gouty episodes in patients who have kidney failure and are receiving cyclosporine. If he is receiving colchicine, this is exactly the setting in which we see colchicine myopathy, an entity that is probably a lot more common than we realize.

The patient had been on peritoneal dialysis for renal failure for 9 months. He had a history of hypertension attributed to cyclosporine, a seizure disorder attributed to an old cerebral infarct, gout, hypothyroidism, chronic anemia, and avascular necrosis of the left hip that had required hip replacement. His medications included cyclosporine 300 mg daily (qd), metoprolol 50 mg twice daily (bid), levothyroxine 0.025 mg qd, colchicine 0.6 mg qd, amitriptyline 50 mg qd, famotidine 20 mg qd, hydroxyzine 25 mg bid, folic acid, multivitamins, ferrous sulfate 325 mg qd, vitamin D$_3$ 0.25 mcg qd, calcium carbonate 1,300 mg thrice daily (tid), and Epogen 4,000 units twice per week.

The peritoneal dialysis clearly puts him a risk for infected dialysate, but the patient usually knows that because the fluid turns cloudy. Why did he have an old cerebral infarct? Was it due to accelerated vascular disease that is common in such patients, or might he have had an embolic episode related to his cardiomyopathy? The history of thyroid disease is interesting because if he were taking too much levothyroxine (although his dose certainly sounds reasonable) he could develop a myopathy and diarrhea. I already discussed a possible contributing role for colchicine. The history of a total hip replacement raises the possibility of an infected prosthesis. I am interested in knowing his CK level.

He did not appear in distress. Blood pressure was 106/72 mm Hg with no postural changes. Pulse rate was 84 per minute and regular, and he was afebrile. Except for a 2/6 systolic ejection murmur, the remainder of the general examination was unremarkable. He was fully oriented to time, place, and person. Cranial nerves were intact. A gag reflex was present. His muscle strength was diffusely 4/5. His pinprick sensation and vibration sense were slightly decreased in his hands and lower legs. Reflexes in the arms and legs could not be elicited.

He appears to have evidence of both a neuropathy and a myopathy. The etiology of these problems could be one of the drugs he is taking, or it could be the disease that resulted in his needing a transplant in the first place—for instance, amyloidosis. I am still interested in knowing if there is any evidence of rhabdomyolysis.

Admission laboratory data: white cell count 4,200, hemoglobin 13.6 g/dL, hematocrit 38%. Sodium 135 mEq/L, potassium 2.9 mEq/L, chloride 97 mEq/L. Total CO$_2$ 23 mEq/L, BUN 37 mg/dL, creatinine 12.0 mg/dL. Sedimentation rate 73 mm/hr. Calcium 7.9 mg/dL, serum albumin 1.8 g/dL. Phosphorus 2.4 mg/dL, magnesium 2.8 mEq/L. Bilirubin 0.5 mg/dL, alanine transaminase (ALT) 43 IU/L, aspartate transaminase (AST) 53 IU/L, lactate dehydrogenase (LDH) 310 IU/L, CK 693 IU/L.

I am assuming his renal disease has no reversible elements. I always want to make sure the possibility of obstruction has been ruled out. The potassium level of 2.9 mEq/L is interesting because severe hypokalemia can be associated with muscle weakness, but it is not associated with muscle breakdown. This patient has some rhabdomyolysis and some myopathy. I think the first thing I would do at this point is discontinue the colchicine. One remote thought I just had was the possibility of lead intoxication, which could cause both renal failure and gout. This would not have any relationship to his heart disease. At this point, a muscle biopsy could be done, but I probably would just stop the colchicine and observe the response.

> Serum potassium was restored to normal without a change in symptoms or physical findings. Upper gastrointestinal (GI) series showed poor peristalsis of the esophagus and some penetration of the barium into the trachea during swallowing. Both the patient's physicians and an infectious disease consultant thought that the patient had either some type of polymyositis or a myopathy. A consultant neurologist thought that the leading diagnosis was Guillain-Barré syndrome.

It may be difficult to distinguish polymyositis from colchicine toxicity without a muscle biopsy. The esophagus appears to be involved, which is not totally surprising since it contains a large amount of striated muscle. It also raises the possibility of something like a mixed connective disease or scleroderma, which could have been the cause of his heart problem. But again, I come back to the possibility I already mentioned. I doubt that he has Guillain-Barré syndrome.

> Electrophysiologic studies showed a mixed picture consistent with an acute myositis superimposed on a longer-standing axonal neuropathy.

The neuropathy could be drug induced, or it could be related to his long-standing kidney disease. The myositis could be caused by colchicine, it could be steroid induced, or it could be an inflammatory myopathy such as polymyositis. But I keep coming back to colchicine as the cause.

> A muscle biopsy from his left thigh showed an acute vacuolar myopathy consistent with colchicine-induced myopathy, and colchicine was discontinued. The patient's muscle pain and weakness gradually improved.

Interesting. In the last case of colchicine myopathy I saw, my initial diagnosis was polymyositis.

Analysis

It took days for the patient's clinicians to come up with the correct diagnosis, and they were not convinced that they had the right one until they had gone as far as they could go, namely to muscle biopsy. By sharp contrast, the discussant, to whom we presented the same clinical information, raised the possibility of colchicine toxicity even before he

knew the patient was taking the drug, and despite opinions to the contrary, he stuck to this diagnosis as Velcro to Velcro. He seemed so confident that he was satisfied not to subject the patient to an invasive procedure, and would have just stopped the drug to determine whether the pain and weakness would vanish. How did he do this?

The discussant is a general internist, not a specialist who regularly looks after transplant patients or patients with chronic kidney disease, but he explained that in his consultation practice, he had seen similar cases. Still, his performance is exemplary. What gave him the clue? Was muscle pain and weakness in association with diarrhea a pattern he recognized? Was he just lucky, and the diagnosis readily came to mind because of his experience with like cases? His diagnostic confidence seems to instantiate the notion that diagnosis is achieved only by quick pattern recognition, in turn based on knowledge and experience.[40,126,136] In other words, if you know about an entity or have experience with it, you will recognize it; if you do not know about an entity or have experience with it, you will not recognize it.

Studies in cognitive science that use physics as a domain have identified several aspects of pattern recognition as a problem-solving technique.[137] These studies propose that knowledge is stored in long-term memory as condition–action pairs. A given condition is a recognizable pattern; the action is whatever concept or act follows from satisfaction of the condition. This concept assumes that when a condition is perceived or identified, the action is evaluated and executed. According to this theory, memory is accessed by an index that contains the conditions. Such condition–action pairs could also underlie the quick recognition of medical entities. Fever in a patient who has no spleen immediately suggests infection with an encapsulated bacterium; hyponatremia with a BUN of 8 immediately suggests the syndrome of inappropriate antidiuretic hormone secretion; chest pain described as "crushing" immediately suggests coronary artery disease. Maybe muscle pain and weakness in a patient with kidney failure should trigger "ask about colchicine."

Alternatively, consider the following possible construct. The discussant certainly realized that this patient had multiple medical problems and was likely on a variety of medications. Quite possibly, he may have thought through a "causal cascade" in which "multiple diseases" triggered "multiple drugs," which in turn triggered "consider drug complication." Or the cascade might have been "kidney failure," which triggered "drugs are poorly excreted," which in turn triggered knowledge such as "colchicine is one such drug and it can cause myopathy." All of this reasoning is more or less instantaneous, and, bingo, the correct diagnosis appears.

Alternatively, perhaps the narrowly focused (and accurate) approach by the discussant is a function of one of the heuristics or short-cuts that we discuss in Chapters 2 and 9. Here, this particular short-cut would be the "availability heuristic," namely a mental process that relies on familiarity with a given clinical entity, usually because a certain pattern of findings evokes a readily recallable, particularly striking clinical entity.[27,28] This mental process seems like a special form of pattern recognition. The use of this rule of thumb can be incredibly accurate, as it was here, but because it has no inherent notion of prevalence (among patients with myopathies, colchicine toxicity is undoubtedly not the most likely cause), such a diagnosis might be wrong more times than it is right.

Pattern recognition, underpinned by knowledge and experience, is almost certainly not the exclusive basis of all clinical problem solving. Hypotheses and inferences are also critical aspects, as they are an established part of the scientific method. We prefer not to accept the opinions of clinicians, some quite distinguished, who have devised concepts of clinical cognition based on their personal theories of how their minds work.[40,138,139] For many years, experts in cognitive psychology and computer science have advised us to be skeptical of personal theories of the mind.

Although modern scholars have been developing extensive theories of how their minds work since the time of Descartes, detailed studies of problem solving in humans show that such theories often are seriously impoverished or grossly incorrect. One modern expert has criticized such theories in these terms: "We often confabulate, we tell unwitting lies and we are often simply in the dark; we have no idea at all."[140]

We and others believe that an experimental approach to the comprehension of clinical cognition, analogous to the experimental approaches that have provided so much understanding of disease mechanisms, provides far more accurate and richer insights than any intuitive approach.[18,19,116,141] Although such experimental studies are not sufficiently advanced to assess what fraction of clinical problem solving relies on pattern recognition and how much on hypothesis generation and testing, these studies demonstrate several features of diagnostic behavior. They show, first, that experts often apply a narrowly focused approach characterized by a "chaining together" of rules.[19,116] Second, they show that hypothesis formulation is used in diagnosis, although they have not yet shed light on how often, by whom, and in what circumstances these alternative approaches are employed. It seems clear, however, that hypothesis formulation and inference are as important in medical diagnosis and medical management decision making as they are in problem solving for simple aspects of logic and arithmetic.[30] Attributing the process of diagnosis simply to knowledge and experience abrogates any attempt to understand and teach it. A detailed elaboration of the process by experimentation has the following major advantages: It provides a deep understanding of the diagnostic process, a format for discussing it, and a language and vocabulary for teaching it.

CASE 4. A QUICK AND ACCURATE SOLUTION

A 38-year-old man with a 12-year history of ulcerative colitis was admitted to a community hospital with bloody diarrhea and abdominal pain. *Campylobacter* was found in the stool. He was treated with erythromycin for 10 days, but the diarrhea worsened. Sigmoidoscopy showed diffuse, erythematous, friable mucosa, and biopsy was consistent with ulcerative colitis. Steroid treatment was begun. Abdominal pain and diarrhea persisted, and an abdominal plain film showed distention of the transverse colon with air-fluid levels. The white cell count was 14,600 with 58 polys and 6 bands.

We are not dealing with an undiagnosed patient. Apparently he has had ulcerative colitis for a long time and then went on to develop a

Campylobacter infection. I assume that this represented real infection because in the adult, *Campylobacter* is simply not a commensal organism. Even though the bloody diarrhea and abdominal pain seem to be correlated with the infection, treatment with appropriate antibiotics did not result in improvement.

With respect to etiology, the first question is whether the *Campylobacter* somehow exacerbated the ulcerative colitis and produced this picture or whether distention of the colon is related directly to the colitis. A third important possible etiology of this exacerbation is antibiotic-related colitis, for example, one associated with *Clostridium difficile* overgrowth. The antibiotic he received—erythromycin—is one that can produce that type of colitis, and we certainly would want to check a stool titer for *C. difficile* to rule out that possibility.

Are we dealing with a toxic megacolon? If so, how should we proceed? First, we need to know how sick the patient is. On examination, how much abdominal tenderness and distention are there? Are bowel sounds present? Is he febrile? How many bands and toxic polys are there? Also, I would be eager for another sigmoidoscopy, to look for pseudomembranous colitis.

Parenteral nutrition was instituted, and he was allowed nothing by mouth. Sharp left upper quadrant pain with shoulder radiation was treated with meperidine.

I am not certain what to make of the left upper quadrant pain because this location is not a dominant site of pain when the bowel is inflamed. Nonetheless, the pattern of the pain worries me because it could be caused by microperforation of the colon at the splenic flexure. I suppose he might only have a large pocket of gas and fluid in his transverse colon, but in the presence of a toxic megacolon, a perforation is of great concern. I really would like to see another KUB (kidneys, ureters, and bladder) radiograph.

The repeat KUB (Figure 13.1) was said to be consistent with toxic megacolon, and the patient was transferred to Tufts Medical Center. On admission, he was afebrile, and vital signs were normal. His abdomen was distended,

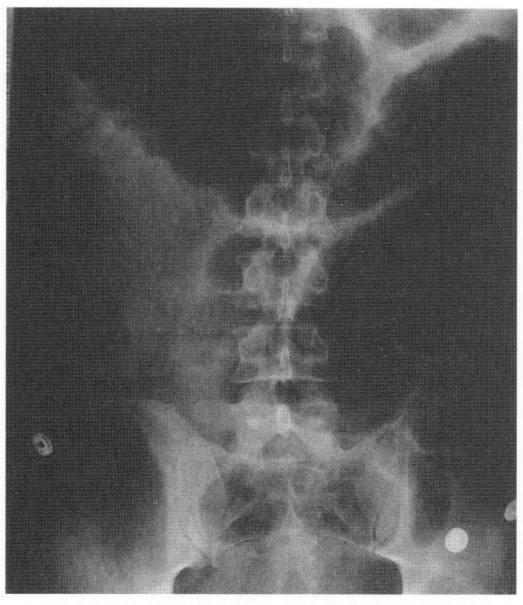

Figure 13.1 • Abdominal plain film; case 4.

with diffuse tenderness. No bowel sounds were heard, but no rebound tenderness was elicited. Rectal examination disclosed liquid brown stool that was guaiac positive, and there was no localized tenderness. Sigmoidoscopy was unchanged.

Well, forgetting the *Campylobacter* for the moment, we are dealing with a patient with toxic megacolon. Our goal here is to save a life. Once toxic megacolon develops, a patient can perforate, develop diffuse peritonitis, and die. The approach should be to direct efforts to maximal intensive therapy, look for improvement, and, if there is no improvement in 24 to 48 hours, recommend surgery. So in my mind this patient will be a candidate for surgery unless he improves in a hurry. My immediate approach would include antibiotics for possible microperforation, intravenous fluids to restore extracellular volume, colloid replacement, and continued steroid therapy.

In relation to operating on this patient for the acute problem, the long history of colitis would lead us toward this option. Any patient with a 12-year history of ulcerative colitis has other factors to be weighed when colectomy is being considered. First and foremost, there is a possibility of malignant degeneration, which occurs at a rate as high as 2% per year once the patient has had colitis for 10 years. We were not told the extent to which the patient has had low-grade morbidity over the 12 years, but to the extent that he has required steroids or felt generally bad, total colectomy might completely restore his health and eliminate both the chance of death from a perforated colon and any anxiety about the development of cancer.

The colon is very dilated, and I do not see air under the diaphragm. Unless there is rapid reversal of the dilation soon, I would get surgeons involved and plan on surgery. I would want the patient and his family to be fully informed of where he stands and of our thinking.

> **The films were thought to show a dilated ascending colon and transverse colon and a "very large" aneurysmal dilation of the splenic flexure with air–fluid levels throughout. Blood pressure was 115/75 mm Hg, pulse 100 per minute, and temperature 38°C. White cell count was 7,200 with 60 polys and 19 bands. An emergency total colectomy was recommended.**

I find it very hard to agree, disagree, or give a strength of agreement in dealing with a patient like this unless I examine him. It is just a thing I have about whether or not to do surgery. The "textbook" response is that immediate colectomy is a safe decision because his risk of dying without surgery is much greater than his risk of dying with early surgery.

What are the clues that I get from examining the patient that are important? First, does the patient look terribly sick or not? Is he sweaty or pale? How tender is the abdomen? How much resistance is there in the abdomen on examination; are bowel sounds present or absent? One must always remember that steroid therapy may mask some of the findings on an abdominal exam. Is there evidence of chronic inanition, which would suggest that he has had a debilitating disease for a long time? What is the personality of the patient like? How can he be expected to respond to the suggestion that he have a total colectomy? Unless some of the tests that we have done demonstrate some unexpected result, on the basis of what I've learned so far, I would not quarrel with the surgeon's recommendation for emergency total colectomy. Toxic megacolon

in ulcerative colitis should be considered a surgical disease unless optimal medical therapy produces improvement within 48 hours.

> **The *C. difficile* assay obtained on admission was reported to be positive. The patient was treated with oral vancomycin (500 mg four times a day) and followed closely. After 2 days of therapy, abdominal pain began to subside, the patient remained afebrile, and there was a decrease in the degree of the left shift in the white count. After 1 week, diarrhea began to diminish, the KUB began to show fewer abnormalities, and the stools became guaiac negative. The patient was discharged after a 3-week hospitalization.**

This case illustrates some important clinical points. First, we always must be on the lookout for reversible causes of extreme colonic dilation in the patient with established ulcerative colitis. I mentioned the possibility of *C. difficile* colitis early, and this diagnosis proved to be correct. In fact, if this diagnosis had been considered highly likely from the beginning, therapy with vancomycin might have been started even earlier. Second, the case illustrates how patients with toxic megacolon frequently are on the verge of requiring surgery and how the presence or absence of certain "soft" clinical findings—such as how the patient looks and how the abdomen feels—can move the choice toward or away from colectomy. Total colectomy cures the problem, but it is associated with risks and postoperative morbidity, and we try to avoid it when possible.

Third, the vigil should not stop in a patient with toxic megacolon if the *C. difficile* assay is positive because those patients too can perforate and require emergency colectomy.

Analysis

In this discussion, we can observe the phenomenon of hypothesis generation, and in particular, we can focus on the part of the clinician's response in which the correct diagnosis was first entertained. In fact, he mentioned *C. difficile* enterocolitis as one of the possible diagnoses in his first response. We know little about how diagnostic hypotheses are initiated, but we can speculate about the process.

One possibility might be that this diagnosis comes up every time as part of a general differential diagnosis of bloody diarrhea. A second, more attractive notion is that this diagnosis is triggered by a pattern (i.e., a constellation) of clues. For example, the onset of diarrhea in a patient previously treated with an antibiotic brings a diagnosis of *C. difficile* enteritis to the fore. This pattern may have been based on a pathophysiologic linkage at one time (antibiotics suppress normal bowel flora and allow *C. difficile*, ever present in the colon, to proliferate and to cause diarrhea), but the experienced clinician may no longer require this return to "first principles" after he internalizes the physiology.

Another possibility is that the triggering process is based on a simple clinical heuristic (i.e., a rule): If a patient has diarrhea and has been treated with an antibiotic, raise the diagnostic possibility of *C. difficile* enteritis. (If that sounds like a statement in a computer program, it is no accident. Some computer programs designed to carry out medical diagnoses incorporate statements remarkably similar to this one.) Other possible explanations for the behavior underlying hypothesis generation are possible, but investigation of this important process has stalled.

A second interesting feature of this diagnostic/patient-management problem-solving exercise is the selection by the clinician of an all-inclusive term for the patient's condition: toxic megacolon. Long before the data given to him provided this designation, the clinician used it in assessing both the diagnosis and the management. Although toxic megacolon is not a specific histopathologic entity, it is a clinical entity. Proposing toxic megacolon as the principal problem permits the clinician to assess whether the patient's findings are consistent with this disorder and to weigh appropriate therapeutic options. "Toxic megacolon" becomes a context for thinking about the problem.

Finally, interesting features of the diagnostic process are readily identified here. One, the use of therapy as a diagnostic test is well illustrated. The clinician is willing to treat the patient with fluids, antibiotics, and steroids for 48 hours and assess his progress during that time. If the patient gets better, surgery is postponed or avoided; if he does not, total colectomy is carried out promptly. This test, like any test, may have false results: The patient may improve initially but relapse later and require surgery (false positive); the patient may fail to improve initially and have a laparotomy but not require colectomy (false negative). By and large, however, response to therapy is often a rather good test.

The clinical assessment of the patient with toxic megacolon is the final subject of this comment. The clinician's assertion that he bases this assessment on how the patient appears to him is somewhat analogous to the concept that many clinical judgments are based on an "overall impression" or on some kind of mysterious and never-to-be-understood "intuition." The clinician's elaboration shows otherwise. In a few sentences, he explicates many, although perhaps not all, of the components of this assessment, including many elements of the physical examination and some psychological features. This kind of experience argues that, if only for didactic purposes, we should endeavor to be as explicit as possible about how we make our clinical decisions.

CASE 5. BETTER LATE THAN NEVER

A 43-year-old woman with a long history of episodic shortness of breath, lightheadedness, and tingling throughout her body was seen in follow-up in the neurology clinic for another episode of loss of consciousness.

A long history of paroxysmal dyspnea brings to mind some form of chronic anxiety or perhaps an arrhythmia. The lightheadedness and tingling raise the question of a seizure disorder, but arrhythmias or anxiety, perhaps associated with hyperventilation, are still possible.

The loss of consciousness puts a different perspective on the history. I would want to know more about the nature of the loss of consciousness. Was it sudden, or was it associated with other symptoms? Did she injure herself when she lost consciousness? I find that kind of information helpful. People do not have protective reflexes during cardiac syncope; thus, if someone recovers from a syncopal episode with a bruise on the nose or a laceration, my suspicion of a cardiac cause increases. The patient with vasovagal syncope commonly sinks slowly to the ground. I also would be interested in knowing if there was any positional component to the loss of consciousness.

> The history disclosed that the patient had been seen frequently for the same complaints in the past. The episodes began 16 years earlier, shortly after her first child, a 7-month-old daughter, died of infantile motor neuron disease (Werdnig-Hoffmann syndrome). When the patient was first seen, she admitted to being nervous. The episodes, then designated "fainting spells," were repeatedly attributed to hyperventilation syndrome, although one neurologist tried to reproduce her complaints by voluntary hyperventilation and was unable to do so.

The fact that at least one neurologist was unable to reproduce the symptoms with voluntary hyperventilation bothers me. Clearly, it is easy to attribute her entire symptom complex to anxiety, but when she actually has loss of consciousness (if that is a new symptom) we have to make sure that we do not ignore the possibility that she has some organic disease.

The question is: What would I have done then? I would be interested in some further cardiac evaluation. I need some information from her physical examination. For example, does she have murmurs? Could she have valvular heart disease or hypertrophic cardiomyopathy? I would want to make sure she does not have an atrial myxoma. I also would want to get an event monitor to make sure she is not having episodic dysrhythmias, either tachyarrhythmias or bradyarrhythmias. If I had to bet on one type of arrhythmia in such a young woman, it would be bradyarrhythmia because supraventricular tachycardias usually do not produce loss of consciousness in young patients without underlying heart disease. I would want to look at her postural reflexes to make sure she is not having autonomic dysfunction with postural hypotension.

> Nine years earlier, after she lost consciousness for the first time, an electroencephalogram (EEG) showed bilateral asynchronous spike foci. Family history disclosed that a cousin had epilepsy. Careful neurologic evaluation dis-

> closed no abnormalities; an MRI scan was normal. The diagnosis was changed to temporal lobe seizures, and she was treated with phenytoin. Phenobarbital and primidone were added early when her episodes failed to diminish in number or severity.

There are EEG patterns that are rather specific for temporal lobe epilepsy, but the findings in this patient, as I recall, were not the classic ones. The most important part of the history is that when she was treated with a variety of antiseizure medications, she did not improve. The lack of response to those drugs diminishes the likelihood that she has temporal lobe epilepsy. We now fall back to thinking that she is just an anxious person, and I do not think we can justify continuing the medications.

> Her usual episodes (shortness of breath, lightheadedness, and tingling throughout her body) recurred approximately once a month between 9 and 3 years ago. During that period, three EEGs showed nonspecific abnormalities, and one done 3 years ago was normal. At that time the antiseizure drugs were discontinued because she had had no new episodes of unconsciousness and because a new neurologist doubted the diagnosis of epilepsy. No new diagnosis was offered to explain her episodic spells.

I do not have any additional thoughts at this point, but I am glad to see that the diagnosis of epilepsy has been challenged. I would like to know what happened to the symptoms when the anticonvulsants were discontinued. Did her episodes change in frequency? Did they still occur once a month?

> Now, 3 years after the antiseizure drugs were discontinued, she returned to the neurology clinic because she had lost consciousness and fallen, injuring her head. She described increasingly frequent episodes of shortness of breath, lightheadedness, and tingling sensations during the previous 6 months. Physical examination and routine laboratory tests were normal. An EEG and electrocardiogram (ECG) were

normal. A Holter monitor study for 24 hours (during which the patient had no symptoms) disclosed no abnormalities. No further studies were done.

Her physical examination and routine laboratory studies are unremarkable. None of the test results are particularly helpful because none of those tests are very sensitive. With an episodic disorder such as this, a routine ECG that represents a 15-second sample of the patient's cardiac rhythm does not tell me very much. An isolated 24-hour Holter monitor reduces the probability of a cardiac cause only slightly, but the patient had no symptoms during the period of testing. We are dealing with a sampling problem. It probably would be necessary to obtain several Holter monitor studies or better yet an event or loop monitor in an effort to pick up an abnormality in the tracing during the time that she has symptoms.

Two weeks later, she began to have one or two of her usual episodes every day without loss of consciousness, and she returned to the neurology clinic. The neurologist ordered another Holter monitor study. During this study, she experienced several of her typical episodes but no loss of consciousness. One segment of the study is shown in Figure 13.2.

Although increasing symptoms are distressing for the patient, their occurrence is a great advantage from the diagnostic point of view. When the frequency of symptoms is high, we are more likely to be able to make an ECG or EEG recording while an event is taking place. The tracing is a case in point. The basic rhythm is normal sinus. However, early on lines 1 and 2 there is evidence of a P wave without a QRS and without a change in the preceding P-R interval. That complex probably represents Mobitz type II atrioventricular (AV) block. Later in the strip, we see a long period of complete heart block. P waves are occurring at the appropriate times, but there is no conduction at all to QRS. An extraordinary thing about the tracing is that during a 10- to 15-second period of AV block, there is no ventricular escape. The patient clearly has intermittent complete heart block, and that could easily explain her symptoms.

The patient was admitted to the hospital, and a DDD pacemaker was implanted. All her episodic attacks ceased, and loss of consciousness did not recur. On several occasions during monitoring, the heart block recurred, but the pacemaker took over, and the patient did not develop any symptoms.

I suspect that they justified using the DDD because of her age. They probably felt that since she is young and active she could benefit from the extra atrial "kick" that the DDD pacemaker provides. I will be provocative. Would it be outrageous to have considered inserting a pacemaker in this patient empirically before it was ever proved that she had a rhythm disturbance? At first blush, that suggestion seems absurd, but it is not, to my mind, illogical, and it raises the more important issue of how certain we must be that a patient has a rhythm disturbance before we recommend a permanent pacer. Conventional wisdom holds that we must fully document a pacemaker-treatable rhythm disturbance before inserting the device, yet a decision-analysis study showed that the indications need not be so stringent because therapy with a pacemaker is quite safe.[142] Indeed, even a moderate suspicion of a pacemaker-responsive disturbance was shown to be a sufficient indication for pacing. In the patient we are discussing, it appears that the suspicion of a rhythm disturbance was so low in the first 15 years that she never would have been considered for such an approach. She is fortunate not to have succumbed to a fatal event before the correct diagnosis was made.

Analysis

In retrospect, although many excellent physicians took care of this patient, they seem quite inept for having missed the diagnosis for 16 years. By contrast, the discussant raised the possibility of a cardiac etiology after he had heard only a few facts. The discrepancy is readily explained by the retrospective approach used in case presentations. Frequently, as in this case, the newest manifestation of a patient's disease is described as a presenting complaint, and it becomes the focus, as it should, for further questioning. The discussant knew that the patient was now being seen for loss of consciousness, whereas the physicians who were seeing the patient

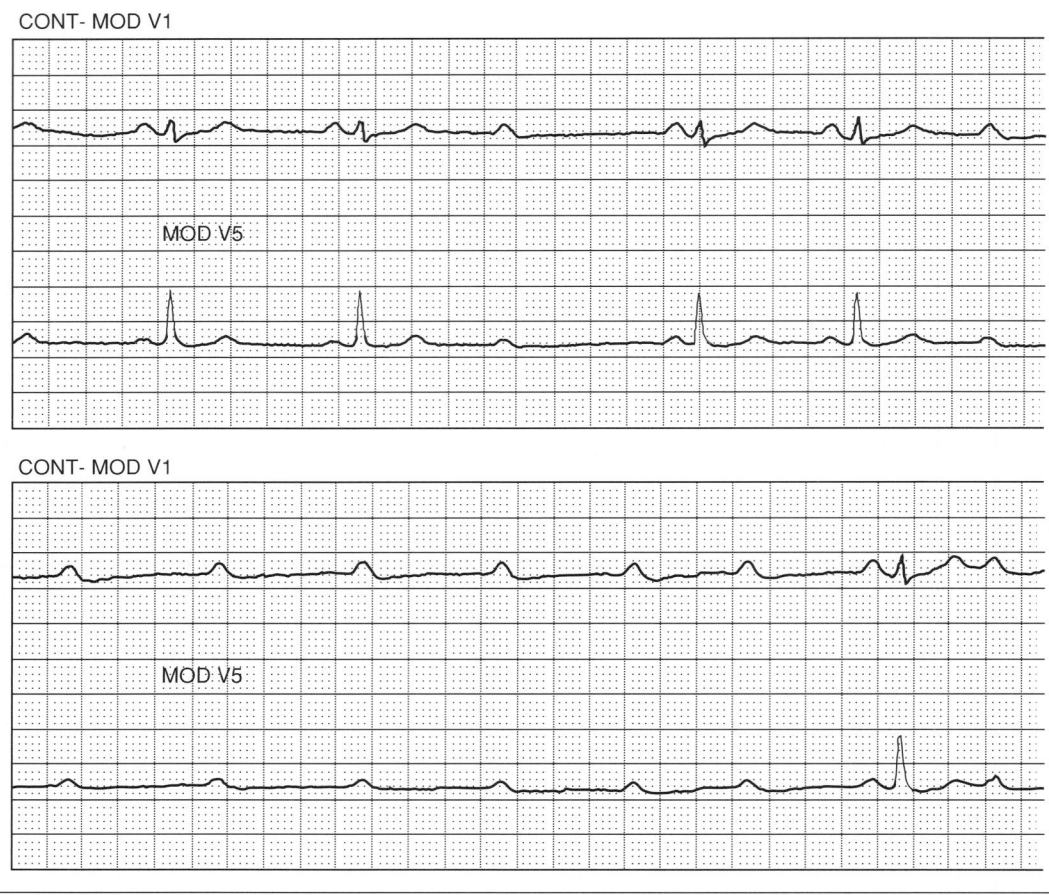

Figure 13.2 • Holter monitor study; case 5. (*continued*)

over the years were evaluating her vague, episodic complaints (shortness of breath, lightheadedness, and tingling throughout the body). Getting the right answer looks easy retrospectively, but it is not so easy prospectively.[143–145]

In fact, one of the principal difficulties in this case was suspecting the correct diagnosis. Because the symptoms were not representative of those seen in patients with heart block and because they were rather vague, they were attributed to either anxiety or seizures. The failure here, probably with little fault on the part of the patient's physicians, is that the correct diagnosis was not "triggered" for years. Failure to raise the possibility of a diagnosis leads, of course, to failure of follow-up questioning and testing. If we do not think of a diagnostic hypothesis, we cannot test it. Albert Einstein said it best: "It is the theory which decides what we can observe."

In this exercise, it is particularly interesting to follow the reasoning processes of the discussant. He is no ordinary clinician. He is an expert decision analyst, and his expertise in this field is apparent from his comments. Although he rarely uses numbers to solve the problem, he describes how he is thinking about the various diagnoses in ways foreign to most clinicians. He uses probabilistic comments extensively ("my suspicion of a cardiac cause increases," "the lack of response to those drugs diminishes the likelihood that she has temporal lobe epilepsy," "none of those tests are very sensitive," "how certain we must be that a patient has a rhythm disturbance before we recommend a permanent pacer"). He also has a way of looking at certain problems. On the basis of decision-analysis data, he raises the possibility that pacemakers may be underused in some patients, rather than overused.[142] In doing so,

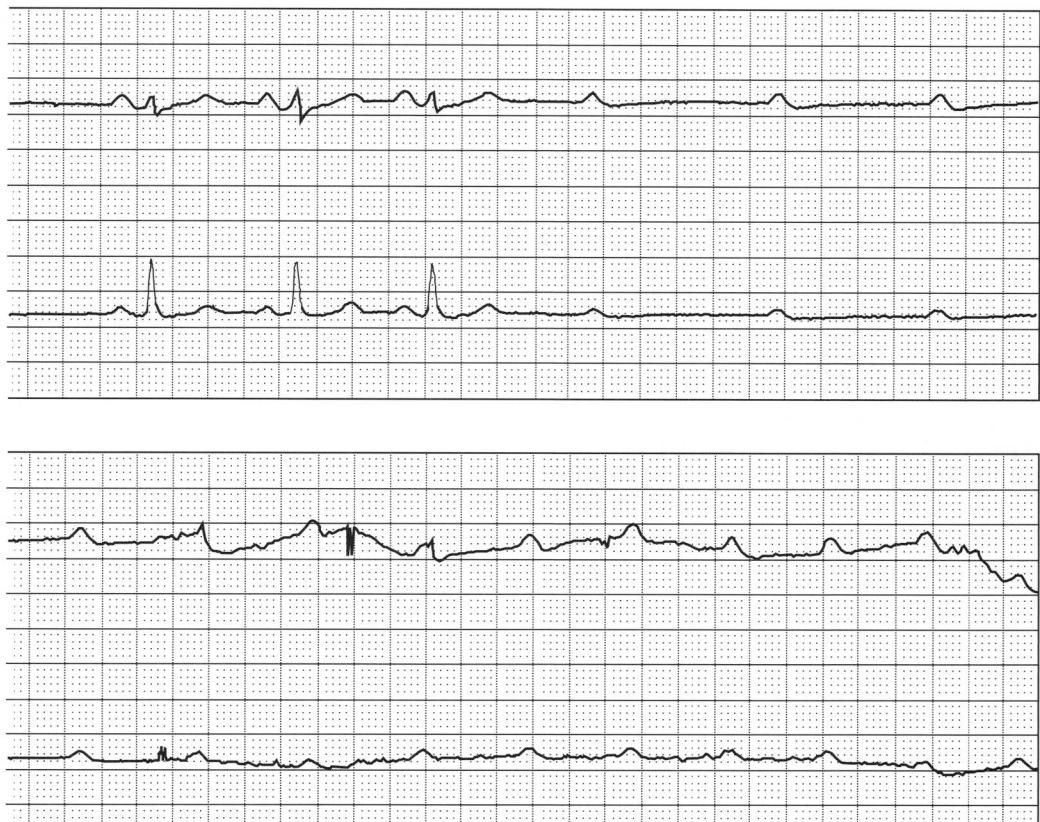

Figure 13.2 • (*Continued*)

he integrates diagnostic uncertainty (how likely is it that the patient has pacemaker-responsive syncope?) with the potential benefits (elimination of the spells) and the potential costs (dollar costs and risk). If a spectrum of clinical thinking can be envisioned with our traditional implicit approach to decision making at one end and formal quantitative decision analysis at the other, the approach used by the discussant lies between those two extremes and leans toward the quantitative approach. For many, it represents a real advance over the traditional, implicit approach.

We prepared this case not only because it provided an opportunity to describe multiple false starts in diagnosis and management, to talk about "triggering diagnostic hypotheses," and to observe a quantitative thinker in action, but also because we were so fascinated by the patient's clinical course. There was enormous inertia in the assumption that her problem was anxiety, hy-

perventilation, or epilepsy that a cardiac cause was not entertained strongly enough and relevant studies were not done. Ultimately, a new staff neurologist, dissatisfied with the earlier diagnosis and suspicious of a cardiac cause, persisted despite two false-negative results (the ECG and the first Holter study) until she uncovered the rhythm disturbance—fortunately for the patient.

CASE 6. A HIT AFTER A MISS

A 38-year-old Vietnamese pastry cook sought medical help for fatigue, stiffness of his arms and legs, and lightheadedness. These symptoms had been worsening for 1 year.

Because he is Vietnamese, one wonders how long he has been in this country. Do we need to consider this background, at least from an epidemiologic standpoint? Second, he has a chronic illness that is rather nondescript in presentation, characterized predominantly by fatigue, some stiffness—not well described—and lightheadedness, whatever that means. This seems to have been a progressive syndrome for 1 year.

> The doctor found no abnormalities on physical examination. Several blood studies were performed. The findings were as follows: hematocrit 33%, mean corpuscular volume (MCV) 89, white cell count 4,600 with a normal differential. Bilirubin 0.2 mg/dL, alkaline phosphatase 33 IU/L, AST 108 IU/L, ALT 53 IU/L, LDH 245 IU/L. Creatinine 2.2 mg /dL, cholesterol 332 mg/dL. Hepatitis A immunoglobulin G (IgG) positive; IgM negative. Hepatitis B surface antigen negative; surface antibody negative. The patient was treated with iron and referred to a medical clinic.

The hematocrit of 33% is low, and an MCV of 89 is within the normal range. AST and ALT are somewhat elevated. The creatinine of 2.2 is elevated, and the cholesterol of 332 also is elevated. He has evidence of exposure to hepatitis A with a positive antibody for IgG and a negative antibody to IgM, which indicates that he had remote rather than recent exposure. His hepatitis B surface antigen and antibody are both negative, which implies that he had no previous exposure to the hepatitis B organism. I would like to know whether the patient is taking any herbal medications. And I think we would need to obtain additional history to explain a chronic syndrome with fatigue, muscle stiffness, and mild anemia. None of these features is particularly characteristic. He does have some evidence of renal insufficiency, which may actually go together with the anemia. (What I mean is that the renal insufficiency might be the cause of the mild anemia.) His liver function tests are abnormal: He has evidence of an active, most likely inflammatory, process in the liver, with an isolated elevation of transaminases. We seem to have excluded at least hepatitis A as an acute cause for these findings and also hepatitis B. Again, it makes me wonder about what this man does in his bakery besides bake. I would like to know whether he has ingested any potential toxins, and I would want to know about his alcohol intake or ingestion of any compounds that may lead to renal failure.

> Through an interpreter the doctor found that the patient also had three-flight dyspnea, a long history of constipation, and occasional low back pain. The patient had a positive PPD (purified protein derivative; tuberculin) test on arrival in the United States from Vietnam 10 years earlier. He thought he had been treated with one drug but could not recall how long he took it. A follow-up chest x-ray was said to be normal. He denied alcohol or tobacco use.

So, working backward, at least one toxin seems to be excluded from the list, namely ethanol, as a cause of hepatic injury. Of interest is the fact that he comes from an area that is endemic for tuberculosis, and he apparently had been treated at least for a positive tuberculin reaction. One has to be concerned about reactivation of tuberculosis in this setting. Although I could perhaps explain the liver function abnormalities, and maybe even the chronicity of the illness and the mild anemia, on this basis, I would be at a loss, given the information we have so far, to relate the elevated creatinine to tuberculosis unless he has renal involvement.

> On examination, the patient's blood pressure was 110/70 mm Hg without postural changes. Pulse rate was 60 per minute lying and 72 per minute sitting. He had no thyromegaly. A 1/6 systolic ejection murmur was present at the apex. Abdominal examination was unremarkable. Neurologic examination was normal, including motor strength. Rectal examination revealed black, guaiac-positive stool (1+).

It seems peculiar that the stool tested only slightly positive for blood, given its color, but this finding does nevertheless indicate a source of blood loss and may explain the patient's anemia.

> Additional tests: hemoglobin 12.7 g/dL, Hematocrit 38%, MCV 98. Direct Coombs negative. Haptoglobin 39 mg/dL. Serum iron 56 μg/dL, transferrin 313 mg/dL. White cell count 4,700, platelet count 172,000. Erythrocyte sedimentation rate 14 mm/hr. Creatinine 1.4 mg/dL.

Urinalysis: normal. Bilirubin 0.9 mg/dL, Alkaline phosphatase 43 IU/L, AST 71 IU/L, ALT 94 IU/L, LDH 263 IU/L, cholesterol 371 mg/dL, Triglycerides 90 mg/dL. Electrolytes, calcium, phosphorus, albumin, and uric acid were all normal. Chest x-ray showed minimal blunting of the right costophrenic angle. Follow-up stool guaiacs were negative.

These findings document a mild anemia. The liver function tests again are consistent with a very mild hepatocellular inflammatory process, but they are not very striking. Follow-up stool tests for blood were negative, which suggests that GI bleeding would have to be intermittent to explain his anemia. Let me think a little about his elevated cholesterol level. It could represent a primary phenomenon, or it could be secondary to a disease process that is causing fatigue, slowing down of activity, and a general feeling of reduced energy. I would be interested in the patient's thyroid function tests.

Because of the hypercholesterolemia, hypothyroidism was suspected. Additional laboratory results: free thyroxine index 1.4, TSH 238.3 μU/mL. Antithyroid antibodies 1:100, antimicrosomal antibodies 1:25,600. Thyroid replacement therapy was started.

So we seem to have come up with an explanation for some of his symptoms of chronic lethargy, slowing down, and stiffness. Namely, the patient is hypothyroid, and there is evidence that there may be an active inflammatory process involving the thyroid gland, with elevation of antithyroid antibodies, as well as of antimicrosomal antibodies. The question is, Does he have an isolated thyroiditis or a more generalized autoimmune process? Perhaps even a vasculitis?

Two months later, all of the patient's symptoms, except for the fatigue, had disappeared. Follow-up laboratory results showed that his free thyroxine index was 9.6, the TSH was 1.1 μU/mL, and creatinine had fallen to 0.9 mg/dL. AST, ALT, and LDH had returned to normal, and cholesterol was 132 mg/dL.

He seems to have responded to thyroid replacement, though the persistence of his fatigue is hard to assess because it is such a vague symptom. So it appears that the patient presented with rather subtle symptoms of hypothyroidism, presumably secondary to an inflammatory thyroiditis.

Analysis

We will pay special attention to only two parts of the clinician's discussion: the segment after the initial serum cholesterol (332 mg/dL) became available and the segment after the second serum cholesterol (371 mg/dL) became available. The first markedly abnormal cholesterol value showed up as part of a panel of screening tests ordered by the patient's physician. Our discussant immediately commented that the cholesterol was elevated, but if his thinking aloud is any reflection of his thought processes, he did not give the abnormal cholesterol value much (if any) consideration. Instead, he focused on the abnormal liver enzymes.

Why did he ignore the cholesterol? One possibility is the limitation of working memory—perhaps because he was incorporating so much new information that the limited capacity of his short-term memory simply could not hold it all (see case 63). A second possibility has to do with how we store information. Some cognitive scientists and artificial intelligence computer experts have proposed that we store compiled information in the form of condition–action pairs or rules of procedure.[21,107]

These rules take the form **if** (a certain observation is made), **then** (a certain action follows). Indeed, it is interesting to speculate that much of the clinical reasoning we do from day to day involves this kind of already compiled, *rule-based (deterministic* or *categorical) reasoning.*[103] If we make this assumption, we can infer that the discussant does not have stored in his memory one of the following rules (or perhaps another quite similar): (1) **If** an adult has a high serum cholesterol value, **then** consider the possibility of hypothyroidism; (2) **if** a patient is a recent immigrant from a country in the Eastern Asia and his or her serum cholesterol is not low, **then** search for a disorder that can explain the discrepancy; (3) **if** a patient who complains of fatigue has an elevated serum cholesterol, **then** consider the possibility of hypothyroidism.

Of course, there are other possible explanations for the failure to consider the diagnosis of hypothyroidism when the first high cholesterol value was observed. The clinician may well have stored the rule, but the information that normally triggers the rule may have been lacking.

No matter what the cause of the failure to recognize the possibility that the patient had hypothyroidism after the first serum cholesterol was observed, the discussant did not fail to make the connection the second time around. This time, however, he did so in an interesting fashion. Having failed to arrive at a diagnosis that was coherent, adequate, or parsimonious (see Chapter 6), he reverted to an examination of each laboratory test or set of tests. He commented on the patient's anemia and on the possibility that intermittent bleeding could be a cause, and then he mentioned the liver function tests. Next, he appreciated that the cholesterol was elevated and—so far—unexplained. Then he connected the high serum cholesterol with one of the patient's presenting complaints—fatigue. The diagnosis of thyroid disease was triggered, and the discussant asked for studies of thyroid function.

Why did the discussant get a hit after he missed the first time? We can only speculate. Presumably, he retrieved the diagnostic hypothesis—hypothyroidism—from long-term memory, checked it against the available data, and found it to be plausible (see case 1). Why then? By the time the second serum cholesterol became available, the discussant had generated many diagnostic hypotheses, but none quite fit the bill. After he was unable to come up with a reasonable diagnostic hypothesis, the discussant seemed to pay more attention to individual test results. Finally, he began to be more analytic about the findings when he was about to strike out, and this careful analytic approach paid off. Although these explanations are reasonable, alternative constructs may be equally cogent.

Some distinguished clinicians have taught that when we are unable to solve a difficult diagnostic problem, it sometimes helps to "start from scratch"—to review the entire record, take the patient's history again, and repeat some (or all) of the laboratory tests. In this case, a second chance was afforded by a second, still-higher, serum cholesterol concentration.

CASE 7. THE CRITICAL ROLE OF CONTEXT IN THE DIAGNOSTIC PROCESS

A 72-year-old woman was admitted to the hospital for abdominal pain, vomiting, and hematemesis.

I am dealing with an elderly adult with an acute illness. I am focused on two things right from the outset: My first concern is to gauge the magnitude of blood loss immediately because I want to stabilize the patient if necessary. Second, I want to learn more about the setting in which this patient presents. Many things come to mind when one hears about abdominal pain, vomiting, and hematemesis. I would want to know about the character of the blood and whether the patient had any previous illness that might give me a clue to the source of the bleeding.

The patient first developed nausea and vomiting 1 week before admission. Three days before admission, middle and lower abdominal pain developed, and immediately before admission, she vomited blood. She had not tried to take antacids to relieve the pain. She did not move her bowels in the 3 days before admission.

I do not know anything yet about the patient's medical history, but I now have a sense of the duration and course of the current illness. This information helps a little but not much because the description is not very specific. If I were at the patient's bedside, I would ask her to localize the pain more specifically: "What do you mean by lower abdominal pain? What do you mean by middle abdominal pain?" I am told that at least it is not epigastric or upper abdominal pain. We do not know anything about maneuvers that would either accentuate or relieve the pain. I do know that the problem is not painless, and maybe there is something going on distal to the duodenum. Again, the thing that brought her to the hospital, despite week-long symptoms, was an acute episode of vomiting blood. We know that she was constipated. But this symptom is not particularly helpful with respect to the cause of her symptoms. So, I am still faced with some of my original concerns. What are the nature, character, and quantity of this blood? We need to localize the bleeding in the gastrointestinal tract.

It helps considerably to frame the diagnosis. In a 72-year-old person who presents with lower abdominal pain, even with vomiting of blood, I would also think of vascular problems, such as aorto-enteric fistulas or ischemic disease of the bowel. I do not think of these when I see a 28-year-old person with similar symptoms. I need to know more history.

> The patient had been treated with aspirin for compression fractures of the vertebrae, and 3 years ago she had been admitted to another hospital for upper gastrointestinal bleeding thought to be secondary to aspirin therapy. In the past several weeks, her back pain had been particularly bothersome; she had been taking increasing amounts of ibuprofen and had been drinking four beers a day. She had also been taking a calcium preparation (1,500 mg per day) for osteoporosis.

I now know that this woman has had a symptom complex similar to what we see now, at least with respect to upper gastrointestinal bleeding. Hematemesis would suggest that she is bleeding from the upper portion of her gastrointestinal tract. Her earlier upper gastrointestinal bleed was attributed to aspirin therapy. The word "thought" makes me question how well that diagnosis was established. Did she have endoscopy with the finding of gastritis and no other bleeding lesion? For the moment, I shall assume that she did have aspirin-induced gastritis.

We know that she has been ingesting three agents that could be noxious to her gastrointestinal mucosa. Nonsteroidal antiinflammatory drugs can induce a defect in the mucosal barrier of the gastrointestinal tract and cause a bleeding tendency. She also is drinking alcohol in sufficient amounts to potentiate gastritis. Finally, she is taking a calcium supplement, and there is clear evidence that exogenous calcium can stimulate acid secretion. Thus, we have a combination of factors that could be inducing gastric irritation.

Many clinicians who have seen patients with upper gastrointestinal bleeding have been led down the garden path of assuming that the gastritis is secondary to alcohol or drugs, only to find

that the patient has some other lesion. I still would not be satisfied with a diagnosis of gastritis and would try to document the cause of the bleeding.

> On admission to the hospital, the patient was lying on her side and was in moderate distress from abdominal pain. Blood pressure and pulse rate were, respectively, 130/70 mm Hg and 116 per minute when lying and 110/60 mm Hg and 132 per minute when standing. Respirations were 30 per minute. Temperature was 37°C. Abdominal examination revealed moderate distention, diminished bowel sounds, and diffuse tenderness. The abdomen was soft, and there was neither guarding nor rebound. Rectal examination showed no tenderness. There was no stool in the rectal vault.

The patient is obviously sick. She has orthostatic blood pressure and pulse changes. She has a distended abdomen with diminished bowel sounds and diffuse tenderness but does not have any of the findings of acute peritonitis.

These findings are disturbing, in that she has lost enough blood or had a sufficient decrease in her fluid intake because of the gastrointestinal symptoms to become dehydrated. On the other hand, we appear to have some time to work out the cause: There is no indication, at least at this moment, that she has perforated a viscus and developed peritonitis. Thus, I think that we can pursue the source of this bleeding. We are not forced to rush in and do something urgent because of a finding of something like free air in her peritoneum.

> Initial laboratory studies: hemoglobin 13 g/dL, hematocrit 44%. White cell count 9,700 with 31 segs, 56 bands, 7 lymphs, 4 monos, and 2 metamyelocytes. Sedimentation rate 20 mm/hr. Amylase 33 U/L, calcium 11.1 mg/dL, creatinine 1.9 mg/dL, BUN 35 mg/dL. Serum electrolytes (mEq/L): sodium 131, potassium 4.0, chloride 82, total CO_2 28. Abdominal plain film showed a nonspecific gas pattern without dilated bowel loops. There was no free air. The film was repeated in the left lateral decubitus position after 200 mL of air was injected into the nasogastric tube, but again, no free air was demonstrated. A nasogastric tube was

inserted and showed material of the consistency of coffee grounds. The drainage was guaiac positive.

Despite her bleeding, she is not anemic. I suspect that she is hemoconcentrated, however, and that once her volume is restored, she will become anemic. She does not have a remarkably elevated white count, but she does have a prominent left shift, with 56 bands. This finding could be a response to acute stress with a demargination of white cells. I am not going to place much emphasis on this finding for now. Despite the abdominal pain and bleeding, her serum amylase is normal. The normal amylase is reasonably reliable evidence that the abdominal pain is not caused by pancreatitis. There are occasional situations in which the serum amylase does not reflect what is going on in the pancreas, but I would expect her serum amylase to be substantially higher with this degree of compromised renal function. Her serum calcium is slightly high. Ingestion of calcium supplements, as I mentioned, can be associated with increased gastric acid secretion. In addition, people with hyperparathyroidism and a high serum calcium may have peptic ulcers and possibly also gastritis. This serum calcium may be telling us something about an underlying condition.

We are given a little more information about the source of bleeding. When we think of coffee grounds, we think of blood that is mixed with acid. We are also told that some attempt was made to determine whether she had perforated a viscus, but I doubt that air injection is particularly reliable. I am still focused on her upper gastrointestinal tract and a possible relationship between her high calcium and gastrointestinal disease, even though I know she has been ingesting several drugs that are toxic to the stomach.

The history and findings were thought to be consistent with gastritis secondary to nonsteroidal antiinflammatory agents. The patient was treated with intravenous fluids. On the second hospital day nasogastric suction continued to yield large quantities of guaiac-positive material. The patient remained afebrile. The abdominal examination remained unchanged. Bowel sounds could not be heard, and she did not have a bowel movement. The abdominal plain film also showed no changes. Repeat blood studies showed hemoglobin was 9.8 g/dL, hematocrit was 38%, and the white cell count was 9,800 with 10 segs, 83 bands, and 7 lymphs. Except for an AST of 116 IU/L, all other liver function studies were normal. Repeat serum amylase was 35 IU/L. Calcium was 9.6 mg/dL. A hydroxy iminodiacetic acid (HIDA) scan was normal. Treatment with clindamycin and gentamicin was begun.

As I mentioned earlier, I am never comfortable invoking the noxious effects of exogenous agents as the cause of upper gastrointestinal bleeding until I am quite sure that other disorders have been excluded. I think that her doctors were similarly concerned. She continued to bleed and was still afebrile, and the abdominal examination remained unchanged. She has no peritoneal signs, and the abdominal plain film does not show any evidence of free air, but she does have a very quiet abdomen. Her white count has not increased much but continues to show a spectacular shift to the left. The finding of 83 bands 2 days into her course is not something that I would easily write off as being due to a stress response to bleeding.

I think her physicians are appropriately concerned that she has sequestered something in her abdomen. They instituted treatment with a regimen of antibiotics directed at a soiled peritoneum. The choice of this particular antibiotic combination, especially the gentamicin, is not optimal, in my view, because of the patient's elevated creatinine. The use of empirical antibiotics for peritoneal soiling is common, but I would have gotten more information before initiating this therapeutic maneuver. In patients who have intraperitoneal soiling from a perforated viscus, one would expect to see some additional clues, such as peritoneal signs, free air in the abdomen, and localized tenderness, but she seems to have none of these. We are told only about a quiet abdomen with an atonic ileus and no localization of symptoms. I do not see much evidence other than the spectacular left shift that makes me think she is infected. I do not have any indication that this woman has an intraperitoneal infectious disease.

> **Gastroscopy showed mild gastritis. A large quantity of brown fluid prevented an adequate examination. The duodenum could not be seen.**

Despite the original assumption that she had gastritis due to the ingestion of multiple noxious agents, gastroscopy did not demonstrate the proximal stomach wall to be the source of bleeding. The blood appears to be coming from the distal part of the stomach. The original diagnosis of gastritis appears to be incorrect. I think the source of her bleeding needs to be pursued further. In the absence of peritoneal signs, I am concerned about a possible vascular etiology. Very often, patients with a communication between the intestine and blood vessels will present with explosive bleeding. Occasionally, such patients have had repetitive small bleeding episodes from such a fistula. My enthusiasm for pursuing the site of the bleeding grows.

> **On the second and third hospital days, the patient remained afebrile. Abdominal tenderness subsided considerably. On the third day, the abdominal plain film was still unchanged. Hemoglobin was 10.2 g/dL, hematocrit was 29%, and the white cell count was 9,200 with 73 segs, 15 bands, 9 lymphs, and 3 monos. Despite the apparent improvement, the patient had no bowel sounds and passed neither gas nor stool.**

The patient is now improving both symptomatically and in terms of laboratory studies. She has less tenderness, and the white count reflects less of a left shift, although it is still present. We have little evidence at this point that she has an intraabdominal infection. She still has obstructive symptoms; she has no bowel sounds, has an ileus, and is not passing gas. Although she is getting better, I continue to be concerned because the source of her bleeding is not yet identified. Attributing her improvement to antibiotics without any documentation of fever bothers me. The shift to the left, with no evidence of peritoneal soiling by peritoneal signs, makes me concerned about what is going on in her abdomen. But I do not think she is infected.

> **Gastroscopy was repeated on the fourth hospital day but showed no more than before. The patient did not aspirate during the procedure,**

> **but later that evening she developed a cough productive of purulent sputum.**

I think that the issue was and continues to be the source of the bleeding. There was sufficient concern to repeat the endoscopy. Although the results reassure us, we really do not know any more. We are told she did not aspirate during the procedure but developed a cough and purulent sputum. Despite the fact that the patient did not aspirate overtly, everybody aspirates with a tube that elevates the epiglottis. The things that come to my mind when someone develops a cough in this setting are, first, aspiration and, second, a communication between the abdominal cavity and the pleural space above the diaphragm. I do not want to invoke an enteropleural connection at this point, and I think that aspiration is most likely. I would also have gotten a chest x-ray.

> **Chest x-ray showed gas underneath the left diaphragm. The gas under that hemidiaphragm moved but not in any pattern consistent with a viscus. CT scan confirmed this finding.**

We now have evidence for perforation of a viscus.

> **The patient underwent laparotomy that evening and was found to have a 3-mm perforation of an anterior pyloric canal ulcer. Purulent material was present throughout the peritoneal cavity. An omentopexy was carried out. After prolonged hospitalization, she recovered and was discharged.**

She indeed had a pyloric ulcer that could not be visualized on gastroscopy and that had perforated. Surprisingly, she had remained afebrile, and the only clues to peritonitis were an ileus and a large shift to the left with bands. She did not manifest most of the other important signs and symptoms seen with peritonitis secondary to a perforated viscus, including rebound tenderness. One could speculate that those symptoms did not occur because of all the antiinflammatory agents she received. I suspect that the aggressive use of empirical antibiotics may well have helped this woman, but they also may have masked some clinical manifestations and delayed the establishment of the correct diagnosis.

Analysis

We intentionally selected this case because the diagnosis of perforated ulcer was missed for days and was discovered only by chance when a chest x-ray was obtained for an unrelated clinical problem. What went wrong? At least in retrospect, the events seem quite clear: On admission, the pyloric canal ulcer was bleeding and probably had already perforated. The abdominal pain, the persistent ileus, and the large number of bands in the differential count would be consistent with this interpretation. Nonetheless, the physicians taking care of the patient and our discussant were fixated on the gastrointestinal bleeding and either ignored or downplayed the possibility of perforation. Why were they blind to the significance of the abdominal pain, the ileus, and the presence of large numbers of bands, and why did they assiduously follow the wrong path and repeatedly study the patient for bleeding by gastroscopy rather than carry out contrast studies?

In this analysis we elaborate on one particular error, namely, incorrect framing of the problem, or an incorrect identification of the "problem space." Less technically, we might describe the error as the commonsense concept of "starting off on the wrong foot and never taking the right step."

What is "framing a problem," and why is it so important? Framing a problem involves selecting the context in which the problem is likely to be solved. Studies of humans solving simple problems have shown that this context, or the cognitive representation of a problem, is an essential element in the process of problem solving. This representation has been called the problem space.[30,31,146] One useful working definition of "problem space" is "the subject's representation of the task environment that permits the consideration of different problem situations and sets limitations on possible operations that can be applied to a given problem."[30] Identifying the correct problem space is not always obvious and simple, but it is a critically important beginning.[75,124,147] Indeed, one study demonstrated that correct identification of the problem space was a major determinant of a subject's subsequent correct responses to a problem set.[32]

Studies of clinicians solving clinical problems show that the problem space, or the context, is selected with only a few clues.[18,19] It consists of a disease entity, a syndrome, or a general operating diagnostic category (e.g., an acute inflammatory disorder). This context serves as a basis for expectation, presumably by configuring a set of findings that should be present and identifying findings that should be absent if a given disease or condition is present. Presumably, it also weighs the importance of each of these findings in confirming or negating the diagnosis. These characteristics of the context thus set the stage for asking further questions and performing further tests that will either confirm or deny that the disease is present. In this case, the initial context appeared to be upper gastrointestinal bleeding—an appropriate choice, given the acute bleeding and the history of this disorder. Since the patient had abdominal pain and had not moved her bowels for the previous 3 days before admission, the context probably should have shifted away from isolated upper gastrointestinal bleeding immediately after this information (inconsistent with this diagnosis) became available.

It is interesting to follow our discussant's logic as he tries to explain the patient's findings. On several occasions, he expresses concern about the possibility of perforation, and he even says on one occasion that "it helps considerably to frame the diagnosis." Yet his conviction in perforation as a diagnosis wavers. After he learns that there are 83% bands but that the abdominal plain film is unrevealing, he says, "We are told only about a quiet abdomen," and he acknowledges that her physicians "are appropriately concerned that she has sequestered something in her abdomen." Still later, he worries again about perforation but dismisses it ("I don't see much evidence other than the spectacular left shift that makes me think she is infected") and continues to focus on the gastrointestinal bleeding. He says, "I don't have any indication that this woman has an intraperitoneal infectious disease."

However, our clinicians and the discussant are not all to blame for this one. Nature, unfortunately, does not always follow the rules that we have derived from repeated exposure to her tricks. One of these useful rules is that "bleeding ulcers don't hurt, and hurting ulcers don't bleed."[148] This heuristic is a valuable one, and it provides a useful guideline for the study of patients with upper gastrointestinal bleeding. However, it is not an invariable rule; it is only a heuristic, a rule that works most of the time.

In this case, it faltered because the patient had an ulcer that not only bled, but induced pain as well. It also faltered because the patient had a perforation without all the classic systemic and abdominal signs that we associate with peritoneal soiling. Unfortunately, many of the patients we encounter do not have "classic" manifestations. It is this variation, among others, that evokes the need for the human problem solver and befuddles attempts to convert all medical problem solving into computer programs.

CASE 8. A MASKED MARAUDER*

A 61-year-old man with seropositive rheumatoid arthritis consulted his rheumatologist because of a 3-week history of pain in the right hip.

My first concern would be to find out whether the hip pain is related to the rheumatoid arthritis. I would want to know whether the man's right hip was involved in the past and whether there was a history of recent trauma. If the patient had been treated with corticosteroids, I would wonder about aseptic necrosis of the hip or infection.

The pain was severe and localized to the right lateral iliac crest, with occasional radiation to the scrotum. At times, the pain increased when the patient lay on his right side, but it was not affected by weight-bearing activities or walking. He had no history of trauma. He had neither pain in his other joints nor gastrointestinal, genitourinary, or constitutional symptoms.

Pain radiating to the scrotum can be a clue to a retroperitoneal or intra-abdominal process, and the localization to the right lateral iliac crest may not be so important. The lack of an effect of weight bearing or walking and the increase in pain when the patient lies on his right side make me think of referred pain. Without a history of trauma, fracture is far less likely. The absence of symptoms in other joints suggests that this is neither an im-

portant flare of his rheumatoid arthritis nor sepsis. Kidney stones seem unlikely without any genitourinary symptoms. We still do not know what medications he may be taking, specifically corticosteroids or other immunosuppressive agents.

The patient had had seropositive rheumatoid arthritis for 3 years, with intermittent synovitis involving both hands, wrists, elbows, shoulders, knees, and ankles. His symptoms had responded to prednisone and hydroxychloroquine. His medical history included a mitral valve replacement, coronary-artery bypass surgery, a septal myotomy for hypertrophic cardiomyopathy, a cholecystectomy, and gastrointestinal bleeding due to peptic ulcer disease. His current medications included prednisone (5 mg per day), hydroxychloroquine (200 mg twice a day), timolol (10 mg twice a day), isosorbide dinitrate (20 mg four times a day), digoxin (0.25 mg per day), nitroglycerin, and warfarin.

Except for the warfarin, I see no obvious direct connections with his current presentation. Patients who are receiving anticoagulants can bleed into the retroperitoneal space, and bleeding into the psoas muscle can certainly cause hip pain or pain referred to the scrotum. The care of patients who have a history of gastrointestinal bleeding and yet need long-term anticoagulation can be extremely difficult and complicated. The prednisone still makes me worry about an infectious complication, although the absence of constitutional symptoms lowers this possibility on my differential-diagnosis list.

There was marked point tenderness over the superior aspect of the right iliac crest with some fullness of the overlying skin. The full range of motion of the hip joint was retained. Initially, mild right-lower-quadrant tenderness was elicited, but this finding was not reproducible. There were no abdominal masses or peritoneal signs. The rest of the examination was unremarkable. X-ray films of the pelvis were normal. The physician was not certain of the cause of the pain and recommended analgesics and local heat.

The point tenderness over the right iliac crest with fullness of the overlying skin cannot be ignored or minimized. On the other hand, the full

*Originally published by Pauker SG, Kopelman RI. *N Engl J Med* 1994;330:1596–1598. For references, see http://content. nejm.org/cgi/content/extract/330/22/1596. Reprinted with permission of the Massachusetts Medical Society

range of motion of the hip joint is somewhat re-assuring, given the possibility of a septic joint or fracture. The absence of abdominal masses or peritoneal signs does not rule out the possibility of a retroperitoneal process. A positive psoas or obturator sign would make me think that a substantial hemorrhage had occurred.

> One week later the pain was unchanged. A bone scan was reported to show "slightly increased uptake in the right hemipelvis and right lower extremity of uncertain significance." Two weeks later the pain was so severe at night that the patient would occasionally have to sleep in a chair. On examination, there was marked tenderness over the right iliac crest with overlying induration, warmth, and erythema. There was slight tenderness in the right lower quadrant. The rectal examination was normal. The right lobe of the prostate was larger than the left, but no nodules were felt. The white-cell count was 6,000 with a normal differential. The erythrocyte sedimentation rate was 43 mm/hr. The results of liver function tests were normal. The physician prescribed oxycodone-acetaminophen and recommended that the patient increase his prednisone dose until a CT scan of the abdomen could be obtained; it was scheduled for 3 weeks later.

If I were concerned about the possibility of retroperitoneal bleeding, I would pursue it more aggressively and not just follow the patient's clinical course. I am not surprised that the pain was unchanged after a week, but I am glad that it had not worsened. The results of the bone scan are not helpful. I am intrigued that the pain later became so severe that he had to sleep in a chair. This suggests that extension of the right leg at the hip is more painful than flexion. The psoas sign extends the hip and should produce discomfort if a retroperitoneal hematoma or appendiceal inflammation is present. Because the patient seems to be more comfortable with his hip in the flexed position, the psoas and obturator muscles are probably involved. The greater prominence of the findings over the iliac crest implies that the underlying process is progressing.

Although both inflammatory and infectious processes can cause these findings, the whole picture is somewhat atypical of infection because the patient has not gotten worse and because systemic symptoms, such as fever, have not developed. The white cell count, again, makes an infectious process less likely, but the sedimentation rate is not very helpful, especially in a patient with rheumatoid arthritis. Although I would need to keep infection on my list, an inflammatory process is now more likely. The slight right-lower-quadrant tenderness is nonspecific but does raise the possibility of an intra-abdominal process.

Three weeks seems to be too long to wait for the abdominal CT scan.

> The CT scan of the abdomen strongly suggested a perforated appendix with a fistulous tract leading toward the anterolateral abdominal wall. On examination, the patient continued to be afebrile. Fullness persisted over the right iliac crest. Only minimal tenderness was elicited over the right lower quadrant, but subcutaneous crepitation was palpable at this site. At surgery, a retrocecal appendiceal abscess was identified and removed. The patient's postoperative course was complicated by angina associated with an unexplained decrease in his hematocrit, but he was discharged on the 16th postoperative day with no residual abdominal or hip pain.

Even in retrospect, I am surprised by this finding, although appendicitis can be chronic and have uncommon, atypical presentations. Fortunately for this man, the process was caught in time.

Analysis

The patient's chief symptom, a few words, or a brief glance can establish the context in which the clinician interprets clinical findings [1] (the reference numbers refer to those in the paper cited in the footnote giving the source of this case). Such contexts are often quite narrow. If they are too broad, even an experienced clinician can find it difficult to sift through large amounts of sometimes irrelevant information and formulate a coherent picture. With the ready access to information that our journals and reference-retrieval services now provide, expert physicians are distinguished from novices mainly by their skill in separating relevant clues from red herrings. That skill depends critically on maintaining the diagnostic focus on a small number of items. However, as with all problem-solving strategies, such a narrow focus can lead us astray. Sometimes the clinician forecloses consideration of important diagnostic possibilities prematurely [2,3] because one hypothesis is especially attractive. When the focus is so narrow, the clinician may consider important clues irrelevant or may misinterpret other findings from the erroneous perspective of presumed diagnostic certainty.

Following different cognitive paths, the rheumatologist caring for this man with appendicitis and the general internist discussing the findings both failed to diagnose an atypical presentation of a ruptured appendix with formation of an abscess that almost produced a disaster. Of interest, neither physician showed signs of premature diagnostic closure in his clinical reasoning [2]. Neither seemed to be in hot pursuit of an overriding alternative hypothesis, yet both were concerned that the patient could have a serious illness, and neither of them could quite get the findings to fit together. Why, then, did both clinicians discount the vague pain in the right lower quadrant and continue to rely on the absence of systemic signs of infection in a patient they knew was receiving corticosteroids?

The patient's new complaint of hip pain with unremarkable x-ray films, the bony tenderness, and the absence of abdominal findings presumably led the rheumatologist, who had been following the patient, to view the problem from the perspective of rheumatologic disease. Once the rheumatologist thought that a fracture or a septic joint had been ruled out, he seemed to consider the patient's illness minor, as we can infer from his actions. Even when the patient's symptoms persisted, the rheumatologist prescribed only symptomatic treatment and a small increase in the dose of corticosteroids; an imaging study was scheduled some weeks in the future, just in case the problem did not resolve with time.

The discussant focused immediately on the potential complications of steroid therapy [4–6] but seemed more concerned with complications caused by steroids than with the possibility that some condition could be masked by steroids. Corticosteroids can mask chronic infections, such as tuberculosis; they can make patients more susceptible to new infections; and, by masking inflammation,

they can make an acute abdomen more difficult to recognize. When it was made clear what drugs the patient was taking, the discussant was sidetracked into considering another set of iatrogenic complications—those related to anticoagulation.

Having raised the possibility of retroperitoneal hemorrhage, the discussant apparently placed complications of steroid therapy in the background. This should not be surprising, given the observation that humans are incapable of juggling a large number of items in working memory simultaneously [2]. When clinical findings or specific hypotheses can be organized into meaningful or "chunked" constructs (so-called working hypotheses), however, the experienced clinician can extend working memory and often can even recall a patient's presentation in surprising detail. When no single hypothesis is available, however, apparently unconnected findings can be dropped (sometimes inappropriately) from consideration. The discussant seemed to reserve a place in the diagnostic list for iatrogenic disease, but he did not seem to keep the complications of two different drugs in mind at the same time.

This patient's clinical course was atypical even for a perforated appendix, probably because it was masked by the long-term steroid therapy and the retrocecal location of the patient's appendix. There were no signs of peritonitis or evolving sepsis; fever and leukocytosis were absent. Most likely, the patient's appendix had perforated early in his course, and the clinical picture was one of a slowly evolving, localized periappendiceal abscess. It is easier to see in retrospect that the severity and the persistence of the patient's pain, its radiation to his scrotum, and the mild right-lower-quadrant discomfort should have suggested appendicitis earlier and should have led the clinician to obtain an abdominal CT scan much sooner.

Abdominal pain, no matter how trivial, cannot be neglected in patients taking steroids [7]. A simple rule —"Lower your threshold for testing in a patient taking steroids who has an undiagnosed illness"—implies that casting a broad net with imaging studies may be an important strategy in helping the clinician overcome too narrow a diagnostic focus. However, selecting an appropriate imaging study is especially difficult if acute appendicitis is the issue at hand, because that diagnosis is made primarily on the basis of the patient's history and by examination of the abdomen. Most imaging studies are unrevealing until late in the clinical course, certainly far later than would be optimal for diagnosis [7–9]. A recent small study suggests that graded-compression abdominal ultrasonography may be useful, but even that test was insensitive in patients with a perforated appendix [10].

Twenty years ago, our diagnostic tools were so limited that the diagnosis of perforated appendix in a patient with such limited signs and symptoms would nearly always have been made at postmortem examination. However, the imaging studies available today allow clinicians to make obscure diagnoses almost by chance. Here, the clinician bumbled into the correct diagnosis when the CT study, performed late in the patient's course, revealed the abscess. He might have insisted that the study be performed earlier if he had given more weight to the possibility that corticosteroids might be masking a lurking disaster.

CASE 9. A SERIOUS LACK OF FOCUS

> A 28-year-old previously healthy man presented in August with a 6-week history of intermittent fever, night sweats, malaise, and diffuse myalgias.

If the 6-week history can be taken at face value, the patient might qualify as someone who has a classic fever of unknown origin. It would be nice to know whether fever was documented. I would be interested in his past medical history, as well as any history of travel or exposures to infectious agents.

> Six weeks previously the man presented to a local clinic with fever, malaise, night sweats, generalized myalgias, sore throat, and a nonproductive cough for a few days. He was given a five-day course of an antibiotic, and his symptoms resolved. Three weeks later while on a train, he developed severe mid and lower back pain, and over the next few days the pain intensified and radiated to both flanks and the abdomen. He also noted a "tingling" sensation on the anterior surface of both thighs. Over the

> next week, the pain became so severe that it prevented him from sleeping.

Depending on the time of year, this common presentation raises many different possibilities, such as mycoplasmal or streptococcal throat infections, or influenza which are relatively minor. Resolution of his symptoms after a 5-day course of antibiotics may be indicative of a bacterial infection. I would not necessarily link the respiratory symptoms with the subsequent development of the back pain. I would want to know if the pain is constant or if it is made worse with coughing or a Valsalva maneuver. In terms of the back pain, I would try to think anatomically. I wonder if he had an underlying illness with a bacteremic episode that then settled into his thoracic or lumbar spine, possibly resulting in an epidural abscess; that would probably be the most worrisome disorder and one that could be easily missed. If the symptoms are not related, he could have had a traumatic event that exacerbated an underlying abnormality of his thoracic or lumbar spine. The tingling sensation on the surface of both thighs could be a marker for the site of the lesion, probably at or around L3. The dysesthesias suggest the possibility of a primary neurologic process, possibly related to a mass lesion in his lower back. I would also consider the possibility of a tumor or a lymphoma. Lymphoma is an interesting possibility in view of his fever, malaise, and myalgias. It is possible that he has Lyme disease: The tingling, the fever, malaise, night sweats, and generalized symptoms are consistent with that diagnosis, although I think that the degree of pain would be a little atypical for that disease.

> Over the next 3 weeks, he again developed fever, night sweats, and malaise. His appetite was poor, and he lost 10 pounds. Myalgias persisted, and he developed diffuse headache, retroorbital pain, and mild photophobia. He also experienced neck tightness and cramping jaw pain. His temperature ranged from 38°C to 38.5°C. He had no gastrointestinal symptoms, joint pain, skin rashes, or productive cough. He had tried ibuprofen and aspirin without relief of his symptoms.

There are some aspects that are causing me to think more about Lyme disease. The diffuse headache, cramping jaw pain, neck tightness, and even the retroorbital pain are consistent with that diagnosis. Having said that, Lyme disease infrequently presents as a classic fever of unknown origin. Vasculitis could also present in this fashion. I am moved a little away from considering an epidural abscess, unless he has a parameningeal focus with tracking. But if that were present, I would have expected more neurologic findings. The degree of pain and fever argues against other primary neurologic diagnoses such as multiple sclerosis. Endocarditis must be considered since it can be a great mimic of many disorders. With the flank and abdominal pain, I would be concerned about an intra-abdominal process, but I have a hard time linking that diagnosis to his headache, retroorbital pain, and photophobia.

His past history was unremarkable. He was self-employed and owned a windsurfing shop in an old converted warehouse in Boston. He had no history of back trauma. He had windsurfed locally, from the Charles River in Boston to Martha's Vineyard. He was heterosexual and had been tested negative for HIV infection during an insurance examination 6 months ago. His only pet was a healthy goldfish. His only travel outside the northeastern United States in the past year was to Georgia.

I suspect that windsurfers probably have frequent unrecognized back trauma. Could he have had some trauma leading to some source of seeding of a bacterial process? He has not been in a climate in which he could have been exposed to an unusual organism such as *Vibrio*. I suppose that he could have encountered *aerophilus* or some unusual gram-negative organism that could have penetrated his skin. Tropical fish fanciers are at risk for atypical mycobacterial infections, especially *Mycobacterium marinum*, which would usually present as a nodular cellulitis. In his travel to Georgia, he could have been exposed to a fungal disease, but his manifestations are not consistent with a fungal infection. Being in Martha's Vineyard and the Boston area would put him at risk for Lyme disease. His findings do not remind me of babesiosis or tularemia. Some viral disorders such as cytomegalovirus infection or Epstein-Barr virus infection can be associated with prolonged fevers

and neuropathies, and tuberculosis should always be considered in the evaluation of a patient with a fever of unknown origin.

On examination he appeared ill, but he was not in acute distress. Blood pressure was 110/72 mm Hg, pulse was 88 per minute, respiratory rate was 14 per minute. Oral temperature was 38.3°C. No skin lesions were noted. One small anterior cervical node was present, as were small axillary lymph nodes. His neck was supple. His masseter muscles were slightly tender. His lungs were clear. Cardiac examination was normal. His abdomen was tender in both outer quadrants, but no organs were palpated. Rectal exam was normal, and stool was guaiac negative. Extremities were normal. His back was diffusely tender over the lower thoracic and upper lumbar vertebrae and flanks. Neurologic examination was normal.

Given his symptoms, I would be surprised if he really had a normal neurologic exam. I would want to know whether the back pain was exacerbated on movement, and whether there really was no sensory deficit. These findings can be subtle. The described findings again suggest that something is going on in his back, such as an epidural abscess or osteomyelitis. The finding of lymphadenopathy is against those diagnoses, unless they are part of systemic response. The enlarged nodes certainly are consistent with Epstein-Barr virus (EBV) or cytomegalovirus infection.

White cell count was 9,200 with 85 polys, 10 lymphs, 4 monos, and 1 eos. Hematocrit was 39%. Urinalysis was normal. Sedimentation rate was 53 mm/hr. Albumin was 3.2 g/L. Glucose, electrolytes, BUN, creatinine, liver function tests, and CK were all normal. Chest x-ray was normal, and KUB suggested a mild increase in liver size. The patient was admitted to the hospital for evaluation of "fever of unknown origin."

Unfortunately, the laboratory results are not very helpful. He has no red cells in his urine or sediment abnormalities that might lead me to consider endocarditis. The fact that his liver function tests are normal argues against a diagnosis of liver abscess. He is not anemic. He does not have any atypical lymphocytes, which leads me away from EBV infection. A retroperitoneal lymphoma is still possible, but it really does not explain findings such as the tightness of the masseter muscles. I would order blood cultures and evaluate his back and abdomen with either a CT or an MRI. If you think of this patient in the context of a fever of unknown origin in conjunction with his constellation of symptoms, you would estimate that infection would constitute 20% to 25% of the cases, and endocarditis and tuberculosis would probably be the leading two infections. Solid tumors, lymphomas, and vasculitis must also be considered.

> Over the next few days his back pain continued to be severe despite oral narcotic administration. Flank and abdominal tenderness and fever persisted. Blood and urine cultures were negative. Throat culture grew beta-hemolytic streptococci group C. PPD was negative. X-rays of lumbosacral spine and sacroiliac joint films were normal. Hepatitis A, B, and C serologies, cytomegalovirus titers, and a monospot test were negative. A Giemsa blood smear showed no evidence of babesial parasites. A right-upper-quadrant and abdominal ultrasound examination was normal.

The presence or absence of group C hemolytic strep in the throat is not helpful diagnostically. The monospot is not a particularly sensitive test for mononucleosis; it is positive in only about one half of the patients. An initial CMV serology does not rule out CMV infection, although if he has the infection, I would have expected a positive serology by now. I would have performed a CT or MRI as opposed to the ultrasound studies. I also would have ordered an aldolase or CK to look for evidence of myositis. Given his history, I would have gotten a Lyme antibody titer for what might be intermediate or late disease. I also would have obtained a neurologic consultation to evaluate the dysesthesias and confirm or deny any subtle localizing findings. One might consider an echocardiogram; culture-negative endocarditis does occur but much less frequently with modern culture techniques.

> Over the next 3 days back pain began to resolve, but flank pain, abdominal tenderness,

and fever persisted. His hematocrit fell to 34%, and the reticulocyte count was low. Studies for hemolysis were negative. An abdominal CT scan showed no adenopathy or organomegaly. Antinuclear antibody (ANA) was positive in a titer of 1:160 in a nonspecific pattern. Antistreptolysin O (ASO) titer was normal. An absolute CD4 count was 471, but all total percentages of T cells were normal. Echocardiogram showed no evidence of valvular abnormalities. A bone marrow aspirate showed reactive hyperplasia with no evidence of lymphoma. EBV IgM was negative and IgG positive. Sedimentation rate remained at 75 mm/hr. No specific diagnosis was made at discharge. He was scheduled for a gallium scan as an outpatient.

The mildly positive ANA in a nonspecific pattern is not helpful. In general, a CD4 count as a screening test for unknown diseases is not useful. We do not have a good idea about the kinetics of CD4 cell counts in most infectious and inflammatory disorders other than to say that patients with bacterial infections often have lymphopenia, which is associated with a reduced CD4 count. The CD4 counts can be reversed and look consistent with HIV infection in patients with CMV and EBV disease and other viral diseases. I doubt that a gallium scan will be useful: The differential diagnosis in this patient is such that no matter what you find on the scan, you will be forced to pursue other kinds of studies. I think a lumbar puncture would have been a reasonable test to perform. This workup appears to be very diffuse.

> Twenty-four hours later the patient returned to the emergency room with a "crooked smile" and difficulty closing his right eye. Examination revealed a right Bell's palsy. Lumbar puncture showed 260 white cells with 70% lymphs, 28% monos, and 2% polys. Cerebrospinal spinal fluid protein was 282 mg/dL, and glucose was 58 mg /dL. Gram stain was negative.

These findings are consistent with Lyme disease. This reinforces the idea that a lumbar puncture could have been performed earlier. These results are also consistent with syphilis or perhaps sarcoidosis, although the normal chest x-ray is against a diagnosis of sarcoidosis. Chronic meningitis is also possible.

> **Serum Lyme titers, obtained on the previous admission, were reported. There was significant elevation of IgM with minimal elevation of IgG. The spinal fluid contained IgG, IgM, and IgA antibodies to *Borrelia burgdorferi*. The patient was treated with ceftriaxone. After 4 weeks, he had full resolution of his symptoms. Six months later, he had suffered no long-term sequelae.**

One must always be aware of the accuracy of the laboratory in which the antibody testing is done since there is great variability in the reliability of testing for Lyme disease. Nonetheless, this appears to be an atypical presentation of Lyme disease. It is clear that patients such as this one need to be treated for a long period of time. A large portion of them will resolve their symptomatic disease, but some people will relapse even with this kind of fairly aggressive approach. I do not think that we know what the optimal therapy is for this disease.

Analysis

You have to sympathize with the discussant, who kindly and gently declares, "This workup appears to be very diffuse." Indeed it is. The physicians taking care of this patient missed the boat for months, seemed bewildered, and ordered every test in the book, including some that had no chance of illuminating the cause of the illness. Using hindsight bias, this diagnostic workup is a classic example of excessive testing, and if the national estimate is correct that about 30% of tests are unnecessary, this patient's evaluation contributed substantially to the excess. Even a prospective examination of the workup suggests that testing was unfocused, and the discussant pinpoints why. The discussant commented early that Lyme disease was possible but complained that the patient's symptoms were not adequately assessed by a careful neurologic examination. It seems quite likely that if the discussant had been in charge, fewer tests would have been done, the diagnosis of Lyme disease would have been made much earlier, the patient would have suffered much less, and his illness would have cost much less. Expertise in this case was sorely lacking.

Nonetheless, this case is representative of the sometimes-frustrating sea of uncertainty in which clinicians often must swim. As we struggle from day to day to discover the cause of a patient's problem, the patient may lose ground, and the need to "get the answer" and give the right treatment becomes increasingly urgent. Imbedded in medical folklore is the notion that the diagnostic insight that gives the "answer" usually appears early and that if one does not have the diagnosis after completing the history, physical examination, and a few well-directed tests, the diagnosis will not surface until much later, if ever. The patient described here is a case in point: Many diagnoses were considered and many were excluded as test results returned, but the diagnosis was missed for weeks. This delay in diagnosis must be considered a medical error; fortunately, the patient suffered no long-term adverse consequences.

Many factors cause delays in diagnosis, and although they have not been studied systematically, several can be identified: (1) The clinician has an erroneous hypothesis, based either on erroneous data or on faulty interpretation of accurate data. (2) The hypothesis is incorrect, and it stays that way because a patient's clinical manifestations are highly atypical. (3) The physician's hypothesis is appropriate, but the choice of the testing sequence is not. (4) The hypothesis and the test selection are reasonable, but one or more test results may be misleading or frankly erroneous—a glitch that may divert the clinician from the right track for days. (5) The hypothesis and test selection are appropriate, but test results are not available for days. (6) The patient has a truly obscure disease, and even the best of us would overlook the correct diagnosis without exhaustive and sometimes unique testing.

It is fair to point out that the patient's manifestations were not typical of Lyme disease. He had no history of a tick bite and no rash, and his neurologic symptoms seemed to appear earlier in his course than usual. Still, atypical manifestations are no excuse for missing the diagnosis for so long. Diseases often do not show up with classic textbook manifestations. Polymorphic manifestations are probably more common than we have been led to believe, and it the clinician's responsibility to appreciate the disorders that are especially protean in their manifestations. Syphilis used to be considered the great imitator; now lupus and Lyme disease have supplanted it.

Many errors can be identified in the care of this patient. The correct diagnosis was not triggered for months; the examination was probably incomplete; the tests seem to be ordered in a blanket, nearly random fashion; and many tests were superfluous. Finally, a Lyme titer was ordered, and if not for a crooked smile, this too might have been overlooked.

CHAPTER 14

Refinement of Diagnostic Hypotheses

CASE 10. WHAT IS A DIFFERENTIAL DIAGNOSIS?

A 34-year-old coal miner from West Virginia was in good health until 4 weeks before admission, when he developed fever (40°C), drenching night sweats, diffuse myalgias, arthralgias, and nasal congestion. He failed to improve after a 5-day course of an oral macrolide antibiotic.

This man's occupation might provide some clues, but given his fever of several weeks' duration, I cannot think of anything to which he might have been exposed. If he had been in an old coal mine where there were a lot of rats, he could have been exposed to leptospirosis. The acute onset of fever and night sweats suggests either an acute viral illness or perhaps bacteremia. He had diffuse myalgias and arthralgias, which are not of particular value in diagnosis because they occur in a variety of systemic infections. If he had some objective sign, such as tenosynovitis, gonococcemia might be an interesting possibility. The nasal congestion suggests a viral respiratory tract infection, but a fever of 40°C seems quite high for that. One would like to know whether this illness occurred in the winter, when influenza A virus was around, because this infection could produce a fever that high. So, at the moment we have a febrile illness of obscure origin.

Two weeks before admission he had a nonproductive cough and pleuritic chest pain. A chest x-ray showed diffuse, small nodular densities and bilateral hilar adenopathy. On examination, his liver was slightly enlarged, and the spleen tip was palpable. The antibiotic was continued, but fever and symptoms persisted. Bronchoscopy showed no abnormality, and transbronchial biopsy material was nondiagnostic.

The development of pleuritic chest pain suggests the possibility of an atypical pneumonia, but the chest x-ray showed small nodular densities and, significantly, bilateral hilar adenopathy. Hilar adenopathy is rather special in relation to respiratory tract infection or in terms of systemic disease because it makes one think of processes like sarcoid, which sometimes can appear acutely with hilar adenopathy and fever. Typically, such patients have the uveoparotid fever syndrome with uveitis, parotid swelling, fever, and small nodular pulmonary densities. Could this man have acquired silicosis as a coal miner and now have miliary tuberculosis as an explanation for the nodular lesions?

Other infections may produce mediastinal adenopathy. For example, does he raise rabbits, which could have exposed him to tularemia? The slight enlargement of the liver and a palpable spleen are both consistent with these possibilities. Of the infections that I mentioned, neither tularemia nor miliary tuberculosis would respond to this antibiotic regimen. I would like to know whether he had parotid enlargement. Could he possibly have Sjögren syndrome with parotid enlargement and respiratory tract involvement? I would also like to know about his joints. For example, if he had tenderness over his costochondral junctions, or if his nasal congestion actually represented involvement of a cartilaginous structure, one could postulate something like polychondritis, but I am not overly impressed by that possibility at present. The unremarkable bronchoscopy is not surprising because the only radiologic abnormalities were small peripheral nodular densities. We still have an unexplained systemic illness with hilar adenopathy. I would want to know at this point about his white cell count because that can help in sorting out a variety of systemic infections. We also certainly want to know the results of blood cultures.

Liver biopsy revealed noncaseating granulomas. Stains for tubercle bacilli were negative. The patient was treated for granulomatous hepatitis with oral prednisone, 30 mg daily. After

> **4 days, he showed no improvement and was admitted to a hospital.**

If we take noncaseating granulomas as a jumping-off point for differential diagnosis, we have to think first about infections. What infections can produce noncaseating granulomas? From a therapeutic point of view, the major concern would be tuberculosis, but the granulomas are not caseating. With miliary tuberculosis, granulomas in the liver are usually not caseating, but in this case, the stains for tubercle bacilli were negative.

What other infections should we think of? A variety of mycotic infections can produce liver involvement with noncaseating granulomas. Epidemiology can be important. In a person from Bloomington, Indiana, one thinks of histoplasmosis; in someone from the Mississippi delta, one thinks of blastomycosis. In someone from the San Joaquin Valley area, one thinks about coccidioidomycosis. This patient comes from West Virginia, and I am not sure which infections are endemic there. I think cryptococcal infections exist there, as in other parts of the country, so I would like to have this histological section subjected to PAS (periodic acid-Schiff) staining.

There are other bacterial agents that produce noncaseating granulomas. If the patient had recently visited Italy or Portugal or if he had eaten unpasteurized cheese or milk, one would have to invoke brucellosis. Tularemia can also produce noncaseating granulomas in the liver, as can secondary syphilis. Some patients actually present with a clinical picture that is consistent with viral hepatitis but turn out to have secondary syphilis. A rash may be a clue to that diagnosis.

Some viral infections have to be considered. Mononucleosis, for example, can produce noncaseating granulomas in the liver. In addition, one has to consider a noninfectious process, such as sarcoid. If he had worked in an old manufacturing plant and been exposed to the material in fluorescent lights, he could have berylliosis. Fortunately, that is not a problem now in the United States.

What are the possible implications of the decision to treat him with prednisone? This strategy encourages me to expand the differential di-

agnosis even further. One can have noncaseating granulomas from malignant disease in the liver. In Hodgkin disease the Reed-Sternberg cells can look somewhat like the giant cells of tuberculosis. We should also consider an uncommon but treatable form of granulomatous hepatitis. This disorder is responsive to corticosteroids and must be considered.

> **At this point additional history revealed that over the last 4 weeks, the patient had severe anorexia, mild dyspnea on exertion, dry eyes and mouth, and a weight loss of 20 pounds. He had smoked one pack of cigarettes a day for 15 years and rarely drank alcohol. There was no history of other drug use. He lived alone on a farm and raised chickens and pigs. He had served in Vietnam. His father had silicosis, and one brother had diabetes.**

The severe anorexia and weight loss make one think of more serious disorders, such as tuberculosis and Hodgkin disease. The dry eyes and dry mouth make one think of keratoconjunctivitis sicca of Sjögren syndrome, which can be associated with a variety of systemic manifestations, including fever. Ultimately, atrophy and lymphocytic infiltration of the parotid and of the sublingual glands occur, and patients also may have recurrent cycles of parotid swelling and shrinking. So I would want to test the capacity of this patient to generate saliva and tears. His joint manifestations could be a feature of the same process.

Are there any diseases that one thinks about in association with exposure to chickens? *Salmonella* infections are transmitted by chickens, though farmers usually do not get salmonellosis. One can have viral infections, such as Newcastle disease, but that disorder primarily involves the eyes and usually has a short course. Swine exposure raises the question of *Brucella*, because one of the forms of brucellosis is *Brucella suis* infection. The history of service in Vietnam might have some significance, possibly because of infection with *Burkholderia pseudomallei*. This was a problem for some of the military in Vietnam in the 1960s, manifested as systemic infection or localized pulmonary lesions that looked like tuberculosis. For a decade or so after the return to the United States, patients experienced relapses of these infections in the context of some other event, such as severe influenza, a thermal burn, or diabetic ketoacidosis. Too much time has elapsed to make this possibility credible. Finally, in any patient these days, one wants to know about the possibility of sexually transmitted diseases and HIV infection, but apparently he is not in one of the high-risk groups.

> On physical examination, he was a thin, ill-appearing white man. His temperature was 37°C, respiration rate 18 per minute, pulse 90 per minute, blood pressure 120/70 mm Hg, and weight 51.6 kg. Skin, HEENT (head, eyes, ears, nose, and throat), chest, and cardiac examinations were all normal. Liver span was 12 cm and not palpable, spleen tip was palpable, and there were no palpable nodes. Chest film showed multiple pulmonary nodules up to 5 mm in diameter, as well as bilateral hilar adenopathy. White blood count was 5,100 with 30 segs, 3 bands, 45 lymphs, 12 monos, 9 eos, and 1 baso. Hematocrit was 37%, mean corpuscular volume (MCV) was 92, and platelets were 362,000. Alkaline phosphatase, lactate dehydrogenase (LDH), aspartate transaminase (AST), and alanine transaminase (ALT) were normal. Serum calcium, 24-hour urinary calcium, and total serum protein were normal. Angiotensin-converting enzyme (ACE) was 133 (normal 44–125).

His chest film could be consistent with a miliary problem of mycotic or mycobacterial etiology. He has relative granulocytopenia, which could be consistent with hypersplenism or an early lymphoproliferative disorder if these are all B lymphocytes. The platelet count does not suggest hypersplenism but does show the expected changes in response to acute-phase reactants. If he had sarcoid, we might expect him to have hypercalcemia or hyperglobulinemia, but he does not have these findings. The ACE level is slightly elevated. One would like to know, in pursuing this diagnosis, whether the patient is anergic.

> The purified protein derivative (PPD) test (5 tuberculin units [TU]) was negative, and sputum produced negative smears for acid-fast bacilli. There were no malignant cells. Culture grew *Candida tropicalis.* Pulmonary function tests revealed mild restrictive lung disease.

His PPD skin test is negative, which could mean that he does not have tuberculosis, but we cannot say that if he is immunocompromised. The culture that grew *C. tropicalis* probably is related to his recent treatment with an antibiotic. So far, this syndrome is suggestive of sarcoid. Could the mild elevation of ACE be due to anything else? We know that ACE levels are increased in pulmonary processes other than sarcoidosis, including various granulomatous processes. So I would be thinking strongly in terms of sarcoid, although, unfortunately, the histologic diagnosis of sarcoid is not specific. Sometimes you stumble on the diagnosis when there are hard granulomas in organs other than the liver. By hard granulomas, I mean noncaseating granulomas with surrounding margins of dense fibroblasts. Those could be seen perhaps in a mediastinal or hilar node biopsy. We should have more tissue to examine at this point.

> Prednisone and the macrolide were discontinued on admission. The patient was afebrile, but his other symptoms persisted. An ophthalmology consultant found no evidence of ocular sarcoidosis but noted slightly decreased tear secretion. Bronchoscopy was normal, and bronchoalveolar lavage showed a slight increase in lymphocytes. Transbronchial biopsy was nondiagnostic. On the sixth hospital day, a thoracotomy was done for lung biopsy and left hilar lymph node biopsy. The lung biopsy revealed noncaseating granulomas with giant cells. With the silver stain, small yeastlike organisms were seen.

Lymphocytes seen on bronchoalveolar lavage might be consistent with sarcoidosis. The lung biopsy results seem consistent with sarcoidosis, but the silver-staining organisms could easily represent *Candida* or, if they are smaller, histoplasmosis. It is important to know if any budding organisms were present.

> The organisms seen on lung biopsy were thought to be *Histoplasma*. Similar organisms were found in the original liver biopsy.

> Cultures of blood and bone marrow were negative for *Histoplasma*. A diagnosis of disseminated histoplasmosis was made. After treatment with a course of antifungal therapy, the patient improved clinically and regained the weight he had lost.

Histoplasma capsulatum in the United States can produce a fungemia that can be identified with special blood culture techniques. In some cases, the organism can be found in bone marrow, but it was not found in this patient. In view of the persistent symptoms and the finding of organisms in the original liver biopsy, I agree with the diagnosis of disseminated histoplasmosis and with the decision to treat with antifungal agent.

Analysis

In this discussion, we consider a single concept, namely a differential diagnosis. We use the term daily, we teach it to our students, and yet a close look uncovers its imprecisions. Indeed, casual conversations with experienced clinicians indicate not only that no universal definition of a differential diagnosis exists, but also that we often use the term to mean different things. Before considering the various usages of differential diagnosis, let us briefly review the diagnostic process. It begins with the evocation, or generation, of hypotheses. Through a sequential approach in which new information is gathered, some hypotheses are refined (specified), some are dropped, and new ones are added. This process proceeds until one or more diagnostic hypotheses are acceptable as the basis for further testing or for taking some therapeutic action.[18,19,103]

If we accept this construct, where does the time-honored concept of a differential diagnosis fit in? Exactly what is a differential diagnosis? How is it defined? What is its purpose? Rather than rely on dictionary definitions, it might be enlightening to describe how the concept is perceived. According to one view, a differential diagnosis is a comprehensive, perhaps exhaustive list of diagnostic hypotheses that could explain a set of salient clinical findings.[41,42,149] These hypotheses could be assembled at any point in the diagnostic process, but presumably not so early (i.e., when only a few of the patient's clinical manifestations are known) that their number becomes unmanageably large. The

list contains all conceivable diagnoses that could apply, no matter how likely or unlikely each one is.[149] Inclusion of exceedingly rare entities in the list ensures that such disorders are not overlooked. Such a list may be formulated informally during a diagnostic exercise, but extensive lists have been compiled to cover all contingencies.[41,150] For example, it is easy to find lists that itemize the differential diagnosis of gynecomastia, hypokalemia, or fever of unknown origin.[149,150] For the most part, such lists are unordered—that is, they are not ranked according to either the probability or the clinical importance of each disorder. Instead, they are usually ordered according to some hierarchical structure, such as pathophysiology.[42,150] No matter what the hierarchical structure of the list (or for any form of differential diagnosis), the list serves as a focus for further diagnostic refinement: to "prove" one diagnosis and eliminate the others.[41]

A second differential diagnostic concept consists of diagnoses formulated in response to each of a patient's relevant clinical findings, including each symptom, physical sign, and abnormal laboratory result.[149] If a patient's manifestations include abdominal pain, fever, and hepatomegaly, for example, a set of possible causes of each clinical attribute is generated. The integration of these sets by the physician is expected to suggest a disease entity or a clinical syndrome.

A third differential diagnostic concept consists of all possible diagnoses that might explain a set of clinical findings, much the same as the first concept, but this list is ordered according to the likelihood that a patient with all the clinical findings observed has each disorder. This list could be used in a Bayesian analysis because, in principle, it should contain the correct diagnosis and because it is already ordered probabilistically.

A fourth concept holds that a differential diagnosis consists of a small set of hypotheses that remain after others have been winnowed out.[42] This small set is the final result of analysis and interpretation of all of the patient's clinical findings. With this short list, the physician must propose tests that can distinguish among the diagnostic possibilities.[42,151] According to this usage, many rare or common diagnostic hypotheses would already have been eliminated before this list is constructed.

With any of these approaches, further refinement of hypotheses could proceed on the basis of probabilistic concepts. As long as the "correct" diagnosis survived on the list, and the list is ordered probabilistically, the correct diagnosis could emerge in a Bayesian analysis as the most likely hypothesis.

How do any of these concepts of differential diagnosis fare in the light of modern cognitive concepts? In Chapter 10, we noted that working memory has a rather limited capacity. The best guess is that ordinarily only five to nine items can be kept in mind at a given time.[23] Although we certainly can recall a list if 15 to 20 disease entities, can we really manipulate such a large number effectively? Various studies suggest that the number of hypotheses kept active at any one time is small; they do not simply pile up into a large list.[18,103] The diagnostic process is an evolving, sequential process of hypothesis generation, deletion, and refinement, not a process that grows a large list of hypotheses for subsequent assessment.[103,131]

The studies also suggest that the dynamics of differential diagnosis encompasses three factors: a drive to find hypotheses that are highly likely and to exclude those that are highly unlikely; a drive to identify diagnoses that represent serious threats to the patient's health; and a drive for efficiency in information gathering and interpretation. If we accept this construction, we might take a radical (fifth) view, namely that a differential diagnosis is an evolving set of diagnostic hypotheses. According to this concept of a differential diagnosis, there is no single set list of hypotheses. Instead, diagnosis is dominated by a flexible, ever-changing set of hypotheses driven by probabilistic reasoning, causal reasoning, and concern for the patient's welfare.[18,103]

Clearly, a differential diagnosis means different things to different people. Some might argue that one should not try to elaborate on these concepts since the term seems to be understood. Instead, we argue, one should be explicit about the value and usage of all parts of the diagnostic process. We have outlined five forms of differential diagnosis: (1) an exhaustive list, not probabilistically ordered, of diagnoses that could explain a set of clinical findings; (2) a list of diagnostic hypotheses for each important clinical attribute; (3) a probabilistically ordered list akin to those used in Bayesian analysis; (4) a short list of diagnoses remaining after a large bulk of clinical data has been digested; and (5) an evolving, sequential list of diagnostic hypotheses. Each has its merits, which we describe here briefly.

The exhaustive list has the advantage that it reminds us to consider some hypotheses that we might otherwise overlook. It is difficult to remember, however, and not readily amenable to further refinement. The probabilistically ordered list is also exhaustive, but it offers a template on which further information can be interpreted. The short list is used primarily for final discrimination among similar clinical entities and serves an important purpose. The evolving sequential concept is a more realistic model of the diagnostic process.

The opening clinical discussion provides an opportunity to view one physician's notion of differential diagnosis firsthand. Over the course of his discussion, his set of hypotheses changes. New hypotheses are added, some are never mentioned again, and some are mentioned several times. Some are not only mentioned but also considered in some detail. Embedded in the evolving process, however, is a traditional "list." When the discussant learns that noncaseating granulomas were found in the liver, he develops a list of diagnostic hypotheses (histoplasmosis, blastomycosis, coccidioidomycosis, etc.) ordered in an informal fashion according to disease prevalence (our third category). Subsequently, he returns to the evolving sequential mode when his original list fails to provide an "answer." Of note, the correct diagnosis was a member of this initial list.

Needless to say, the discussion here is only a single example of the one clinician's differential diagnosis. It illustrates, however, the rather fuzzy and incomplete nature of our concepts of a differential diagnosis. One expert in cognitive psychology characterizes the need to embrace common but fuzzy concepts:

> The fuzzier the concept, the more readily it seems to be used. The fact that these terms are employed so frequently is a good indication that they indeed fill a need, which would be better served if the term were more clearly delineated, broken down, and its connections with related concepts made more explicit.[152]

We need to determine what place each concept of differential diagnosis has in our day-to-day diagnostic encounters.

CASE 11. AN ORDERLY, SEQUENTIAL APPROACH

A 64-year-old man with valvular and coronary heart disease documented previously by cardiac catheterization developed increasingly refractory cardiac failure and was admitted to the hospital for aortic and mitral valve replacement. He had abused both alcohol and cigarettes and was known to have chronic pulmonary disease. His medications included digoxin, diuretics, hydralazine, and nitrates. On admission, he was in moderately severe respiratory distress. Temperature was 36.5°C, blood pressure was 180/70 mm Hg, pulse was 60 per minute (irregularly irregular) with a collapsing quality, and respiratory rate was 24 per minute. He had rales bilaterally to mid-scapula and percussion dullness in the right chest. Cardiac examination disclosed a right ventricular heave, a 3/6 diastolic murmur at the upper right sternal border radiating to the apex, and a soft systolic murmur at the apex. No S_3 or S_4 was heard. The liver was moderately enlarged, and there was no edema.

The patient clearly has congestive heart failure and valvular heart disease. With cardiac surgery being considered, some important questions need to be addressed on admission. First of all, I want to know if the failure is due solely to the natural history of his underlying heart disease. As a corollary, I would question whether he might have a superimposed problem that is contributing to his decompensation—for example, thyrotoxicosis (particularly in a patient with atrial fibrillation), endocarditis (especially given his valvular disease), multiple pulmonary emboli, dietary indiscretion, or noncompliance with his medications. I also worry about the possibility of poor control of his ventricular rate, with a rhythm I assume to be atrial fibrillation. Although his rate is slow at rest, it might increase with moderate exertion to such an extent that he is unable to maintain sufficient cardiac output.

Second, we need to determine the patient's risks for valvular surgery and then maximize his medical therapy beforehand. We also need to assess whether his myocardium is strong enough to maintain an adequate cardiac output once the valves are replaced. We want to be quite confident that he does not have some sort of cardiomyopathy secondary to chronic volume overload, ischemia, or alcoholism.

To ensure that his cardiac status is optimal preoperatively, I would do the following: Check to see that his electrolytes are normal, determine whether he has undergone maximal diuresis, and reduce his cardiac work as much as possible. I assume that the hydralazine and nitrate combination was being used for afterload and preload reduction. I would change his vasodilator therapy to an ACE inhibitor. Finally, because of his history of tobacco abuse, I would ascertain whether he needs bronchodilator therapy. In summary, efforts must be directed at maximizing his medical status before any surgical intervention.

Laboratory results: hematocrit 38%, white cell count 6,100 with 79% segmented neutrophils, 13% lymphocytes, 7% monocytes, 1% eosinophils. Sedimentation rate 68 mm/hr, electrolytes normal, creatinine 1.5 mg/dL, and blood urea nitrogen (BUN) 27 mg/dL. Stool guaiac was negative. Urinalysis: specific gravity 1.021, no protein, no red or white cells or casts. Liver function studies were normal. Electrocardiogram (ECG): atrial fibrillation, rate 52, QRS 0.08, ST-T changes compatible with ischemia, strain, digitalis effect. Chest x-ray: cardiomegaly, moderately large right pleural effusion, vascular redistribution with Kerley B lines.

Most of those studies confirm the physical examination findings of congestive heart failure. I think the finding that needs further consideration is the sedimentation rate of 68. An elevated value is unusual in uncomplicated congestive heart failure. In fact, patients with congestive heart failure classically have a low sedimentation rate. I am interested in his heart rhythm because his resting rate with atrial fibrillation is a little slow. I would want to be certain that he does not have regularization of the rate or some other ECG findings that would suggest digitalis intoxication.

I would also obtain an echocardiogram to evaluate his cardiac status. I would probably get some blood cultures somewhere along the line, given his elevated sedimentation rate.

The patient was given intravenous diuretics and increasing doses of hydralazine. His weight fell, the chest findings improved, and his breathlessness abated, but 24 hours after admission his temperature rose to 38°C. Examination was otherwise unchanged, and the white count was unchanged.

In terms of his fever, one of the first things to come to mind is endocarditis. The fever increases my desire to get blood cultures. Other things to be considered are multiple pulmonary emboli, not an uncommon problem in a patient with advanced congestive heart failure. Pulmonary emboli sometimes can present with fever but without significant respiratory symptoms. The more common causes of fever must also be considered. We would want to get another look at his chest x-ray and also see if there is any sputum available to rule out a superimposed pneumonitis. His urine should be examined. Finally, one must consider whether or not he has a drug fever or a lupus-like syndrome secondary to the hydralazine.

The resident asked the intern to obtain cultures of blood (several sets), urine, and pleural fluid. The next morning the attending physician suggested that this testing approach might have been a bit overzealous.

I think that when one seriously entertains the diagnosis of endocarditis, one must get several sets of blood cultures. Most patients who have culture-positive endocarditis have consistently positive blood cultures; although in some patients multiple blood cultures are required before one culture turns up positive, this pattern is clearly the exception rather than the rule. Nonetheless, given the seriousness of the infection and its therapeutic import, it is my practice to get four or five sets of blood cultures when I think endocarditis is a real possibility. The necessity of culturing the urine would depend more on what was in the urine sediment. If the sediment examination was unremarkable and if a Gram stain of the urine was negative, the yield from a urine culture would be low. I agree with the decision to tap the pleural fluid and send some of it for culture.

Twelve hours later all blood cultures were reported to contain gram-positive cocci in pairs. Echocardiography disclosed no vegetations on the cardiac valves. Treatment with ampicillin and gentamicin was initiated.

The lack of vegetations does not dissuade me from the diagnosis of endocarditis. Some time ago, there was great enthusiasm for the prognostic significance of such vegetations. Patients who have echocardiographically visible vegetations seem to do worse than patients whose echoes do not show them, but the absence of vegetations certainly does not rule out endocarditis. I have no objection to the combination of ampicillin and gentamicin, pending sensitivity studies. This choice of antibiotics is reasonable, especially because the combination is effective even against resistant organisms such as *Enterococcus*.

One day later the organisms in the blood were identified as *Streptococcus bovis*. Other cultures were sterile.

Strep. bovis is an interesting organism. Because of its unusual association with gastrointestinal adenomas and malignancies, any patient who has *Strep. bovis* endocarditis requires studies of the gastrointestinal tract for malignancy.

The resident next ordered a colonoscopy. The attending physician pointed out that the procedures posed some risk to this patient and that the stool guaiac had been repeatedly negative.

I do not think that the attending physician is correct here. I think the presence of *Strep. bovis* endocarditis requires evaluation of the patient's gastrointestinal (GI) tract. I think the attending physician is correct, however, with regard to the risks of the procedures. Cardiac patients occasionally have worrisome arrhythmias during these tests. In addition, there is at least a theoretical risk of bacteremia from the procedures. But in a patient who is already receiving ampicillin and gentamicin, the latter risk from GI studies is minimal. Therefore, I think that when the patient's cardiovascular status is stable, he should undergo this workup.

> Colonoscopy disclosed a 2-cm, nonobstructing lesion in the distal sigmoid colon. Biopsies showed a villous adenoma with no evidence of malignancy.

I think that before the patient undergoes surgery for his colonic lesion, an upper GI series should be considered to ascertain that no other lesions are present. In deciding whether to do the cardiac surgery or the bowel surgery first, I would be strongly influenced by the degree of cardiac compensation after his endocarditis has been treated and his medical management optimized.

Analysis

This problem-solving process exemplifies an orderly, sequential diagnostic approach. The clinician senses immediately that the patient is not in optimal medical condition and sets out to find out why. He initially considers a wide range of possibilities that might explain the absence of optimal cardiac function. Endocarditis, the actual cause, is included. After he receives the next chunk of data, he focuses on the high sedimentation rate, which is highly atypical of patients in cardiac failure, and he requests blood cultures. Clearly, endocarditis has become the leading diagnostic possibility. When he learns that the patient has fever (quite moderate, in fact), his interest in endocarditis continues, but he cautiously considers other common causes of fever, including pneumonia and a drug reaction. A comment by another physician, who is not convinced of the need for so many studies, fails to dissuade him from thinking that the blood and other cultures were appropriate. Although the blood cultures are positive, the echocardiogram discloses no vegetations; even this fact does not dissuade the clinician from his growing suspicion of endocarditis.

The orderly process continues after the clinician learns that the organism recovered from the blood is a *Strep. bovis* strain. Knowing that *Strep. bovis* endocarditis is highly correlated with bowel lesions, he immediately considers the possibility of such a lesion and recommends studies to determine whether one exists.

To recapitulate, the initial diagnostic hypothesis was "some condition that worsens cardiac failure." This hypothesis became further specified as

"endocarditis," and the remainder of the diagnostic encounter encompassed further efforts to refine the endocarditis hypothesis, down to identifying a tumor in the bowel responsible for the particular bacterium on the valves. This highly directed approach is strongly dependent on a substantial base of knowledge and experience.

Experiments in the game of chess illustrate the importance of knowledge in the problem-solving process. When novice players and chess masters are shown a chessboard with pieces arranged in a random fashion, both groups do equally well (or poorly) in recalling the positions of the pieces on the board. However, when both groups are shown a board with the pieces distributed as they might be in a real game, the masters recall the positions of the pieces far better than do the novices. Presumably, the positions represent known strategies that the masters recognize readily.[118,153] The correlation between such behavior in chess and the clinical behavior observed here should be evident.

CASE 12. WEAK REASONING: DIAGNOSIS BY DRUG REACTION*

> A 40-year-old Haitian woman who had never smoked had respiratory distress at work and was taken to the emergency department by ambulance.

The first things that come to mind are the usual causes of respiratory distress, such as pneumonia, congestive heart failure, or a pulmonary embolus.

> Two days before admission she noticed chest congestion, a cough productive of yellow sputum, and shortness of breath, which progressed until she could no longer talk. While receiving oxygen in the Emergency Department, she could communicate with difficulty; she said that she had not previously had any similar symptoms, chest pain, or asthma. She did report a lump in her throat and occasional difficulty

*Originally published by Pauker SG, Kopelman RI. *N Engl J Med* 1993;328:336–339. For references see http://content.nejm.org/cgi/content/extract/328/5/336. Reprinted with permission of the Massachusetts Medical Society.

swallowing. Two weeks earlier, a doctor had told her that she had an enlarged thyroid but that her thyroid function was normal. Otherwise, she said, she was in good health.

There is nothing to suggest a chronic illness. The congestion and shortness of breath make me think of a lower airway problem, but the sensation of a lump in one's throat, especially if stridor is present, would localize the cause of the respiratory distress to the upper airway. The difficulty in swallowing makes me wonder about an esophageal abnormality causing aspiration or an enlarged thyroid, but this would not fit the acute onset. Viral thyroiditis and myocarditis might tie the symptoms together, but the thyromegaly and the respiratory distress may be totally unrelated.

The woman was sitting bolt upright, gasping in obvious respiratory distress. Her blood pressure was 120/80 mm Hg, her pulse rate was 120 per minute, and her respirations were labored at 40 per minute. Her temperature was 36.9°C. No stridor was noted. There was mild, diffuse thyromegaly. Coarse, harsh rhonchi and bronchial breath sounds were heard throughout the chest. No crackles or wheezes were heard. There was no evidence of thrombophlebitis. The rest of the examination was unremarkable.

The rhonchi and bronchial breath sounds both suggest large-airway lower respiratory tract disease. The absence of stridor makes me think that the thyromegaly is unrelated to the shortness of breath. The physical findings do not suggest a primary cardiogenic problem.

The laboratory results included the following: hematocrit 32%, hemoglobin 10.7 g/dL, white cell count 8,000 with 82% polys, 11% lymphocytes, and 7% monocytes. BUN 7 mg/dL, creatinine 0.6 mg/dL, sodium 138 mEq/L, potassium 3.2 mEq/L, chloride 103 mEq/L, total CO_2 22 mEq/L. An electrocardiogram appeared normal, revealing no acute changes. The chest film was normal, demonstrating no infiltrates. With the patient breathing oxygen at 10 L/min by face mask, the arterial blood gas values were pH 7.39, partial pressure of oxygen (PO_2)

63 mm Hg, and partial pressure of carbon dioxide (PCO_2) 38 mm Hg.

Her slightly low hematocrit could be due to many things. I am surprised that her partial pressure of carbon dioxide is 38 mm Hg in the face of respiratory distress and severe hypoxia. She should do a better job of blowing off carbon dioxide with that respiratory rate. She may well have an element of alveolar hypoventilation. There is no evidence of pneumonia or upper-airway obstruction, but asthma can produce substantial air trapping without wheezing. She probably has an element of airway disease, and perhaps her chest film is normal because she is dehydrated. We may be dealing with an infectious process, possibly viral, because the white cell count does not suggest a bacterial problem. *Legionella* infection is possible. Finally, she could have thromboembolic disease in spite of the absence of overt thrombophlebitis. Given the severe hypoxemia and a substantial alveolar–arterial gradient, I am inclined to put pulmonary embolus at the top of my list.

Because she had progressive respiratory distress, the patient was intubated in the Emergency Department. Direct laryngoscopy was negative. Gram staining of the secretions revealed moderate polymorphonuclear neutrophils, with some gram-positive diplococci. A ventilation-perfusion lung scan, obtained during the trip from the Emergency Department to the medical intensive care unit, was interpreted as indicating a low probability of pulmonary embolism. Her temperature rose to 39.7°C. Ceftriaxone and erythromycin were administered intravenously.

I assume she was intubated because of exhaustion. There is no evidence of upper-tract obstruction. Given the magnitude of the alveolar–arterial gradient, if she had had a pulmonary embolus, I would have thought that the scan would have been abnormal. The Gram stain raises the possibility of diplococcal pneumonia and even early adult respiratory distress syndrome, not yet visible on the chest film. I agree with the choice of antibiotics. Ceftriaxone would give good broad-spectrum coverage, and erythromycin would cover the possibility of *Legionella*.

> Over the next 18 hours the patient's condition improved. Her temperature fell to 37.8°C. On 40% inspired oxygen, her arterial blood gas values were as follows: pH 7.40, partial pressure of oxygen 189 mm Hg, and partial pressure of carbon dioxide 38 mm Hg. Her respiratory mechanics were thought to be adequate: Her inspiratory force was −24 cm of water, and her vital capacity was 0.63 L. The ventilation tube was removed, but over the next hour, she had difficulty coughing and clearing her secretions, and she was intubated again. Her diaphragm was noted to move paradoxically with deep breaths.

Paradoxical movement of the diaphragm could be due to a mediastinal mass affecting her phrenic nerve. After reintubation, I would get a computed tomography scan. The low inspiratory force would go along with the abnormal diaphragm movement. We do not have any evidence that she has a neurologic disorder to account for these findings.

> Two hours later, the patient was noted to have bilateral ptosis and was slumped forward in bed. Because these new findings suggested a neuromuscular disorder, the house officer questioned the patient's sister about earlier episodes of weakness. The sister then stated that 5 years earlier the patient had had an episode of severe weakness in her arms and difficulty swallowing, clearing her throat, and drinking through a straw. The weakness had waxed and waned over the next few years. At times, she was unable to pick up a baby.

With her potassium level of 3.2 mmol/L, hypokalemic periodic paralysis comes to mind, but I doubt that is the problem here. At this point, the picture looks more like a neuromuscular disorder with a superimposed acute event, something like a myasthenic crisis. Considering the history of dysphagia, I am now most concerned about myasthenia gravis, multiple sclerosis, or even amyotrophic lateral sclerosis. The waxing and waning of her previous symptoms could certainly be seen with myasthenia gravis.

> A neurologist observed that the patient had moderate muscle weakness in her extremities, more proximal than distal. With repeated testing, fatigue was noted in all muscle groups. The reflexes were intact.

With her enlarged thyroid and the possibility of a mediastinal mass interfering with phrenic nerve function, I might wonder about Eaton-Lambert syndrome, but this sounds like myasthenia gravis to me.

> An edrophonium test was positive, and an electromyogram was consistent with myasthenia gravis. Acetylcholine-receptor antibodies were present. Erythromycin was discontinued, but the course of ceftriaxone was completed for a presumed bacterial superinfection of viral bronchitis. The patient was treated with neostigmine, prednisone, and plasmapheresis. She underwent a thymectomy, but no thymoma was found. After the patient's condition improved with treatment, she admitted that she had been ignoring her symptoms because she was afraid of losing her job if she lost time from work because of illness. In the anxious moments in the Emergency Department, she had neglected to mention her previous episodes of weakness. Several months later she had no weakness, and plans were made to taper the steroid therapy.

Analysis

Although an image is sometimes said to carry far more information than thousands of words, clinicians have long recognized that the physical examination, even when supplemented by x-ray images, is far less effective in establishing a context for diagnostic reasoning than a detailed history. We teach students to take the patient's history first; we begin every presentation with the patient's chief complaint and a history of the present illness; as consultants, we doggedly ask patients to retell their stories and sometimes uncover nuances that clarify their diagnoses. However, medical emergencies demand rapid and effective therapy. Whether patients are threatened by pulmonary insufficiency, hemodynamic instability, arrhythmia, hemorrhage, or metabolic chaos, we must quickly stabilize the situation, often before the diagnosis is clear. Acute respiratory distress is particularly problematic because effective therapy—intubation—can impair communication and make gathering additional historical information from the patient difficult and sometimes almost impossible.

In the case of this woman, the recent onset of respiratory distress and dysphagia led both her physicians and the discussant to focus tenaciously on pulmonary parenchymal and upper-airway disease despite several inconsistencies. The patient was breathing 40 times each minute, but her partial pressure of carbon dioxide was nearly normal [1] (the reference numbers refer to those in the paper cited in the footnote giving the source of this case). She had severe hypoxemia despite clear lung fields and the absence of cardiomegaly on the chest film. Although there was no overt thrombophlebitis, the large alveolar–arterial gradient strongly suggested a pulmonary embolus. That diagnosis was abandoned, however, when the lung scan was interpreted as indicating a "low probability" of embolism. When the patient became febrile, early pulmonary infection was invoked to explain the hypoxemia in the face of a normal chest x-ray film.

With the development of fever and results of Gram staining consistent with pneumococcal infection, broad-spectrum antibiotic coverage seemed appropriate because the short-term risk of using ceftriaxone and erythromycin was considered to be low. When the patient's condition improved with antibiotic therapy, the presumptive diagnosis of early severe pneumonitis seemed correct. The woman's frightening downhill course seemed to reverse, and the standard gambit of early extubation was chosen. The clinicians seemed to make little of her somewhat low inspiratory force and vital capacity. Something appeared awry only when pulmonary insufficiency recurred. The discussant remarked that the paradoxical movement of the patient's diaphragm could reflect either systemic neuromuscular disease or local involvement of the phrenic nerve; both would explain her low inspiratory force and the need for reintubation. Without either a history of the patient's earlier episodes of weakness or the striking bedside picture of ptosis and abnormal posture, which became evident soon thereafter, the discussant pursued the more likely cause—phrenic nerve disease—with computed tomography.

Once the bedside image suggested generalized neuromuscular disease, a focused history allowed the house officer to recognize the clinical picture of myasthenia gravis [2,3], which was then confirmed by the neurologic testing. Until the patient's presentation raised flags that could not be ignored, there was little reason to doubt her initial statement that she had had no similar episodes in the past. Perhaps with a clinical picture so littered with inconsistencies, the house officer should have returned to the patient or her family for a more detailed history, but the combination of intubation and a language barrier raised the threshold for such pursuit.

Within the first day after her presentation to the Emergency Department, this woman's myasthenia waxed and waned, at first requiring tracheal intubation for respiratory support, then allowing extubation, and finally requiring reintubation. When the diagnosis became evident, the clinical picture of bilateral ptosis, a slumped posture, and paradoxical diaphragmatic movement was far more suggestive of neuromuscular disease than was the woman's presentation in the Emergency Department. If the house officer had seen these more typical findings initially, the diagnostic context would probably have been quite different, and the definitive diagnosis would almost surely have been made far sooner.

Although myasthenia appears in most textbook discussions of respiratory failure [4] and although many physicians, when pushed hard enough, would add that possibility to the differential diagnosis, the relative infrequency of that cause as compared with pneumonia, obstructive and parenchymal pulmonary disease, heart failure, or even pulmonary embolism would place myasthenia near the bottom of the list, especially for patients not already known to have neuromuscular disease. It would not be a diagnostic contender unless some quite specific aspect of the patient's presentation raised its likelihood above that of other possibilities. In retrospect, there were several clues in this patient's clinical picture (dysphagia, an unexpectedly near-normal partial pressure of carbon dioxide, hypoxemia despite a clear chest film and a low-probability lung scan, a low inspiratory force, and a sudden need for reintubation), but none was sufficiently specific in its effect on the clinicians' intuitive diagnostic process until the overt signs of neuromuscular disease became apparent.

If none of the earlier inconsistencies were specific enough to elevate neuromuscular disease into active diagnostic contention, why was the cumulative effect of these cues also insufficient? The explanation lies in the incremental nature of clinical reasoning. On the basis of a patient's initial presentation, clinicians formulate an array of diagnostic hypotheses, which can vary from broad categories (such as airway obstruction) to rather specific disorders (such as *Legionella* pneumonia). As additional clinical data appear, clinicians modify their estimates of the likelihoods of those hypotheses, often categorizing a new finding as being either consistent or inconsistent with each hypothesis. Sometimes specific new findings bring new possibilities to mind; for example, this patient's severe hypoxemia in the face of a normal chest film suggested pulmonary embolic disease, and the development of ptosis suggested myasthenia gravis. However, sometimes we merely place rather nonspecific inconsistencies on a mental list of items requiring later attention.

Many physicians learn to keep their diagnostic focus quite narrow, using specific cues to shift from one hypothesis to another. Even for experienced clinicians, the cognitive task of abandoning all current hypotheses and going back to square one can be so daunting that we usually avoid it. Our working memories are limited, making it hard to manage all but the simplest case descriptions as isolated findings. Perhaps to compensate for this limitation, we quickly formulate hypotheses, which serve as contexts for reasoning and provide a format for recalling the patient's findings. Although these reasoning contexts can obscure the broader diagnostic horizon, we cannot abandon this approach to diagnosis because our working memories are so limited. Realizing the danger of prematurely foreclosing consideration of additional possibilities [5], we try to validate our diagnoses carefully and sometimes use rules of thumb or refer to textbooks and review articles to widen our view. When a case just does not hang together, we consult colleagues; they sometimes bring more specialized knowledge, but more often just a fresh perspective—a new diagnostic context. Occasionally, simply organizing the case sufficiently to refer it to a colleague or creating lists of findings and differential diagnoses allows us to see the patient from a new perspective. At times, we need only to consider the findings in a different sequence.

Why did this woman's muscle weakness progress so markedly during her first hospital day? She was not exposed to aminoglycosides, muscle relaxants, pesticides, tainted food, or other substances known to impede neuromuscular transmission. Fever can occur with either myasthenic crisis or infection, and under the stress of infection, myasthenia gravis is often exacerbated [3]. The consulting neurologist offered the most likely explanation. He recalled several reports that suggested that intravenous erythromycin can uncover or exacerbate myasthenia gravis in children [6] and adults [7,8]. This rather recent observation is not yet reflected in standard pharmacology references [9–11].

As this patient's clinical course evolved, intubation was not the only iatrogenic risk. Empirical antibiotic therapy with relatively benign drugs exacerbated her myasthenia in a way that few physicians would anticipate or recognize. However, with careful reasoning and consultation about the patient's progressive weakness, that unexpected drug reaction actually led to the correct diagnosis.

CASE 13. NARROWING DOWN THE DIAGNOSTIC OPTIONS

> A 37-year-old postman, a military veteran, was seen in the Emergency Department for mid-abdominal pain, nausea, vomiting, and watery diarrhea that had persisted for the previous 11 hours.

The sudden onset of mid-abdominal pain, nausea, vomiting, and watery diarrhea brings to mind gastroenteritis that could be viral, bacterial, or protozoal in origin. Unless the patient appeared extremely ill, had severe abdominal pain, or required fluid replacement, I most likely would not put him through a vigorous diagnostic workup. While he was being evaluated, however, a few studies would be useful. I am a believer in the rule that anybody who complains of diarrhea should have a stool specimen examined both grossly and microscopically for blood, polymorphonuclear leukocytes, and parasites. Polys in the stool would suggest inflammatory disease of the colon or possibly the lower ileum—which could be caused by a variety of disorders, including inflammatory bowel disease, protozoal disease, *c. difficile* colitis, and infection with *Shigella*, *Salmonella*, or *Campylobacter*. Of course, a hematocrit and white cell count would be in order.

> The patient had thalassemia minor and a long history of depression, and he had been seen many times at the hospital for various musculoskeletal complaints. Two years before admission, he had an episode of nausea, vomiting, and diarrhea but without abdominal pain or fever. Those symptoms resolved without treatment.

I am not sure what to make of this information. The fact that he had a single episode of nausea, vomiting, and diarrhea 1 year ago does not influence me in any way. Does he have any risk factors for diarrheal diseases? Has he traveled recently? Any unusual food exposures? Is he infected with HIV? Is he on any medications? Once again, the extent of my workup for those common symptoms would depend on how sick he appeared to be.

> On the evening before the gastrointestinal symptoms began, he ate some hamburger of questionable freshness. When he awoke at 1:00 a.m., the pain was severe but not crampy; it did not radiate. Neither the vomitus nor the stool contained obvious blood. The patient began to feel chilly while he waited in the Emergency Department. He had taken no medications for several days before the onset of symptoms. He had no turtles or any other pets.

The fact that he had eaten some food that was possibly contaminated would alert us to the possibility of bacterial diarrhea, which can be associated with toxin production. Organisms responsible for that kind of diarrhea include clostridia and staphylococci.

> On examination, the patient was curled up in the fetal position. Blood pressure was 120/84 mm Hg, pulse was 100 per minute, respiration was 18 per minute, and temperature was 40°C. Abdominal examination disclosed normal bowel sounds and diffuse lower abdominal tenderness without rebound tenderness. There

> were no masses and no palpable organs. The stool was guaiac negative. The remainder of the examination was unremarkable.

His significantly elevated temperature would argue for some form of bacterial gastroenteritis. I would still be interested in the quality of his stool, and the high fever would prompt me to obtain some blood cultures to look for *Salmonella*, for example.

> Initial lab studies revealed the following: hematocrit 43%, white cell count 16,300 with 74 segs, 6 bands, 8 lymphs, 11 monos, and 1 basophil. Amylase 85 IU/L, creatinine 1.1 mg/dL, BUN 15 mg/dL. Serum electrolytes (mEq/L): sodium 141, potassium 4.4, chloride 105, total CO_2 23. Four blood cultures were obtained.

The leukocytosis with a slight shift to the left suggests infection. His diarrhea apparently was not severe enough to cause much volume contraction or electrolyte imbalance. I await the results of the blood cultures with interest.

> Chest x-ray was normal, and abdominal plain film showed no abnormalities. There was gas throughout the colon. Viral gastroenteritis and inflammatory bowel disease were the leading diagnoses. The patient was treated with intravenous fluids, and by the next day, he had stopped vomiting. Fever, diarrhea, and diffuse abdominal pain persisted, but on examination, the abdomen was soft and there was neither guarding nor rebound tenderness. Bowel sounds were hypoactive at some times and hyperactive at others.

I do not see anything unusual about this case so far. The patient improved with intravenous fluids, vomiting resolved, but the other symptoms persisted. I would continue to watch the evolution of his symptoms, observe his temperature and white blood cell count, examine his abdomen repeatedly, and obtain the results of the blood cultures as soon as they were available.

> On the second hospital day, all blood cultures were found to contain *Escherichia coli*. The urine was sterile. The infectious disease consultant wondered if the clinical picture might

> be consistent with either biliary tract disease or a pathogenic toxin-producing *E. coli* infection. Treatment with antibiotics was initiated.

This finding of *E. coli* bacteremia forces me to reevaluate my differential diagnoses. I suppose one must consider biliary tract disease, although I should think that a young person with biliary tract disease would have some suggestive manifestations. I am not familiar with the clinical entity in which a pathogenic toxin-producing *E. coli* causes bacteremia. I wonder about a couple of other things: One is retrocecal appendicitis or a retrosigmoid ruptured appendix. Both could cause an irritative diarrhea and bacteremia. The other is whether the patient was a drug user and had a bacteremia for another reason, with coincidental diarrhea. We would also have to consider diverticular disease, although he is rather young for that.

> Bilirubin 3.3 mg/dL, AST 40 IU/L, ALT 20 IU/L, and alkaline phosphatase 98 IU/L. Ultrasound of the biliary tract revealed no dilated ducts; the gallbladder and pancreas appeared to be normal.

The minimally elevated alkaline phosphatase would argue against obstruction. An elevated bilirubin in the presence of other normal liver function tests raises the possibility of Gilbert syndrome or low-grade hemolysis. My approach to that bilirubin would be to ask for a breakdown of direct and indirect fractions. I doubt that the hyperbilirubinemia is significant, given the meager evidence for biliary tract or liver disease.

> Over the course of the next 2 days, the patient began to feel better. The diarrhea subsided, and the vomiting did not recur. His temperature fell to normal, and his appetite improved. Although abdominal pain decreased, abdominal tenderness persisted; an intern thought that tenderness was localized just to the right of midline. Despite the improvement, a gastroenterologist thought that the patient should have further gastrointestinal studies.

I agree with this plan. When considering a possible septic source due to a perforation, we cannot exclude a lower ileitis—although when bacteremia is due to a perforation, it is usually from the colon rather than the small intestine.

> On the morning of the fifth hospital day, abdominal pain recurred, requiring meperidine for relief. A social worker noted that the patient was angry and that he felt that, as usual, nothing was going well for him. An abdominal computed tomography (CT) scan was consistent with acute appendicitis. The patient underwent surgery and was found to have retrocecal appendicitis. He recovered uneventfully.

One of the points to be made here is that in the differential diagnosis of diarrhea, appendicitis should be on the list because a retrocecal appendix can cause an irritative diarrhea, thus making the presenting manifestations atypical for appendicitis. In addition to atypical symptoms, the physical examination can also be misleading; that is, the abdominal findings may not localize to the right lower quadrant over the McBurney point. Most important, retrocecal appendicitis is a disorder you do not want to miss. In practical terms, how far would you proceed beyond getting the blood cultures? You are certainly not going to get a CT scan on every patient with diarrhea.

My experience with this disorder goes back to the second week of my internship. The surgeons were discussing a young man whose temperature had been 103°C to 104°C for 4 days, and I, fresh out of medical school, naively suggested a diagnosis of retrocecal appendicitis. I got a lot of sneers and scorn, but when they finally operated, they were nice enough to invite me up to the operating room, because that is just what it was. The lesson is that this diagnosis should be entertained when fever, diarrhea, and abdominal pain persist into the third and fourth days. In addition, when I see *E. coli* bacteremia in that setting, I ask this question: What in the bowel can perforate and produce diarrhea? My first thoughts are the appendix and a diverticulum.

Analysis

Several features of this problem-solving session are worthy of consideration: (1) the "case-building" process employed by the discussant; (2) the diagnostic value of a "gestalt picture" of the patient; (3) the approach to diagnosis of a disease in evolution; and (4) the use of heuristic solutions to clinical problems.

The process of taking the history of the present illness is an unstructured problem-solving task that involves generating diagnostic hypotheses, testing them, rejecting weak ones, and refining the surviving hypotheses into coherent diagnoses. The initial diagnostic hypothesis is critically important because it forms a context in which data gathering takes place. Indeed, the data-gathering process is guided by predictions—based on the initial hypotheses—of which the cardinal clinical features are likely to be either positive or negative. If these concepts sound arcane and nonspecific, they are illustrated clearly by the discussant's approach to the patient in this exercise.

His initial reaction to the patient's presenting complaints is that the patient has gastroenteritis. However, he quickly qualifies his remarks by explaining that if he thought that the patient was quite ill, he would be more vigorous in his workup. We interpret this qualification as his real hypothesis: that the patient may have a serious gastrointestinal disorder, as yet unspecified. As information accumulates, it strengthens his conviction that this hypothesis is correct (i.e., the probability increases that the patient has a bacterial infection), and when he learns that the patient has a high fever, he asks for the results of blood cultures. This request does not simply come "out of the blue"; it is presumably based on the prediction that if the patient has a perforated viscus, blood cultures are likely to be positive. It is also presumably driven by a new but tacit hypothesis that whatever has produced the initial symptoms has also produced sepsis.

The impression that the discussant suspects a septic process gains credence when he repeatedly asks for the blood culture results, and his suspicion that the sepsis is originating from a bowel perforation is evident from his assertion that he will examine the patient's abdomen repeatedly. His suspicion of a perforated viscus is enhanced when he learns about the positive blood cultures, and the strength of his conviction is evidenced by the fact that he is not dissuaded by the incorrect opinion of an infectious disease consultant or by the transient improvement in the patient's clinical condition. Finally, the CT scan provides the "smoking gun"— that is, the penultimate evidence that the appendix is the source of the problem. In this sequence, the problem-solving features of hypothesis activation, prediction, data acquisition, and hypothesis revision are clearly evident.

The second interesting feature of this session is the reliance of the discussant on a general clinical impression of how sick the patient is, a concept we described before as a gestalt picture of the patient. In some cases, the gestalt picture can be broken down into its component parts, such as the patient's demeanor and the presence or absence of sweating or pallor, which could provide specific clues to the nature of the problem (see case 4). Whether there are clues from the "gestalt picture" of a patient that a clinician uses is a subject for further study.

Another feature of this session that deserves comment is the evolutionary nature of some diagnostic entities. Many disease processes attain relatively steady states: Both the disease and its clinical manifestations remain relatively constant over time. Chronic renal failure, chronic hypertension, and stable angina pectoris might be examples of such disorders. For those conditions, the diagnostic process might be viewed as a relatively static one, which does not require that the manifestations of the patient be assessed repeatedly. On the other hand, diseases in evolution do not attain a steady state, and the affected patient's clinical manifestations may change abruptly. In such disorders—for example, unstable angina, septic shock, and acute pericarditis—the patient's clinical state must be assessed repeatedly, and the diagnosis may have to be revised as often as manifestations change. A static approach to diagnosis is simply not appropriate in such cases—exemplified by the one presented here—and the clinician has to be willing to re-examine, reassess, and revise the diagnosis and the therapeutic approach at a moment's notice.

Finally, the discussion also shows the importance of one's previous experience in the approach to problem solving. Many of us, when we read about disease entities, remember them in the context of our experience. We can recall the typical as well as the atypical features of particular cases. In the case under discussion, the discussant clearly is familiar with the manifestations of retrocecal appendicitis, but his recall is greatly influenced by his earlier experience with a similar patient. In solving this problem, the discussant relies on a common heuristic (a mental aid to the solution to a problem), known to cognitive psychologists as the "availability" heuristic.[27,28] It is based on the concept that recall of events is biased toward items that stand out particularly strongly in our memory. Sometimes it produces errors because what we remember most clearly may not be relevant to the problem at hand. Often, however, as in the case discussed here, the approach produces dramatic results.

CASE 14. A PICTURE IS WORTH A THOUSAND WORDS

The flow sheet shown in Figure 14.1 on a 53-year-old man was left on the desk in the intensive care unit. What are your impressions?

Well, this is not the usual way we look at clinical information, but let us see what we can learn

New England Medical Center, Inc.
LABORATORY SHEET
Page _____

H.R.S.
53 ♂

DATE	2/2	2/3		2/5	2/7	2/9	2/11				
Hgb/Hct	32	31		28	29	25	30				
WBC ×1000	29	22		29	27	23	22				
GENTAMICIN	✕	✕	✕	✕	✕	✕	✕	✕	✕		
CEFOXITIN				✕	✕	✕	✕	✕	✕	✕	
CLINDAMYCIN				✕	✕	✕	✕	✕	✕	✕	
WEIGHT (KG)	79.6	79.2		85.6	86.1	86.7	87.7				
U Na					4	6					
U SP. GR.	1.016			1.025			1.025				
ART. pH		7.42		7.46	7.43	7.45	7.40				
Pa O2		64		62	66	58	78				
Pa CO2		34		29	28	32	36				
Sodium 135-145 mEq/l	147	144		147	145	145	146				
Potassium 3.5-5.0 mEq/l	5.0	4.4		3.9	3.3	3.4	3.5				
Chloride 97-107 mEq/l	116	114		108	107	107	106				
Total CO2 22-33 mEq/l	21	22		21	22	24	24				
Anion Gap (Δ) 6-12 mEq/l Na -(Cl+CO2)											
Urea N (BUN) 8-20 mg/dl	31	32		45	60	77	94				
Creatinine 0.6-1.2 mg/dl	1.0	1.0		1.9	2.6	2.8	3.7				
Total Protein 6-8 g/dl	6.3										
Albumin 3.5-5.0 g/dl	2.8			2.4	2.4						
Calcium 8.5-10.5 mg/dl	8.9			8.1	7.7	8.0	8.0				
Phosphorus 2.5-4.5 mg/dl	2.5			3.8	5.3	6.1	6.7				
Uric Acid 2.0-7.5 mg/dl											
Total Bilirubin 0.1-1.0 mg/dl		7.5		6.1	6.4	6.3	6.1				
Alkaline Phosphatase to 90 u/l	129			134							
SGPT(ALT) to 30 u/l	27			28							
CPK (CK) to 120 u/l											
SGOT(AST) to 40 u/l	115			80							
LDH to 225 u/l											
P.T.	14.6	14.5		15.6	15.2		14.3				
P.T.T.	45.2	39.4		44.0	58.6		39.4				
Amylase to 110 u/l	82			57							

(Arrow labeled: HYPOTENSIVE EPISODE)

M1-042-1 (8-81)
318861

Figure 14.1 • Flow sheet of patient data; case 14.

from the data (Figure 14.1). Events described here occurred over a 10-day period, from February 2 through February 11. I will start at the top of the page and interpret changes in the parameters over time. His hematocrit was low but relatively stable, and his white count was elevated, in the range of 22,000 to 29,000. He initially received cefoxitin and gentamicin, but on February 4, that regimen was changed to one that included clindamycin, ampicillin, and gentamicin. On February 4, he had a hypotensive episode.

The patient's weight increased dramatically, roughly from 79 to 85 kg by February 5 and to 87 kg by February 11. There was obviously a lot of fluid retention. The urinary specific gravity on February 2 was 1.016, but later it was 1.025 on two occasions.

Initially, arterial pH was 7.42 with a PO_2 of 64 mm Hg and a PCO_2 of 34 mm Hg. The PO_2 changed some: it fell as low as 58 and rose as high as 78. The PCO_2 also was initially low and generally remained low. The patient's pH fell a bit from 7.46 at its highest to 7.40 in conjunction with a modest increase in arterial PCO_2. Serum sodium was elevated and remained moderately high. Serum potassium started out at 5 mEq/L and fell to 3.3 to 3.5. Serum chloride was elevated initially and then fell. Total CO_2 was persistently low normal. BUN initially was 31 to 32 mg/dL with concomitant creatinine of 1. On February 5, the creatinine increased to 1.9 mg/dL and continued to rise. The BUN increased to 94 mg/dL. The patient was hypoalbuminemic, and the serum calcium was about normal for his serum albumin. Serum phosphate increased progressively. Total bilirubin was quite high, and alkaline phosphatase was slightly elevated, but ALT was normal. AST was elevated, however, and both prothrombin time and partial thromboplastin time were prolonged.

Now that I have a feel for the data, let me try to summarize my thoughts. This 53-year-old man had a hypotensive episode and obviously was thought to have some kind of infection. I will come back to that issue in a minute. Given the high bilirubin, the low albumin, and the elevated prothrombin time, liver disease is a virtual certainty. His low arterial PCO_2 and his slightly elevated blood pH suggest that he is hyperventilating. The hyperventilation could be related to liver disease and some abnormality of hepatic function, but because endotoxemia also can produce respiratory stimulation, it could be related to sepsis.

He had a high white cell count and probably was infected. The question is, What kind of infection would we worry about in a person who has liver disease and who may be septic? Obviously, I think we would be concerned about infection in the biliary tree or the gastrointestinal tract. The urinary tract is another obvious site of infection, although we have no evidence for or against that possibility. If we assume that he had cirrhosis and probably ascites as well, he could have had spontaneous bacterial peritonitis. The fact that he was treated with clindamycin suggests that his physicians were concerned about devitalized bowel or sepsis involving fecal flora.

Now let me turn to his renal problem. He was given gentamicin for a few days, and he had a hypotensive episode. Subsequently, he had acute renal failure, a complication that could be related to the gentamicin or the hypotension or some other factors we have not yet heard about. The picture could be consistent with acute tubular necrosis, but his urine sodium concentration was quite low and his urinary specific gravity remained quite high. I will presume that specific gravity measurements were checked with a measurement of urine osmolality and that the urine actually was quite concentrated. I would want to make sure that we were not being fooled into thinking that the urine was concentrated when, in fact, he had received contrast material, which simply increased the specific gravity. I will assume that he had a highly concentrated urine. We have a clinical picture consistent with progressive retention of salt and water; the concentrated urine and virtual lack of sodium in the urine are simply manifestations of fluid retention. One would be worried that his urine volume was probably falling simultaneously, although no such data are given. The one disorder consistent with all of these findings is the hepatorenal syndrome. I suspect that this disorder was the cause of the renal failure. I think I have gone as far as I can with the available data.

Case Summary

The patient had a long history of alcohol abuse with resultant cirrhosis, ascites, and esophageal varices, and he was admitted to the hospital for management of upper gastrointestinal tract bleeding. On admission, in addition to the finding of chronic liver disease, he was found to have right upper lobe pneumonia, for which he was treated with the antibiotics listed on the flow sheet. He was also given a benzodiazepine for impending delirium tremens. Initially, all cultures, including those of the urine and peritoneal fluid, were negative. His condition stabilized until February 4, when, as shown on the flow sheet, he experienced a hypotensive episode. Hypotension was accompanied by respiratory arrest, from which he was successfully resuscitated. Because of unexplained hypotension and the rise in his white blood cell count, on February 4 his antibiotic therapy was changed. All subsequent cultures also were negative. His urine output declined markedly after the hypotensive episode, and in spite of adequate hemodynamic support, his creatinine rose inexorably. He was thought to have hepatorenal syndrome. Supportive care was maintained, but he had a fatal cardiorespiratory arrest on the 20th hospital day.

ANOTHER SET OF NUMBERS:

> **A 66-year-old woman was brought to the Emergency Department from her assisted living facility. She was stuporous and tachypneic. She was not febrile, and her blood pressure was 160/90 mm Hg. The admitting physician drew blood but was called away immediately for another patient with massive bleeding. By the time, she returned to this patient, the following tests were available: creatinine 1.5 mg/dL; electrolytes (mEq/L): sodium 140, potassium 4.1, chloride 106, total CO_2 10. pH 7.54, partial pressure of carbon dioxide in the arterial blood ($PaCO_2$) 12 mm Hg. The resident immediately made the diagnosis and began treatment.**

There are only a limited number of disorders that present with these findings. The patient has a mixed acid-base disorder. Let me start with the most abnormal result. The bicarbonate of 10 mEq/L is unequivocal evidence of metabolic acidosis because plasma bicarbonate never gets that low in respiratory alkalosis, and the calculated anion gap of 24 mEq/L is increased by about 14 mEq/L. These findings, in the face of a moderate increase in creatinine, are the hallmark of an organic acidosis.

At the same time, her $PaCO_2$ is much lower that I would have expected for someone with a plasma bicarbonate of 10 mEq/L (it should be around 22 to 24 mm Hg if she had only metabolic acidosis), and her blood pH is on the alkaline side. I conclude from this analysis that she has an independent ventilatory stimulus, therefore a concomitant respiratory alkalosis. To summarize, she has an "anion-gap metabolic acidosis" and superimposed respiratory alkalosis. What could cause these abnormalities? Salicylate intoxication and sepsis with lactic acidosis are the two leading contenders, though other complex mixed acid-base disorders are also possible.

The first thing I would do is find out whether she left any medication bottles behind in her apartment. The fact that that she is not hypotensive argues against sepsis, although her blood pressure could drop precipitously at any time.

I would get a salicylate and lactate level immediately.

Case Summary

Salicylate level was 82 mg/dL. Treatment consisted of saline, mannitol, and cautious alkalinization of the urine. The patient's fingers were not deformed, but she had been taking large amounts of aspirin for arthritic pains. She recovered completely.

Analysis

We anticipate that some educators will object to the format of this exercise. In both cases only fragments of clinical data were presented to a discussant, and he was asked to "think out loud" as he studied the laboratory data. The sequence of data presentation is quite unconventional, especially to those who believe that all diagnostic evaluations should begin with the chief complaint, followed in lockstep fashion by the history of the present illness, review of systems, social history, family history, and physical examination. Here we provided no complaints, and in the first case, the only clinical information available was the patient's age and sex, the notations that he had a hypotensive episode on the third hospital day, and that he had been given various antibiotics. Despite those meager clues, the discussant interpreted the 100 or so laboratory results and arrived at the correct diagnosis, that is, hepatorenal syndrome. In the second case, with only 14 bits of data (the patient's age, sex, her living arrangement, two symptoms, two physical findings, and seven laboratory tests), the discussant narrowed the diagnostic possibilities to only one.

How concerned should we be about this unconventional presentation of clinical material? Will it give students and house officers the wrong idea about how to approach the evaluation of a patient? Will they believe that it is okay to "look at the numbers and not at the patient"?

By teaching the lockstep approach to diagnostic problem solving, we ignore what good physicians actually do when they are engaged in this process. Studies of clinical problem solving show that physicians frequently skip around during a history-taking session and that they feel quite comfortable about asking for data "out of sequence." In addition, some of our more successful teaching conferences are based on sequences of data presentation that are totally different form those that we use to teach our students. X-rays are sometimes presented first at clinical gastrointestinal conferences, echocardiograms at cardiology conferences, and electrolytes at nephrology conferences. In each case, clinical historical data are sometimes withheld until after a clinician interprets the laboratory results.

Perhaps we should stop asking students to "do as I say," and instead ask them to "do as I do."[1] This is not to say that we should stop teaching a systematic approach to history taking and diagnostic inquiry, but simply that we should explain why we recommend that students follow certain parts of the "routine" examination. Instead of insisting that somehow the data derived from the history, the physical examination, and the laboratory are different and distinct types of information, we should admit that all of those sources merely supply data, essentially without risk. Whether we begin to incorporate laboratory data first or clinical data first seems quite irrelevant, at least with respect to the processes of diagnostic hypothesis formulation and testing.

If we are willing to approach diagnostic problem solving in this manner—that is, by incorporating any available data into our thinking—what do we tell students about the need for the routine parts of the history and physical examination? We should tell it as it is: Some are designed to obtain baseline information (the neurologic examination in patients without neurologic symptoms), some to prevent complications (the history of drug allergies), some to screen for disorders low in prevalence but disastrous in outcome (breast examination for cancer), some to identify predisposing or risk factors (family history of diabetes or heart attack), and some to alert the physician to psychological factors that may affect the patient (social history). Indeed, the exact reasons for many of the questions asked during the traditional routine history have not been fully explicated.

Our principal point is that the sequence in which data are interpreted is not important; as long as they are obtained without risk, it is reasonable to interpret data from the history, the physical examination, and the laboratory in order of availability. Thus, we should always gather any laboratory results that are available and interpret them even before we examine the patient. Indeed, if we know beforehand that a patient has been found to be hypercalcemic by a laboratory screening test, we are likely to ask far-more-intelligent questions and to examine the patient far more specifically than if we were merely searching without direction for causes of weakness and joint pain. Accordingly, we felt justified in asking a clinician to interpret a panel of laboratory tests and justified in displaying his responses even if this exercise is shown to medical students who are being taught to narrowly follow the rules—that is, to ask all the questions and to do a complete physical examination before even thinking about which laboratory tests might be appropriate. Of course, not all physicians would agree with our view.[154]

The interesting approach followed by the discussant in the first case of this exercise provides evidence that interpretation of laboratory data alone has great value. The clinician spent considerable time first simply describing the data. He defined whether certain values were high or low and whether there were trends over time. In the early part of the session, he offered little in the way of diagnostic hypotheses. However, after he had integrated the levels and the trends, he launched into a brief but superb differential diagnosis. He inferred that the patient had liver disease from the liver function tests and bolstered this view by the patient's acid-base status. He built a case for infection and suggested sites of possible sepsis. He appreciated that the patient had acute renal insufficiency, toyed with the possibility of tubular necrosis, but—noticing the high urine specific gravity and low urinary sodium concentration—came up with the (correct) diagnosis of hepatorenal syndrome. And he did so knowing only a few standard items of clinical data.

The discussant in the aspirin intoxication case seemed to follow a "diagnostic prescription," or algorithm. He zeroed in on the low bicarbonate, decided it had to represent metabolic acidosis, then decided that the disorder must include an organic acidosis when he found that the anion gap was increased and could not be explained by kidney failure. Then, appreciating that the patient was hyperventilating more than expected from acidosis, he diagnosed a mixed acid-base disturbance, which he then inferred would be caused only by a small number of disorders. Was his analysis algorithmic, or is it something simpler? Both of these discussants are seasoned nephrologists, which probably explains their rapid and expert problem-solving abilities in their domain. The discussant in the aspirin intoxication case seems to be describing his sequential reasoning, but it is uncertain whether his theory of how he solves problems is correct. More than many specialists, nephrologists deal with sets of numbers every day and, like seasoned chess players, probably recognize typical patterns. It certainly is possible that the striking pattern of the patient's chemistries evoked the representativeness heuristic rather than leading to a sequential reasoning process, instead yielding a simpler process that might be described as "it looks like salicylate intoxication, so maybe that's what it is."[135]

Is it appropriate to ignore the patient and attend only to the laboratory results? Never. Is it sometimes appropriate to scrutinize the "numbers" as diagnostic clues even before completing a full history and physical examination? Sure.

CASE 15. STRATEGIES OF INFORMATION GATHERING

NOTE Our goal in this exercise is to consider a neglected aspect of diagnostic problem solving, namely the strategies that physicians use to gather data as they confront a diagnostic dilemma. First, we analyze the rationale for individual questions and for the sequence of questions that a general internist used when taking the history from a previously ill physician. Then, we review some of the studies that bear on the experimental approach to information gathering.

Patient: **I am a 34-year-old physician. I sought medical attention because of the 5 days of fever, chills, myalgias, and periumbilical cramping pain, followed by 3 days of profuse watery diarrhea. I have been a resident of Boston for the past 2 ½ years. I traveled to Texas for a meeting 2 ½ weeks before symptoms developed.**

Discussant: 1. Did you feel well before that time and upon returning from Texas?

Patient: **Yes.**

Discussant: 2. What were your general activities upon returning to work? What kind of exposures did you have?

Patient: **During that period, I was not working with patients but had been in the laboratory, working mainly on studies of leukocytes.**

Discussant: 3. Did you have any exposure to animals?

Patient: **No.**

Discussant: I am obviously worried about an exposure to some infectious agent. Of course, there are many other things to consider. The patient apparently had not been sick before. I am wondering whether he had traveled somewhere where he may have come in contact with enteric pathogens or whether he was exposed to such agents in the course of his practice, his laboratory work, or his social life. Apparently, the fever preceded the diarrhea, beginning at the same time as the abdominal pain.

Discussant: 4. When the diarrhea began, was it bloody? Was it watery?

Patient: **It was watery, nonbloody, and at its peak occurred about 16 to 17 times a day.**

Discussant: That description makes me worry more about some kind of toxin-producing agent or something that is invasive, producing a mucoid type of diarrhea.

Discussant: 5. Were you taking any medications at the time your symptoms developed?

Patient: **I had been exposed to tuberculosis and had converted my PPD, and I had been taking isoniazid and pyridoxine for 3 months before this illness.**

[Discussant: I would like to know more about the medical history.]

Discussant: 6. Have you ever had inflammatory bowel disease, ulcer disease, biliary tract disease, or any similar problems?

Patient: **I had none of those problems. Before coming to Boston, I spent a year on the Cambodia–Thailand border as a refugee worker.**

Discussant: 7. Did you have any significant illness during that time?

Patient: **I had dengue fever. I had no problem with malaria, but I took malaria prophylaxis.**

[Discussant: The diarrhea seems rather extensive. At this point, I need to know more about the physical examination.]

Discussant: 8. What were your vital signs? Did you have postural blood pressure changes? Did you have any skin rashes or lymphadenopathy? Did you have any heart murmurs? What was your abdominal examination like? What did the rectal examination show?

Patient: **I did not appear ill, and my blood pressure was 120/80 mm Hg with no postural changes. My pulse was 70 per minute, and temperature was 37.5°C. I had no skin rashes or lymphadenopathy and had no heart murmurs. My abdomen was nontender with normal bowel sounds. Rectal exam was normal. The stool was guaiac-negative and minimally greenish.**

[Discussant: It appears that we have a patient with a history of fever and diarrhea who looks pretty well. With the history of frequent watery diarrhea, I am somewhat surprised that he does not have any evidence of volume depletion. It seems to me that the patient has most likely been exposed to some type of infectious agent.]

Discussant: 9. Did anyone look at the stool? What did routine tests show?

Patient: **The stool was not examined then, but a sample was taken for culture. Laboratory data showed a white blood cell count of 7,000 with 66% polys and 12% bands. The hematocrit was normal, as were liver function tests. Serum electrolytes and urinalysis were normal.**

[Discussant: These data do not help me much, except that they do not give any evidence of any major chronic disease. His electrolyte loss did not appear to be very dramatic. I would still like to know what was found in the stool.]

Discussant: 10. Did they look for parasites?

Patient: **No parasites were found. Over the next 3 days my illness quieted down, and the diarrhea subsided somewhat. At that point, the stool culture was negative for *Salmonella* and *Shigella*.**

Discussant: 11. Were other organisms looked for in the stool? For instance, was there any evidence of *Clostridium difficile?* Were cultures obtained for *Yersinia?*

Patient: **The physician who was taking care of me was concerned about the possibility of *Campylobacter* as well as *Salmonella,* although the first stool culture had been negative for *Salmonella.***

Discussant: We probably should think a little more about why this patient had watery diarrhea. Could he have an infectious agent that produced an invasive lesion of the bowel wall, which in turn produced sloughing of the cells and leakage of fluid? This does not sound very likely. Could he have had something that was producing a toxic effect on the bowel? Such an agent could cause watery diarrhea by stimulating excessive secretion of intestinal fluid. Did he have an organism that was producing watery diarrhea but would not show up in a stool examination or culture? Some such organisms are recovered only from an upper gastrointestinal aspirate. As for endogenous materials causing a diarrheal state, there is no reason to think the patient has a vasoactive intestinal polypeptide-producing tumor. Furthermore, there is no reason to think that the patient suddenly developed inflammatory bowel disease, which is giving him this type of picture.

Discussant: 12. Did any of the other people who attended that meeting develop similar problems? Were any other results of stool cultures available? Were any toxins searched for?

Patient: **Nobody else was ill, as far as I know. No toxin had been looked for. Cultures for *Salmonella* and *Shigella* were negative at this point. No result had been obtained from the *Campylobacter* culture.**

Discussant: If I thought that the patient had *Campylobacter,* I would consider giving a macrolide antibiotic because of some evidence that the treatment could shorten the illness. Nonetheless, that infection usually resolves on its own. The question is, which organisms would cause an infection that is not self-limited? Could he have acquired any organisms from seafood obtained from the Gulf of Mexico? There have been reports of *Vibrio* infection in that area.

Discussant: 13. Did you eat raw seafood while in Texas?

Patient: **No, I ate nothing out of the ordinary. By the eighth day of the illness, I began to feel worse again. My temperature was as high as 38.5°C, and chills, myalgias, periumbilical pain, and diarrhea returned. I was seen again by my physician at this time, and except for the elevated temperature, my physical examination was again unremarkable. My white count had not changed. The rest of the laboratory tests showed only a slightly elevated AST. I was seen again on the 10th day of my illness. At that time, abdominal examination revealed mild tenderness in the periumbilical area with pain referred to the right lower quadrant. At this point cultures were again negative for *Salmonella*, *Shigella*, and *Campylobacter*. Cultures were obtained for *Vibrio* and for *Yersinia*. The white blood cell count on the 10th day of the illness was 10,000 with 70% polys and 8% bands.**

Discussant: In an adult with fever, abdominal tenderness, and negative stool cultures, one must also think of an endogenous source of inflammation. One obvious possibility is appendicitis.

Discussant: 14. Have you had your appendix removed? Is the examination of the right lower quadrant abnormal?

Patient: **I've had no surgery. On palpation of the right lower quadrant, there was only minimal tenderness, more as a referral from the periumbilical area. Rectal examination was still negative.**

Discussant: A retrocecal appendicitis is still possible. I would be interested to know whether a surgeon had looked at the patient. We certainly need to keep appendicitis in mind, but I am still wondering whether there are other kinds of infection that we should be thinking about. I'm curious to know why we are having this much trouble culturing some of these organisms.

Discussant: 15. What happened to you next?

Patient: **On the 11th day, I was given a macrolide antibiotic to cover *Campylobacter*. Over the next day, I developed orthostatic hypotension, and on the 12th day of my illness, I was hospi-**

talized. By then diarrhea had decreased to approximately six watery stools a day. I was given intravenous fluids, and the antibiotic was continued.

Discussant: 16. What did the physical examination, especially the abdominal examination, show now?

Patient: **Upon admission, my temperature was 37.8°C. Once again, I had some right lower quadrant tenderness. The white blood cell count was unchanged, and the sedimentation rate was 40 mm/hr.**

Discussant: This really seems like too long and too severe a course for the standard type of infection. Localization of pain to the right lower quadrant is bothersome to me. We were told that the patient had a positive PPD. I guess we should wonder whether or not he could have tuberculosis, although nothing suggests active tuberculosis in other parts of his body. I would be more concerned about appendicitis at this point.

Patient: **On the same day, a stool culture submitted 10 days earlier was found to be positive for *Yersinia enterocolitica*. My convalescent sera later agglutinated *Yersinia* in a high dilution. When the result of this culture was obtained, the macrolide was discontinued, and a 10-day course of doxycycline was started. After 3 days, my abdominal symptoms abated, and my bowel function returned to normal and stayed normal.**

Analysis

Rationale and Sequence of Questions

The discussant asked 16 questions (or combinations of questions) during the diagnostic appraisal. Each question is numbered for the reader's convenience in tracing our line of reasoning. The principal hypothesis, reflected as early as the discussant's second question, is infectious diarrhea. Questions concerning this hypothesis (the correct one) dominate both early (questions 2 and 3) and late (questions 9 to 13) in the transcript. Enhancing the hypothesis of infectious diarrhea appears to be the goal of these questions. Early questions and even two later ones (12 and 13) concern historical features, namely various exposures, that might increase the probability of an infectious cause, whereas later questions (9 to 12) seek information from the laboratory to differentiate one infectious cause from another.

Even a brief perusal of the transcript reveals, however, that the discussant strays from the line of questioning about infectious diarrhea. Her interest seems to get diverted repeatedly from the main theme, that is, from her main hypothesis. Why this diversion? Many explanations come to mind. (1) Changing to questions that explore other hypotheses could be only an artifact of the method of the case presentation. (2) The switch might be related to the discussant's desire to consider the implications of new data she had uncovered. (3) Perhaps the discussant is only "marking time" because she is temporarily stymied and needs to think of a useful line of questioning. (4) Perhaps the discussant is simply bound to tradition and is only asking questions in the sequence expected of her (first historical questions, then those about the physical examinations, etc).

There are other possible explanations for failure to pursue a single line of reasoning. The discussant seems unwilling to dismiss entirely the hypothesis that the patient is suffering from a recurrent illness, and in questions 6 and 7 she returns to this notion and seeks further information. She also interrupts questioning about infections to assess how sick the patient is, and after receiving some data from the physical examination, she concludes that the patient "looks pretty well." The latter tactic is well known.[19]

However, are there explanations for questions that go beyond these and at the same time provide clues to her strategies of information gathering? Possibly so. We think it is reasonable to interpret some of the diversions from the "infectious diarrhea" hypothesis as attempts to quickly rule in and rule out competing diagnostic hypotheses. Consider questions 4, 5, and 14. For each of these questions, answers different from those obtained would have drastically altered the discussant's diagnostic hypotheses. These questions can be likened to "surgical strikes"—quick and clean ways of clearing the field of existing, potentially important hypotheses. Examination of one of these questions (14) is particularly noteworthy. The discussant asks whether the patient had an appendectomy, but in the same breath, she asks what the examination of the right lower quadrant shows—presumably to confirm or deny the hypothesis of appendicitis if the patient's appendix is still in place.

In any diagnostic encounter the questions asked have multiple, complex goals. In this transcript, we have tried to isolate primarily those questions designed to gather information relevant to the diagnostic dilemma at hand. We identify not only what seems to be a hypothesis-directed line of reasoning as a principal strategy but also interpolated, seemingly spotty questioning directed at multiple hypotheses other than the principal one. The relation of these findings to experimental studies of information gathering is considered next.

Comments on Information Gathering

Some physicians seem to arrive at diagnostic conclusions after asking a patient only a few questions, whereas others are unable to come to the same conclusion without extensive questioning. Being efficient in diagnostic information gathering and processing is one of those cognitive skills we prize, yet we do not understand it very well. How does the efficient diagnostician choose which question to ask at a given time? If we knew, perhaps we could all become more efficient, and we would have a basis for teaching this trait to our students.

Early in the diagnostic encounter—after the patient voices his or her principal complaints—physicians often face a bewildering array of diagnostic possibilities, and they could ask many hundreds of questions to elucidate the cause of the complaints. At this early point in the diagnostic process, the diagnostic uncertainty—that is, confusion or entropy—is high. In fact, uncertainty is highest when all possible diagnoses are equally likely. A diagnostic hypothesis, however, is not a single entity; it can be likened more to a motion picture than to a snapshot. It is a pattern of probabilities that evolves as information is requested, obtained, and digested.

Take a 30-year-old man with crushing chest pain. Initially, the probability of coronary disease might be considered quite low and the probability of noncardiac pain might be quite high—say, 0.01 and 0.99, respectively. With a family history of myocardial infarction at an early age, the probabilities of the two disorders might shift to 0.4 and 0.6, respectively; and if a history of a previous, well-documented myocardial infarction were next revealed, the revised probabilities might shift to 0.7 and 0.3, respectively. Revising these probabilities, given the new information, can be accomplished according to Bayes' rule.[155–157] But Bayes' rule, as useful as it may be, merely elaborates on the meaning of a given piece of information; it does not help decide which of many questions to ask and thus which of the many pieces of information to gather.

The goal of selecting a given question at a given time is to obtain data that will reduce diagnostic uncertainty and point to a working diagnosis that is both coherent and adequate.[158] Here we explore two approaches to the selection of questions. One is a prescriptive method based on signal theory and decision theory, and the other is a descriptive, experimental approach used in medicine in studies of clinical problem solving[18,157] and in psychology in studies of social information gathering.[35,37,38]

The Prescriptive Approach

In one computerized application of the prescriptive approach, an exclusive set of attributes of patients known to have a given clinical syndrome (acute renal failure) was identified, and all questions that could be asked to explore these attributes and thus diagnose a specific cause of the acute renal failure were specified.[159] To establish which question was optimal, the computer program first used Bayes' rule to calculate the posterior probabilities of every possible answer to each question. This process yielded multiple sets of diagnostic probabilities; each of these probabilities was then converted into a numerical index of diagnostic uncertainty. Decision analysis was then used to select the best of many possible questions. For each question, the chance of getting a positive (or negative) answer was computed, and the reduction in uncertainty achieved by the answer was used as the utility. Calculating the expected utility for each question in this fashion yielded the optimal expected utility among all the questions and thus identified the best questions. To summarize this complex calculation, the best question was an integrated combination of the one that was most likely to be positive (or negative) and the one that would most reduce diagnostic uncertainty. This prescriptive model contains many assumptions and has not been used much to solve clinical problems.

The Descriptive Approach

The descriptive approach utilizes observations of problem solvers as they select questions to ask. In an early study of the clinical problem-solving process, we identified several tactics that were used in this process of information gathering.[157] We described a confirmation strategy—a method by which a clinician apparently attempted to prove a hypothesis by matching the patient's characteristics to a model of the disease. We also described an elimination strategy—a method by which questions were directed at excluding hypotheses that competed with the leading one or ones.

Studies in psychology have elaborated considerably on these information-gathering processes. Although they are designed principally to probe the information-processing strategies of people attempting to identify certain personality traits in others, the insights from these studies may well be applicable to the diagnosis of medical problems. The studies identified two strategies for gathering information: a "hypothesis-confirming" strategy and a "diagnosing" strategy.[35,37,38] The hypothesis-confirming strategy focuses only on the hypothesis under current consideration. In this strategy (which is analogous to the "confirmation" tactic described before), one seeks information that is probable, given the working hypothesis. When a question is asked to elaborate on the hypothesis under consideration, a positive response thus enhances the likelihood of the hypothesis. Some psychologists argue that this kind of confirmation strategy is a reasonable and efficient one. These researchers argue that, rather than gather evidence that disconfirms a hypothesis (the "elimination" strategy described before) and thus require that negative evidence be brought to bear, people prefer to request positive confirming information that is familiar and presumably carries more weight than disconfirming data.

The diagnosing strategy is an alternative approach to information gathering that involves collecting data about features that are most differentially probable, given both the hypothesis and its alternatives. When using this strategy, people gather information that will help them best distinguish among hypotheses, whether or not the response confirms their current hypothesis or an alternative one. The diagnosing strategy, a mathematical formulation based on Bayes' rule, assumes that a given question's value is a function of the probability of getting a response to that question (similar to that described before for the prescriptive approach to the diagnosis of acute renal failure) and the conditional probabilities of the attribute being assessed. Studies suggest that people making social diagnoses use the diagnosing strategy far more frequently than the hypothesis-confirming strategy.[35,38] In addition, those studies tell us not only that people tend to request data that will maximally separate two or more hypotheses, but also that given a choice of questions, people appear to select those that tend to produce the greatest possible separation of hypotheses.

The finding that people select a rational strategy that can be approximated by a probabilistic model when making social inferences is interesting. Whether physicians use the diagnosing strategy is uncertain; however, such an approach is probably less likely to introduce bias into information gathering than the hypothesis-confirming strategy. We have little information as to whether either the hypothesis-confirming or the diagnosing strategy is used in medical diagnosis. In the foregoing case discussion, it appears that both strategies were used in the same diagnostic encounter. It seems quite likely that both (or possibly even more than two) strategies are used in the process of medical diagnosis, depending on the kind of information being sought. Perhaps diagnosing, confirmation, and elimination strategies are only some of the tactics used to decide which question should be asked next.

CASE 16. A FATAL FLAW IN SUTTON'S LAW

A 35-year-old woman was admitted to the hospital with right-upper-quadrant abdominal pain and watery diarrhea for the previous 3 days.

A long list of diagnoses comes to mind. First, any of the infectious diarrheas, particularly the bacterial diarrheas, could induce right-upper-quadrant abdominal pain and watery diarrhea. A second group of diseases to consider are the inflammatory bowel diseases: ulcerative colitis and— more likely with watery diarrhea—Crohn disease. Disease of the gallbladder also could present in this manner. In addition to bacterial infection, one particular parasitic infection could account for these symptoms: giardiasis. The patient's travel history might be interesting.

The patient was in good health until 1 month before admission, when she became anorectic; since then she had lost 5 pounds. The pain was worse on inspiration and radiated to the right shoulder. It diminished when she sat and leaned forward. She was nauseated and reported having night sweats. The diarrhea was not accompanied by tenesmus or bleeding, and she had not vomited.

Anorexia and weight loss could be nonspecific consequences of her underlying disease, whatever it is. The pattern of her pain—worse on inspiration and radiating to the right shoulder—suggests some process under the right diaphragm. It could be in one of the spaces below the diaphragm or in the liver. When I see a patient whose chief complaints are diarrhea and right-upper-quadrant pain radiating to the shoulder and that patient has traveled to areas in which parasitic infections are endemic, one of the first things I think of is an amebic liver abscess. If she had experienced a previous episode of abdominal pain, I would wonder if in the past she had had either biliary tract disease or acute appendicitis and was now presenting with a right subphrenic abscess. The night sweats also suggest that she has some type of infection, possibly in or around the liver. The diarrhea might be only an accompanying symptom.

I suppose she also could have pericarditis, since an inflammatory process below the diaphragm could involve the pericardial area. I must admit that although pericarditis could conceivably present with anorexia, night sweats, and diarrhea, this diagnosis would be low on my list. She could have pancreatitis, however. I should have included that diagnosis earlier when I raised the possibility of biliary tract disease. I think I would need a little more history and findings from the physical examination.

Three months earlier, after she had been in Portugal for a month, the patient and several of her

traveling companions had developed an illness characterized by fever, nausea, and watery diarrhea. Those symptoms subsided over a few days without specific therapy. She previously had been well. She was taking no medications and did not use drugs or alcohol. She had had no exposure to hepatitis, and none of her friends or family members had been ill recently.

She was previously healthy, which leads me to think that she acquired one of the "traveling" types of diarrhea in Portugal. I am not sure of the organisms that you can pick up there, but *Salmonella* and amebae are among them. I am sure you also can pick up a lot of the other infectious diarrheal diseases as well. In most cases, traveler's diarrhea is caused by one of the classic bacterial or parasitic pathogens, but it can be caused by a virus. In fact, up to 80% of people traveling to any of a number of different countries can get severe diarrhea. I suspect she has one of the bacteria- or parasite-caused diarrheas because of the complications that developed subsequently.

The physical examination revealed a thin woman who was experiencing considerable discomfort. Blood pressure was 110/70 mm Hg, pulse was 80 per minute, respiration was 16 per minute, temperature was 37°C. She was not icteric. Chest examination showed no abnormalities. Abdominal examination disclosed marked guarding in the right upper quadrant, but there was no rebound tenderness. No masses were present, and bowel sounds were normal, as were rectal and pelvic examinations.

Once again, the findings focus our attention on the right upper quadrant, and some of the diseases I mentioned earlier are the ones that continue to concern me: biliary tract infection with a stone in the common bile duct, with or without pancreatic inflammation; acute pancreatitis; liver infection; and, if she did have amebiasis, an amebic liver abscess. She could well have an abscess in the right upper quadrant that does not involve the hepatobiliary tree, and such a lesion could have resulted from a previous intestinal perforation. Of course, her diarrhea and other symptoms that developed in Portugal could be the consequence of inflammatory bowel disease or even appendicitis.

The one other thing we should do is ascertain that her lungs are normal. On examination, at least, there was no fluid or evidence of consolidation. I am cautious about this issue because it is bad practice to plan surgery and then find on chest x-ray a right-lower-lobe pneumonia that presented with intraabdominal manifestations. At this point, I would like some laboratory data, including a complete blood count and a microscopic examination of the stool.

Laboratory studies revealed the following: hemoglobin 11 g/dL, hematocrit 33%, white cell count 11,500 with 81 polys, 13 bands, 5 monos, and 1 atypical lymphocyte. The sedimentation rate was 44 mm/hr. Stool guaiac was negative, and no polys were seen on the stool smear. Electrolytes, BUN, creatinine, liver function studies, and amylase were normal. On urinalysis, the specific gravity was 1.026, pH 5.0, ketones 3+; 2 to 5 white blood cells (WBCs) and 2 to 5 red blood cells (RBCs) per high-power field (hpf) were found in the sediment. Chest x-ray and upright KUB (kidneys, ureters, and bladder) radiograph were unremarkable.

Her hemoglobin and hematocrit are slightly low, her white cell count is increased, and there is a shift to the left. She has one atypical lymphocyte, but I really cannot make much of that. Her sedimentation rate is high, which also suggests the presence of an inflammatory process, and the shift to the left suggests that it is a pyogenic infection. The urinalysis is not very revealing, although the combination of two to five white blood cells and two to five red blood cells is probably abnormal. I would want to have this finding confirmed, and if the specimen was a good clean-catch urine, we would have to make sure she did not have something going on either in the kidney or in the bladder. She could have an inflammatory process in the abdomen with extension around the bladder. Minor urine sediment abnormalities can be found even with an infection outside the bladder; such findings can occur in patients with appendicitis, for example. Incidentally, the normal amylase reduces the chance that she has pancreatitis.

Because I suspect a collection of pus in or around the biliary tree or in the subphrenic space, I would like to go right to that area to study it.

The most direct method, when physical examination and routine x-rays are negative, is to do a CT scan, which is more effective in detecting intra-abdominal abscesses than an ultrasound. If CT were not available, ultrasound would be my second choice. Interestingly, when ultrasound is done in addition to CT, no additional diagnostic information is obtained. A gallium scan would be of little value in this situation, since both false-positive and false-negative rates are high.

> **The initial diagnosis was either acute chole-cystitis or an intestinal infection. A hydroxy iminodiacetic acid (HIDA) scan and stool specimens for *Giardia, Yersinia, Entamoeba histolytica, Shigella, Salmonella*, and *Campylobacter* were ordered.**

The advantage of the HIDA scan is that it can be done in a couple of hours, and it may tell you whether the gallbladder is working well. If it is negative, we would still have to get a CT scan. If the HIDA scan is positive, I would suspect cholecystitis, but because of the atypical presentation, I would still want to know what the anatomy was. In particular, I would want to make sure that there was not a collection of fluid above or in the liver, so I would end up doing a CT scan anyway. Direct observation of a stool smear might have been revealing. If the smear was negative, we could pretty much exclude a diagnosis of amebiasis. We are going to have to wait for the *Yersinia, Salmonella, Shigella*, and *Campylobacter* cultures for at least 24 to 48 hours. I think I also would obtain blood cultures at this time.

> **The HIDA scan could not be performed, and the radiologist did a right-upper-quadrant ultrasound study instead. The gallbladder was normal, but the right lobe of the liver showed multiple hypoechoic masses, some of which appeared to be confluent. No subphrenic collection was present. The revised diagnoses, given these new findings, included liver metastases or abscesses, and discussions were held with the echographers about needle aspiration of one of the lesions.**

At this point, I would like a little more history. I would want to make sure she had not been in an area endemic for echinococcosis, such as the Rocky Mountains, Greece, or Turkey. I am not sure whether this parasite is indigenous to Portugal. I would also want to re-examine the x-rays to make sure that there are no calcifications in the liver. One would not want to insert a needle into an echinococcal cyst and spill its contents.

You might attempt to aspirate this patient's lesion if it is accessible. The ideal location of a lesion for percutaneous aspiration is the surface of the liver, but the real decision to go ahead with this procedure has to be made in conjunction with the echographer who performs it.

We are faced with a previously healthy woman who has multiple defects in the liver revealed by ultrasound. There are no clues that she has a carcinoma anywhere. We are told that the pelvic examination was normal and that there are no genitourinary symptoms, so I think I'd home in on the liver and search for an infectious process—especially an amebic abscess—because she has been in an area where she might have developed amebiasis. She does have many symptoms that could be indicative of a pyogenic infection of the liver. On the basis of the finding of multiple small lesions, I would say that the likelihood of amebiasis goes way down and the likelihood of a pyogenic infection goes way up.

> **The next morning, the patient's abdominal pain was less severe and diarrhea had not recurred. Her abdomen was less tender. Repeat hematocrit was 27%, and the white cell count was 7,100 with 80 polys, 1 band, 14 lymphocytes, and 5 monocytes. Repeat urinalysis was normal.**

The fall in her hematocrit from 33% to 27% might be only the consequence of hydration, but I would want to make sure that she was not losing blood somewhere or hemolyzing. Her white count has dropped to 7,100, and she still has a shift to the left, although it is not as impressive as it was a day earlier.

We have to find out what those lesions are in the liver. We should either try to aspirate them or do some other studies to find out what they are. Using *Sutton's law*, if the patient has defects in an area in which she is having all of those symptoms and there is strongly suggestive evidence of infection,

I'd want to get a specimen and decide what this lesion is so I could recommend specific therapy.

> On the second hospital day, both an abdominal CT scan with contrast and a technetium scan showed a single large lesion (9 × 12 cm) in the right lobe of the liver, which had the characteristics of a cavernous hemangioma. Clots were thought to be present within the lesion. All stool cultures were negative.

So she has a cavernous hemangioma that bled. This lesion could account for her pain and the fall in hematocrit, but I do not understand how a bleeding hemangioma causes diarrhea.

> Nothing further was done. The diarrhea ceased, and the patient recovered uneventfully. The nature of her lesion was explained in detail, and a MedicAlert bracelet was ordered for her. Two months after discharge she was asymptomatic. Her hemoglobin and hematocrit had returned to normal.

We still have not explained the diarrhea.

Analysis

It is worth contrasting the tactics used in this problem-solving exercise with those used in an earlier example (see case 2) because in both cases the patient had an obscure disease. In that case, the patient was a young Chinese man who complained of weakness, and after only a few manifestations were described, the discussant—an endocrinologist—immediately reached the conclusion that the patient had periodic paralysis with hyperthyroidism, which was the correct diagnosis. He then spent the remainder of the session confirming the diagnosis. The presentation of weakness in an Asian male patient represented a pattern that the endocrinologist recognized immediately.

In the foregoing session, the discussant followed no such highly directed approach. Instead, he selected an erroneous etiologic category (infection) and spent the remainder of the session proposing one infection after another without making the correct diagnosis. He is in good company. The clinicians taking care of the patient also were confused and stumbled on the correct diagnosis almost by accident.

Although the correct diagnosis was never even entertained by the discussant, many valuable lessons can be derived from his broad consideration of the possible diagnostic hypotheses because the process he used is representative of the approach that characterizes much diagnostic problem solving: consideration of multiple competing hypotheses. Newell and Simon's studies of people as they solved simple problems in chess, cryptarithmetic, and logic, as well as several studies of medical problem solving, show that the diagnostic process frequently proceeds in much the same fashion as the process of scientific inquiry.[18,19,30,160] The initial approach, to paraphrase Karl Popper, is not simply to accumulate facts and then build theories about them, but to start out with some conjecture that goes beyond the available facts and either proves or disproves the hunch.[161]

Indeed, the discussant made liberal use of conjectures and hunches as he evaluated the data in this case, and it is possible to enumerate many of his competing hypotheses and to rank them progressively from the most general to the most specific. As shown in Table 14.1, he offered more than 30 separate and distinct diagnostic hypotheses throughout the session and repeated some of them several times. At least seven categories of hypotheses are discernible, some quite general and some more specific.

In order of progressive specificity are the following (rather arbitrarily chosen) categories and examples: a general diagnostic category (inflammatory process); diagnoses that consider only disease location (collection in liver, something in kidney); unclassified diseases of specific organs (gallbladder disease, biliary tract disease); a kind of disease of an organ (Crohn disease, pancreatitis); general etiologic hypotheses (infectious diarrhea, liver abscess); specific etiologic hypotheses (amebic liver abscess, *Salmonella* diarrhea); and finally—presumably the most specific—causally related diagnoses (subphrenic abscess caused by previous appendicitis, pericarditis caused by inflammatory process below the diaphragm).

Although the discussant wavered a lot and offered a large number of competing hypotheses as more information became available, eventually he did home in on a space-occupying process in the liver, a rather specific entity. It was at this juncture that he invoked Sutton's law, and, in our view,

TABLE 14.1	
Diagnostic Hypotheses Proposed for a 35-Year-Old Woman with Right-Upper-Quadrant Abdominal Pain and Diarrhea	
General hypotheses	Inflammatory process
"Location" hypotheses	Something under diaphragm
	Something in kidney
	Collection in liver
	Collection above liver
Disease of an organ	Gallbladder disease
	Biliary tract disease
Kind of disease of an organ	Inflammatory bowel disease
	Crohn disease
	Ulcerative colitis
	Pericarditis
	Pancreatitis
	Biliary tract infection
	Cholecystitis
General etiologic hypotheses	Infectious diarrhea
	Subphrenic abscess
	Traveler's diarrhea
	Liver abscess
	Pneumonia
	Pyogenic infection
	Inflammatory process around the bladder
	Pus in biliary tree
	Pus around biliary tree
	Carcinoma
Specific etiologic hypotheses	Giardiasis
	Amebic liver abscess
	Salmonella diarrhea
	Amebiasis
	Yersinia diarrhea
	Echinococcosis
	Viral diarrhea
	Parasitic diarrhea
	Bacterial diarrhea
Causal hypotheses	Subphrenic abscess caused by appendicitis
	Pericarditis caused by inflammatory process below the diaphragm

his discussion aptly illustrates a serious flaw in this law.

Willie Sutton, for readers who have not heard his "law" quoted before, was a notorious bank robber who, when asked why he robbed banks, is said to have replied, "That's where the money is." Many are fond of quoting Sutton's law in medical contexts: If the patient has a diffuse pulmonary process,

biopsy the lung; if the patient has evidence of liver disease, biopsy the liver. The notion is, "go where the money is."

Certainly, there are situations in which following that clinical dictum is appropriate. But we have serious reservations about invoking it uncritically as a diagnostic strategy. Clinicians sometimes use Sutton's law to convince less experienced physicians that if they had only "gone where the money is" instead of ordering less useful tests, the correct diagnosis would have surfaced sooner. Unfortunately, such discussions often are held only *after* a test has identified a lesion. The point here is that Sutton's law frequently is confounded by substantial retrospective bias, a problem we comment on in other discussions (see cases 5 and 46). In fact, we suspect that this law is applicable principally in retrospect.

Why is Sutton's law less applicable prospectively? Because this concept implies that the answer to a diagnostic dilemma is predestined. If you are confident that a patient has a right-upper-quadrant abscess, for example, go after it. Unfortunately, because of the unstructured nature of the process of diagnostic inquiry and because usually so many diagnoses are possible, we often do not know precisely "where the money is." Typically, we make some good guesses and some bad guesses; we make some false starts, we backtrack, and sometimes, as here, a chance occurrence makes us (and the patient) lucky. The flaw is exposed when our confidence encourages us to "go where the money is" but the "money" simply is not there; then the patient pays a penalty for the erroneous approach. That flaw is illustrated vividly in the case discussed here. Following Sutton's law could have wrought a disaster: The act of puncturing a hemangioma might have produced a life-threatening hemorrhage. This example should be humbling to those who frequently rely on that old clinical saw.

Sutton's law is not always faulty. In two examples in this series, we present cases in which it worked (see cases 24 and 45). In one case, the chance of a specific diagnosis (pulmonary embolism) was extremely high, and the clinician proposed bypassing intermediate, less accurate (and minimally risky) diagnostic tests (ECG and blood gases) for a more accurate one (lung scan). Thus, we can safely invoke Sutton's law from time to time, at least when the risk of doing so is minimal and when we are sure that there is "money in the bank."

CASE 17. HOW TO DISREGARD RED HERRINGS

A 70-year-old man presented with a 4-week history of intermittent fever.

First, I would need to know whether or not he has already undergone any diagnostic workup and would fall into the classic category of a fever of unknown origin. In young patients, the major causes of fevers of unknown origin are infections, tumors, and vasculitis, more or less in that order. In older patients, malignancy occurs with greater frequency. Giant-cell arteritis must always be considered in the evaluation of fever in an elderly patient.

The patient recently returned from a weekend trip to the Oregon coast. While there, he purchased raw oysters at a roadside stand and ate them fully cooked. Two days later, he developed intermittent fever as high as 102°F, anorexia, and mild nausea. These symptoms persisted, and he went to see his physician.

When I think of diseases associated with oyster ingestion, I think of bacterial infections such as *Vibrio vulnificus* and *Listeria*, as well as viral hepatitis. Because fever came on relatively soon after the oyster ingestion, viral hepatitis becomes a less likely possibility. Of course, ingestion of oysters may be totally unrelated to the fevers.

He had no abdominal pain, change in bowel habits, headaches, jaw pain, skin rash, arthralgias, or other symptoms, but he had lost 6 pounds since the illness began. Two years previously, he had coronary bypass surgery, and he also suffered from atrial fibrillation, congestive heart failure (currently stable), gout, and hypothyroidism. Medications included hydrochlorothiazide, captopril, levothyroxine, allopurinol, and warfarin.

The weight loss is bothersome. The absence of headaches and jaw pain is against the possibility of temporal arteritis, although this diagnosis can exist without the classic symptoms. If he had a typical bypass surgery with a median sternotomy, the possibility of a chronic occult infection with an agent such as *Mycobacterium chelonae* must be entertained. The presence of atrial fibrillation raises the possibility of multiple emboli. Gout can present as a febrile illness, but usually would be accompanied by acute inflammatory joint symptoms as well. Any medication can cause a fever, and in this case, allopurinol would be the most likely culprit.

Perhaps the oysters are in fact the molluscal equivalent of a red herring. I wonder if they are unrelated to the presenting symptoms.

> **The patient lived on a farm with his wife. He recently slaughtered a pig for his own consumption (he does so once a year). He drinks well water. He traveled to Mexico 18 months previously and Hawaii 6 months ago. He drank two beers a day until his illness began and had smoked cigarettes, but not for decades. His wife was not ill.**

People living on a farm can be at risk for developing brucellosis, Q fever, or tetanus. The slaughtering of a pig raises the possibility of trichina infection. I would expect that if this man and his wife cooked the oysters completely, then they would have been just as diligent in cooking the pig. Although well water could have exposed the patient to a variety of toxins, including mercury or selenium, fever is not usually a manifestation of heavy metal intoxication. People traveling to Mexico can get infections with *Salmonella* or malaria, but an 18-month interval before the infection manifested itself would be quite unusual. I do not know of any unusual illnesses endemic to Hawaii. His lack of interest in drinking beer makes me wonder about the state of his liver. Although he gave up smoking cigarettes, he probably is still at increased risk for lung or bladder cancer. If his wife is well and also ate the oysters, his symptoms are less likely to be related to that meal.

> **On examination, he appeared elderly. He was in no distress. Vital signs were normal. He was afebrile. A few ecchymoses were noted on his extremities. HEENT examination was normal. There was no lymphadenopathy. A few rales were heard at the left lung base. Cardiac examination revealed an irregularly irregular pulse with a 2/6 systolic ejection murmur at the apex. There was no organomegaly or abdominal tenderness. There was no peripheral edema.**

He is now afebrile and does not appear "toxic." The ecchymoses could be related to warfarin therapy. I assume that there was no temporal artery tenderness and that the funduscopic examination was unremarkable. The absence of lymphadenopathy is important in considering the possibility of lymphoma. The rales could be chronic due to his underlying lung disease or could reflect a new process. He appears to be in atrial fibrillation but not in congestive heart failure. The murmur raises the issue of endocarditis. With these symptoms and findings in a chronic smoker, he could well have lung cancer with a postobstructive infection. The other historical information may be irrelevant.

> **The initial white blood cell count was 24,000 with 50% eosinophils.**

He has an absolute eosinophilia. Eosinophilia has a long differential diagnosis and often is nonspecific unless it gets to extreme levels such as these. When I encounter eosinophilia of this magnitude, I always recall the phrase, "worms, wheezes, and weird diseases." Invasive parasitemia can certainly do this. An allergic reaction can also give rise to marked eosinophilia. This man takes a number of drugs, of which allopurinol is a potential culprit. There are a variety of tumors associated with eosinophilia, including lymphomas and cancer of the lung. Vasculitis, especially of the Churg-Strauss variety, could do this. He could have one of the eosinophilic pneumonias or the hypereosinophilic syndrome with infiltration of the heart, lung, or other tissues. Eosinophilic fasciitis from L-tryptophan ingestion is possible. Eosinophilia does not occur with intraluminal parasite infection or with sequestered parasites such as an amebic abscess, but it does bring us back to the recently slaughtered pig and the possibility of trichinosis. Nonetheless, trichinosis usually is associated with myalgias, swelling of the eyelids, and splinter hemorrhages. He has none of these findings.

> **Captopril, allopurinol, warfarin and hydrochlorothiazide were stopped, but fever persisted, and 1 week later the patient was admitted to the hospital. Physical examination was unchanged. Laboratory data: white cell count 17,800 with 35% neutrophils, 13% lymphocytes, and 52% eosinophils. Hemoglobin 14.6 g/dL. Platelet count 280,000. Electrolytes were normal. BUN was 77 mg/dL, creatinine 1.9 mg/dL. Urinalysis was normal. Total bilirubin 0.8 mg/dL. Alkaline phosphatase 211 IU/L (normal 32–110), ALT 130 IU/L (normal**

6–42), AST 95 IU/L (normal 11–39), LDH 440 IU/L (normal 100–240). Albumin 3.6 g/L. Chest x-ray was unremarkable.

His medications were stopped on the assumption that his symptoms and eosinophilia could be a drug reaction, but that thought did not pan out. He returned clinically unchanged, with persistent fevers and eosinophilia. He is not anemic. His BUN and creatinine are high with a normal urinalysis. He could have some prerenal azotemia. The elevation of his alkaline phosphatase and the mild transaminitis suggest a hepatic process, but viral hepatitis does not usually cause eosinophilia. Maybe he has hepatic congestion from congestive heart failure. Does he have tumor in his liver, either from a gastrointestinal source or from a pulmonary lesion not seen on the chest x-ray? A medium- or large-sized vessel vasculitis, such as polyarteritis nodosa, can produce hepatic dysfunction, as well as eosinophilia. Or perhaps he has the hypereosinophilic syndrome with infiltration of his liver. I am beginning to think of vasculitis as a major possibility or idiopathic eosinophilic syndrome acting like a malignancy. Lymphoma remains a possibility, as does a solid tumor. Parasitemia seems less likely to me, given the clinical state. Trichinosis seems less likely, although *Strongyloides* infection is remotely possible.

Stool for ova and parasites contained a few *Blastocystis hominis*. Three sets of blood cultures were negative. Abdominal CT scan without contrast was unremarkable. An echocardiogram demonstrated global hypokinesis with an ejection fraction of 20%. Moderate mitral regurgitation was present, as well as inferior and posterior akinesis. *Trichinella* antibody was negative.

Blastocystis hominis is a relatively harmless commensal organism. The negative blood cultures are against bacteremia. The abnormal echocardiogram makes me wonder about infiltrative cardiac disease. I think the *Trichinella* antibody test is a reasonably good test and probably rules out trichinosis. One other disease that I have not mentioned and just came to mind is Addison disease, but the eosinophilia in that disorder is low grade. At this point, I wonder about the primary hypere-

osinophilic syndrome and would consider a myocardial biopsy. I am not sure the abnormalities seen on the echocardiogram can all be ascribed to his coronary artery disease. One might empirically try him on steroids, but I would like a closer look at his heart.

Bone marrow biopsy revealed an anaplastic large-cell lymphoma. The patient was started on a chemotherapy regimen.

The lymphoma was probably producing an eosinophil chemotactic factor.

Analysis

Internists love diagnostic challenges. The initial context for diagnostic problem solving in this case was "fever of unknown origin," a favorite of all internists. This diagnosis conjures up a long list of possible causes and necessitates an exceptionally detailed history, including an extensive travel history, exposure history, and medication history. This patient's history was dotted with intriguing possibilities and false leads, including his exposure to raw oysters, consumption of well water, slaughtering of a pig, and travel to Mexico and Hawaii. When the eosinophilia was discovered, the number of possible diagnoses narrowed and attention was focused on "worms, wheezes, and weird diseases." The job of the clinician was to find the overlap between fever of unknown origin and "worms, wheezes, and weird diseases." Although she mentioned lymphoma more than once and even suggested the possibility of eosinophilic syndrome acting like a malignancy, ultimately she never made a firm diagnosis of lymphoma.

One possible explanation is that she lost sight of several critically important findings, some of which she actually mentioned, namely cardiac dysfunction, renal insufficiency without abnormalities of the urinary sediment, and an elevated alkaline phosphatase (possibly a manifestation of liver infiltration by tumor). It is not easy keeping every finding in mind, given the limitation of working memory, and for this reason, it always makes sense when trying to solve a diagnostic quandary to go back to the data, review all the pertinent positive and negative findings, and summarize them. In this case such a list might include weight loss, fever, severe eosinophilia, evidence of infiltration of the liver, and possibly also the kidneys and heart. When you put it this way, diagnoses of lymphoma and/or the hypereosinophilic syndrome almost jump out of the page.

Why the reference here to red herrings as false clues? Smoked herrings, otherwise known as red herrings, have a strong odor, and in 19th-century Britain, some unscrupulous hunters sometimes dragged these fishes behind their horses to divert rival hunters' oncoming hounds onto a false path. Although Mother Nature does not act unscrupulously, she frequently does strew false-positive clues across our diagnostic path. Chapter 4 describes how to recognize and deal with such false leads.

CASE 18. DISCRIMINATION: THE PROBLEM OF LOOK-ALIKES

A 53-year-old man transferred to the medical center for treatment of persistent chest pain following an acute myocardial infarction experienced severe abdominal and back pain 10 hours after admission.

My first concern is whether he is hypotensive and might have developed ischemic disease of his small intestine. I would wonder if, on physical examination, there was anything to suggest that he had an abdominal aortic aneurysm as a complication of his arteriosclerosis. I need to know his blood pressure on admission to the hospital and would like more data about his hemodynamic status in the face of his persistent chest pain. I would like to know what his gastrointestinal status is by physical examination and whether his nasogastric contents and stool are guaiac positive. Mostly I am worried about two catastrophes: ischemic bowel disease and rupture or leakage of an abdominal aortic aneurysm. Either of these could be related to or somehow coincidental with the acute myocardial infarction.

Three days earlier, the patient had been admitted to another hospital with chest pain and paroxysmal atrial fibrillation, and he was found to have a non–Q-wave myocardial infarction. He had a history of diabetes mellitus, recurrent deep venous thrombosis, and pulmonary emboli. Medications on admission to the hospital included insulin, heparin, intravenous nitroglycerin, furosemide, and diltiazem. On examination he was in no distress. Blood pressure was 130/80 mm Hg, pulse was 72 per minute, irregularly irregular, and temperature was 36.7°C. The rest of the examination was remarkable only for bibasilar rales. Admission laboratory data: WBC 10,300, hematocrit 36%, electrolytes normal, creatinine 1.4 mg/L, bilirubin 0.8 mg/dL, alkaline phosphatase 86 IU/L, AST 18 IU/L, ALT 76 IU/L, amylase 139 IU/L, International Normalized Ratio (INR) 1.7, partial thromboplastin time 67.4 seconds, and platelet count 147,000. Chest x-ray showed mild vascular redistribution.

The myocardial infarction has been characterized as nontransmural. The patient has a history of pulmonary emboli, but I do not believe that helps us with his current problem. He does have a history of paroxysmal atrial fibrillation, which raises the possibility of an embolic event. We are told that the initial examination was remarkable only for basilar rales in addition to atrial fibrillation. We are not told specifically what his abdominal findings were and whether he had bowel sounds or what his stool guaiac was, so I shall presume that his initial abdominal examination was normal.

I am still interested in knowing whether there was any evidence of an aortic aneurysm. His age is somewhat against his having an aneurysm, but he does have severe vascular disease. I would at least like to see whether he had evidence of vascular calcification and whether his aorta was palpable. With the information we have so far, I am still concerned about ischemic or embolic disease in his gastrointestinal tract. I would like to know where the back pain is and how it relates to his abdominal complaints.

His chest pain subsided shortly after admission but was replaced several hours later by severe, dull, constant upper abdominal pain, which later became sharp. The pain was in a bandlike distribution across his upper abdomen with radiation to the back. He complained of excessive belching but no nausea, vomiting, fever, or chills. On examination, he was still afebrile. He had right-upper-quadrant tenderness with guarding and decreased bowel sounds; Murphy's sign was positive. There was no costovertebral angle tenderness. Laboratory findings were unchanged. His stool was guaiac negative. A right-upper-quadrant ultrasound revealed gallstones and a thickened gallbladder wall. The bile ducts and pancreas appeared normal.

We now have an exceedingly difficult situation: a patient who has some findings consistent with an acute abdomen. There is evidence on right-upper-quadrant ultrasound of chronic biliary tract disease with gallstones and a thickened gallbladder wall in a man who had an acute myocardial infarction only a few days ago. Operating on such a patient carries a prohibitive mortality risk. I would simply observe the patient for now. I would monitor his abdominal findings carefully over the next 24 hours. I would also follow his white count, hepatic enzymes, and amylase. One could occasionally miss kidney stones in this kind of situation, so I would check his urine for any red cells.

One of the things we could do is to further evaluate the possibility of an acute embolic event would be to perform echocardiography to assess left atrial size. I believe there are some data suggesting that the larger the left atrium, the greater is the likelihood of clot formation and subsequent emboli. Since the patient just had a myocardial infarction, one could also look at his left ventricle to see if there is a hypokinetic area with intraventricular clot formation. That is another possible source of an embolus. I would not do anything further at this time except follow him closely over the next 24 hours.

The patient was treated for presumed acute cholecystitis with intravenous fluids, analgesics, and ampicillin/sulbactam. Cardiac catheterization on the third day after transfer showed occlusion of the right coronary artery but no other significant disease. Ejection fraction was 40%. Abdominal pain persisted on the night of the catheterization, and the patient became febrile for the first time (40°C). Physical examination was unchanged. WBC was 12,000 with a slight left shift. Liver function tests were unchanged. HIDA scan was normal. Antibiotic coverage was broadened, and heparin was stopped.

I am stuck now. The presumed acute cholecystitis would have a terrible prognosis if any surgical intervention were required in the face of an acute myocardial infarction. The cardiac catheterization is interesting in that the patient had only one-vessel disease but a reasonably poor ejection fraction. I assume that there were no clots in the ventricle or atrium. I would continue to follow the patient. I am still concerned about his gallbladder, as well as his pancreas. I would like to know whether there had been any change in his serum amylase. I should have asked earlier if he had any history of alcohol intake, which would make acute pancreatitis a more likely diagnosis. The medications he is receiving are not helpful to me in attempting to make any kind of diagnosis.

On the next day pain and abdominal findings persisted, and an exploratory laparotomy was performed. Nonocclusive vascular ischemia of the distal third of the small bowel was diagnosed, but there was no perforation or peritonitis, and a postoperative abdominal arteriogram was normal. Over the next few days fever (38° to 39°C) and abdominal pain persisted. White cell count was 12,000 to 13,000. INR was 1.8, partial thromboplastin time was 41.6 seconds, platelet count was 56,000, thrombin time was normal, and fibrin split products were elevated. Other laboratory findings were unchanged. Cultures from multiple sites (including blood) were negative. Blood pressure required pressor support. The cause of the fever, abdominal pain, and hypotension was unclear.

I am not sure I would have performed a laparotomy, but that decision would obviously depend on seeing the patient and evaluating his pain. At this point, it seems reasonable to discuss the hypotension further. I do not think that hypotension is cardiogenic. In spite of the recent myocardial infarction, his ejection fraction is 40%, which in the absence of any other abnormalities should not result in this degree of hypotension. Even if he had cardiogenic hypotension (and I do not believe that this is the case), that would not account for the fever and abdominal pain. Furthermore, there is no evidence of hypovolemic shock, which also would not adequately explain the fever and the abdominal pain.

I am left with a septic type of shock as the most likely cause of the hypotension, fever, abdominal pain, reduced platelet count, and the elevated fibrin split products. The specific site of infection is not clear. It still seems to me that vascular disease of the small bowel could be inferred. Although there was no perforation initially, one could have occurred since then. The gallbladder could be a source of infection, but I heard nothing about the gallbladder in the report of the exploratory laparotomy, so I shall assume that it was unremarkable. The pancreas is another possible site, but it would have been examined during the laparotomy as well.

In a febrile postoperative patient, all the conventional causes of infection would have to be considered: pulmonary infection, sepsis related to an indwelling vascular catheter, and urinary tract infection. Undoubtedly, by this time, the patient had a Foley catheter in place. I would carry out a detailed workup to identify any infectious cause. I would be interested in his urinalysis, his urine and blood cultures, and whether he was having any deterioration in his renal function because of the prolonged hypotension. I am still concerned about doing the exploratory laparotomy in the first place. In retrospect, it was not helpful and could have been harmful in this high-risk patient.

> On the eighth day, laparotomy was repeated because abdominal pain and tenderness persisted. A localized, sealed-over perforation of the ileum was described, and a closed ileostomy and cholecystectomy were performed. The gallbladder was not inflamed. Postoperatively, the patient continued to appear severely ill. His temperature was 39.3°C, and his blood pressure required pressors. Cardiac output was 10 L/min. Systemic vascular resistance was low (432). White cell count was 8,500 and platelets were 36,000. INR was normal. Antibiotics were changed to allow for more anaerobic coverage. The patient was given intravenous hydrocortisone empirically.

The patient apparently did not have cholecystitis, although I believe that it was appropriate to treat him for this disease earlier in the hospital course. We still have a patient who appears to have sepsis and is not improving after two laparotomies. The only possible site of infection we have so far is the perforation of ileum, but I am a little worried about blaming all of the patient's problems on a localized, sealed-over perforation. Was there any evidence of true abscess, and if so, how big was it? Did it need to be drained? On the other hand, was the tiny perforation clinically irrelevant? I do not believe we have a diagnosis at this point. The intravenous hydrocortisone is being given either for gram-negative sepsis on the minimal evidence that it works or for the remote possibility of adrenal insufficiency. I have heard nothing to make me suspect adrenal insufficiency. I do not have a diagnosis. I would still be following his abdominal examination to see what happens.

> Over the next 24 hours, the patient's blood pressure was more easily controlled with pressors. His systemic vascular resistance increased, and his temperature started to fall. The value for plasma cortisol in blood drawn before the second operation (when the patient appeared septic) was reported to be 0.6 μg/dL.

Given that the patient was hypotensive and appeared septic, this cortisol level is inappropriately low. Adrenal insufficiency still surprises me, but much of this patient's complicated course could be explained by relative or absolute adrenal insufficiency. I do not remember any comments about his electrolytes. Adrenal insufficiency has such a low prior probability these days that I do not think of it even when I should. When I was giving the list of reasons for hypotension earlier, I did not even list it.

> CT scan of the adrenal glands was consistent with bilateral adrenal hemorrhage. Retrospectively, the patient's abdominal pain, fever, and hypotension were attributed to acute adrenal hemorrhage, probably related to anticoagulant therapy. The patient had a prolonged hospital course. He was discharged approximately 2 months after admission, on cortisol and mineralocorticoid replacement. When seen by the endocrinologist 2 months later, he felt well and was recovering uneventfully.

Obviously, I missed it cold, and if I had another 3 hours to think about it, I do not think I would have come up with bilateral adrenal hemorrhage as the cause of his pain and hypotensive episode. In retrospect, I would be even more interested in the electrolytes to see if they were helpful in any way. The risk of bilateral adrenal hemorrhage and insufficiency from anticoagulant therapy must be exceedingly low.

Analysis

The cause of this patient's clinical manifestations remained obscure for many days to the physicians responsible for his care, and our discussant also had considerable difficulty in deducing that hypotension had resulted from adrenal hemorrhage. Such difficulty in diagnosis is not surprising: Except in patients previously treated with steroids, acute adrenal insufficiency is rare, and adrenal hemorrhage is a reportable complication of anticoagulant therapy.

One of the interesting features of this patient's course is a clinical conundrum that has received scant attention: namely, the close resemblance of one clinical entity to another. In the patient presented here, both physicians responsible for his care and the discussant focused appropriately on the possibility that the patient was septic: Certainly, sepsis is a far more likely in-hospital cause of hypotension than acute adrenal hemorrhage. Indeed, the clinicians and the discussant agreed on treating the patient for sepsis, and we suspect that many others also would have acted similarly. If not for a resident who spent time going through a long differential diagnosis of persistent hypotension, the correct diagnosis may have gone unnoticed.

Let us explore the error of confusing one disorder with its "look-alikes"—namely, disorders with clinical manifestations that are quite similar. For clarity in the discussion, we shall consider disorders that closely resemble each other but differ sufficiently in their prognosis or their response to treatment so that differentiation between the two entities is worthwhile.

How often do we confuse two look-alikes? What is the nature of this error? Do we already have effective mechanisms for dealing with the problem? No catalog of look-alikes exists, yet many come to mind: Constrictive pericarditis resembles restrictive cardiomyopathy, diuretic abuse

resembles Bartter syndrome, exogenous insulin administration resembles an insulinoma, atheroembolism resembles vasculitis. In many of these examples, considerable energy has been poured into developing methods to distinguish one from another.

Not surprisingly, diagnostic computer programs based either on Bayes' rule or on the artificial intelligence/expert systems approach would be expected to make the same error. In one case a probabilistic computer program for the diagnosis of acute renal failure confused the renal disease of scleroderma with malignant nephrosclerosis.[159] In another case an artificial intelligence computer program designed to identify the causes of edema confused constrictive pericarditis with severe cardiac failure.[162]

If we have two disorders that resemble each other both clinically and in the results of common laboratory tests, how do we distinguish between them, and under what circumstances is it important to do so? Transcript analysis of physicians engaged in the diagnostic process has identified a discriminating strategy for dealing with syndromes with similar findings.[19] First, we should search the clinical findings with great care for subtle differences that might distinguish one disorder from another. Second, we should pay close attention to differences in prevalence between the two disorders: Geese are more common than swans (at least in the United States), and if a given creature resembles both, it is more likely to be a goose than a swan.

However, just because one disorder is considerably more prevalent than another (e.g., diuretic abuse vs. Bartter syndrome), there is no guarantee that a patient with all the clinical manifestations of the more common disorder actually has that disorder. Because prevalence alone often is not an adequate discriminator, tests other than the "routine" laboratory tests may be required. Curiously, the guidelines for carrying out such tests relate as much to the characteristics of the treatments for both conditions as they do to the characteristics of the test. Certainly the accuracy and risks of the test are important determinants of the decision to use it, but the efficacy of treatment and the consequences of not treating are equally critical. If a test is highly sensitive and highly specific but is somewhat risky, we may be willing to use the test if identifying the current diagnosis allows us to (1) use a highly effective treatment, (2) avoid a highly risky treatment, or (3) avoid missing the opportunity to treat a treatable disorder. Thus, the accuracy and risks of further testing (perhaps also the cost of further testing) and the therapeutic efficacy of approaches to both the common and rare look-alikes need to be considered.

As a practical matter, we may be willing to subject a patient to cardiac catheterization to distinguish between constrictive and restrictive cardiomyopathy despite the substantial risk of cardiac catheterization and pericardiectomy because the benefit of surgery is substantial if the patient has constrictive pericarditis. The lost opportunity of treating such a reversible disorder is far too costly. Although considerable attention has been paid to the diagnostic procedures required to separate one look-alike from another, we have paid less attention to the more difficult task of weighing the tradeoffs between the risks and accuracy of invasive tests and the risks and benefits of alternate therapies.

Finally, the process of identifying look-alikes could be vastly improved. Rather than search our experience to come up with examples, it might be beneficial to compile lists for each medical domain. At the very least, such a compilation might warn us that we may be missing a disorder for which there is an effective treatment. Replacement steroid therapy for acute adrenal insufficiency certainly is one such example.

CASE 19. LOCATION, LOCATION, LOCATION

> A previously healthy 5½-year-old boy suddenly developed malaise, headache, abdominal aches, and shortness of breath. These symptoms occurred at the end of April, in Massachusetts.

This is a fairly nonspecific presentation. Even though it is almost May, an influenza-like illness could account for all of these symptoms. Respiratory syncytial virus could also give a similar presentation in a child. I would like to know more about his epidemiology, including sick contacts in his family or school. What is his travel history? Are there ticks out yet?

> The patient had finished playing soccer and complained to his parents of dyspnea and tiredness and he said he was sick to his stomach. He had a poorly characterized headache and said his stomach and legs hurt. When he got home, his oral temperature was 39°C. He had no cough, nausea, vomiting, or diarrhea. His past history was unremarkable. His immunizations were up to date. He was not taking any medications. No one else at home had been sick.

This is still pretty nonspecific. Headaches in a 5-year-old are not that common. Things that I would think of in that context which could be serious would include the early onset of bacterial meningitis. In a child, that would mean organisms such as meningococcus, *Haemophilus influenzae*, and, less commonly, pneumococcus. Bacteremia without an obvious focus could present with a headache as well. Being on a soccer team means that he obviously has been in contact with other children. I am specifically interested in knowing if he had the vaccinations against meningococcus and *H. influenzae*, which cannot be assumed from the statement that his immunizations were up to date.

> His parents (both are internists) initially thought that he had a viral infection. His father, however, remembered that 10 days earlier during their trip to the Smoky Mountains in Tennessee, the boy's mother had pulled a nonengorged tick from the boy's hair. Since both parents had gone to medical school in North Carolina and had seen critically ill patients with Rocky Mountain spotted fever, they became alarmed about this possibility.

I would like to know what kind of tick this was. A dog tick could be the vector for Rocky Mountain spotted fever. Certainly North Carolina is a hotbed for Rocky Mountain spotted fever, but I am not certain about Tennessee. This is a reasonable thought. The incubation period seems appropriate. He has part of the triad of fever, headache, and rash that is seen in about two-thirds of patients with the disease. Obviously, I want to hear about his physical examination. Does he look toxic? Is there a rash? Making a diagnosis can be difficult. Serology takes too long to be practical in making the diagnosis acutely. If you really think this is the diagnosis, you should start treatment. The usual treatment would be doxycycline, which is problematic in a youngster due to the potential toxicity to his developing teeth.

> The boy was seen by a pediatrician, who noted him to be somewhat fatigued and withdrawn. Physical examination was unremarkable. No rashes were noted. White cell count was 10,800 with a normal differential. Hematocrit, platelet count, electrolytes, and liver function tests were all normal.

The lack of rash and the normal platelet count are somewhat against the diagnosis of Rocky Mountain spotted fever. The presentation here is still quite nonspecific. If it were a deer tick, I would also think of Lyme disease and ehrlichiosis, although I'd have to check on the incidence of Lyme disease in Tennessee. Babesiosis could also be transmitted by a deer tick, and, once again, I would have to check to see if it is found in that part of the county. The normal laboratory tests are a little against ehrlichiosis and babesiosis, but I would keep these diagnoses in the back of my mind. A non-arthropod disease must be kept in mind.

> Two infectious disease consultants both agreed that Rocky Mountain spotted fever could not be ruled out at this early stage. They agreed that tetracycline was contraindicated because of the child's age, and both recommended treatment with oral chloramphenicol for 5 to 7 days.

I agree that if you think Rocky Mountain spotted fever is a reasonable diagnosis, then it should be treated, but I would also want to do additional workup, including blood cultures, chest x-ray, and urinalysis. One could look at a blood smear for evidence of *Babesia* or *Ehrlichia*. A Lyme titer could be sent, but even if he had Lyme disease, it may be too early for him to have seroconverted.

> It took the pediatrician 45 minutes to find a pharmacy that could mix an oral suspension of chloramphenicol. When the parents arrived to pick up the prescription the pharmacist told them that his only use for the suspension for the previous 3 years had been for veterinarians who used it in bird feed. In fact, he pointed out

that the drug company no longer made the oral suspension. The parents began to have second thoughts about this course of action.

So what do the parents want to do? It would be really important to me to see the patient and get a better sense of how sick he looks. I still do not think we have ruled out meningitis because early on in meningitis, meningismus may not be present. Of course, in early meningitis, the cerebral spinal fluid may not be overly abnormal. I would like some more data before deciding on what course of action might be most appropriate.

> A pediatric infectious disease expert from the father's institution returned an earlier page and when told about the case he stated that he never used oral chloramphenicol because of evidence that the oral form had greater risk of the drug's known toxicities. He stated that if he felt that the child really had Rocky Mountain spotted fever, he would admit the patient for parenteral chloramphenicol. He agreed with not using tetracycline. The parents decided in consultation with the initial pediatrician and the last infectious disease consultant not to administer an antibiotic and to follow the child closely.

This is a dilemma. I feel uncomfortable that we do not have a complete enough workup. I might be inclined on what I know to empirically treat the patient for Rocky Mountain spotted fever, if not meningitis.

> The patient did fairly well over the next 24 hours as long as his fever was suppressed with acetaminophen. No new symptoms developed. At one point, 24 hours after the onset of the symptoms, his axillary temperature was 40°C. Observation was continued.

It is good that he is at least stable. We still have not ruled out a viral process. He could have acute cytomegalovirus or Epstein-Barr infection.

> Over the second 24 hours, his temperature fell. He received his last dose of acetaminophen 48 hours after the onset of his symptoms. His mother called the park ranger in the Smoky Mountains and was told that they had not had any documented cases of Rocky Mountain

spotted fever in recent years. The child recovered uneventfully from his presumed viral illness. The parents wondered if their medical background had been an asset or a nuisance in this case.

It certainly worked out okay for the patient and the parents were right that he probably had some type of viral infection, the exact etiology of which we will never know. Did the parents interfere? Yes. I still think it would have been better to be more aggressive in the workup and possible use of empiric therapy. Intravenous chloramphenicol is not to be taken lightly, but neither is Rocky Mountain spotted fever.

Analysis

It's a good bet that any 5-year-old child in Massachusetts (or just about anywhere else in the United States, for that matter) with a bellyache, fever, and lassitude has a self-limited viral illness, but many parents fear the worst when a little one gets sick. Physicians, like the parents in this case, are especially likely to worry that their child has a dread disease. Surely, from an objective viewpoint, not only the parents, but the various consultants must have appreciated that, in terms of prevalence, a viral illness was overwhelmingly likely, yet they were sidetracked into worrying about a rare (but potentially fatal) disease.

Their trip into "Rocky Mountain spotted fever land" was initiated by two recalls: the discovery of a tick in their child's head and a salient memory of patients they had seen with the disease. It is well known that memory is facilitated by strong emotional experiences, and it is not surprising that

the parents' memories of serious cases of the disease evoked this diagnosis, despite the low prevalence of the disease anywhere in the United States (there are only 250 to 1,200 cases in the United States a year, according to the Centers for Disease Control and Prevention).[163] Even more interesting is how the consultants seemed to be drawn into the same domain, even going so far as to recommend hospitalization and the intravenous use of a fairly toxic antibiotic. It is as if the parents and the consultants were caught up in a bizarre epidemiologic delusion. Fortunately, Mom kept a cool head, checked the incidence of Rocky Mountain spotted fever in Tennessee, and found a cipher. Mom saved the day.

Although we have made light of this experience, we quickly point out that assessing the incidence of disease is a fundamental diagnostic strategy. Given the extent of world travel, we must be aware of the incidence of infectious diseases in countries other than our own. When foreign citizens arrive in our country with febrile illnesses, we must be aware of diseases in the countries from which they came. When our own citizens travel abroad, the same holds. A febrile illness in a traveler could be malaria, dengue, or (epidemiologically) something much worse.

Regions of a country do matter, of course. Connecticut is infamous for Lyme disease, Martha's Vineyard for babesiosis, the San Joaquin valley in California for coccidioidomycosis, and North Carolina and Oklahoma for Rocky Mountain spotted fever (most cases are seen in these two states; curiously, few cases are seen in the Rocky Mountain states.) However, common diseases are still most common, and we might save ourselves much grief if we keep that in mind.

CHAPTER 15

Use and Interpretation of Diagnostic Tests

CASE 20. INTERPRETING A NEGATIVE TEST RESULT

A 72-year-old woman with a history of mitral valve prolapse presented with a 3-week history of almost daily fevers and night sweats.

In a patient like this with 3 weeks of fever, acute infections seem unlikely. Disorders such as pneumonia or a urinary tract infection (UTI) would present much sooner than that. I would lean toward a chronic infection or a malignancy as the cause of her fever. The history of mitral valve prolapse by itself does not strike me as overly important at this time unless it was associated with significant mitral regurgitation, which might increase her risk of bacterial endocarditis.

We begin the history of her present illness on May 4, when the patient had a normal routine examination by her primary care physician. On May 9, she developed a self-limited "intestinal flu" with 2 days of diarrhea and abdominal cramps. Shortly thereafter, she developed nightly fevers, flushing, drenching night sweats, and bifrontal headaches. On May 22, she again saw her physician, who obtained the following studies: white blood cell count (WBC) 6,000, hematocrit 30%, platelet count 405,000, sedimentation rate 115 mm/hr. Two blood cultures were negative. She also saw her dentist because she thought her symptoms might be due to a dental abscess. She received prophylactic cephalexin. No abscess was found.

The recent history of diarrhea raises the possibility of a lingering gastroenterologic infection from an organism such as *Salmonella*. That organism can be associated with mycotic aneurysms, and hence I would wonder about some type of endovascular infection leading to persisting fevers. The elevated sedimentation rate is striking. It is not characteristic of any specific diagnosis, but levels above 100 make me think of diagnoses such as endocarditis, osteomyelitis, tuberculosis, nephritic

syndrome, and certain cancers. Other than the mild anemia, the complete blood count (CBC) is not very helpful. The differential does not suggest something like a lymphoma, where one might see more of a lymphocyte predominance, and the slightly elevated platelet count is probably consistent with an inflammatory process. Blood cultures are usually a good way to pick up a bacteremia, especially if they are collected and plated properly. The negative cultures could be compatible with a fastidious organism such as one of the HACEK organisms (*Haemophilus* species, *Actinobacillus actinomycetemcomitans*, *Cardiobacterium hominis*, *Eikenella corrodens*, and *Kingella kingae*). *Salmonella*, if present, should be relatively easy to culture from the blood. The visit to the dentist is always interesting, but it appears that her fevers predated her visit to the dentist. Since the blood cultures were done before she got the antibiotics from the dentist, a partially treated endocarditis with negative cultures is pretty much ruled out.

She had a long history of mitral valve prolapse with an associated murmur of mitral regurgitation. Her right eye had been enucleated decades ago for a malignant melanoma. She was on no medications at the time of the illness. There was no history of recent travel or unusual exposures.

The previously known murmur makes the mitral valve prolapse more bothersome. Until the recent practice guidelines were published, mitral valve prolapse with a murmur was considered to be an indication for prophylactic antibiotics, but it no longer is. However, many physicians still like to give prophylaxis in patients with these findings. Drug fever seems unlikely unless the patient is taking some type of medication we are not aware of, such as herbal medications. We have nothing to suggest a travel-related infection.

On May 24, she was seen at a hospital clinic for further studies. Questioning revealed that she also had diffuse muscle aches, decreased

energy, and mild nausea. On examination, she was in no distress. Oral temperature was 38°C. Blood pressure was normal. No temporal artery tenderness was noted. Lungs were clear. Her systolic click and murmur were unchanged. No petechiae were noted. There was no lymphadenopathy. Repeat laboratory studies were as follows: WBC 8,200 with a normal differential. Hematocrit 32%, sedimentation rate 121 mm/hr (1 year previously, her hematocrit was 40%, and the sedimentation rate was 17 mm/hr). Liver function tests were normal. The leading diagnoses at this time were subacute bacterial endocarditis, giant cell arteritis, and polymyalgia rheumatica.

Diffuse muscle aches are not very specific, but if there was localization to the hips or shoulder girdle, I would certainly be suspicious of polymyalgia rheumatica. The temporal headaches raise the possibility of temporal arteritis, although the temporal arteries were not tender. We must remember, however, that they are not always tender in that disorder. We now have confirmation of fevers, although she does not yet meet the classic criteria for a fever of unknown origin, given the minimal workup to date. She has no skin manifestations of bacterial endocarditis, although these findings are not very sensitive.

At this point, I would repeat blood cultures and obtain an echocardiogram. A transesophageal echo would be more sensitive than a transthoracic echo, although most clinicians would start with the latter, given its noninvasive nature. If the workup for endocarditis were negative, I would proceed with a temporal artery biopsy. Given the lack of tenderness on one side, however, we may need to ultimately do biopsies on both sides.

On May 24, a transthoracic echocardiogram showed mild mitral valve prolapse. A small echo density was noted on the anterior mitral leaflet. The report said that if endocarditis was "clinically suspected, a transesophageal echocardiogram was recommended."

The finding of the small density of the mitral leaflet does merit further evaluation. I agree with performing a transesophageal echo.

On May 25, a transesophageal echocardiogram showed no evidence of endocarditis. The working diagnosis was polymyalgia rheumatica, and prednisone 10 mg daily was begun.

Given the negative transesophageal echo, it appears that endocarditis has been ruled out although another endovascular source of infection such as a mycotic aneurysm is still possible. I think the initiation of steroid therapy at this point is reasonable, given the possibility of temporal arteritis and its associated risk of blindness. The dose of 10 mg is more appropriate for polymyalgia rheumatica than temporal arteritis. I think she should have a temporal artery biopsy. We still have not ruled out an underlying malignancy, and further studies, including CT (computed tomography) scans would be reasonable. The clinicians taking care of the patient also seem focused on polymyalgia rheumatica at this point, although we should consider other diagnoses as well.

On May 31, the patient reported that the fevers, myalgias, and headaches had persisted. Two more blood cultures were drawn. A chest x-ray was negative. The patient was scheduled for a temporal artery biopsy.

I agree with drawing more blood cultures. I would want to make sure that the microbiology lab was holding on to the cultures long enough to make sure that we are not dealing with fastidious organisms. The utility of placing a PPD (purified protein derivative skin test) is questionable. The normal chest x-ray would make tuberculosis extremely unlikely. It also makes a thoracic lymphoma less likely.

On June 1, the patient had an ophthalmologic examination and a 0.5-cm biopsy of the right temporal artery. The eye examination was normal, and the biopsy showed no evidence of giant cell arteritis. On that day, it was reported that one of two bottles from one of her blood cultures contained gram-positive cocci. The patient was admitted to the hospital for further evaluation.

The right temporal artery biopsy does not rule out temporal arteritis. Even though it was negative, there is always the potential for sampling error. The positive blood culture, once again, raises the possibility of endocarditis, if that culture is not a contaminant, which will depend on the organism that is cultured. If the organism is an anaerobic one, I would wonder about a dental infection that had spread. My previous thought about *Salmonella* seems even less likely since that is a gram-negative organism.

> The patient's physicians thought that the blood culture result was probably a contaminant, and no antibiotics were given. Her physicians and a rheumatology consultant continued to be concerned about temporal arteritis. A daily dose of 60 mg of prednisone was started, and another temporal artery biopsy was requested.

I think further blood cultures should be drawn to make sure the initially positive one was a contaminant. I agree with the rheumatologist that a negative temporal artery biopsy on one side does not rule out the presence of arteritis.

> A 1.3-cm segment of the left temporal artery showed disruption of the internal elastic lamina with associated neointimal fibrosis. Although no giant cells were seen, the changes were considered to be consistent with healed arteritis. Prednisone was continued. The final blood culture results showed a coagulase-negative *Staphylococcus*.

In light of this biopsy, the diagnosis of temporal arteritis is the most likely one. Treatment with high-dose prednisone is appropriate.

> The patient responded to the therapy. Her symptoms all resolved. One month later, her hematocrit was 40% and her sedimentation rate was 7 mm/hr on a tapering course of steroids.

The patient's course is certainly consistent with the diagnosis of temporal arteritis. A chronic infection would not respond to steroids in this fashion. Some malignancies, such as a lymphoma, might show a response to steroids, but it does appear that this patient has temporal arteritis.

Analysis

In this case, we focus again on the interpretation of laboratory test results. To preface this commentary, it is worth noting that one diagnosis dominated the clinicians' thinking throughout, and that they persisted in pursuing this diagnosis even when the "gold standard" diagnostic tests for the condition failed to disclose characteristic findings of the disease. This directed approach is the hallmark of clinical expertise.[19,36]

We use the transcript here to illustrate principles of interpreting negative test results. In other cases, we discuss the importance of the prevalence of a disease (the prior probability in a given patient) when interpreting test results. We have described the pitfalls of overinterpreting positive test results when the prevalence of the disease is low. In one of our examples, the possibility of a pheochromocytoma was raised when vanillylmandelic acid (VMA) excretion was found to be elevated, even though the prior probability of a pheochromocytoma was extremely low. The high urinary VMA excretion ultimately was found to be a false-positive result (see case 23).

We selected this case because although a positive test result on the first biopsy would have been extremely important and meaningful, yet the first biopsy result was negative. The posttest probability of a disease after a negative test is a function of the test's sensitivity. By definition, the greater the sensitivity, the lower is the false-negative rate.[155,156]

Although neither the treating physician nor the discussant commented specifically on the sensitivity of a temporal artery biopsy for temporal arteritis, they ignored the negative test and recommended a second biopsy, implying that the test is not highly sensitive. If it were, in a patient strongly suspected of having the disease, a negative result would have virtually excluded arteritis as the cause of the patient's manifestations. All these physicians knew that arterial inflammation can be spotty even in patients with severe manifestations of temporal arteritis, that a random biopsy could miss an involved site, and that a negative result could be a false negative. Let us try to be more specific here. Assuming that the prior probability of temporal arteritis in this patient was approximately 0.65 and the sensitivity of temporal artery biopsies is 0.75, the false-negative rate would be 0.25. Assuming that the specificity is 0.99, the false-positive rate would be 0.01. Despite a negative biopsy, the probability of temporal arteritis would still be approximately 0.3, and at that likelihood further study would be warranted, given that the disease is risky (i.e., untreated it can lead to blindness) and treatable with corticosteroids.

Although histologic evaluation generally is highly sensitive, sensitivity is eroded and the false negativity increases when the sample is a small fraction of the lesion, when the histologic changes are not always evenly distributed, and (in other instances) when analysis of the sample is preliminary or incomplete. In this case, the patient's doctor and the discussant both recognized that the biopsy findings had only a modest sensitivity, continued to operate on the strength of their convictions, and arranged another biopsy.

Why was their conviction so strong that the patient had temporal arteritis? We posit that a constellation of findings, namely fever, headaches, muscle aches, and a very high sedimentation rate in an elderly woman, is a characteristic pattern of temporal arteritis. True, other disorders mentioned in the transcript could have caused all these manifestations, yet as disorders such as endocarditis and salmonellosis became less and less likely, temporal arteritis became more and more likely. And physicians are always searching for reversible disease.

The "take home" lessons: When the clinical suspicion of a disorder is strong, the sensitivity of a test determines the impact of a negative result on the therapeutic approach. If the test is highly sensitive, a negative result can exclude the disease from consideration and argue against treatment for that disease. If the test is not very sensitive, a negative result only slightly lowers suspicion of the disease, and plans for treatment can proceed unchanged. The management of a patient is most likely to be affected by a negative test result when the pretest probability is neither very high nor very low and the pretest suspicion of a disease is close to the threshold probability for treatment.[58,59] In such circumstances, a negative result will provide sufficient evidence that the optimal choice is to withhold therapy.

CASE 21. DIAGNOSIS AND THE RISKS OF THE PRIMROSE PATH

A 54-year-old man with a history of smoking, hypertension, Graves disease, and chronic back pain presented to the Emergency Department with hemoptysis.

Hemoptysis in a patient with a history of tobacco use raises the possibility of cancer. Hypertension can be associated with hemoptysis if a patient has concurrent severe heart disease. I cannot find a way to attribute hemoptysis to Graves disease. Chronic back pain also raises the possibility of malignancy. The commonest cause of hemoptysis in the United States is probably bronchitis, sometimes associated with bronchiectasis.

The patient was in his usual state of health until he awoke one morning and began coughing. He coughed up bright red blood, about the size of a quarter, mixed with sputum. He had several similar episodes throughout the day and came to the emergency department. He had no history of upper respiratory infection, nasal trauma, fever, chills, or night sweats. He had had no contacts with ill people. His last episode of bronchitis was 6 months previously.

I wonder if he has a daily cough because of his smoking or whether there was something acute that caused the cough and hemoptysis such as a pulmonary embolism. Perhaps he aspirated and now has a lung abscess that eroded a pulmonary vessel. The bright red blood could be coming from anywhere from the nose down to the alveoli. Each anatomic site would have its own differential diagnosis. Hemoptysis could even be a manifestation of gastrointestinal bleeding with some degree of aspiration, although in this instance I would not have expected the blood to be bright red. At this point, bleeding does not seem to be massive, but I always worry that it could change. The patient could have a coagulopathy or some type of systemic bleeding disorder. He could have mitral stenosis, one of the classic causes of hemoptysis. The history is not suggestive of infection such as tuberculosis. The previous history of bronchitis could have given rise to bronchiectasis that might cause hemoptysis periodically. Goodpasture syndrome and Wegener granulomatosis are other rare causes of hemoptysis.

He had a history of chronic back pain and had had four laminectomies with chronic arachnoiditis and spinal stenosis. He was on disability

for this condition. He had smoked one to two packs of cigarettes a day for 30 years. He previously worked removing lead paint. His Graves disease had recently been treated with I-131 ablation. His medications on admission were atenolol, hydrochlorothiazide, ranitidine, and one aspirin a day.

The history of heavy cigarette smoking brings up any of a number of tumors located from the oropharynx to the lung. The disability is interesting to me because it appears that people who do not work seem to get sicker than people who do. I do not think I can tie in the exposure to lead paint with hemoptysis. His medications should not cause hemoptysis, although aspirin use may affect his platelet function and exacerbate whatever bleeding occurs.

On examination, he appeared in no distress. Vital signs were normal. Head, eyes, ears, nose, and throat (HEENT) examination was unremarkable. There was no lymphadenopathy. He had decreased breath sounds bilaterally without wheezes, rhonchi, or rales. His cardiac exam was normal. The rest of the examination was normal. Electrolytes and liver function tests were normal. White blood cell count was 9,200, hematocrit was 36%, and mean corpuscular volume (MCV) was 77. Platelet count was 267,000. His electrocardiogram showed no acute changes. His arterial blood gases on room air were as follows: pH 7.47, partial pressure of oxygen (PO_2) 72 mm Hg, partial pressure of carbon dioxide in the arterial blood ($PaCO_2$) 42 mm Hg.

His lack of distress presumably means that he is not having massive hemoptysis. He appears to have no obvious bleeding source in his head and neck. There is no evidence of petechiae or ecchymoses. The decreased breath sounds could be a manifestation of chronic obstructive pulmonary disease. The absence of wheezes, rhonchi, or rales is not helpful. Although his cardiac examination was described as normal, one can easily miss an opening snap. He is anemic, which appears to be particularly pronounced since I would have expected a patient with this smoking history to have a hematocrit as high as 50% or 55%. His MCV

is slightly low, raising the possibility of iron deficiency or even lead toxicity. The hypoxia reinforces my expectation that his hematocrit should have been higher.

His chest x-ray showed a right-upper-lobe bulla with an air–fluid level.

It is not clear to me if this is a new finding. An abscess could be possible with erosion of a vessel. It could be a tumor. An upper lobe cavitary lesion always raises the suspicion of tuberculosis. At this point, I would put the patient in respiratory isolation until I rule out tuberculosis. *Aspergillus* and *Actinomyces* infection are other infectious possibilities. Vasculitis with pulmonary involvement such as occurs in Wegener granulomatosis must also be considered. At this point some clinicians may opt to go right ahead and perform a bronchoscopy or consider a percutaneous aspiration if feasible.

On the night of the admission, he was given ceftriaxone for a possible bacterial infection. Sputum was sent for acid-fast bacillus (AFB) smear. A chest computed tomography (CT) scan showed a right apical thin-wall bulla with an air–fluid level. A 4-cm right-upper-lobe mass located 4 cm above the carina adjacent to the bulla was noted. Patchy air space disease in the right upper lobe, possibly representing a postobstructive pneumonia, was present. Small mediastinal nodes were noted. The working diagnosis was bronchogenic cancer.

A tumor certainly seems to be the most likely diagnosis. The anemia could be a manifestation of his tumor or could represent metastatic disease. I think a biopsy would be revealing.

AFB smears were negative. Bronchoscopy showed bleeding from the right upper lobe with minimal secretions. An endobronchial biopsy showed no evidence of malignancy. Routine cultures were negative, as were stains of the specimen for acid-fast bacilli and fungi.

These findings do not mean that he does not have a cancer. He still could have a malignancy or a chronic infection. Sarcoidosis would be extremely unlikely in this setting. I think the house officers and attending caring for this patient probably believe that these results represent a sampling error and that a malignancy is still the most likely diagnosis.

> The patient underwent a CT-guided needle biopsy. He developed a pneumothorax, and a Heimlich valve was inserted. The fine needle aspirate only showed fibrous tissue, skeletal muscle, and occasional histiocytes. A second needle biopsy provided insufficient tissue for diagnosis.

This man is on the slippery slope of iatrogenic disease. How far are we going to go to make this diagnosis? Fibrous tissue could just represent scar tissue. Could he have reactive hyperplasia that can occur with a gumma? Skeletal muscle and fibrous tissue make one wonder about a hamartoma. The histiocytes raise the possibility of a disorder called malignant histiocytosis X, which can be a devastating illness. An examination of the bone marrow could help make that diagnosis by showing erythrophagocytosis. At this point, I would stop and reevaluate whether to go any further.

> The patient was continued on ceftriaxone. He was presented at tumor conference. The decision of the group was to proceed with a right upper lobectomy, but with surgery to be preceded by a cardiac evaluation. Pulmonary function tests were normal.

Now he undergoes a cardiac evaluation. They wanted to make sure he could survive his right upper lobectomy. Are they going to find occult mitral stenosis? I am surprised the pulmonary function tests were normal, in view of his smoking history.

> An echocardiogram was unremarkable. During a dobutamine stress test, the patient reached 67% of his maximum predicted heart rate and developed chest pressure. The scan showed a medium-sized, moderately severe, reversible inferior defect.

This endless workup continues. Is all this going to benefit the patient? He is on a slippery slope of one complication after another. Is he now to undergo a cardiac catheterization? One could opt to watch and wait. If he has a primary malignancy of the lung with possible mediastinal metastases, the chance of a cure is low. If he has a lymphoma, maybe he can be helped. We are treating him for

a bacterial infection and have looked for tuberculosis. If he is doing well, we could continue our current treatment and let time show us what is going on.

> Cardiac catheterization revealed a 20% left anterior descending lesion and a 60% to 70% large first obtuse marginal lesion. Medical therapy was recommended.

At least he did not suffer a complication from the procedure. Fortunately, his cardiac disease does not seem to be serious.

> The patient returned 1 week later for a wedge resection of his right upper lobe. The specimen revealed subapical scarring and an emphysematous bulla (7 × 7 × 3 cm) containing a blood clot. There was no evidence of malignancy. The patient's postoperative course was uneventful.

So he just had benign disease, and he went through all those tests and procedures at considerable expense. This gentleman did get onto the slippery slope. One of the other things we have to do, not only because of cost containment, but also for better-quality medicine, is not to ask what a test will show, but whether the test and the result will benefit the patient. Do we have to know the answers right away? The main reason to know right away is if it is going to make a difference in the therapy or well-being of the patient. Sometimes just knowing the facts does make a difference in the well being of the patient even if he or she has incurable disease. On the other hand, there are a number of people who do not urgently need to know the diagnosis and who can tolerate the wait until the answer surfaces.

Analysis

Here we have a prime example of the losing battle against excessive diagnostic testing. Looked at from a standpoint of diagnostic efficiency and cost, we would have to conclude that there was much waste in the workup of this patient. He ended up having a benign lesion, but to come to that conclusion his physicians carried out a bronchoscopy, bronchoscopic biopsy, chest CT, two CT-guided biopsies, an echocardiogram, a stress test, a cardiac catheterization, and finally a wedge resection of the lung. The hospital bill must have been enormous. Fortunately, in the process, the patient suffered only one potentially serious complication. You can nearly hear the frustration of the discussant as she complains about the testing decisions along the way.

In retrospect, of course, all this testing seems superfluous, yet even in retrospect, it is difficult to know when to have stopped the testing cascade in this patient. Diagnostic problems do not present retrospectively, and that is why in virtually all of the cases in this book, we present the clinical story as it unfolded to the physicians in charge of the patient. Where could the diagnostic cascade have been shortened or interrupted? It is hard to argue that no tests should have been done; after all, the man was relatively young, and even though bleeding was modest at the beginning, it might have become life threatening. Should they have stopped testing after the first bronchoscopy was unrevealing? No, not if the test was thought likely to reveal the cause. The same logic would apply to the CT-guided biopsies: Once the physicians decided that the test was likely to provide a definite diagnosis, repeating the biopsy seemed rational. Could the cardiac evaluation have been dispensed with? This decision is clearly a judgment call, but it is at least understandable, given the nature of the proposed surgery and the patient's risk factors such as hypertension and smoking. Lastly, there is the critically important question that the discussant asks. What disease could be found that would be treatable? The working diagnosis was lung cancer, and if this were the only possible diagnosis, we might have argued from the beginning that no testing was worthwhile, given the marginal improvement in life expectancy and quality of life from treatment of such cancers. However, here is the trap that we all fall into: Suppose it is not a lung cancer, but a treatable infection or a lymphoma for which treatment is quite effective? This reasoning is what drives us to "go down the primrose path," as some call it. The discussant was not sure that continued testing was the right choice. She wondered whether a more appropriate strategy would have been to cease the testing, follow the patient, and, as she describes it, "let time show us what is going on."

Many physicians are reluctant to give up on a 54-year-old man with a potentially treatable lesion. Sometimes they go too far, basing their contin-

ued diagnostic exploits on miniscule probabilities of a long-term positive outcome. With respect to the cost of all this testing, our health care system puts no skids on test ordering. Given that no such constraints exist, decisions such as these ultimately come down to difficult judgment calls. If the patient had been older and sicker and was highly likely to have lung cancer, choosing to do no tests might have been right. But he was not.

CASE 22. SEARCHING FOR A PONY

A 62-year-old man was admitted to the hospital with a 4- to 6-month history of progressive changes in mental status, emotional lability, gait disturbance, and visual impairment.

These symptoms make me think of central nervous system disease, and I would like to think of reversible central nervous system diseases. Could he have nonobstructive hydrocephalus? The patient has a gait disturbance, but there is no history of urinary incontinence. I will have to keep that diagnosis in the back of my mind. Unfortunately, normal-pressure hydrocephalus is analogous in certain respects to emboli of the small bowel; by the time you diagnose it, it is usually too late to treat it. In this case, we would have to think of a gamut of central nervous system disorders: mass lesions, degenerative disorders, and inflammatory processes. Incidentally, manifestations of 4 to 6 months' duration would be a bit long for the last. Vascular disease such as multiinfarct dementia, however, could produce this picture. I am not sure what to make of the visual impairment.

The patient had a 6-year history of insulin-dependent diabetes mellitus. He had not used over-the-counter medications or illicit drugs. He drank alcohol on weekends. He denied homosexual contacts. Family history was negative. Medications on admission included NPH insulin, furosemide, and potassium chloride. He was wheelchair bound with a stooped posture. He had poor comprehension and cried frequently. Vital signs were normal. Visual acuity was 7/200 in both eyes. There was no retinopathy. The rest of the examination was negative except for a wide-based slow gait with ataxia

on turning. He swayed on standing with eyes open and closed. Motor strength and reflexes were normal. Babinski reflexes were absent. Fine movements were curtailed because of a terminal tremor.

Over the last 4 to 6 months, the patient apparently has gone from engaging in normal activity to being wheelchair bound. We have a progressive, serious neurologic disorder associated with emotional lability and a variety of abnormal neurologic findings. I cannot relate much of this to central nervous system complications of diabetes, which usually involve cranial nerves. There is no evidence of diabetic retinopathy; if it is carefully looked for, that is the best sign of microvascular disease outside of a biopsy. This condition looks like an acute degenerative process of the central nervous system that is rapidly progressive and needs to be investigated aggressively. Let us try again to think of reversible disorders, enumerating the screening tests for medical causes of abnormal mental status. Vitamin B_{12} deficiency is always a possibility, but the poor visual acuity perhaps is a little atypical for this. How about hypothyroidism or even myxedema madness? Some of the findings are compatible, but some are not. Again, the poor visual acuity is disturbing to me.

Electrolyte disorders? I do not think so. Neoplastic disorders? Syphilis or other infections of the central nervous system? Possibly. Lupus? I do not think so. Lupus is possible, but the patient is male, and this presentation would be unusual. In a patient with lupus, the sudden deterioration of higher cortical functions could be ascribable to central nervous system lupus. So vitamin B_{12} deficiency is an interesting thought. Again, there are features here that do not fit, such as the emotional lability and the decreased visual acuity. It certainly would be worth at least looking at a CBC (complete blood count) and a peripheral smear and also getting thyroid function tests.

Laboratory results were hemoglobin 14.4 g/dL, hematocrit 41%, white blood cell count (WBC) 7,500 with a normal differential; indices and blood smear were normal. Fasting blood sugar was 131 mg/dL, and blood urea nitrogen (BUN) was 24 mg/dL. Other studies were

normal, including electrolytes, liver function tests, thyroid function tests, cerebrospinal fluid, serology, arterial blood gases, chest x-ray, head CT, and magnetic resonance imaging (MRI) scan.

He has a normal hemoglobin and hematocrit with a normal differential and indices, without an elevated mean corpuscular volume, without hypersegmented polymorphonuclear leukocytes, and without macrocytosis on the blood smear. I think we probably can exclude vitamin B_{12} deficiency. His blood sugar is under good control. There is no uremia, which is another potentially reversible cause of altered mental status. The other studies are normal, and this finding addresses many of the diagnoses I just considered.

The diagnosis of exclusion is Alzheimer disease. The gait disturbance would imply something more than that, but some degenerative diseases of the central nervous system may be in the category of Alzheimer disease. I am bothered that the MRI is normal. Does it show anything? In any of the other disorders, we would expect to see white-matter dysfunction, but none is visible here. I would ask my neurology colleagues for some help. I am concerned that we are looking at irreversible or idiopathic dementia associated with a motor disorder, but I cannot pin a diagnosis on it.

Additional laboratory studies included serum B_{12} level 67 mg/L (normal >190 mg/L) and serum folate level 15.6 mg/L (normal 2–16 mg/L); homocysteine and methylmalonic acid levels were elevated.

This patient's problem defies the rational approach. It troubles me that we could not have gotten here without ordering a vitamin B_{12} level. I am surprised to see a case of vitamin B_{12} deficiency without hematologic manifestations. I would be interested to know what happened to the patient after vitamin B_{12} replacement.

Outcome: After 2 months of vitamin B_{12} therapy, the patient's mental status was normal, and he was walking without help. After 4 months, his emotional lability was almost gone. His visual acuity had improved, and he was again able to drive a car.

Analysis

Works of art, literature, and music endure when they continue to provide society with special meaning or value. The same can be said for common aphorisms and even jokes. At first blush, a clinical dilemma such as that described above seems a far cry from a joke, yet the analogy strikes us as a sound one. The joke, which has endured for decades, describes a young boy toiling for hours, digging happily into a deep pile of manure. When asked why digging knee-deep in manure seemed to be such an enjoyable task, the boy replied, "With all this manure, there must be a pony around somewhere." In case the analogy is lost on the reader, the common thread, we propose, is the combination of a low-probability outcome (cobalamin-responsive dementia; finding a pony in a pile of manure) with an outcome that is exceptionally valuable (cure of dementia; discovery of a pony).

In the patient presented here, the issue is how far to proceed in diagnostic testing for reversible causes of neuropsychiatric symptoms. In particular, the question is whether to study patients for cobalamin (vitamin B_{12}) deficiency if their hemoglobin is normal and if the morphology of their red blood cells also is normal. This patient teaches us at least one thing about the answer to the question: namely, that at least in one instance, cobalamin deficiency can cause reversible dementia in the absence of any obvious abnormalities of hemoglobin concentration and red cell morphology. Other reports of similar cases confirm the existence of this clinical phenomenon, although we have little information about its frequency.[164]

Should we test all patients with unexplained neuropsychiatric symptoms for cobalamin deficiency? Taking it a step further, should all patients with unexplained neuropsychiatric symptoms be given an empiric therapeutic trial of cobalamin? Well-defined principles underlie testing decisions. The accuracy of the test is one important consideration. Unless a diagnostic test is exceptionally specific (i.e., the test gives normal results in virtually all people who do not have the disease in question), it will produce a large number of false-positive results if used in populations with a low prevalence of the disease. Even for tests that are not exceptionally specific, the test still might be useful if it is applied in a population with a high prevalence of the disease in question. The cost of the test and its risks are other factors, as is the availability of other confirmatory tests.

In the case of the cobalamin assay we are considering, risk is not a factor, and for the sake of discussion, we shall assume that cost also is not a factor in making the decision to use the test. Aside from accuracy, cost, risk, and the availability of confirmatory tests, a critical element in the decision to use a test is its therapeutic implications. Here we return to the possibility that there might be an exceptionally valuable payoff (such as a pony in the manure). Given that cobalamin deficiency is acknowledged to be a rare cause of dementia, and given that normal red cell morphology is rare among patients with cobalamin deficiency, we must be dealing with a low-probability event. One could argue, therefore, that unless the test is nearly perfect, we should not use it.

In a situation such as the one described here, however, one can make a convincing case that the test still should be used. First, even if many positive tests are not true positives, the associated tests (plasma levels of methylmalonic acid and total homocysteine, response of these plasma concentrations to cobalamin therapy) will be helpful in weeding out the false results. Second, given the exceptionally high payoff of finding a case of reversible dementia and the effectiveness and safety of cobalamin in reversing neurologic abnormalities, we should be willing to accept even a rather high number of false-positive results. Thus, one could easily make a case for testing all patients with new dementia and other neuropsychiatric symptoms for plasma levels of cobalamin.

One has to have considerable admiration for the general internist who discussed this case. He raised the possibility of cobalamin deficiency twice but dismissed the diagnosis when the hemoglobin and blood smear were reported to be normal. Although he did not request either a cobalamin level or other related tests, he gave thoughtful consideration to the possibility of dementia secondary to cobalamin deficiency. No doubt he learned the same important lesson as anyone who reads the transcript.

Finally, should every patient with newly discovered dementia or other neuropsychiatric symptoms be given therapeutic doses of cobalamin to assess its possible effect? Should we even bother testing? Is the therapeutic threshold so low that we should treat without testing? Given the low cost and virtual absence of toxicity with cobalamin, such an approach would be hard to criticize.

CASE 23: INTERPRETING HOOFBEATS: CAN BAYES HELP CLEAR THE HAZE?*

The physician of a 59-year-old man with a long history of mild, labile hypertension became concerned when, despite drug therapy, the patient's blood pressure remained persistently elevated, reaching levels as high as 180/120 mm Hg. He ordered a test of urinary vanillylmandelic acid (VMA) excretion and was surprised when he received a report of 20.9 mg/day, a value twice the upper limit of normal.

VMA is the end product of catecholamine metabolism, and its excretion is increased in a large proportion of patients with pheochromocytomas. When we collect 24-hour urine samples for VMA in hypertensive patients, especially those under some stress, we frequently get values above the upper limit of normal. Most often, when we evaluate those patients, they do not have pheochromocytomas. In addition, when we do urinary catecholamine or metanephrine studies in hospitalized patients, we may find somewhat elevated values because such patients are not in a basal state. But a urinary VMA of 20.9 mg/day is very abnormal.

With this high value, there is ample reason to suspect that the patient does have a pheochromocytoma. The question is what to do next. We could repeat the VMA, obtain urinary catecholamine or metanephrine studies, or perform a clonidine suppression test. This may sound heretical, but I wonder whether doing that makes sense. Should we just get a CT scan of the abdomen? Even though such tumors are rare, in a patient with a VMA excretion this high the chance of a pheochromocytoma might be as great as 40%. Of course, we must keep in mind that laboratory errors do occur.

*Originally published by Pauker SG, Kopelman RI. *N Engl J Med* 1992;327:1009–1013. Reprinted with permission of the Massachusetts Medical Society.

Except for the hypertension and mild osteoarthritis, the patient had been in good health. He described himself as highly stressed and compulsive. He regularly monitored his blood pressure at home. His drugs had included enalapril, diltiazem, and nifedipine. With each drug, his blood pressure fell but then gradually returned to pretreatment levels. Over the previous several months, he had reported mild diffuse headaches but no excessive sweating or palpitations. Physical examination revealed a strong, well-muscled man with a blood pressure of 162/90 mm Hg and a pulse of 82 per minute. The fundi were normal. There were no carotid, thoracic, or abdominal bruits. The heart was normal, without murmurs. The kidneys were not palpable. Pulses in the arms and legs were strong. There was no edema.

All of this is consistent with anxiety and essential hypertension, but I am still worried about the possibility of a pheochromocytoma. I would try to find out whether the patient is taking anything that would increase the excretion of VMA, although I admit that most laboratory tests for VMA are fairly specific now and are not affected by drugs, bananas, or the like.

Laboratory results included the following: BUN 13 mg/dL, creatinine 1.1 mg/dL, sodium 141 mEq/L, potassium 4.6 mEq/L, chloride 104 mEq/L, total CO_2 30 mEq/L, calcium 9.2 mg/dL, phosphorus 3.1 mg/dL, and glucose 96 mg/dL. The 24-hour excretion of both catecholamines (51 pg) and metanephrine (220 pg) was normal. The physician was concerned about the severity of the hypertension and the possibility of a pheochromocytoma. Despite the normal values for catecholamine and metanephrine excretion, he started the patient on 20 mg of phenoxybenzamine per day.

As the patient's doctor appreciated, we now have a problem: The VMA excretion is elevated, but both the catecholamine and metanephrine excretions are normal. A patient with a pheochromocytoma can have some elements of this picture because the mix of VMA and catecholamines excreted in the urine depends on the extent of catecholamine metabolism by the tumor. If the rate of conversion of catecholamines to VMA and metanephrines is relatively low, norepinephrine and epinephrine, the two principal catecholamines, will be released from the tumor. In that case, the clinical diagnosis of pheochromocytoma is likely to be made early because the catecholamines produce symptoms, severe hypertension, or both. If the conversion rate is relatively high, then the major products of the tumor will be inactive metabolites. When this occurs, the pheochromocytoma may escape early detection and grow quite large. Urinary catecholamines will then be low, and VMA excretion may be disproportionately high.

In this patient, however, there are two discrepancies—namely, hypertension with normal catecholamine excretion and high excretion of one metabolite while excretion of another metabolite is normal. This brings the VMA analysis into question. Could one of the drugs he has taken produce a falsely elevated VMA? How reliable was the laboratory in which the tests were performed? I would repeat the tests before I did anything further. On the basis of this flimsy evidence of a pheochromocytoma, starting phenoxybenzamine seems premature. Phenoxybenzamine, a long acting alpha-blocker, is very effective in controlling hypertension in patients with pheochromocytoma, but I would not use it unless I was quite confident of the diagnosis.

> While he was taking phenoxybenzamine, the patient's blood pressure was approximately 130/90 mm Hg at home, but it was 142/103 mm Hg on a follow-up visit to the doctor's office several days later. At that visit, the patient mentioned that both his brother and his father had had "adrenal tumors."

This is a diagnostic roller coaster. Early evidence argued against the diagnosis of pheochromocytoma, but the patient's response to phenoxybenzamine and the additional family history argue in favor of it and raise the possibility of a familial form of pheochromocytoma.

> An abdominal CT scan was unremarkable, showing normal adrenal glands.

From 90% to 95% of pheochromocytomas are in the adrenal gland. If the CT scan was care-

fully done and read, then the probability of his having a pheochromocytoma drops quite substantially. Needless to say, the patient could have a small tumor in the adrenal or a pheochromocytoma in locations other than the adrenal, such as the chest, bladder, or paraganglionic region. Pheochromocytoma is less likely, but the question is how much less likely. I would review the CT scan with an expert.

> Because of this confusing picture, the patient was referred to an endocrinologist. Careful inquiry by the endocrinologist disclosed that neither the patient's brother nor his father had had a pheochromocytoma. On close questioning, the patient indicated that his initial urine collection included the first morning voiding on both the day the collection began and the day it ended. The total creatinine in that specimen had been 3.3 g for this 102-kg man. A repeated 24-hour urine test revealed normal excretion of fractionated catecholamines (epinephrine <5 pg, norepinephrine 41 pg, dopamine, 327 pg). The total creatinine in that specimen was 2.3 g. The endocrinologist believed that urinary catecholamines offered the best screening test for a pheochromocytoma and, given his low level of suspicion, thought that no further testing was necessary. The urinary VMA test was not repeated.
>
> Given the patient's labile blood pressure and inconsistent response to drugs, the endocrinologist thought that there was a substantial degree of "white-coat hypertension." A trial of behavior modification therapy was suggested. The patient seemed pleased with this and returned to his referring physician for follow-up.

If you look back at the discrepant laboratory studies, the negative CT scan, and the accurate family history, the likelihood of a pheochromocytoma becomes remarkably small. Imagine what a better history taking would have accomplished in this patient! Both the abnormal VMA excretion and the pseudo family history could have been discovered, saving substantial expense and aggravation.

> The patient's blood pressure remained labile. One year later, it was 140/80 to 140/85 mm Hg

> when taken by a nurse, but it was as high as 150/100 mm Hg when taken by a physician. No medications were prescribed.

Analysis

Hypertension is ubiquitous, affecting about 15% to 40% of the population.[165] Identifying a reversible cause is a prize obtained in only 1 or 2 of every 100 hypertensive patients, but finding a pheochromocytoma, an entity with a prevalence of 14 per 10,000 hypertensive patients,[166] carries for the patient a chance of curing a potentially fatal condition and for the physician the intellectual thrill of "bagging a big one." Most primary care providers may see only a couple of adults with pheochromocytoma in their professional lifetimes. When the armamentarium of antihypertensive drugs was smaller, less potent, and far more likely to produce intolerable side effects, we often searched for secondary hypertension beneath every blood-pressure cuff. For the last 2 decades, however, we have been more selective in our workups, reserving screening for young patients, those with severe or poorly controlled hypertension, and those with symptoms, signs, or routine laboratory evidence that points strongly to a secondary cause.[167] The triad of headache, sweating, and tachycardia occurs in 90% of patients with pheochromocytomas but in only 6% of other patients with hypertension.[168]

Although experts may disagree about the optimal way to screen for a pheochromocytoma, labile blood pressure that is poorly controlled by a variety of agents is sufficient justification to begin the search. Here, urine was collected for VMA testing, and a level more than twice the upper limit of normal was found. Although urinary VMA levels are less likely to be falsely elevated by drugs and diet than are urinary catecholamine levels, no test is perfect, and one must pause to reflect on the implications of an abnormal result, even a very abnormal one. The interpretation of any imperfect diagnostic test (or for that matter any clinical information) depends both on the characteristics of the test (its sensitivity and specificity) and on the probability of disease before the test result is revealed. Because the probability of pheochromocytoma in a patient with poorly controlled hypertension who does not have weight loss, paroxysms of sweating, or palpitations is not precisely known, the clinician often makes an intuitive estimate. However, the heuristics (rules of thumb) we use to judge the likelihood of diseases such as pheochromocytoma may well produce a substantial overestimate because of the salient features of the tumor, its therapeutic importance, and the intellectual attraction of making the diagnosis. Even with a markedly elevated level of VMA excretion, confirmation is essential because many other diseases mimic pheochromocytoma.

When a relatively unexpected (but not urgently abnormal) laboratory value is obtained, the clinician has several confirmatory strategies available: The test can be repeated (as suggested by the discussant), a supplemental or confirmatory test can be performed, or treatment can be initiated, either as a diagnostic or as a diagnostic and therapeutic maneuver. The choice of strategy depends on urgency, risk, cost, and even the clinician's style. In most scientific endeavors, measurements are replicated, and measured responses are calculated as means and variances. In individual patients, however, physicians must often react to single values, and they respond, more often than not, by ordering expensive and perhaps even risky tests and therapies. Leaving aside life-threatening abnormalities that require urgent action, when should one simply repeat a test with an abnormal result and when should one move down the diagnostic or therapeutic path? The answer depends on the information the various alternatives could provide in a patient known to have an abnormal test result, as well as on the risks and costs. The most likely result of simply repeating the urinary VMA test would be either a similar value, although one perhaps not quite as abnormal because of the sampling phenomenon of regression toward the mean,[169] or a normal result, suggesting that the initial abnormality may have been a laboratory error. Even if the repeated VMA test was normal and the prevalence of disease low, the physician might still feel compelled to examine a third collection or perform another test to "break the tie." On the other hand, a confirmatory test whose results are linked to whether a pheochromocytoma is present and not to the results of the initial VMA test (e.g., an abdominal CT scan) can sometimes provide much more information whether it confirms *or* refutes the VMA determination. The choice of diagnostic

TABLE 15.1

Characteristics of Tests for Pheochromocytoma

Test	Sensitivity (%)	Specificity (%)	Likelihood Ratio[a] Positive Result	Likelihood Ratio[a] Negative Result	Reference
Vanillylmandelic acid excretion	81	97	27	0.20	Young et al.,[173] Kaplan[170]
Catecholamine excretion	82	95	16.4	0.19	Bravo,[168] Kaplan[170]
Metanephrine excretion	83	95	16.6	0.18	Young et al.,[173] Kaplan[170]
Abdominal computed tomography scan	92	80	4.6	0.10	Kaplan,[170] Feldman,[171] Stewart et al.[172]

[a] The likelihood ratio for a positive result is the sensitivity divided by 1 minus the specificity; the ratio for a negative result is 1 minus the sensitivity divided by the specificity.

strategy can be problematic, however, because confirmatory procedures are often more expensive and more risky than simply repeating the original test. Here, the confirmatory urine-chemistry tests are riskless and are in fact hardly more expensive than a second VMA test, each costing less than $30. Neither the urinary catecholamine tests nor the abdominal CT scan (which costs substantially more) confirmed the diagnostic hypothesis of pheochromocytoma.

As each new clinical fact is uncovered, the physician should ask two questions. First, does the new information increase or decrease the likelihood of each diagnostic hypothesis? Second, how much does the new information change the likelihood? The information provided by a test result can be summarized as the ratio of two conditional likelihoods: the likelihood of that result in patients who have the disease under consideration and the likelihood of that result in patients who do not have the disease. Likelihood ratios can range from zero to infinity. Ratios greater than 1 indicate an increased likelihood of disease; the larger the ratio, the greater is the increase. Ratios less than 1 indicate a decreased likelihood of disease; the smaller the ratio, the greater is the decrease. A ratio of exactly 1 implies that the test result provides no diagnostic information. The probability of a positive test result in patients with disease is, of course,

the sensitivity of the test. The probability of a positive test result in patients without disease is, similarly, the false-positive rate, or 1 − specificity. For a positive test result (i.e., one that increases the likelihood of disease), the likelihood ratio is then (sensitivity)/(1 − specificity). For a negative result (i.e., one that decreases the likelihood of disease), the likelihood ratio is (1 − sensitivity)/(specificity). In Table 15.1,[170−173] we summarize the sensitivity, specificity, and likelihood ratios for each of the four tests that presented the diagnostic problem.

The joint likelihood ratio for a combination of test results is simply the product of the separate ratios,[174] assuming that the likelihood of one test's being positive in patients with disease is not affected by whether another of the tests is also positive.[175] For the three urine tests that presented the problem here, there are eight such combinations, and the joint likelihood ratios are shown in Table 15.2. In this case, the ratios are roughly related to the number of abnormal test results. If all three tests are positive, the joint likelihood ratio is 7,400, which would make the presence of a pheochromocytoma virtually certain. If two tests are positive, the likelihood ratio is between 53 and 85, which would raise the likelihood of disease substantially. If only one test is positive, the joint likelihood ratio is between 0.6 and 0.92, which would

---

TABLE 15.2

Likelihood Ratios Favoring Pheochromocytoma for Combinations of Urine-Test Results

Vanillylmandelic acid Excretion	Catecholamine Excretion	Metanephrine Excretion	Number of Abnormal Results	Likelihood Ratio
Elevated	Elevated	Elevated	3	7,400
Elevated	Normal	Elevated	2	85
Elevated	Elevated	Normal	2	79
Normal	Elevated	Elevated	2	53
Elevated	**Normal**	**Normal**	**1**	**0.92**
Normal	Normal	Elevated	1	0.6
Normal	Elevated	Normal	1	0.6
Normal	Normal	Normal	0	0.007

Boldface type indicates the results in the patient under study.

---

lower the likelihood slightly. If not one of the tests is abnormal, the joint likelihood ratio is 0.007, which would make pheochromocytoma approximately 150 times less likely.

One can interpret tests—combining the likelihood ratio of a test result with the prior likelihood of disease—using Bayes' rule, which states that the likelihood of disease in a patient with a given set of findings can be estimated as the proportion of patients with the same findings who also have the disease. This sequential process is most easily accomplished by constructing a small table,[176] as shown in Table 15.3. Column A contains the prior likelihoods—in other words, the chances of disease before the test result is known, which, in the absence of clinical information, is the prevalence of disease. Column B contains the likelihood ratios, in this case relative to the chance of the observed result in patients without disease. By definition, the entry in column B corresponding to the absence of pheochromocytoma is 1. For each row in the table, column C is the product of columns A and B.

TABLE 15.3

Using Bayes' Rule to Interpret Diagnostic Tests

	A. Prior Likelihood of Disease	B. Conditional Likelihood of Finding	C. Product (A × B)	D. Revised Percent Likelihood (C/Sum × 100)
Typical patient with hypertension				
Pheochromocytoma	14	27	378	**3.6**
No pheochromocytoma	9986	1	9,986	**96.4**
Sum			10,364	
Patient under study				
Pheochromocytoma	1	0.92	0.92	**0.9**
No pheochromocytoma	99	1	99.00	**99.1**
Sum			99.92	

For the typical patient with hypertension, the finding is an elevated vanillylmandelic acid (VMA) level; for the patient under study, it is an elevated VMA level plus normal catecholamine and metanephrine levels.

Also in column C are the sums of these products. Finally, column D contains the quotients of each product and that sum. Each quotient represents the revised probability of the diagnosis—that is, the probability based on both the prior information and the test result. The first part of Table 15.3 demonstrates how this technique can be applied to interpreting an elevated 24-hour VMA level in a population of unselected hypertensive patients, among whom the prevalence of pheochromocytoma is 14 in 10,000 (0.14%).[166] The joint likelihood ratio (27) is greater than 1, and, as seen in column D, the chance of pheochromocytoma increases from 0.14% to 3.6%. Incidentally, if the urinary VMA excretion were normal (with a likelihood ratio of 0.20), the chance of pheochromocytoma would be less than 3 in 10,000 (0.03%).

In the patient described here, both confirmatory urine tests failed to support the diagnosis of pheochromocytoma. As seen in Table 15.2, the joint likelihood ratio for the three results is 0.92, a value very close to 1, implying that the two negative confirmatory tests together balance the effect of the elevated VMA level. The prevalence of pheochromocytoma among patients referred for scintigraphy or CT scanning is approximately 6%.[173] The chance that this far-less-typical patient has a pheochromocytoma must be lower. For the sake of illustration, in Table 15.3 we assume a prior probability of 1%, a value higher than the prevalence of pheochromocytoma in unselected hypertensive patients. As seen in column D, the revised likelihood is approximately 0.9%. Had the clinician performed this calculation, he would probably not have prescribed phenoxybenzamine. As the case evolved, the negative abdominal CT scan (with a likelihood ratio of 0.1) reduced the likelihood of pheochromocytoma even further, to 0.09%. Finally, the normal fractionated catecholamine excretion made the chance of a tumor virtually zero.

With these likelihood ratios and Bayes' rule in hand, we are now in a position to consider the diagnostic implications of simply repeating the VMA test and obtaining a normal value on the second determination. Many physicians might reason that the positive and negative results would cancel each other out, leaving simply the initial low likelihood of pheochromocytoma. However, such reasoning would be wrong. As seen in Table 15.1, the like-

lihood ratio for an elevated VMA level is 27, and the likelihood ratio for a normal VMA level is 0.20. If we consider the two collections to be independent tests, the joint likelihood ratio is 5.4 (27 × 0.2), not 1.0, and the combination of a normal and an abnormal result makes the chance of pheochromocytoma some five times higher than before the VMA determinations were performed. In general, if a test is repeated and the two results differ (one positive and one negative), the results cancel each other out only if the test's sensitivity and specificity are equal.[177] The simple heuristic method of counting the number of positive and negative results is incorrect because it assumes that sensitivity and specificity are equal.

Astute clinicians will recognize some sleight of hand in the foregoing calculations. The patient's VMA excretion was more than double the upper limit of normal, not simply above that limit. Values of more than 20 mg/day were found in 25% of one series of patients with pheochromocytoma.[178] Such values are almost six standard deviations (SDs) above the mean of the normal range, making their chance occurrence in a patient without pheochromocytoma seem most unlikely. Obviously, errors in urine collection must occur more frequently than one time in a billion, and the likelihood of a result so far above the mean of a normal distribution is a substantial underestimate of the chance of this finding in a hypertensive patient without a pheochromocytoma. The explanation for this discrepancy is that patients with either inadequate or, as was the case here, excessive urine collections do not appear in published series. We rarely acknowledge this important omission.

The incorrect urine collection only partially explains this urinary VMA level. In a 100-kg man, creatinine excretion should be 2.0 to 2.6 g/day[179] (as was found in the second collection), suggesting that the initial collection was perhaps 50% too large. If we adjust the VMA excretion for the creatinine (assuming that both excretions are in the same proportion throughout the day), we have a VMA excretion of approximately 14 mg/day, a value still above the upper limit of normal. However, that level would not be markedly abnormal, and the Bayesian analysis performed here would be even more comforting and consistent with the consulting endocrinologist's decision not to repeat the study. Had that not been the case, the next step in the diagnostic evaluation would perhaps have been a clonidine suppression test or another imaging study, such as iodine-131 metaiodobenzylguanidine scintigraphy,[180] to attempt to localize the tumor.

Although the most common causes of unusual test results are random variation and laboratory error, clinicians should continue to hunt for unusual and therapeutically important game. Hoofbeats usually signal the presence of horses, but the judicious application of Bayes' rule can help prevent clinicians from being trampled by a stampeding herd that occasionally includes a zebra.

CASE 24. SHORT-CIRCUITING THE DIAGNOSTIC PROCESS

> A 63-year-old man sought medical attention for anorexia, abdominal pain, and weight loss. Six months before, he had begun to have diffuse, burning abdominal pain that was associated with nausea and early satiety and was aggravated by eating. During this period, he lost 40 pounds. He also noted increased frequency of defecation and occasional bloody diarrhea.

Diffuse, burning abdominal pain associated with nausea and early satiety suggests a gastric problem, although we are not told where the pain is localized. Early satiety is one of the early symptoms of gastric cancer, but that, of course, is not the only possible explanation.

In addition, he has occasional bloody diarrhea. We are not told how many bowel movements a day he has, which might give us a clue as to whether this is a secretory type of diarrhea. We might be making a case for pancreatic disease here. We clearly need to examine the patient at this point.

> Vital signs were as follows: blood pressure 145/75 mm Hg with no orthostatic changes, pulse 122 per minute, respirations 18 per minute, temperature 37°C. The patient was cachectic but not in acute distress. His abdomen was slightly distended and diffusely tender. Bowel sounds were normal. There was voluntary guarding, but no organs or masses were palpable. No bruits or pulsations were detected.

> The rest of the examination was normal. Stool was guaiac positive.

So now I think we have clearly focused on the possibility that this man has a primary abdominal problem, probably located somewhere around the pancreas. I guess you worry a great deal about carcinoma of the pancreas in such a patient, with a gradual downhill course over a period of months and a lot of weight loss. You rarely feel such a tumor. The guaiac-positive stool might make sense if he had a lesion of the ampulla, but it may also be a red herring. We see a lot of positive stool guaiacs. If you routinely test the stool for blood in all patients who do not have any symptoms, approximately 2% of them are positive, so false-positive results are fairly common.

> Laboratory data: hemoglobin 12.2 g/dL, hematocrit 36%, WBC 35,000 with 85 polys, 3 bands, 8 lymphocytes, and 4 monos. Platelet count was 812,000, and blood glucose was 135 mg/dL. BUN and creatinine were normal, and electrolytes were normal except for serum potassium of 3 mEq/L. Calcium was 6.3 mg/dL, phosphorus 1.7 mg/dL, and albumin 1.9 gm/dL. Liver function studies were normal except for an alkaline phosphatase of 204 IU/L. Serum amylase was 64 IU/L.

His hematocrit is slightly low, and his white count is quite high: It almost qualifies as a leukemoid reaction. He also has a marked left shift. I will assume that the cells are normal and that he does not have a myeloproliferative disorder. Remember that this man is afebrile, he has had a chronic course, and he looks chronically ill, so it is hard to believe that such a white count reflects active infection. For these reasons, I suspect this is most likely a leukemoid reaction. My suspicion of malignancy is very high, but we will go on.

His serum calcium is a little low, but he clearly has marked hypoalbuminemia caused by either dietary factors or protein loss. We have to find out which. Protein could be lost either through the gastrointestinal tract or perhaps through the kidney. I will assume his urinalysis is normal and, therefore, that he either is losing albumin in the gut or has marked malnutrition secondary to a poor appetite, which may be more likely.

The liver function tests are within normal limits. Alkaline phosphatase is mildly elevated. His amylase is normal. The alkaline phosphatase is helpful because it suggests some ductal obstruction, although his other liver function studies are normal. I think at this point that we have focused the problem to the mid-epigastrium, probably to the pancreas, in a man who certainly seems to have malignancy. My first diagnosis is cancer of the pancreas.

> **Results of the initial studies: abdominal ultrasound normal (no masses or aneurysm); abdominal CT, distended stomach with partial obstruction; upper gastrointestinal (GI) series, pyloric narrowing.**

The ultrasound and CT really have not helped us very much. It is a bit of a disappointment if we are considering carcinoma of the pancreas, although I would not be dissuaded from that diagnosis on the basis of these studies if I really felt that that was what he had. Some pancreatic cancers are hard to see. CT, in my experience, is much better than ultrasound in making this diagnosis, so a negative study is a point against the diagnosis of pancreatic cancer. Pyloric narrowing probably is an important clue, especially given his symptom of early satiety. Could this man have a gastric carcinoma or perhaps a pancreatic carcinoma involving that area? Given these findings, I would do a gastroscopy.

> **Gastroscopy revealed an infiltrating adenocarcinoma of the stomach.**

That is interesting because I cannot remember the last time I saw a patient with gastric carcinoma. That disease is rare now in the United States, and I think the decline in incidence is continuing. On the other hand, the incidence is very high in Japan.

Analysis

Willie Sutton, the infamous bank robber, would have shaken his head in disbelief over this patient's workup. Sutton, when asked why he robbed banks, replied, "That's where the money is." Sutton was anathema to the police but has become a cult hero to those who prize diagnostic expertise. Sutton's law, although fallible, assumes that a physician should be able to order the test most likely to reveal the correct diagnosis (see case 16). Its adherents would argue that the right test, virtually from the beginning of the history, would have been a gastroscopy and that most of the other tests were superfluous. They would decry the diagnostic strategy in this case as the "shotgun" approach.

On review of the patient's workup, it is difficult to deny that some unnecessary tests were done. Yet, aside from the expense, the patient really was not exposed to substantial risks. So why the fuss? Is the concern for excessive testing in this patient simply making a mountain out of a molehill? Is it much ado about nothing? We think not. Our vigilance in deterring excessive testing must be maintained not only to control costs but also to avoid possible complications.

First, let us review the diagnostic strategy and consider how it might have differed. In particular, how might a more direct approach have evolved? The discussant raised the possibility of gastric cancer with a minimum of clinical data, including symptoms of anorexia, burning abdominal pain aggravated by eating, and early satiety. Yet he dismissed the importance of the guaiac-positive stools and focused instead on the possibility of pancreatic cancer. Probably neither the discussant nor the physicians responsible for the patient should have bypassed that diagnosis so readily, because the alternative diagnoses suggested did not explain the findings in the patient nearly as well. Gastric cancer would have explained all the patient's findings; pancreatic cancer would be a far less likely explanation.

Given a reasonable suspicion of gastric cancer at the outset, what would constitute an appropriate workup? Let us take a radical viewpoint for the sake of having a target at which to shoot. Let us argue that the first, most appropriate step was immediate gastroscopy. This strategy is the essence of Sutton's law: Go for the money. Although it strikes us as eminently reasonable, its appropriateness is principally a function of how strongly one believed, on the basis of the patient's initial complaints, that gastric cancer was a likely possibility. We get some indication at the end of the transcript why the discussant abandoned his provisional diagnosis of gastric cancer, even though the clinical manifestations were classic. In an afterthought, once he has been told of the correct diagnosis, the discussant explains that he cannot remember having seen a patient with gastric cancer in some time and that the tumor has become uncommon.

Although his decision to drop the diagnosis of gastric cancer may seem appropriate in view of his correct assessment of its low prior probability, the characteristic symptoms and findings (bleeding) probably should have been sufficient to keep that diagnosis active; gastroscopy might then have been an appropriate next step. Indeed, one could even raise the question of whether this procedure should have been carried out before all the routine tests were available (except, perhaps, for the hematocrit). Too often, we are locked into our traditional diagnostic strategies (first take a complete history, then do a complete physical examination, then do the routine laboratory tests, then choose the nonroutine tests). We should be willing to give up this traditional approach when it is opportune to do so. In this case, the risk of gastroscopy is very small, and its ability to diagnose gastric cancer is quite good. Because of those advantages, the threshold—that is the diagnostic suspicion of gastric cancer required to recommend gastroscopy—is quite low; even with a rather low level of suspicion, gastroscopy would have been an appropriate choice.[59]

What would immediate gastroscopy have accomplished? Many of the tests that were done would have had to be performed eventually to assess the extent of the patient's malignant disease. Specifically, routine blood tests, liver function studies, and CT scan would have been required, but some tests might have been avoided, and the patient and his family would have known the answer a little sooner. It is difficult in this case to imagine any therapeutic gain from this short-cut in the workup, although such a gain certainly is conceivable in other situations.

In the patient described here, the correct diagnosis was made after his physicians ordered a "battery" of tests designed to uncover an unknown abdominal ailment: ultrasound, CT scan, upper GI series, and, finally, gastroscopy (when the upper GI series and CT scan focused attention back to the stomach). The patient did not sustain any untoward consequences of excessive testing, but in this respect, we simply can consider him fortunate. In case 29, we describe a patient who was led on a diagnostic wild goose chase by a series of vague, slightly positive radiologic images. That patient experienced considerable anxiety about the several "positive" tests. In other cases, the consequences of unnecessary diagnostic tests might be even more distressing.

If our discussant and the patient's physicians had accepted the initial complaints and clinical findings as credible, a more direct approach might have been adopted, even though, admittedly, the prior probability of gastric cancer was low. The prevalence of gastric cancer may be declining rapidly in the United States, but as we have seen here, the disease has not disappeared.

CASE 25. THE BYPASS ON THE WAY TO THE BYPASS

> A 47-year-old man consulted a physician for heartburn brought on by exertion and relieved with rest or burping. He had experienced the symptoms for 3 months.

This patient is the appropriate sex and age to be a prime candidate for coronary disease, but he could have gastrointestinal disease. It is interesting that the sensation is described as "heartburn" because the word obviously suggests the possibility of a problem with either the heart or the gastrointestinal tract. Nonetheless, the fact that the discomfort is exertional and relieved by rest makes angina more likely. Burping can be a function of upper gastrointestinal distress, such as gastroesophageal reflux, but it also can be related to cardiac disease. I would lean toward a cardiac origin.

> The discomfort did not radiate and was not associated with shortness of breath or palpitations. It had not occurred at rest. There was no apparent relationship to food intake. The patient had no history of heart disease, but he did have long-standing hypertension that recently had been brought under control with an angiotensin-converting-enzyme (ACE) inhibitor, a beta-blocker, and a diuretic. Evaluation of the hypertension had revealed a physiologically insignificant right renal artery stenosis. The patient had smoked one pack of cigarettes a day for many years. His father had died at age 49 years during open-heart surgery.

His mother and two of his three siblings had myocardial infarctions at early ages.

The lack of radiation of the pain and the lack of dyspnea and palpitations slightly diminish the likelihood that the pain is cardiac in nature, but we must remember that the characteristics of angina can be extremely variable. Pain did not occur at rest. Angina at rest could be a sign of instability or impending infarction. The lack of apparent relation to food intake does not rule out gallbladder disease, pancreatic disease, gastroesophageal reflux, or ulcer disease, but it does make them less likely.

Even though we are told that the patient has no history of heart disease, it is my guess that he does have it. I view any history of hypertension, be it long-standing or of short duration, as a positive cardiac history. Control of his hypertension required several drugs, including the ACE inhibitor, which suggests that the hypertension was moderately severe. It would not surprise me if he had both significant coronary disease and left ventricular hypertrophy. The fact that he is on a diuretic also raises the issue of hypokalemia, although ACE inhibitors tend to raise serum potassium.

The patient is a smoker. Too bad, because that adds the worst risk factor for coronary disease to the second nastiest, hypertension. Even without a family history, this fellow has at least a six-to-eight-fold greater risk of coronary disease than do subjects of the same age, sex, and weight who are normotensive and do not smoke.

His father died at age 49 years during open-heart surgery, but I would consider that history relevant only if it were coronary surgery. However, the fact that his mother and two of his three siblings had myocardial infarctions represents an extremely strong family history, even if his father did not die as a consequence of coronary disease. Now we have to wonder why there is so much coronary disease in this family at such an early age. We need to know whether there is a predisposition, such as hyperlipidemia or diabetes.

Given his suggestive symptoms, the strong family history, and his hypertension and smoking—even before any further diagnostic tests—I would estimate the probability of his having coronary disease to be 70% to 80%, maybe even

90%. Whether it is significant coronary disease is another issue, which would need to be evaluated.

On physical examination, blood pressure was 120/90 mm Hg, pulse was 66 per minute and regular, and weight was 110 kg. Lungs were clear. Cardiac examination was normal, with no murmurs or gallops. Soft bilateral carotid bruits were noted. The abdomen was benign. The rest of the examination was normal. Complete blood count, creatinine, electrolytes, glucose, and cholesterol were normal. Urinalysis was also normal. Electrocardiogram revealed normal sinus rhythm with nonspecific ST and T-wave changes.

The physical examination adds another risk factor to our patient—namely, obesity—and the carotid bruits raise the possibility that he has diffuse vascular disease. The rest of the examination was unremarkable, although I would have expected him to have an S_4 gallop. I did not expect to gain much information from the physical examination because it often is normal in patients with extensive coronary artery disease.

The initial laboratory evaluation also is not very helpful. He does not have overt diabetes, and his cholesterol is normal. The electrocardiogram is nonspecific, but I still think the patient has coronary artery disease.

What should be done next in this case is an interesting question. Many physicians would reflexively order an exercise tolerance test and, if it was positive, proceed to cardiac catheterization. If the test was negative, they would do a more elaborate exercise study. Finally, if all tests were negative, they would sit around and worry about what to do. As I interpret this patient's findings, I think his chance of coronary disease is so high that I might well skip the exercise tolerance test and recommend coronary angiography directly. I probably would do a coronary angiogram even if all the noninvasive studies were negative. Despite all the criticisms of coronary surgery, I believe it to be highly effective—and I am not even a surgeon! So we really should find out whether this patient has an operable lesion.

A stress test was carried out. During stage 1 of the test, the exercise reproduced the patient's

substernal burning, but there were no electrocardiogram (ECG) changes (65% target heart rate). The patient exercised for 5 minutes and stopped because of fatigue. During the first 2 minutes of the recovery period, 1-mm ST depression in leads II, aVF, and V$_{4-6}$ developed and persisted for 3 minutes. Neither arrhythmias nor hypotension occurred.

I am not surprised that the patient's heart rate did not increase much, since he was receiving beta-blockers, and exercise never proceeded beyond stage 1. The fact that his pain was reproduced in stage 1 is enormously significant and indicates that he does have angina. I am not quite sure what to make of the lack of early ECG changes, again because he was tested while on beta-blockers and achieved only stage 1 exercise. However, he did have ECG changes during the recovery period, and they persisted for a long time. Sometimes one sees changes during the exercise period and sometimes during recovery. Clearly, the test was positive, and cardiac catheterization certainly is in order now. I still think we wasted hundred of dollars by doing the stress test.

Cardiac catheterization revealed 95% midright coronary artery stenosis, 50% mid-left anterior descending artery stenosis, 25% proximal first obtuse marginal artery stenosis, and 100% proximal second obtuse marginal artery stenosis. Ventricular function was normal.

The 25% lesion is not significant, and the 50% lesion is marginal, so basically we can consider the patient to have two-vessel coronary disease and normal ventricular function. What should be done? I am not sure I know.[181] If he had symptoms that were not responsive to medical therapy, I would do an invasive procedure. Notice that I said "medical therapy," not maximal medical therapy. Maximal medical therapy is likely to make the patient so miserable and symptomatic that it might compromise his lifestyle sufficiently to push us toward more invasive therapy, that is, either percutaneous coronary intervention or bypass surgery. My first choice would be stenting if the lesions were approachable, but I would have to get the advice of an expert in this procedure.

If the lesions are not accessible to percutaneous approaches, the question is whether to perform bypass surgery. If he were symptomatic, there is no doubt that I would recommend surgery. If medical therapy controlled his symptoms with only minimal side effects, the decision would be problematic. In terms of survival, mixed results have been documented in such patients. A 2007 meta-analysis suggested that there is no significant gain,[182] but other studies report some gain in surgically treated patients.[183] This is not an easy choice. If you wished to define what he has as single-vessel disease, a bypass graft would not be indicated to prolong survival. If he had three-vessel disease, left main disease, two-vessel disease with a severe left anterior descending lesion, or a proximal left anterior descending lesion (the so-called widowmaker), I would recommend bypass surgery. But the choice in two-vessel disease involving the mid-right coronary artery is not easy to make. If his symptoms were readily controlled, I probably would go no further.

The patient was treated with long-acting nitrates, with marked improvement in his symptoms. The lesions appeared to be accessible to coronary stenting, and if angina increased despite medical therapy, coronary artery stenting was planned.

I think that plan is reasonable. I suspect that if one presented the same patient to many different cardiologists, opinions as to how to best manage his coronary artery disease would not be uniform.[184] In fact, although many would decide "on paper" not to recommend invasive therapy, in practice the great majority would recommend stenting or surgery. Because the decision is a close call, many physicians bow to societal pressures and to patients' preferences in making the final choice. None of us is particularly pleased about the ambiguity that surrounds the treatment of this kind of patient. But decisions still have to be made.

Analysis

Of the many interesting features of the problem-solving process illustrated by this session, one of the issues raised involves the decision to perform a common diagnostic test, namely, whether to conduct a stress test before resorting to cardiac catheterization. The physicians responsible for the patient's care performed the test: The discussant would have bypassed it. Some reasons for the difference in approach form the basis for this commentary.

Many factors drive the decision to conduct diagnostic tests, including the accuracy of the test results, the clinical suspicion that a patient has the condition being sought, the value of the therapeutic choice dictated by the test result, the risk of the test, and the cost of the test. Which of those elements apply here? The discussant raised cost as an issue, but only to bolster his view that the test was unnecessary. He did not cite risk as a serious concern, and he hardly mentioned the accuracy of the test. Indeed, the main issues here are the clinical suspicion that a patient has the condition being sought and the value of the therapeutic choice dictated by the test result. We have no way of knowing whether the physicians caring for the patient had a different view from that of the discussant about the probability of coronary disease in this patient. The fact that they proceeded with stress testing and catheterization certainly illustrates that their suspicion was high. But how high? Not high enough, we might presume, to convince them to proceed directly with cardiac catheterization.

Is that the only reason for the different approach? We think not. We think that a major factor is the attitude of the discussant toward the efficacy of therapy for coronary disease. Consider two physicians—one who believes that a treatment is highly effective, and the other who believes that the same treatment is only moderately effective. The first should be willing to treat when the suspicion of the disease is only moderately high, and the second should be willing to treat only when he or she is quite sure that the patient has the disease.[59] In this case, recommendation of cardiac catheterization is tantamount to a treatment decision because the results of catheterization dictate whether to proceed with surgery. (Admittedly, there are differences of opinion about the value of bypass grafts for some lesions,[185,186] as brought out in the discussion of this patient, but for purposes of exposition, we will assume that no difference of opinion exists with respect to surgical indications.) It is our presumption, therefore, based on the strong statements by the discussant favoring surgery for coronary disease, that his view of therapy is a commanding issue.

He proceeds directly to cardiac catheterization not only because he has an extremely high suspicion of coronary disease (and would not be dissuaded by a negative stress test from his decision to catheterize), but also because he thinks that the patient who does have a surgically treatable lesion will derive considerable benefit from coronary artery bypass. Presumably, the same principles apply to coronary angioplasty, which is an alternative therapeutic approach considered briefly.

CASE 26: IT IS WHAT YOU BELIEVE THAT COUNTS

> **A 70-year-old man presented with new exertional shortness of breath and substernal chest pressure for 5 days.**

We have a new pulmonary and chest symptom in a 70-year-old man. He has two things against him, first, he is a man, and second, he is 70 years old. We are not told any other medical history, including risk factors for heart disease or lung disease, but at the top of the list would be exertional angina. In his differential diagnosis, exertional angina would be at the top of the list in terms of likelihood, but in addition, I would consider other lung pathology or even esophageal reflux disease and other common entities.

> **The patient was a retired policeman and usually took long walks two or three times a week. These new symptoms occurred after walking 25 to 30 yards and were relieved with rest after a few minutes. The pain did not radiate. He felt slightly dizzy during these episodes. He had no nausea, vomiting, diaphoresis, nocturnal dyspnea, orthopnea, or pain at rest.**

The exertional nature of these symptoms and the fact that they were relieved with rest after a few minutes are consistent with angina. Since he had previously taken long walks without any difficulty, it is suggestive that he has developed progressive stenosis of his coronary arteries. The absence of the other symptoms except for slight dizziness does not necessarily lower the likelihood of the cardiac diagnosis.

The patient had a history of diabetes mellitus with peripheral neuropathy, hypertension, hypercholesterolemia, benign prostatic hypertrophy, gout, and nephrolithiasis. Five years ago, he was admitted to a hospital for syncope, which was attributed to hypoglycemia. At that time, his echocardiogram was normal; ejection fraction was 60%. Four years ago, he had a normal nuclear stress test.

The top ten diagnoses now are all exertional angina given his history of diabetes, hypertension and hypercholesterolemia. The only thing missing here is a smoking history. At least some of these common risk factors are seen in the vast majority of patients with coronary artery disease. The negative nuclear stress test 4 years earlier suggests that he probably did not have disease at that time, at least not hemodynamically significant disease. The stress test has a sensitivity of approximately 80% to 85% and a specificity of about 90% in a man. However, he could have had less than 70% stenosis at that time that has now progressed to more than 70% stenosis, leading to his exertional angina. These findings would represent slowly progressive atherosclerotic disease, as opposed to what is seen with sudden death or an acute myocardial infarction. At this point, I would perform another nuclear stress test.

Review of systems was otherwise noncontributory. He did not smoke. He had a remote history of excessive alcohol consumption. Medications on admission included insulin, atorvastatin, lisinopril, terazosin, pioglitazone, and aspirin.

The absence of smoking helps a little bit, but as I mentioned before, he has all the other important risk factors for coronary disease. Given these risk factors, his target LDL (low-density lipoprotein) cholesterol should be less than 100 mg/dL—some would say less than 70 mg/dL—given the fact that he is diabetic.

Aspirin is obviously indicated because he is in the high-risk group for heart attack and stroke, given his diabetes and hypertension.

On physical exam, he was in no distress. Blood pressure 158/60 mm Hg and nonpostural. Pulse

72 per minute and regular. Respirations 20 per minute. O_2 saturation was 98% on room air. General physical examination was unremarkable. Lungs were clear. Cardiac examination showed a soft 1/6 systolic murmur, which he had had before.

The physical exam is notable for systolic hypertension. In someone with diabetes and a history of hypertension, you would aim to have a systolic blood pressure goal of 125 or even 120. The remainder of his exam is pretty much noncontributory. At this point, I am looking forward to other laboratory tests and probably an exercise test.

Laboratory data: Electrolytes, BUN, creatinine, and CBC were normal. Electrocardiogram was normal. Chest x-ray was unremarkable. Recent cholesterol was 185 mg/dL with high-density-lipoprotein (HDL) cholesterol of 51 mg/dL. Recent hemoglobin A1c was 7.6%. Initial creatine kinase (CK) and troponin levels were normal.

There are no acute ischemic changes on his ECG. His biochemical markers CK (MB presumably) and troponin were also negative. His hemoglobin A1c of 7.6% reflects only moderately well controlled diabetes. Ideally, we would aim for an A1c of less than 7%. We are not given his LDL cholesterol, but he is probably pretty close to an LDL cholesterol of 100.

The patient's doctor was concerned that this man was presenting with new onset angina pectoris. Three sets of cardiac enzymes were negative. An exercise stress test was ordered for the next day.

One issue would be whether to order the exercise stress test with or without imaging. In this particular case, given the high suspicion for the presence of new angina, I would likely order the test with imaging, increasing the sensitivity of the exercise test from perhaps 60% up to as high as 85%.

The patient exercised for 7 minutes on a Bruce protocol to a heart rate of 120 per minute, which was 80% of his predicted heart rate. He had no chest pain or ECG changes during the test. The

> **perfusion scan was normal with no defects. Left ventricular ejection fraction was 56%.**

So this man has clinical symptoms that are highly suggestive of exertional angina, but he has a "negative" exercise test. Factors that are under-appreciated about exercise tests are the duration of exercise and the implications for prognosis. In particular, he only achieved 80% of his predicted heart rate. Based on his symptoms and his risk factors, I would still have a very high suspicion for exertional angina. The issue at this point could be summarized as follows: Would I treat the patient for presumed exertional angina with medications or would I recommend cardiac catheterization? I would probably feel comfortable enough saying that this is exertional angina even with a relatively negative exercise test. I would probably attempt to manage his new angina medically. I would probably add a beta-blocker to his regimen. In addition, I would probably drive his LDL cholesterol lower, toward 70 if he could tolerate statins without myalgias or hepatitis. And I would probably prescribe nitroglycerin and warn him to present promptly with recurrence of his symptoms if they recurred and were unrelieved by rest and/or nitroglycerin. But if I had to guess, he probably will get a cardiac catheterization.

> **The doctor was concerned that the scan could be a false-negative test in this high-risk individual and asked for a cardiologist's opinion regarding cardiac catheterization.**

The issue here is whether the cardiac catheterization would change management and benefit this 70-year-old man. I feel comfortable with a diagnosis of angina. Because he has diabetes, his risk of complications from revascularization is rather high. Patients with diabetes who require revascularization benefit more from coronary bypass surgery than from percutaneous revascularization. The benefit from bypass surgery in these patients is probably mostly for symptomatic relief, and I would think that this patient has not had an adequate trial yet of medical therapy to try to prevent the occurrence of exertional angina. In addition, the revascularization itself carries risk for stroke and heart attack. From a survival standpoint, he would benefit only if he had left main or three-

vessel disease with depressed left ventricular function. He has a normal ejection fraction. I still feel comfortable enough with the diagnosis of exertional angina to manage this patient medically.

> **Cardiac catheterization revealed a 70% stenosis of the left main coronary artery and 40% lesion of the proximal right coronary artery. Ejection fraction was normal. The patient underwent an uncomplicated coronary artery bypass surgery. In the short term, his chest discomfort did not recur.**

Left main coronary disease was the first coronary anatomy for a survival benefit with coronary revascularization which was found. It is worth noting that there is generally a misconception about the understanding about stenoses and causes for myocardial infarction that has evolved over time, with the initial concept of the disease being one of gradual progressive obstruction of coronary arteries. Over the last 15 years, our understanding of the disease has evolved toward the development of unstable or vulnerable plaques. Many friable plaques that can lead to heart attacks are obstructions that are less than 50% to 70% of the lumen. In fact, the risk of a heart attack from those lesions is actually greater than from arteries that are completely occluded or those that are occluded 70% and higher. So if the goal of therapy were to prevent heart attacks, revascularization does not help, and medical management does that more often. In this particular case, left main disease is one of the findings in which there is clearly a survival advantage for patients who undergo revascularization. To get that advantage, however, patients have to be willing to subject themselves to the risk of coronary bypass surgery, which includes surgery-related mortality, stroke related to the surgery, heart attack at the time of surgery, and also sternal wound infections.

Analysis

Chest pain is one of the most common symptoms encountered by clinicians, and the choice of diagnostic tests represents a critical aspect of making the right choices. In this discussion, we focus on the ordering and interpretation of the exercise tolerance test. When this patient, who had multiple risk factors, presented with new exertional chest pain, both the clinicians caring for him and the discussant felt that he had classic exertional angina pectoris. After all, we are all taught that angina in most cases is diagnosed from the history, and that coronary artery disease is more common in the presence of typical angina as opposed to atypical or nonanginal chest pain. Indeed, in a 70-year-old man with typical angina, the prevalence of coronary artery disease exceeds 90% based simply on age, gender, and characteristics of the chest pain.[187]

What to do next is the challenge. Which patients should undergo exercise testing or cardiac catheterization? Which patients might benefit from either percutaneous or surgical intervention, and which might do just as well with medical therapy? Even "front-line" cardiologists differ in their testing and treatment approaches: Some only adopt new technology cautiously, some are the first to employ it, and some are just more aggressive ("invasive") than others. Just as cardiologists vary, patients and their primary care physicians also may have particular attitudes, beliefs, or preferences about the risks and benefits. Often there may not be an absolute right or wrong. From one vantage point, one choice of treatment may be best; from another, a quite different treatment looms as most desirable. From the perspective of overall benefit to the patient, the choice of one approach or another might not matter because the two approaches would be equally beneficial.[60]

In this instance, there was no disagreement about diagnosis. Neither the clinicians nor the discussant felt that the patient had unstable angina that would necessitate urgent catheterization. Nor had the patient had a trial of medical management, so catheterization for medically refractory angina was not indicated. Therefore, the principal choice about additional testing, namely, the decision to order a stress test, was made to stratify prognosis. The aim of the stress test was to use a noninvasive test to stratify risk—in other words, to identify whether the patient might fall into one of those high-risk categories for which surgical intervention would improve life expectancy.

If the clinicians were going to have the patient undergo definitive anatomic testing (cardiac catheterization) regardless of the exercise test result, there would have been no justification for the stress test. Instead, they chose to do the stress test because it would have helped direct their next step. Cardiac catheterization would have been the optimal choice if the stress test had been markedly abnormal (e.g., if it showed exercise-induced global ischemia or substantial left ventricular myocardium at risk). Medical management would have been preferred if the test had shown reproduction of symptoms with a reasonable workload and only a small area of noncritical ischemia. In fact, the stress test showed no evidence of ischemia. It is here that the clinicians and the discussant varied in their approach.

The clinicians may have felt uncomfortable with the normal result since they were confident that the patient had coronary disease and they considered the negative test "nondiagnostic" in providing prognostic information, hence their request for cardiac catheterization. The discussant, on the other hand, did comment that the patient may not have exercised sufficiently since his heart rate only increased to 80% of predicted, thus compromising the sensitivity of the test, but at the same time, he recognized that a shortened exercise duration increased the risk for subsequent cardiac events. Nonetheless, it appears that the discussant thought that the patient had exercised enough so that if he had the severe lesions he was looking for, it still would have some degree of positivity.

Yet it is hard to fault the discussant, who, while recognizing the limitation of nonmaximal testing, may have interpreted the test as sufficiently lowering the likelihood of potentially life-prolonging surgical disease so that catheterization was not pursued. The discussant considered all of these issues meticulously as he tried to decide whether to recommend medical therapy or proceed to cardiac catheterization. He says that he probably would treat the patient medically, yet before he is informed of the results of cardiac catheterization, he raises all the right issues, including his conviction that the patient does have coronary disease and the possible benefits and risks of surgery. He even states that cardiac catheterization would not be an inappropriate choice. The decision whether or not to proceed with cardiac catheterization in this patient is clearly a close call,[60] and examining it prospectively as we did shows how difficult it was and how highly qualified physicians can come to different conclusions from the same or nearly the same clinical information.

This case illustrates the use of testing not for diagnosis but for prognostic risk stratification. It also demonstrates the importance of test interpretation and how clinicians presented with identical information may arrive at alternative clinical approaches. Finally, despite all of the elements of the clinical problem-solving process that this case provides, one is left wondering about the basis for the discrepancy between the clinician and the discussant recommendations. Is it what they perceive about the patient, what they know about the disease or patient, or what they believe about the benefits and risks of treatment that counts?

CASE 27. RENAL RESCUE BY REVEREND BAYES

> A 75-year-old woman who had been treated with warfarin for 3 weeks in preparation for conversion from atrial fibrillation to sinus rhythm was seen in the Emergency Department for gross hematuria.

This common problem raises a number of important issues. Because the risk of systemic embolization is increased in patients with atrial fibrillation, anticoagulants typically are prescribed. The risk of embolism is a function of the underlying heart disease, and the greater that risk, the more urgent is the need for anticoagulation. Restoration of sinus rhythm reduces the likelihood of systemic embolization. The risk is not eliminated because the patient can still revert to atrial fibrillation, but usually it is low enough to avoid the need for long-term anticoagulant therapy. The risk of long-term anticoagulation is quite high in elderly patients. As I recall, annual mortality from treatment alone is 1% to 2%. So my preference would be to cardiovert her for that reason.

Since there is always some risk of embolism during cardioversion, the patient ideally should be anticoagulated for 2 to 3 weeks beforehand. During that time, all loose clots presumably will become fibrosed and bound down, and the conversion will not generate emboli. The optimal duration of anticoagulation is not clear. The usual 2- to 3-week period is not derived from solid data. Furthermore, how long to maintain anticoagulation after conversion is not well substantiated.

The patient under discussion had developed a problem that may or may not require withdrawal of anticoagulation. Two important questions come to mind immediately. First, why did she develop hematuria? When a patient on anticoagulants has a bleeding complication, one must wonder if some underlying pathology is being revealed. I need to know the patient's INR (International Normalized Ratio) and whether it is in the therapeutic range. If it is, I would be more inclined to work up the hematuria aggressively, looking for such things as a tumor of the genitourinary tract. The second critical issue is whether we can proceed with cardioversion. Assuming that the anticoagulants have not yet been withdrawn, can we proceed with the cardioversion while she is still protected, rather than stopping warfarin, working up the hematuria, and then facing the issue of anticoagulation all over again? If we must stop the warfarin, should we try emergency cardioversion? I should add that everything I say about chemical cardioversion applies equally to electrical conversion. There is no difference in the risk of embolization from either modality.

> Three years earlier she first developed atrial fibrillation after an uncomplicated emergency appendectomy. Antiarrhythmics were given, and sinus rhythm was restored. Several months later, the drugs were discontinued, and the patient remained asymptomatic. Her cardiac rhythm was not monitored closely. Three weeks before the Emergency Department visit her physician found that atrial fibrillation had recurred at a rate of 92 per minute. Thyroid function tests and an echocardiogram were normal. The doctor prescribed diltiazem and warfarin; the warfarin dose was regulated in outpatient visits.

It is not clear why this patient developed atrial fibrillation initially. Was it the stress of surgery? Was she in congestive heart failure? Did she have a myocardial infarction or underlying heart disease, such as mitral stenosis? Did she have a pulmonary embolus, or was she thyrotoxic? I would be interested in the answers to those questions.

The current treatment and plan strike me as appropriate and reasonable. Diltiazem was started to control the ventricular response, and warfarin was prescribed to decrease the risk of embolization at the time of cardioversion.

> On the day of the Emergency Department visit, gross hematuria developed, and the patient was admitted to the hospital. Examination disclosed no abnormalities other than the atrial fibrillation at a rate of 120 per minute. The urine was grossly bloody and contained clots. INR had increased from 2.3 one week earlier to 6.3. Hematocrit was 35% (it had been 44%). Stool was guaiac negative. Creatinine was 1.3 mg/dL. Sedimentation rate was 90 mm/hr (the value 4 years earlier was 43 mm/hr). The INR promptly returned to normal when warfarin was discontinued.

What impresses me about this examination is that the patient now has atrial fibrillation at a rate of 120 per minute. As I recall, her heart rate was 92 three weeks ago, and now, during treatment with diltiazem (which would be expected to lower the heart rate), it is even faster. I wonder why. Perhaps she bled a fair amount and is hypovolemic. Heavy bleeding from the kidney is unusual, but her urine was grossly bloody and contained clots. Her hematocrit is now 35%, down 9 points. There could be a further dilutional drop.

She was overtly overanticoagulated, but it is not clear why that happened. Could she have taken the wrong warfarin dose? Did she start taking any new medications that could accentuate the anticoagulant effect of warfarin? Did she change her diet or contract a viral infection? Does she have liver disease? The fact that her INR promptly returned to normal implies that her liver function was grossly intact. I am impressed that there was no evidence of gastrointestinal bleeding even with the excessive anticoagulation.

The sedimentation rate of 90 mm/hr is very high; the value of 43 four years earlier also is high. Sedimentation rates increase with age, but a value of 90 raises the possibility of infection, vasculitis, collagen diseases, polymyalgia rheumatica, or malignancy. I am not sure what to make of that finding.

Should we work up the hematuria now? I do not think I would. I am not convinced that hematuria occurring in the presence of an INR of 6.3 has the same implications as hematuria occurring with a therapeutic INR. I think we have some time here for observation. I would continue to take care of her

initial problem, that is, the conversion of her atrial fibrillation, and follow her urinalyses. If the hematuria persists when her INR is in the therapeutic range, I would investigate her genitourinary tract.

> CT scan of the abdomen showed a left intrarenal mass in the mid lower pole that indented the pelvis; otherwise, the collecting systems were unremarkable. Further studies confirmed the left renal mass and were considered to be consistent with a renal cell cancer. Two urine cytology studies were negative for tumor cells.

So, she was studied—and the imaging procedures suggested renal cell cancer. Nonetheless, two urine cytology studies were negative for tumor cells.

I think this is an interesting issue. We know there is a mass in the kidney that is big enough to be displacing the renal pelvis, and we have to consider whether it is a cystic mass or a solid mass. Urine cytology is not a very sensitive test, and given that all three radiologic tests were thought to be consistent with a solid tumor, I think there is a reasonable chance that the lesion is indeed a renal cancer. I am not totally at ease about that diagnosis, however. I would want to do a Bayesian analysis, although we would have to look up the data. We could calculate the likelihood of renal cancer in a 75-year-old woman who has a lesion with these radiologic characteristics and two negative urine cytology studies.

The point is that we have two conflicting sets of diagnostic studies—findings consistent with renal cell cancer and negative cytology examinations. To understand the significance of normal cytology examinations, I would need to know beforehand the likelihood that there would be no cancer. First, what are the data on elderly women with renal bleeding with excessive anticoagulation? How many have a cancer, and how many have other lesions? Second, we are not told specifically what the arteriogram showed, and I do not know what "considered to be consistent with a renal cancer" means. Consistent could mean that the likelihood is 30% or that it is 90%. I need to know where she is in that range. If there is a very strong suspicion of a tumor, I think one has to consider doing a biopsy or exploring to see what's there.

> **Radical left nephrectomy was carried out with-out complications. No tumor was present. The specimen showed only focal necrosis and hem-orrhage within the hilar fat and the submucosa of the renal pelvis.**

Interesting. The surgeons obviously felt so confident that the patient had a renal tumor that they performed a radical nephrectomy. As I stated, a careful Bayesian analysis before surgery might have put the likelihood of a renal cancer in a dif-ferent light and hence affected the choice of pro-cedure. I am assuming that a thorough analysis of the pathology specimen was performed. We must be certain that we are not dealing with a sampling error if we are to accept the pathology report as the gold standard.

> **The patient recovered uneventfully. When seen 4 months later, she was in sinus rhythm on antiarrhythmic drugs. Anticoagulants were not restarted. Her sedimentation rate was 36 mm/hr.**

It is not unreasonable, once she is converted, not to put her back on anticoagulants. However, she has had paroxysmal fibrillation at least twice, and I am not sure that I would leave her off an-ticoagulants. With no bleeding diathesis or other bleeding problem, my major concern would be to keep her carefully controlled on some anticoagu-lants for a few months and make sure that she is not slipping in and out of atrial fibrillation. I would obtain serial Holter monitor studies because, even in the absence of underlying heart disease, parox-ysmal atrial fibrillation represents a great risk for precipitating embolic events.

Analysis

In this case, we will focus only on a single statement. When the discussant first learned that the findings of the CT scan and other studies were thought to be consistent with a renal cancer, he observed, "I'm not totally at ease about that diagnosis." Now that we know that the patient had no tumor and that she lost her kidney unnecessarily, we need to explore his reaction and ask ourselves whether this unfortunate (but not disastrous) outcome could have been avoided.

The discussant provides some important clues to his reasoning processes. He acknowledges that the radiologic findings might well be representa-tive of a renal cancer, but even with the vague recol-lection that the sensitivity of urine cytology studies is not very high, he is concerned about the discor-dance. He wonders about the prevalence of the var-ious lesions that could produce urinary tract bleed-ing as a result of excessive anticoagulation. The statement that he might not "work up" a patient for renal bleeding if it occurred with an extremely high INR implies that he considers the probability of a serious renal lesion to be low. Finally, with these suspicions heightened, he begins to wonder about the interpretation of the radiologic studies: What does "consistent with a renal cell cancer" mean? What kind of concept is that? He wonders whether that assessment represents a very high (90% likely) or only moderate (30% likely) suspicion of a cancer. Finally, he says that he might be able to resolve his diagnostic concern by a Bayesian analysis.

Many clinicians, we suspect, will be confused by his interest in using Bayes' rule because it is commonly assumed that Bayesian arithmetic is re-served for binary (i.e., positive and negative) test results and that unless test results can be expressed in terms of sensitivity and specificity, the Bayes formulation cannot be applied. That assumption is incorrect. Bayes' rule can be used to calculate the likelihood that a given disease is present from any number of relevant clinical characteristics, in-cluding laboratory test results, radiologic studies, and clinical attributes. In fact, any test or clini-cal attribute need not be represented by a positive or negative result and can be denoted in grada-tions, such as blood pressure between 90 and 104, between 105 and 119, and greater than 120 mm Hg. A Bayesian diagnosis of acute renal failure published at a time when Bayes' rule was first in-troduced in medicine, for example, considered 14 clinical states and 31 clinical characteristics, many of which were distributed among more than two attributes.[159]

What would have been required to perform a Bayesian analysis in the patient described here? First, we would need data on the prevalence of the various renal lesions that bleed during exces-sive coagulation. If possible, such data would best be age specific—that is, based on data not from the general population but from elderly patients.

Those data would provide the prior probabilities. We also would need as complete a set of diagnostic possibilities as is feasible. In particular, it would be essential to have as one of the possible disorders "no significant pathology." Without that "diagnosis," the analysis could never identify the correct answer, no matter how much evidence built up to support it. Next, we would need interpretations from the radiologists. Instead of a blanket opinion about whether the studies were consistent with renal cancer, we would collect their opinions about each of the studies that were performed. We would inquire about the probability of the specific findings of each test in each set of diagnostic possibilities.[155,188] Those assessments would be the conditional probabilities. For example, among 100 patients with renal cell cancer, how often would you expect them to have this particular CT scan appearance? Such language avoids the overinterpretation of descriptions such as "consistent with cancer" or "cannot exclude the possibility of cancer" and highlights the importance of reviewing radiographic findings with a radiologist. Then, with the data assembled, we could use Bayes' rule to calculate the posterior probabilities.

Suppose the calculation had been done—How would we have used the data? If the result showed an overwhelmingly high likelihood of renal cancer, we would probably have proceeded precisely as the patient's physicians did. With a near certainty that the patient had a renal cancer, the reasonable choice would be not to disturb the lesion and risk spreading tumor cells with further diagnostic studies but to remove the tumor en bloc. What, on the other hand, would we have done if the analysis had demonstrated that renal cancer was still quite likely but nowhere near a certainty? We would have wanted additional confirmation of the diagnosis before proceeding with nephrectomy. The consequences of losing a kidney are not extremely serious, but we cannot be willing to sacrifice a kidney lightly, and we should not subject a 75-year-old woman to unnecessary major surgery if we can avoid doing so. In this situation, we would discuss with the radiologists, the cytologists, and the urologists how to get the additional data.

A Bayesian analysis was not done preoperatively in this case. Nonetheless, the mathematics formulated by the Reverend Thomas Bayes more than 200 years ago[189,190] might well have heightened the suspicion that the bleeding lesion was benign and might have inspired a more conservative approach.

CASE 28. A DIAGNOSTIC FLUKE

During his yearly routine examination of a symptom-free, 52-year-old advertising manager with recurrent colonic polyps, a physician palpated what he thought was an abdominal aortic aneurysm. To the physician's surprise, abdominal ultrasound showed a solid echodense lesion in the liver but no aneurysm.

So we are faced with an unexpected finding in an asymptomatic man. The major concern would be that he has a quiet colonic neoplasm and metastases to the liver.

The patient had a history of peptic ulcer disease, and he was known to be hepatitis antibody-positive but antigen-negative. He had not traveled abroad in more than 30 years, and he had no known exposure to vinyl chloride. The results of the physical examination were normal, and all laboratory tests, including all liver function studies, were normal. Stool guaiac was negative.

In terms of history, primary hepatoma is not likely; note the lack of vinyl chloride exposure and the hepatitis serology profile. The peptic ulcer disease is not particularly relevant. We are not told what hepatitis antibody this is, whether it is hepatitis A, B or C, and I think that would be of interest. If it is hepatitis B, he has undoubtedly been exposed to this agent, but the fact that he's surface antigen-negative and not a chronic carrier lowers the index of suspicion that this could be a primary hepatoma.

Blood pool scan showed no accumulation of isotope and was thought to exclude a hemangioma. CT scan of the liver was done next (Figure 15.1).

The contrast CT scan shows what appears to be a contrast-enhanced mass in the center of the right lobe of the liver. My concern is that this would be consistent with a neoplasm in this patient

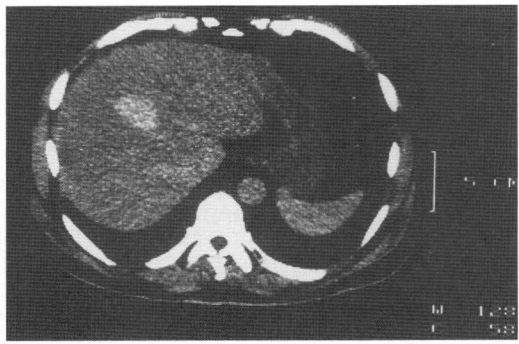

Figure 15.1 • Computed tomography scan of the liver; case 28.

with a history of colonic polyps. A fine-needle, CT-guided biopsy of the liver would be indicated.

CT-guided biopsy of the liver disclosed eggs of *Paragonimus westermani* (Figure 15.2). When this parasite was discovered, additional questioning revealed that the patient had been stationed in Japan in 1952. Because *Paragonimus* typically does not produce a mass lesion in the liver, the CT scan was reviewed. It was reinterpreted as consistent with fatty liver, with

a central island of normal liver. The patient was treated with praziquantel, 75 mg/kg in three divided doses over 24 hours.

In this case, a diagnostic procedure was done for the right reasons, and a surprise was found. The finding illustrated how long this organism can survive in the human body.

Analysis

In the case described, a diagnostic fluke led to the diagnosis of a fluke! Was the discovery worthwhile or important? This one is hard to call: Either the physician responsible for this patient was on a wild goose chase with no clinical relevance, or he was lucky to stumble on a finding that eventually would have caused considerable morbidity. This patient's medical problem illustrates how several common clinical dilemmas can intersect in a single patient.

These issues are as follows: how to interpret unexpected and surprising results of diagnostic tests (see case 29); how to decide how far to proceed with diagnostic testing when the potential payoff is almost certain to be quite small[191]; how to decide whether to use a particular drug for a given clinical problem, with respect to the specific tradeoffs between toxicity and the potential benefits of therapy[58,59]; and how to revise our hypotheses, given new data that are at odds with our current hypotheses.[19]

The first decision by the patient's physician—to obtain an abdominal ultrasound examination when he mistakenly identified an abdominal aortic aneurysm during a routine physical examination—cannot be faulted. Missing such a lesion has an extremely high disutility, palpation for such aneurysms has a low sensitivity,[192] ultrasound has an exceptionally high sensitivity,[192] and the test is risk-free (though obviously not cost-free). The second decision was to obtain a blood pool scan. Because liver hemangiomas are frequently asymptomatic and because of the danger of proceeding with invasive studies in such cases (see case 16), the blood pool scan is warranted, even though hemangiomas of the liver are rare.

Once the physician was convinced that the lesion was solid, he faced an interesting problem, namely, whether to proceed further with the elucidation of this unexpected finding. The principal

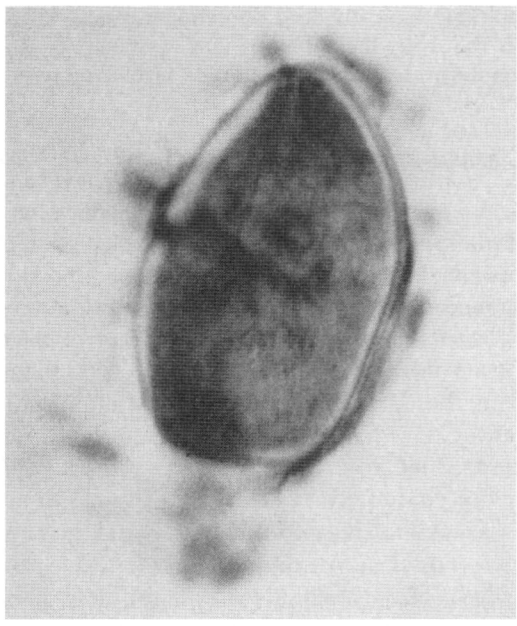

Figure 15.2 • Liver biopsy specimen; case 28.

issue he faced was to assess the likelihood that the lesion was significant in terms of the patient's outcome. In this assessment, the following questions had to be considered: How likely is it that I will find a lesion that will cause future morbidity? (It certainly was causing no morbidity at present and had not in the past.) How risky will it be to find out what it is, and how likely is it that I can find a treatment that will cure the disorder without hurting the patient?

Although this reasoning process is correct, the first procedure that will be needed is a liver biopsy. Liver biopsy is not risk-free, although the risk of a serious complication is extremely low. Given even a small chance of a safely treatable and potentially correctable disorder, therefore, biopsy seems an appropriate choice, even though the patient is basically healthy. We must recognize, however, and we must inform the patient, that we may end up in a succession of tests without any benefit at all. Indeed, the decision to test or not to test in these circumstances should be made by a fully informed patient whenever possible.[193]

The next decision was to treat or not to treat. The patient had had an asymptomatic parasitic infestation for more than 30 years. Chances are that he would not have experienced any complication of this parasitic infection in the future. Because praziquantel, the drug used for this infection, is highly effective against flukes and because its toxicity is low and dose is proportional to the degree of infestation (presumably mild in this case), therapy was administered.

Finally, we see how diagnostic hypotheses are revised in the light of new data. Because this parasitic infestation does not produce the kind of picture seen on CT scan, the radiologist reassessed the interpretation and decided that the findings were most consistent with fatty liver. Indeed, if this interpretation had been the original one, no further studies would have been done, and the patient would still have his parasite.

CASE 29. SURPRISE!

A 50-year-old, previously healthy business consultant and decision analyst saw a urologist for epididymitis. The urologist detected mi- **croscopic hematuria and recommended further studies.**

The information that we have here is scant. I will have to take the epididymitis at face value. Most patients with epididymitis complain of pain, swelling, or dysuria. The microscopic hematuria is of concern because the new onset of hematuria raises the possibility of a number of urologic diseases. A malignant disease anywhere from the bladder to the ureters to the kidneys could present with microscopic hematuria. In addition, many nonmalignant diseases, including interstitial cystitis, nephrolithiasis, tuberculosis or another infectious disease, and benign recurrent hematuria with proteinuria would be possible. I would like to know whether proteinuria was detected. Then a series of other tests needs to be done to look at kidney structure and function.

I would be interested in the patient's physical examination, including his blood pressure. Does he have an enlarged prostate or prostatic nodule on rectal examination? As for tests of renal function, I would like at least a BUN and creatinine. I would like a urinalysis, looking for red cell casts, a CT scan to look for stones or a mass lesion, and probably a cystoscopy.

Cystoscopy was negative. The CT scan of the kidneys, liver, spleen, adrenal glands, gallbladder, and the body and tail of the pancreas was unremarkable. The head of the pancreas, however, appeared "generous and bulbous, and there is poor definition and loss of sharpness of the medial aspect of the head of the uncinate process. On one or two cuts, there is a question of whether there was some extrinsic pressure on the lesser curve aspect of the second portion of the duodenum. A good cleavage plane between the vena cava and the pancreas is not appreciated. We are mildly concerned about the appearance of the head of the pancreas."

Let me ignore the pancreas for a moment and look at the information about the kidneys, because that is where we started. We have a patient with apparent epididymitis who has microscopic hematuria. I would be more concerned if there were 50 to 100 red cells on sediment examination rather than only 5 or 10 red cells. I would like to know something about his urinary protein excretion, but for the moment, I will assume it is normal. The kidneys appeared unremarkable on CT scan, so I would not evaluate the genitourinary tract further.

Now we have a new problem that has been raised by the CT scan. The report described the head of the pancreas as "generous and bulbous," and the radiologist was "mildly concerned about the appearance of the head of the pancreas." All we know from the history is that his only symptom was epididymitis. Pancreatic cancer certainly can appear out of the blue without much in the way of any prodromal symptoms. Does this patient have any risk factors that would increase the likelihood of cancer of the pancreas? Is he a smoker? Does he consume six alcoholic drinks per day, which might increase the risk of cancer of the pancreas?

Assuming that none of those risk factors is present, I would not go any further. I would first have the CT scan reviewed by an expert. If we are still left with the same information that we are given here, I would repeat the CT scan in 3 months or some other reasonable period to see if there has been any change. I think one can go overboard with this kind of interpretation and wind up even performing exploratory surgery in a patient whose pancreas is perfectly normal.

The patient's only other complaints were "sinus trouble," occasional discomfort in his right knee, and some low-back discomfort after heavy exercise (he is a runner). He had no previous history of gastrointestinal or liver disease. He had no abdominal complaints or change in bowel habits. He consumed little alcohol, and he was a nonsmoker.

The essence of this information is that the probability of pancreatic cancer in this man is not very different from that in the average asymptomatic 50-year-old person. Beyond pushing for a better interpretation of the CT scan, I still would not do anything for three months.

The following laboratory results were obtained: hemoglobin 15.4 g/dL, hematocrit 46%, WBC 6,200, bilirubin 0.6 mg/dL, cholesterol 211 mg/dL, albumin 4.3 g/dL, globulin 2.7 g/dL, alkaline phosphatase 60 IU/L, lactate dehydrogenase 112 IU/L, aspartate transaminase 16 IU/L,

alanine transaminase 22 IU/L, INR 1.4, and amylase 74 IU/L and lipase 4 IU/L (normal ranges, 10–85 and 0–19, respectively). Urinalysis was normal except for 10 to 15 red cells per high-power field.

I should have commented previously on the laboratory data. My assumption was that in a nondrinker they were going to be normal. I still would not change my opinion regarding further workup, and I would still watch him for 3 months.

The patient was referred to a gastroenterologist, who noted that there was moderate enlargement of the pancreas on the CT scan that was "significantly abnormal to justify further evaluation." He raised the following possibilities: subclinical inflammatory disease of the pancreas, stenosis of the pancreatic duct, pancreatic tumor, and pancreas divisum. The gastroenterologist recommended an endoscopic retrograde cholangiopancreatography (ERCP).

I remain dubious about this recommendation. I am at a disadvantage because I have not seen the CT scan or had an opportunity to review it with a radiologist. I would still stick to my guns.

The patient was skeptical about the recommendation. After discussing the problem with two physicians, he assessed the base rate of cancer of the pancreas and adjusted this rate for his status as a nonsmoker. He used Bayes' rule to calculate the probability of a treatable lesion and then made a calculation of the average gain in life expectancy if any treatable lesion was found. This calculation included a sensitivity analysis of the conditional probability of a large pancreas in an otherwise healthy person. The patient concluded that the maximum gain in life expectancy (given the assumption of the prevalence of a slightly enlarged pancreas in otherwise healthy people) was as little as 5 days or as much as 50 days. He argued that the procedure was unnecessary.

I am impressed that a layperson could make these calculations; most physicians would not be able to do so. I agree with the decision analyst. I think a repeat CT scan in 3 months would be a reasonable compromise between the aggressiveness of the gastroenterologist and the skepticism of the decision analyst toward not doing anything.

> The physicians thought he was "nuts." They both opined that the chance of cancer was much higher than the patient had concluded.

The concept of probability, unfortunately, has not gotten into the brains of some physicians. I am dismayed that some primary care clinicians do all the histories and physicals and obtain the baseline information and then relinquish their power to the next consultant, the gastroenterologist or the radiologist in this case.

> The patient reluctantly agreed to have the ERCP. The study was uncomplicated, and no abnormality was found. The patient continues to be well 15 years later. Hematuria has disappeared. He wrote, "The cost of this was lost time doing the tests and about $2,500 of medical bills, which I paid myself." The biggest cost, he wrote, "was strain and anxiety associated with the possible diagnosis of pancreatic cancer, which I knew was very serious. The perceived seriousness was heightened by the fact that I had lost my father just a year before to cancer (lung metastasized from bowel) after watching him painfully waste away over a six-month period. More than anything, I had the ERCP to eliminate the anxiety. I doubt that I would have been anxious with good data and a sound analysis."

Analysis

What a surprise! This unfortunate man went to his physician for scrotal pain, and a few days later, he was informed that he might have cancer of the pancreas. Being an intelligent fellow, experienced in decision making under conditions of uncertainty, the patient doubted this conclusion. However, having been rendered anxious by the abnormal finding on CT scan and cowed by the insistence of two physicians that he undergo further diagnostic evaluation, the patient submitted to having a study he considered unnecessary.

Did the patient go to see the wrong physician? Clearly, if our discussant had been his physician, the ERCP would not have been done. What are the diagnostic principles underlying this common

clinical problem? What can we learn from this kind of experience that would help us make the optimal decision the next time we are surprised by an unexpected result of a diagnostic test? Should the ERCP have been recommended? Instead of an ERCP, was it even necessary to repeat the CT scan in 3 months, as recommended by our discussant? Should the patient simply have been told that the chance that the CT scan findings represented anything serious was small enough to warrant ignoring the finding entirely?

Probability theory provides a framework for a rational approach to this problem. As we explained before, the probability that a patient has a given disease when a certain kind of abnormality is found on a diagnostic study is a function of two variables: (1) the probability of the disease before the test and (2) the probability that the same test result occurs in the disease under question and the probabilities that the same test result occurs in all other possible "diseases"—even in normal subjects.

Let us consider surprises analogous to the one faced in this example by the business consultant's physician. That is, we will consider cases in which the probability of a disease before testing is small. Cancer of the pancreas in this patient is such an example; cancer of the kidney in one of our other cases is another such example (see cases 23 and 27).

Consider this patient: Given his age and the lack of any manifestations even remotely related to pancreatic disease, it is overwhelmingly likely that he has no serious disease of the pancreas. To simplify our consideration of the problem, we will assume him to be in one of two states: Either he has pancreatic cancer, as suggested by the result of the test (CT scan), or he is healthy. Because he seemed healthy and had no predisposing risk factors or clinical manifestations, the pretest (i.e., pre-CT scan) probability of pancreatic cancer is quite low (roughly equivalent to the prevalence of pancreatic cancer in his age-, sex-, and race-matched population); the pretest probability that he is normal is correspondingly high.

What characteristics of the CT result determine whether we sustain our belief that he is normal or whether we begin to believe strongly that he has pancreatic cancer? Given the low pretest probability of cancer, the extent to which the test result deviates from normal provides the critical clue. A *slightly abnormal test result* will increase the posttest probability of cancer only minimally because the likelihood of this result in healthy persons may be high, or, at worst, quite similar to that in patients with cancer, making the posttest probability at best identical to the pretest likelihood of cancer. By contrast, a *dramatically abnormal test result* will increase the posttest probability of cancer substantially because the likelihood of this result in pancreatic cancer is high and in healthy persons it is quite low.

In the case we are discussing, the result is a radiographic finding, but the principles for interpreting such findings are not different for other test results. A sedimentation rate of 40 in an apparently healthy 60-year-old woman probably has little significance, whereas a sedimentation rate of 120 in the same woman is highly likely to be a manifestation of some serious disease.[194]

This explanation, although it satisfactorily answers how to interpret an unexpected and surprising abnormal test result, fails to illuminate the process for dealing with the interpreted result. Suppose we correctly interpret such an abnormal test result. What action should we take based on this result? In the patient considered here, what approach should we follow to decide whether to cease testing or to test further (i.e., perform an ERCP?) Except when the probability of disease is virtually zero, the probability of disease alone clearly is insufficient.

Instead, to make this decision, one needs to assess the consequences of each possible action, which in this case is either further ERCP testing or no further testing. The consequences of further testing include the frequency of false-positive and false-negative results, the risk of the ERCP tests, and the therapeutic benefit of finding a presumably true-positive, early, potentially curable cancer. The important consequences of no further testing are principally those that follow from ignoring a potentially curable lesion.

The process of combining these data is now a standard one and is accomplished by decision analysis to calculate a no-test/test threshold[59] (see Chapter 4). The testing threshold is first calculated by decision analysis. This threshold is the probability of disease at which the benefits and risks of either no further testing or of testing are equivalent, so for likelihoods of disease below this threshold, no further testing is preferred (i.e., has a higher value, or

expected utility because the risks of the tests exceed the benefits of testing) compared to testing. For any disease probability greater than the threshold, however, further testing has a higher expected utility than no testing, and thus the choice to test is optimal. To make a choice, then, we must compare the probability of disease at any stage of the patient's workup with the derived value for the threshold.

To illustrate further for this patient: Suppose that the pretest (before CT scan) probability of pancreatic cancer in this man was 1 in 1,000 (0.0010) and suppose that the no-test/test threshold was found to be 5 in 100 (0.05). Then, if the probability of pancreatic cancer after the abnormal CT scan was still judged to be lower than 0.05, no additional ERCP testing would be warranted. However, if the probability was thought to be greater than 0.05, an ERCP would be indicated. In this framework, the significance of the degree of positivity of the CT scan can be understood. Note that the post-CT scan probability of pancreatic cancer becomes the pre-ERCP probability of pancreatic cancer. The more abnormal the CT scan, the higher will be the posttest probability. Presumably, a slightly abnormal result would not raise the probability of cancer above the threshold and an ERCP would not be indicated, whereas after a markedly abnormal test, the post-CT scan probability of pancreatic cancer would exceed the testing threshold and the clear choice would be to carry out the ERCP.

Finally, how can we account for the discrepancy between the recommendations of the patient's physicians and our discussant? The patient's physicians insisted that he have the ERCP; the discussant would not have done it. The patient's physicians may have overinterpreted the positivity of the CT findings and thus may have in their own minds exceeded the testing threshold.[57] They may have been following a common but imperfect clinical dictum that abnormal findings must always be followed up, no matter how unlikely they are to indicate a treatable disorder. They may have been concerned about their vulnerability to a malpractice action if some, even unrelated, disorder showed up later. They may have been in the "regret" mode, in which missing a lesion is perceived as far more egregious than testing inappropriately, even if testing complications ensue.[81,139] It is even conceivable that a financial incentive may have tipped them over the testing threshold if their suspicion of cancer was at or near the threshold value. Without further information on their reasoning processes, however, we can only speculate.

Medical surprises abound in day-today practice, especially as routine imaging studies for common complaints become more widespread. Sometimes they are important to the care of the patient, and sometimes they send us down blind or even dangerous trails. How can we tell when a finding is not clinically important? As described here, we must have a framework for assessing the significance of surprises and taking the appropriate action. To expect perfection—always ignoring misleading test results and always following up surprises that are clinically relevant—is unrealistic. However, thoughtful consideration of the probability of the diseases, the test results in question, and the consequences of our clinical choices is essential in making the fewest testing errors.

CASE 30. TRIPPING OVER TECHNOLOGY

Case 29 describes a patient in whom technological advances in diagnostic testing yielded suboptimal medical decisions. The patient was a 50-year-old business consultant who presented with epididymitis; in the initial workup, his physician discovered microscopic hematuria (in retrospect, probably the consequence of long-distance running). The patient had no abdominal or gastrointestinal symptoms or abnormal physical findings, and an abdominal CT scan showed no abnormalities in his kidneys. However, the scan yielded an unexpected finding in the pancreas. It was described as follows: The head of the pancreas is "generous and bulbous, and there is poor definition . . . of the uncinate process. On one or two cuts there is a question of whether there was some extrinsic pressure on the lesser curve aspect of the second portion of the duodenum . . . We are mildly concerned about the appearance of the head of the pancreas." This surprising finding led a consultant gastroenterologist to recommend ERCP to rule out pancreatic cancer. In the discussion, the editors argued, using nonquantitative reasoning, that the chance of cancer of the pancreas was so small that the decision to perform ERCP was incorrect. Here we present a quantitative analysis of the same problem.

A Succinct Description of the Dilemma

The patient had no manifestations of pancreatic disease: He had no weight loss, gastrointestinal symptoms, or abdominal pain. The likelihood that he has a silent pancreatic carcinoma, identified almost by chance by a CT scan done for hematuria, is remote. If by some chance he does have pancreatic cancer, however, it would probably be an early lesion; the chance of cure might be considerably higher than it would for a lesion that presented with typical symptoms. The equivocal CT findings alone do not make the diagnosis.

If ERCP is performed, an early cancer might well be diagnosed; but if no cancer is present, the patient will have been exposed to the small risk and moderate discomfort of the ERCP. Accordingly, the decision is a tradeoff between potential life expectancy gained if cancer is present and the morbidity and inconvenience of ERCP. In our reanalysis of the problem, we used decision analysis to obtain a quantitative answer to the same question: How high must the probability of pancreatic cancer be, given the results of the CT scan, to justify proceeding with ERCP?

The Decision Tree

We structured the problem as a decision tree that defined two competing strategies; either perform ERCP or observe without ERCP (Figure 15.3). The tree represents false-positive and false-negative results of the CT and ERCP and examines the probability that pancreatic cancer is either present or absent. Although the gastroenterologist considered several other diagnoses, the most important possible diagnosis is pancreatic cancer.

The schema represents the choice between ERCP and observation. If the patient undergoes ERCP, he may or may not survive the procedure. If he survives, he may have a positive or negative test, depending on whether or not disease is actually present. If the ERCP is positive, we assume that an exploratory laparotomy will be performed; the patient may or may not survive the procedure. If he survives, his subsequent life expectancy is modeled according to a *Markov process*[195] (a given outcome is estimated by calculating the number of life-years a patient can be expected to spend in various health states). If the choice is to observe, the patient's subsequent life expectancy is again modeled according

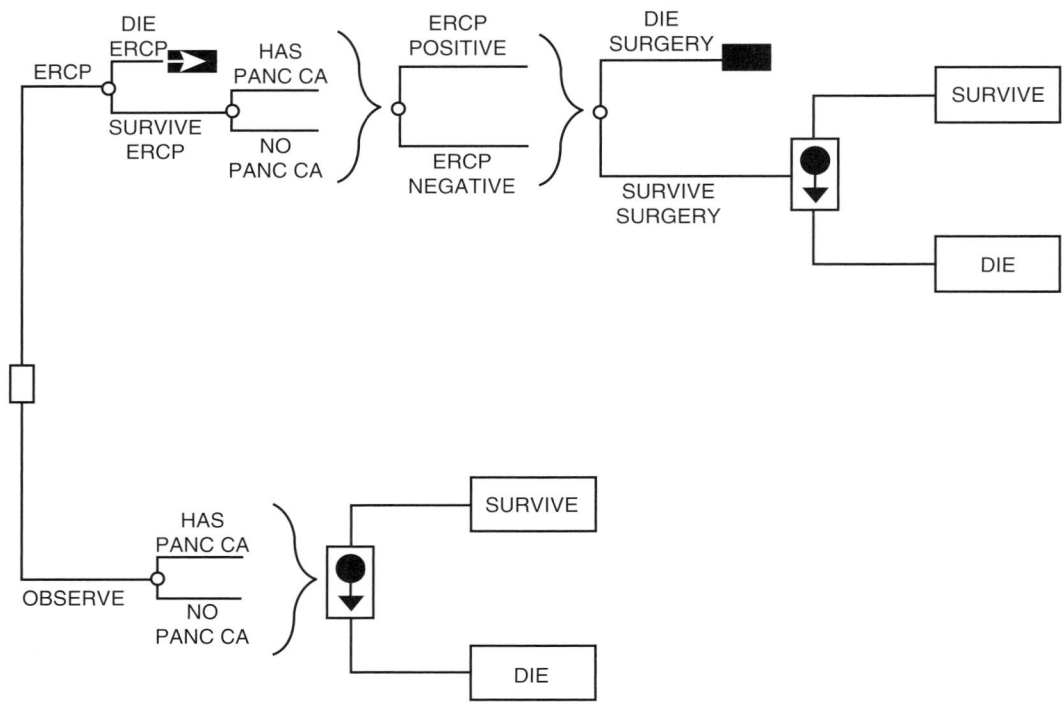

Figure 15.3 • Decision tree for case 30. The vertical rectangular node at the left denotes the choice that must be made between carrying out the endoscopic retrograde cholangiopancreatography (ERCP) or not. The nodes to the right of the brackets attach to each of the end branches to the left of the brackets. The arrow-circle symbol represents a "Markov" node. All horizontal rectangular symbols denote outcomes. PANC CA, pancreatic cancer.

to the same process; the pertinent probabilities reflect survival with or without untreated pancreatic cancer.

The Data

To analyze this problem, we need the following critical data: the probability of pancreatic cancer before any tests were done, the sensitivity and specificity of the CT scan in detecting pancreatic cancer, the risk of ERCP, the probability of a cure of an early pancreatic cancer if one is present, and the risk of surgery for pancreatic cancer. First, we elaborate on these data (summarized in Table 15.4).

The Prior Probability of Pancreatic Cancer

The probability that the patient had pancreatic cancer was assumed to be very low because he had no symptoms or physical findings referable to the pancreas. The annual incidence of pancreatic cancer is approximately 11 per 100,000 for white

males, and only 14% of patients are alive 1 year after diagnosis.[196] These data can be used to estimate the prevalence of pancreatic cancer in a patient cohort, and our calculations yielded an estimate of about 13.3 per 100,000 (0.000133). Because some pancreatic cancers may go undiagnosed, we assumed the prevalence to be somewhat higher and used a "baseline" prevalence of 0.0002 for our calculations. (To the extent that this value overestimates the likelihood of cancer, it biases the analysis toward ERCP.)

The Sensitivity and Specificity of CT Scan and ERCP

We culled estimates of false-positive and false-negative rates for "equivocal" CT findings that suggest pancreatic cancer. Two reports give false-positive rates for an equivocal CT scan in the diagnosis of pancreatic cancer of 55% and 73%, respectively.[197,198] CT sensitivity for pancreatic cancer is about 80% when unequivocal findings are

TABLE 15.4

Data Used in the Decision Analysis

Baseline probability of pancreatic cancer	0.0002
CT scan: false-positive rate for "equivocal" result	0.64
CT scan: true-positive rate (sensitivity)	1.00
ERCP: true-positive rate (for cancer)	0.90
ERCP: false-positive rate (for cancer)	0.03
Probability of ERCP-associated mortality	0.002
Probability of operative mortality associated with pancreatic cancer resection	0.20
Probability of a resectable pancreatic cancer	0.26
Monthly probability of death with unresectable pancreatic cancer	0.06
Monthly probability of death with resected pancreatic cancer	0.03

CT, computed tomography; ERCP, endoscopic retrograde cholangiopancreatography.

used to define a positive result.[199,200] If equivocal findings are included as positive diagnosis criteria, however, the sensitivity approaches 100%.[197] We used 100% for the sensitivity, a value that also biases the analysis toward the ERCP strategy. The sensitivity of ERCP for pancreatic cancer is approximately 90%,[201–203] and the ERCP false-positive rate is approximately 3%.[204]

The Risk of ERCP

The most common complications of ERCP are pancreatitis and cholangitis, which occur in approximately 3% of examinations. ERCP mortality is approximately 0.2%.

The Curability of Pancreatic Cancer

For testing to be worthwhile in this patient, the potential gain in life expectancy consequent to early diagnosis of the cancer must be greater than the risks associated with evaluating and inappropriately treating false-positive test results. No data are available regarding treatment outcomes for incidentally found, asymptomatic early pancreatic cancers. Approximately 10% of pancreatic cancers are resectable. There is some evidence that pancreatic malignancies that appear localized preoperatively may have a higher resectability, possibly as high as 26%. Resectability does not mean curability, however; the 1-year mortality of patients who have undergone successful resection still is approximately 30%. If further evaluation is to yield substantial gain in life expectancy, compared with

simple observation, the curability of an early cancer found with ERCP must be higher than usual to justify the inaccuracies of ERCP, the morbidity and mortality of ERCP, and the operative risks of laparotomy if the ERCP is positive.

The Risk of Pancreatic Surgery

Operative mortality for pancreaticoduodenal resections averages 20% in most series. These procedures are also associated with high complication rates: Fistulas, hemorrhage, infection, or other complications occur in more than half of those patients. The mortality for an exploratory laparotomy is approximately 0.5%. We assumed a similarly low operative mortality for patients who undergo laparotomy for evaluation of a positive ERCP.

The Analysis and Interpretation

As we explained in our earlier discussion of this case, the analysis proceeds in three steps. First, we assess the posterior probability of pancreatic cancer given the CT findings; next we calculate—from the benefits and risks of treating pancreatic cancer—how high the probability of cancer would have to be before proceeding with further testing (the testing threshold); and then we compare the two probabilities. If the posterior probability of cancer is less than the testing threshold, the net benefit of further observation exceeds the net benefit of testing, and we would not recommend ERCP.

It if is greater than the threshold for testing, ERCP would be the optimal choice.[59]

Calculation of the Post-CT Probability of Pancreatic Cancer

The first value we need is the post-CT probability that the patient has pancreatic cancer—that is, given the results seen on CT, what is the probability that a cancer (CA) is present? This calculation is made by straightforward application of Bayes' theorem.[10,11] In this situation, in which we are primarily interested in the presence or absence of cancer, Bayes' theorem can be written as follows:

$$P\,(\text{CA}|\text{CT result}) = \frac{P(\text{CT result}|\text{CA}) \times P(\text{CA})}{P(\text{CT result}|\text{CA}) \times P(\text{CA}) + P(\text{CT false-positive rate}) \times [1 - P(\text{CA})]}$$

where $P(\text{CA}|\text{CT result})$ is the probability that cancer is present, given the CT findings; $P(\text{CT result}|\text{CA})$ is the sensitivity of CT for pancreatic cancer; and $P(\text{CA})$ is the baseline probability of pancreatic cancer in an asymptomatic man. According to the values from the table, the patient's likelihood of having pancreatic cancer is

$$\frac{(1.00) \times (0.0002)}{(1.00) \times (0.0002) + (0.64) \times (0.9998)} = 0.0003$$

Thus, with an equivocal finding as described on his CT scan, the patient's likelihood of harboring pancreatic cancer still is approximately 1 in 3,000.

Calculation of the Testing Threshold

The testing threshold (the probability of disease at which the net benefits of not testing and testing are equal) was calculated by a computer program using the decision tree shown in Figure 15.3 and the data in the table. The probability of pancreatic cancer would have to exceed 0.025 before the ERCP strategy would outweigh the observation strategy (Figure 15.4). After the CT scan, the probability of pancreatic cancer in the patient (0.0003) was considerably lower than this threshold value. Thus, avoiding ERCP is the optimal strategy.

Expected Utilities

When the baseline assumptions shown in the table are used, the expected utility (in this case, life expectancy) of proceeding with ERCP is 26.53 years, and the expected utility of avoiding ERCP is 26.59 years. The difference between these choices is extremely small.

Sensitivity Analysis and Interpretation

The calculations were based on fairly pessimistic estimates for the resectability and curability of a pancreatic cancer found early in its course. Nonetheless, the choice in this case is quite insensitive to the data used in the analysis. As the probability of successful resection approaches 100%, the threshold for proceeding to ERCP decreases to only approximately 0.024. In addition, as the cure rate improves, the threshold for proceeding to ERCP drops further. If we assume that a successfully resected cancer is cured and the probability of successfully resecting the early-identified cancer is approximately 0.70, the probability of cancer for which ERCP should be undertaken drops to approximately 0.022. In our patient, the probability of his having pancreatic cancer remains far below this threshold. Thus, not testing remains superior to testing.

Analysis

The results of this analysis confirm our decision that ERCP was unnecessary; yet, the choice to avoid the test is only marginally better than the choice to perform the test. The reader now can appreciate the complexity of the assumptions that were weighted in this analysis. Some assumptions were unobtainable from any source in the literature. Should that lack of data deter us from carrying out such analyses? Admittedly, we must be careful not to be seduced into thinking that our numerical estimates are "hard numbers," but if we avoid this trap, the estimates form a basis for examining how variations in these values influence the results of the analysis. As it turned out, extensive sensitivity analyses disclosed that the choice of ERCP was not the better one, even though it trailed only marginally in expected utility behind the choice of avoiding the test.

Here we have an illustration of advanced technology yielding confusing and equivocal results, which in turn leads to excessive and risky testing. However, how "wrong" were the patient's physicians in recommending ERCP? Could factors other than those we considered in our analysis

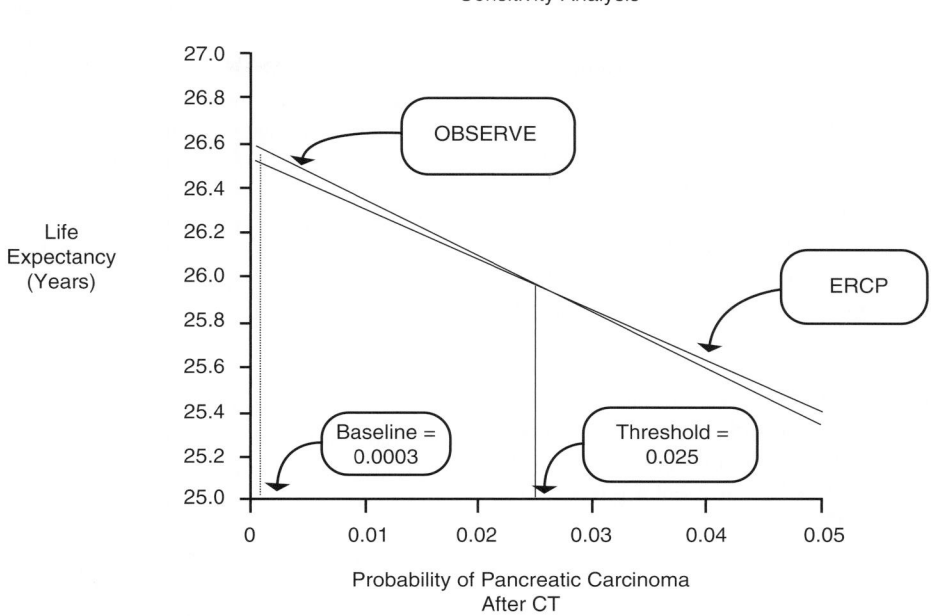

Figure 15.4 • One-way sensitivity analysis for case 30. At low probabilities of pancreatic cancer, the optimal choice is not to test, and at high probabilities, the optimal choice is to carry out the test (endoscopic retrograde cholangiopancreatography [ERCP]). The threshold denotes the probability at which the two choices are equal with respect to the patient's life expectancy. Note that the baseline probability (the estimated probability in the patient) is well below the threshold, suggesting that the optimal choice in the patient is not to test. CT, computed tomography.

have influenced their decision? If we assume that there was no financial motivation for doing the test and that concern about a malpractice claim was not an issue, what other motivation could there be?

We suggest that reduction of uncertainty is one possibility. Physicians are so accustomed to reducing uncertainty before embarking on a course of therapy that they have become compulsive about "knowing for sure." In one cognitive study of decision making under conditions of uncertainty, physicians were confronted with a patient who had an unidentified pulmonary infiltrate. Required to choose between gathering further information by invasive testing and treating the patient empirically, they selected the invasive tests and never even considered empiric therapy.[205] They chose to test even though a formal decision analysis disclosed no substantial difference between the expected utility of testing and treating empirically.

Further research into the intrinsic value of information above and beyond its value in making

choices about testing and treatment is warranted. Such research may help explain why we sometimes stumble over peculiar results of diagnostic tests.

CASE 31. THE PROBABILITY OF A PROBABILITY

A 67-year-old man presented to the Emergency Department with diffuse, burning abdominal pain. During his evaluation he was found to be in atrial fibrillation; serum sodium was 124 mEq/L.

Some intraabdominal process is presumably going on to explain the burning pain. I would like to know how long he had the complaint and how long he has had the atrial fibrillation. I do not know why his serum sodium is low. It could be caused by sodium depletion, water intoxication, adrenal insufficiency, the syndrome of inappropriate antidiuretic hormone (SIADH), or a variety of other causes. I am not sure I can tie these findings together.

> The patient had had diffuse, burning abdominal pain for 3 weeks. He reported no nausea, vomiting, weight loss, hematemesis, melena, or change in bowel habits. He had a remote history of peptic ulcer disease. He denied recent alcohol use but had smoked one to two packs of cigarettes a day for several years. His only medication was an occasional aspirin. On physical examination, he was not in distress. His blood pressure was 150/88 mm Hg, and his pulse rate was 130 per minute and irregularly irregular. The lungs were clear. No murmurs were heard. The abdomen was benign. Stool was trace guaiac positive. The rest of the examination was normal.

In view of the seemingly benign history and findings, I do not know why he came to the hospital at this time complaining of pain, unless an acute onset of atrial fibrillation caused some new, unexplained symptoms. I still do not know how that would relate to the finding of the low serum sodium.

> Additional laboratory data: WBC 15,200, hemoglobin 15.5 g/dL, hematocrit 42%, glucose 128 mg/dL, sodium 124 mEq/L, potassium 3.7 mEq/L, chloride 91 mEq/L, total CO_2 20 mEq/L, BUN 6 mg/dL, and creatinine 0.9 mg/dL. Urinalysis: specific gravity 1.020 and pH 7; dipstick and sediment examination were unremarkable. ECG showed atrial fibrillation with frequent premature ventricular contractions. Chest x-ray was compatible with chronic obstructive pulmonary disease. A retrocardiac hiatal hernia was present.

The high white cell count suggests the possibility of an infection, but the differential isn't given, and it could be helpful. The high specific gravity of the urine is inappropriate for the hyponatremia. Since the patient was a smoker and lung cancer is a frequent cause of SIADH, I thought he might end up having a lung nodule. Apparently, one was not seen on the chest x-ray.

> The patient was admitted for evaluation of atrial fibrillation and abdominal pain. The atrial fibrillation reverted to sinus rhythm spontaneously, and the patient was treated with diltiazem. Myocardial enzymes were not elevated. Thyroid function tests were normal. An echocardiogram showed normal valves and ejection fraction and a left atrial size of 3.7 cm. The gastrointestinal symptoms resolved, and his stool became guaiac negative.

The pain is gone without treatment. These findings are compatible with many things, but I would be interested in knowing what gastrointestinal workup he had. The atrial fibrillation appears to have been adequately evaluated, but the low serum sodium appears to have been lost.

> One month later, the patient returned with recurrent atrial fibrillation and abdominal pain. Once again, the stool was guaiac positive. Sodium was 128 mEq/L, and serum osmolality was 268 mOsm/kg, with a simultaneous urine osmolality of 384 mOsm/kg. His cardiac rhythm reverted to sinus rhythm with antiarrhythmic therapy after initial heparinization. The stool remained guaiac positive. The possibility of an occult gastrointestinal lesion was suggested as the cause of the apparent syndrome of inappropriate ADH secretion.

The osmolality studies are certainly compatible with SIADH. I am not sure about an association with gastrointestinal lesions. I am much more familiar with the association with pulmonary lesions.

> Colonoscopy revealed multiple adenomatous polyps with no evidence of malignancy. A barium swallow revealed right-upper-quadrant calcification and a large hiatal hernia with gastrointestinal reflux. Follow-up serum sodium was 132 mEq/L.

I suppose his abdominal burning could be related to the hiatal hernia with reflux, but I do not see an explanation for his low serum sodium and apparent SIADH. If there were no evidence of malignancy (and I assume all the polyps were removed and examined microscopically), I would not do any further gastrointestinal workup. I would consider getting a CT scan of his chest to make sure he does not have an occult neoplasm in his lung.

> The patient was seen at follow-up 4 months later. He complained of poor appetite and a 12-pound weight loss. Chest x-ray revealed a 2-cm mass in the right hilum with collapse of the right lower lobe. Serum sodium was 122 mEq/L. Biopsy of the lesion on bronchoscopy showed a poorly differentiated squamous cell cancer. Hyponatremia was treated successfully with demeclocycline, and a workup for metastatic disease was negative. A right pneumonectomy was performed; 2 of 13 carinal nodes were positive for tumor. The patient was given radiation therapy.

I wonder if the mass could have been hidden on the chest x-ray by the hiatal hernia. I would be interested in reviewing that with a radiologist. In retrospect, should SIADH have been worked up more aggressively earlier? I might have gotten the chest CT earlier because I am not familiar with gastrointestinal lesions causing SIADH. The colonic polyps just did not make sense to me as the cause of the hyponatremia.

Analysis

In the patient presented here, the correct diagnosis was missed for 5 months, and a "far-out" erroneous diagnosis was made instead. In retrospect, the physicians responsible for the patient's care seem foolish. The patient was a heavy smoker, his chest x-ray showed evidence of chronic lung disease, and he had SIADH. Lung cancer, especially small-cell cancer, should have been strongly considered, and the physicians should have been unwilling to give up on this diagnosis—despite the "negative" chest x-ray—until they had performed all reasonable tests (such as bronchoscopy or CT scan). Instead, when the chest x-ray showed no obvious tumor and an unrelated finding (intestinal polyps) was uncovered in the process of an investigation for guaiac-positive stools, the SIADH was attributed to "an occult gastrointestinal lesion." Undoubtedly, the physicians knew with confidence and with little ambiguity how high the likelihood of lung cancer was in a male smoker with SIADH. However, how confident were they of the likelihood that an occult gastrointestinal le-

sion could account for these findings? One might guess that they had little confidence.

This case raises an issue that we have not explored—confidence in probability judgments. Therefore, we shall discuss the concept of ambiguity. We think that the patient's physicians failed to consider this concept in their diagnostic hypotheses.

A busy clinician makes dozens, perhaps hundreds, of probability assessments each day on an array of probabilities: that one or more diseases may be present; that a patient will have a positive or negative (or some other) result of a diagnostic test; that, given a certain test result, one or more diseases are present or absent; that there might be an adverse reaction to a test or a treatment; that the patient might or might not respond to a regimen; and the probability of survival. Typically, each assessment is made without reference to a numerical value for the chance of the outcome. Instead, the probability is either categorical (high, very small, and practically nil) or ordinal (higher than, lower than, safer than).[61]

Even given the implicit categorical and ordinal descriptions of likelihood that we use every day, on the surface all probability assessments seem to be similar. Each requires the physician's judgment about the chance of some future event, and each is presumably grounded not only on personal experience, but also on the physician's understanding of the pertinent medical literature. To be sure, they are beliefs about the state of a given patient rather than "hard data," and they all require a judgment based on medical data.

However, are all assessments of probabilities really the same? Even if we were to state our views of the likelihood of several different outcomes in numerical terms, would we have the same confidence about all of our judgments? If the initial reaction is that all probabilities have similar meaning to us, ponder this: Suppose we can choose between two treatments for a given disease. One treatment has been used for years, and considerable data show that it cures 65% of patients. A second treatment has been introduced recently—only two studies have been published, each a small series—but the success rate is 70%. Are the two probabilities, 65% and 70%, comparable?

Most would agree that they are not. Large experience with the first treatment gives the physician confidence in a 65% probability of success. In the second treatment, there may be much uncertainty about the probability of 70% success, given limited data. Any probability needs to have a built-in factor that determines the confidence in which the value is held. The confidence in a probability often is described in terms of ambiguity. Ambiguity is uncertainty about a given probability. It sometimes is thought of as a "second-order" probability, or as a probability of a probability.

A certain amount of ambiguity characterizes all assessments of chance outcomes. Nonetheless, considerable ambiguity is likely to exist when available information is scanty (e.g., when the sample size is small), when data are unreliable (e.g., when the credibility of the source is questionable), or when facts or opinions of putative experts are conflicting.[206] All of these are encountered regularly in medicine and may contribute to variation in care.[207]

How to express ambiguity in probability assessments has yet to reach consensus. Some argue that the uncertainty of a probability should be expressed in terms used for characterizing outcome uncertainty, namely, as a probability range. This would require establishment of a range for a given set of probabilities (hence, the probability of a probability). Finally, a measure of confidence has been applied by some to rate the degree of ambiguity.[208] Although a confidence rating seems superior in experimental settings for expressing uncertainty in a probability, its relevance to the real world is uncertain.

Many experts in probability have figuratively thrown up their hands when it comes to assessing ambiguity. Some have suggested that we simply ask people to state their views directly.[209] Some argue that such verbal answers may or may not reflect beliefs and judgments.[5] Some suggest that the only way to be sure how a person feels about a problem is to observe what action he or she takes.[209] Others point out that many probabilities for observable events cannot be identified simply by observing behavior.

Does it matter whether we recognize ambiguity in assessment of likelihoods? It probably does because people generally try to avoid ambiguity.

Many reasons have been advanced to explain this: (1) People may reason that it is better to have more information than less; (2) they may be concerned that if not all information is available, they will have less control; (3) they may be concerned that their judgment will be evaluated by others (or even themselves after the fact); and (4) they may wish to avoid uncertainty.[210,211] Although some of these seem to predominate in experimental settings in which subjects are asked to participate in monetary lotteries, we suspect that all or at least most obtain in day-to-day decision making.

Thus, we are left with an unresolved problem: Ambiguity in assessing likelihood in clinical practice certainly exists. It influences how we think about a given disease, test, or treatment, but we have not yet learned how best to express the uncertainty in our probabilistic beliefs. What do we do in the meantime? We can identify situations in which ambiguity is likely to be greatest (few data available, unreliable data, conflicting data) and appreciate that confidence in judgments about the probabilities of medical outcomes in these situations may not be unshakable.

When undertaking formal decision assessments, we can test the most ambiguous variables by multivariate sensitivity analyses. Or we can even use the so-called *Monte Carlo simulation*, which carries out sensitivity analysis on all variables simultaneously.[10,212] At the very least, an understanding of the roots of ambiguity should make us aware of the potential limitations of our assessment of probabilistic clinical data.

Perhaps the diagnosis of lung cancer would have been made sooner in the patient presented if the concept of ambiguity had been considered. Perhaps the extreme "softness" in the probability of an occult gastrointestinal lesion as the cause of the SIADH would have led his physicians away from this hypothesis toward others. Given the type of the patient's tumor, earlier diagnosis and treatment probably would not have extended his life by much, if at all. Yet because a similar error could well have substantial implications for a patient's survival or even for a patient's quality of life, we should be alert about how avidly we accept our numerous probability assessments.

CHAPTER 16

Causal Reasoning

CASE 32. JUDGING CAUSALITY

> A 55-year-old man with cancer was admitted to the hospital for progressive jaundice.

Progressive jaundice in a man with cancer has many possible causes. His jaundice could be due to excessive red cell breakdown. Some cancers, particularly the B cell lymphomas, may produce immunoglobulins that cause a Coombs-positive hemolytic anemia. More often, cancers infiltrate the liver and cause either hepatocellular disarray or obstruction. In addition, he could have an unusual cholestatic jaundice, such as that which rarely occurs with renal cancer. The other question that always should be raised is, What therapy has he been on? Has he been on any hepatotoxic therapy? Has he been to a "specialist" in complementary and alternative medicine who is giving him hepatotoxic drugs? Among these are two vitamins that are hepatotoxic in high doses: Excess vitamin A can lead to cirrhosis, and high doses of niacin can cause inflammatory hepatitis. One would want to take a careful history not only about the cancer, but also about the cancer therapy.

> Twenty-four months before admission, the patient had a left hemicolectomy and local irradiation for Dukes' C_2 adenocarcinoma of the sigmoid colon. Five months before admission, a wedge resection of the liver was performed for recurrent tumor. A catheter was inserted into the hepatic artery, an infusion line was implanted, and a course of intra-arterial floxuridine (FUDR) was begun.

The use of intra-arterial chemotherapy for tumors is controversial. The goal is to provide the drug through the hepatic artery and to perfuse the tumor in the liver without necessarily affecting the rest of the liver or organs perfused by the systemic circulation. In theory, other organs can be spared because the liver extracts these toxins and prevents their access to the general circulation. The success rate of intrahepatic infusion (and I am not that familiar with this particular technique) has been variable to the best of my knowledge, although experts might argue with me.

We need to find out if the patient indeed has recurrent tumor in his liver or if there is something hepatotoxic about this chemotherapeutic agent. Clearly, a major hepatotoxin would not be the best chemotherapeutic agent to choose for intrahepatic infusion. The other possibility, since he has cancer and an implanted catheter, is an infection, either bacterial or viral.

> Over the next 4 months, the patient received FUDR by continuous infusion for 2 weeks, alternating with saline for 2 weeks. During this interval, he felt well. Serial studies showed the following (ALT, alanine transaminase):

Months before Admission	Bilirubin (mg/dL)	ALT (IU/L)	Alkaline phosphatase (IU/L)
18	0.5	—	83
5	0.9	208	64
4	0.3	23	135
3	0.4	16	154
2	1.6	—	630
1	3.5	155	588

> One month before admission, he complained of low-grade fever, and right infrascapular pain developed 2 weeks later. Pain persisted, and jaundice became clinically apparent two days before admission. He was admitted for studies.

Serial studies show a gradually rising bilirubin associated with an initial elevation of ALT, which subsequently fluctuated. His alkaline phosphatase, on the other hand, is rising steadily along with his bilirubin, which suggests that something is stimulating those cells within his biliary radicles to produce alkaline phosphatase. Obstruction would be the most common cause of this picture. I wonder who was looking at him 1 month before admission. With a bilirubin of 3.5, most jaundice is clinically apparent, but subtle jaundice is not always obvious to those who are seeing a person regularly. In retrospect, some obvious malfunction was occurring 1 month before admission or even earlier. The patient had infrascapular pain and already had

169

abnormal liver function studies. In fact, he was almost certainly clinically jaundiced at that time.

Why is jaundice occurring? Is it hepatotoxicity from the infusate? Is it a complication of the instrumentation? One might wonder about hepatic artery occlusion, but thrombosis of the hepatic artery usually is not a serious problem because the portal vein is the major route of blood supply to the liver.

Does he now have an infection? The right infrascapular pain suggests that some process in the dome of the liver was irritating the subdiaphragmatic surface, causing that classic referral of pain. Could he have recurrent tumor to account for low-grade fever? All of these possibilities come to mind.

> **On admission, the patient was overtly jaundiced. The liver width was 14 cm by percussion and was palpated three fingerbreadths below the costal margin. No other abnormalities were noted on physical examination. Laboratory studies showed hematocrit 32% and white cell count 6,600; normal electrolytes, blood urea nitrogen (BUN), and creatinine; bilirubin 8.0 mg/dL, ALT 230 IU/L, and alkaline phosphatase 735 IU/L.**

The normal white count argues against infection. The bilirubin is now 8.0, so it has gone up rather precipitously from 3.5 one month before admission. His ALT is now high, which suggests hepatocellular damage, and his alkaline phosphatase is high. If I were dealing with this patient, I would seek the help of chemotherapy experts as to whether the drug could be doing this. If the drug is not the likely cause, could his hepatic artery be occluded? Would there be some value in opacifying the infusion line to see whether the hepatic artery is patent? I would also like to visualize the liver by scan to look for recurrent tumor or infection.

> **Both computed tomography (CT) scan and ultrasound revealed dilated intrahepatic ducts but a normal-sized common bile duct. Residual tumor, not in a position to obstruct major bile ducts, was demonstrated on the CT scan.**

So he has residual tumor, but we do not know if it has been reduced in size in response to therapy. He has dilated intrahepatic ducts but evidently

does not have biliary tract obstruction of the usual sort.

Now, what could do this? Is there a biliary cirrhosis-like phenomenon occurring with this drug? Frankly, I do not know. I would have to look it up. Could he have another cause of a dilated intrahepatic ductular system, such as a sclerosing cholangitis or a rare condition called a Klatskin-type cholangiocarcinoma, which can produce a similar picture? Perhaps he has a history of inflammatory bowel disease predisposing him to cancer of the colon. I raise this possibility because ulcerative colitis is associated with a sclerosing cholangitis. Again, one would have to demonstrate what precisely was going on there. In this circumstance, I would ask the oncologists whether the drug could do it.

> **Transhepatic cholangiography revealed multiple stenoses within the intrahepatic ducts and at the bifurcation of the intrahepatic and common hepatic ducts.**

Well, something is stenosing those ducts and producing sclerosing cholangitis.

> **The findings were considered characteristic of FUDR-associated sclerosing cholangitis. Chemotherapy was discontinued, and a drainage tube was left in the biliary tree. A repeat cholangiogram 2 weeks later showed progressive stenosis; serum bilirubin and alkaline phosphatase increased to 10.2 mg/dL and 923 IU/L, respectively. Subsequently, the patient was stricken with biliary sepsis, *Pseudomonas* endocarditis, and massive hematobilia. He died approximately 3 months later from uncontrollable biliary sepsis.**

In some cases, it is possible to reduce obstruction surgically in patients with sclerosing cholangitis; that is, it is possible to relieve some of the most obvious of the obstructive lesions. Theoretically, if the stenoses are relieved, survival can be extended. Evidently, that was not possible in this patient, presumably because of the multiplicity of his lesions and his other medical problems.

Analysis

Here a general internist, unarmed with experimental evidence that the chemotherapeutic agent floxuridine induces toxicity to bile duct epithelium and unaware that the intraarterial infusion of this drug in the hepatic artery already has been solidly implicated on clinical grounds as a cause of sclerosing cholangitis, invents the correct causal connection, and then becomes convinced that FUDR is the cause of obstructive jaundice.

Causality of clinical events or clinical entities is an essential ingredient in clinical cognition.[44,45,47] A useful framework for provisionally attributing causality includes these components: a causal field, cues to a causal relation, and factors that influence causal strength. A *causal field* is a context or problem space in which reasoning and judgments about probable cause occur. In this instance the causal field could be construed as a chain consisting of multiple intermediate steps (drug causes arterial damage, which in turn causes ischemia of the lining of bile canaliculi, which in turn causes fibrosis of canaliculi, which in turn causes biliary obstruction, which in turn causes reduction of bile excretion, which in turn causes bile retention, which in turn causes jaundice). Or it might be viewed at a lower level of understanding—a shunted version with only a few links (drug causes biliary obstruction, which causes jaundice). Which of these contexts is selected is determined largely by the purpose. The causal field also is important in setting the number of alternative explanations for an event or finding. For example, in the cause we are considering, the presence of cancer in the liver offers an obvious alternative explanation for jaundice, at least before the CT scan result was available. If the patient had been an acknowledged alcoholic or if he had received several blood transfusions in the preceding months, other alternative explanations might also have been appropriate. In the case of our patient, there was concordance between stimulus and effect. Chemotherapeutic agents are certainly known to have multiple toxic effects. The infusion of FUDR directly into the liver over the time interval immediately preceding the development of jaundice provides evidence of concordance both in space and in time. Thus, the cues all point to a causal relation between the FUDR and the jaundice. Necessarily, this relation is a probabilistic one: On the basis of the cues alone, we would be justified only in being suspicious that the drug caused obstructive jaundice. As with most judgments about the state of the world, our assessment

of the cause-and-effect relation between the drug and the jaundice yields only a probability that an effect is linked to some cause.

Several measures make it possible to test the *strength* of the link between a cause and an effect. Many of these measures were satisfied in our jaundiced patient, particularly the relation in time and space between the stimulus (intrahepatic FUDR) and the response (cholangitis). Of course, these relationships are only correlations. Indeed, care must be taken to avoid using spurious correlations to enhance causal strength.

Finally, the strength of a given causal hypothesis must stand the test of alternative possible explanations. The fact that a single causal explanation appears to account for all of the observed findings does not ensure that this causal chain is the correct one. Alternative constructions of the chain must be sought deliberately and tested for their strengths. The discussant raises many alternate causal explanations for the jaundice: At various points she considers hemolysis, tumor infiltration, tumor-related cholestasis, vitamin overdose, drug-induced hepatocellular damage, catheter-related pyogenic infection, catheter-induced hepatic artery occlusion, and viral hepatitis—but close scrutiny fails to enhance the causal strength of any of these entities.

Reversion to "first principles" sometimes pays off, but assigning causality is fraught with difficulties. Multiple approaches, as used here by the discussant, are minimal criteria for beginning such assessments.

CASE 33. POST HOC, ERGO PROPTER HOC

> On her sixth hospital day, a 26-year-old woman on the urology service gradually developed a flaccid quadriplegia and required intubation for hypercapnia.

That is a dramatic development. I am going to the bedside to try to find out about the catastrophe that has just happened to this young woman, and I am wondering why she was in the hospital in the first place. How did this whole illness start? I have to make that assessment quickly because there is a sense of urgency here if we are to have any hope of reversing the process and avoiding a further catastrophe.

The first two questions that come to my mind are, Why is she in the hospital on the urology service, and what would cause her paralysis? I have three basic pigeonholes that I will use to explain the origin of this patient's flaccid quadriplegia and flaccid diaphragm. One is an intrinsic lesion of the spinal cord, such as a vascular event or possibly a transverse myelitis. A cord lesion would have to be fairly high, at about C2, to give her a flaccid diaphragm as well. The second is an external lesion compressing the cervical spinal cord, and I may learn something more about that from her history. The third is some metabolic reason for flaccid quadriplegia—that is, a disorder in which the spinal cord and its pathways are all intact but for some reason end-organ sensitivity has been lost. Those are the three broad categories I would be thinking about as I was running to the patient's bedside.

> The patient had had a gastric bypass operation for morbid obesity, and she has a history of recurrent *Proteus* urinary tract infections complicated by struvite stones. An abdominal CT scan showed a large right staghorn calculus with partial obstruction and scattered calcifications in the left kidney. The patient was admitted for treatment of the staghorn calculus.

Now I know why she is in the hospital. Patients with certain types of intestinal bypass operations have a variety of metabolic imbalances, which I may hear more about in the upcoming laboratory studies. She also had *Proteus* urinary tract infections complicated by struvite stones. That kind of stone is common with urea-splitting organisms such as *Proteus*, which alkalinize the urine and promote the crystallization of struvite.

Can I make a connection between the information that she had a partially obstructed kidney with some calcifications in the contralateral side and her subacute to acute neurologic deterioration? It certainly makes me think less strongly about a vascular compromise, and it gives me no clue that a mass lesion is responsible. I am inclined to think that this clinical picture falls under the rubric of metabolic causes. I want the results of

the physical examination and some laboratory data pretty quickly.

> On admission, the patient was alert and oriented. She was not febrile. Physical examination was unremarkable except for massive obesity. She had normal muscle strength. All laboratory studies were normal except the urine sediment (which showed 15 to 20 white blood cells per high-power field) and the urine culture (which contained more than 100,000 colonies per milliliter of *Proteus mirabilis*). Treatment with gentamicin was begun on the second hospital day. On the second day, a nephrostomy tube was inserted into the right renal pelvis. Saline was infused for 3 days, and on the fourth day, the saline was replaced by an antilithic solution, intended to dissolve the stone.

Again, I need to focus on the cause of her quadriplegia because that is what is jeopardizing her life at the moment. I now know that she had a normal neurologic examination when she was admitted. She had significant bacteriuria, for which she received gentamicin. Four days before the onset of the acute neurologic event, an invasive procedure was carried out, and on the day before the event, she received the antilithic infusion.

I am still convinced it is not a vascular event or a compressive lesion. I am concerned that it might be a problem of neural transmission. I have not been told anything about her mental status; if I knew whether she was awake and alert, I would know whether or not she has cortical dysfunction. From what I have been told so far, there is no indication that there is cortical dysfunction. She received some drugs in the hospital. Gentamicin has various kinds of neurotoxicity, most commonly involving the eighth nerve; it probably causes direct toxicity to nerve cells. In addition, like all the aminoglycosides, gentamicin has been associated with disruption of neural transmission. That complication has usually been observed with intraperitoneal infusions. In these cases, patients are suddenly unable to breathe because the aminoglycoside interrupts neural transmission to the diaphragm.

However, I have never heard of flaccid quadriplegia developing on the fifth day of intravenous gentamicin therapy, so I do not think that drug is the culprit. Nevertheless, it is an intervention that preceded the development of paralysis, and knowing that the drug can be neurotoxic, I must keep it in mind.

I am not sure what the antilithic agent is. I am concerned that anything that preceded this sudden neurologic event could be related to it. I would get more information about the agent. What is it, and, specifically, does it pose a risk of acute neurotoxicity?

> The patient did well on day 5, but on the morning of day 6, she complained of increasing fatigue and weakness. Neurologic examination disclosed no abnormalities, and the remainder of the physical examination and the laboratory findings were unremarkable. Aside from the antilithic and gentamicin, the patient was also receiving alprazolam and an antacid.

I guess the problem developed subacutely, with increasing fatigue and weakness. I am still very much concerned about these medicines, especially the gentamicin and the antilithic. I am not aware that antacids and alprazolam are associated with acute neurologic abnormalities such as this.

> Over the next several hours, she became more lethargic and later had no spontaneous respirations. Blood pressure was 110/70 mm Hg, pulse 80 per minute and regular, temperature 35°C. Neurologic examination disclosed that she had a flaccid quadriparesis with areflexia; she was able to open her eyes and blink on command.

The areflexia is important. If she had an upper motor neuron lesion, she would have been hyperreflexic instead of areflexic. What I am left with is one of my earlier hypotheses: that she has a problem with neural transmission. I am concerned now that she has drug-induced neuromuscular blockade. Either she cannot secrete acetylcholine or she is unresponsive to it on the other side of the neuromuscular junction.

> Laboratory findings: hematocrit 37%, white cell count 28,000; sodium 132 mEq/L, potassium 3.6 mEq/L, chloride 79 mEq/L, total CO_2 38 mEq/L, and creatinine 1.5 mg/dL. Blood gases (on room air): pH 7.32, partial pressure of oxygen (PO_2) 49 mm Hg, partial pressure

> of carbon dioxide (PCO_2) 79 mm Hg. Blood glucose (after two ampoules of 50% dextrose) 460 mg/dL.

The most striking abnormality here is the hypercapnia. She has a PCO_2 of 79 and a pH of 7.32 with a bicarbonate of 38. That is somewhat surprising. As I recall, this patient had normal baseline chemistries. She now has a strikingly high bicarbonate level. She could not have retained all that bicarbonate that fast in response to an acute rise in PCO_2. Derangements of the serum potassium, especially hypokalemia, can sometimes cause flaccidity. This woman does not have that. The white count of 28,000 is not readily explained. She recently had a urinary tract infection, but that is an awfully high white count for that. Could she have developed an acute infection? The glucose of 460 shortly after two ampoules of 50% dextrose is what I would have expected. I do not see a clear explanation for her flaccid paralysis, and I am still not sure what is happening. I would still be hot on the trail of drug-induced disease.

> Serum magnesium values were being checked daily. On the day of the respiratory arrest, the laboratory called to report that the patient's serum magnesium was 19 mEq/L. They also had rerun the magnesium level from the previous day, reported originally to be 1.7 mEq/L, and found the value to be 12 mEq/L. A nephrostogram disclosed that the catheter had slipped out of the renal pelvis. Contrast material extravasated into the retroperitoneal space.

Well, that is a spectacular finding! A magnesium level of that order of magnitude is higher than I have ever heard of. Extremely high levels of divalent cations can inhibit neural transmission. I think we should now focus on the hypermagnesemia as being causally related to her quadriplegia. How did she get so hypermagnesemic? Looking at input and output, she either has taken in a lot of magnesium or has not excreted it—or a combination thereof—to get to that level.

I need to know whether the antilithic has magnesium in it. We know that her serum creatinine is slightly increased, and she may not be excreting much magnesium. I think she must be getting a large amount of magnesium and is not excreting much. Could hypermagnesemia in any way be associated with the gastric bypass? I do not believe that such patients have spontaneous hypermagnesemia, so I would say that this occurrence represents some kind of infusion and inability to get rid of it. There must be some relationship between this infusion, which is now not being retrieved from the nephrostomy irrigation, and absorption of an exorbitant amount of magnesium. I want to find out the composition of the antilithic.

> **The antilithic, which contains high concentrations of magnesium carbonate, was being administered at a rate between 30 and 90 mL per hour. She received a total of approximately 2 L of a standard solution over a period of 45 hours. The magnesium concentration of that solution is 550 mEq/L.**

It is now clear that the hypermagnesemia resulted from the retroperitoneal infusion of the antilithic and caused a failure of neural transmission, thus producing the quadriplegia.

> **The antilithic was discontinued. Quadriplegia, respiratory paralysis, and hypercapnia were attributed to magnesium absorption from the retroperitoneum. Metabolic alkalosis was attributed to alkali (carbonate) overload. She was treated with mechanical ventilation, intravenous fluids (including hydrochloric acid), and furosemide. She had a large diuresis and improved remarkably over the next 12 hours. Serum magnesium fell progressively to normal over a 72-hour period. She also was treated for an aspiration pneumonia, extubated the next morning, and discharged on the 14th hospital day.**

Well, the proof of the pudding is in the eating. The major therapeutic intervention was directed at lowering her serum magnesium and correcting her metabolic derangements. The fact that she improved with this treatment validates the hypothesis that hypermagnesemia caused the failure of neural transmission.

> **Note: The patient described here was treated more than a decade ago, and the intravenous antilithic solution is rarely used today. Nonetheless, because intravenous magnesium salts are**
>
> **still given today for a variety of indications, including acute myocardial infarction, asthma, and severe headaches, we have preserved this case from an earlier edition. The following analysis remains relevant.**

Analysis

Two key methods of clinical problem solving are evident in this transcript: assessing causality on the basis of antecedent events and reverting to first principles to establish diagnostic hypotheses. Because both of those approaches are aspects of the process of "case building," or hypothesis revision, we introduce them briefly by considering how physicians construct, reject, and reconstruct diagnostic hypotheses as they gather and interpret clinical findings.

After generating one or more hypotheses, clinicians select those questions most likely to add to or detract from those hypotheses.[18,19] In doing so, they identify existing findings that tend to confirm that the patient has a given disease. Subsequently, they search for additional findings that their hypotheses lead them to believe should be either present or absent. The findings that are assessed in this process are many and varied. They include simple clinical manifestations (historical features, physical findings, and laboratory results), predisposing factors, known complications of the disease, and certain temporal relationships. In other cases in this book, we have considered some of the techniques physicians use to combine those findings and build a case for one or more diagnostic hypotheses. Here, we focus on only one of the findings they use to make that assessment: namely, the temporal relationship between clinical events.

Every experienced clinician uses antecedent temporal relationships as a diagnostic tool. In confirming a diagnosis of acute tubular necrosis, we look for a preceding hypotensive episode; in evaluating a new rash, we inquire about the recent addition of new medications; in confirming a diagnosis of worsened cardiac failure, we look for excessive sodium intake or a preceding infection; in confirming a diagnosis of gout, we look for recent initiation of diuretic therapy. Each medical specialist knows and uses those temporal relationships, often without making a special mental effort.

The identification of disease antecedents probably represents one of the most useful tools for case building, and in the foregoing transcript, we can appreciate the power of that strategy. The discussant correctly assumed that the patient's paralysis was the consequence of some untoward event that occurred during the hospitalization, not an event that just happened by chance while she was hospitalized. Furthermore, he believed that the paralysis could be related to some antecedent therapeutic maneuver. Initially, he considered the possibility that gentamicin might be responsible but quickly dismissed it. Subsequently, he focused on the antilithic as a cause, even though he was unaware of its composition. The temporal association between the administration of the antilithic and the onset of quadriplegia was so compelling that it became the basis for a causal explanation of the paralysis.

Admittedly, temporal associations alone cannot be taken as ironclad proof of causality. The phrase *post hoc, ergo propter hoc* (after this, therefore because of this) is often cited to warn the uninitiated not to assume that a clear antecedent is necessarily causally implicated. The importance of antecedent events in a case-building strategy is one of the underdeveloped and untested aspects of clinical problem solving and has been under investigation for some time.[44,47] How often we interpret antecedents appropriately and how often we are led down the garden path by relying on temporal associations alone is an interesting subject for further research.

A second significant aspect of the problem-solving exercise in this case is the discussant's reversion to "first principles." As noted, he correctly associated the antilithic administration and the paralysis temporally, but he was unable to extend that relationship further. He did, however, exclude structural neurologic disorders as the cause and hypothesized that the disorder was metabolic in origin. That judgment in itself is not particularly impressive because many neurologic diagnoses are frequently considered "toxic" or "metabolic" by exclusion alone. However, in this instance, the discussant came closer to a true functional classification of the neurologic disorder by identifying the disturbance as one that affected neuromuscular

transmission. Unable to establish a precise etiologic diagnosis, he reasoned that some agent had either interfered with secretion of acetylcholine or had blocked the ability of the neurotransmitter to react with its receptor. In this circumstance, the discussant precisely identified the site of the neuromuscular derangement, even though the correct diagnosis escaped him. This is one instance in which reliance on "precompiled" diagnostic and therapeutic decisions would have faltered badly.

It is reasonable to assume that had our discussant actually been responsible for the care of this patient, his identification of the antecedent cause of the disorder and his capacity to reason back to first principles and determine the nature of the paralysis would have led him quickly to the correct etiology and the correct treatment.

CASE 34. THE CASE FOR CAUSAL REASONING

> A 71-year-old man consulted his physician for swelling of his legs and feet and a 30-pound weight gain over the previous 2 months.

We have a man with weight gain and lower-extremity edema, but no mention of shortness of breath, so there is no definitive evidence of biventricular cardiac failure. If he had dyspnea, I would worry about a cardiac basis for the edema. Of course, he could have predominant right-sided failure secondary to left-sided failure without dyspnea, but that is clearly uncommon. If we explore the history of a patient who presents with right-sided failure, there usually are some symptoms or signs consistent with left-sided failure. This patient also has no manifestations that suggest pulmonary disease, which argues against the possibility that cor pulmonale is the cause of the edema.

Finding no obvious immediate explanation, I would examine the mechanisms that could explain edema of the legs. I would think about four considerations. First, he could have increased hydrostatic pressure in the leg vessels, with consequent fluid accumulation in the tissues. Second, he could have decreased oncotic pressure secondary to a low serum albumin. If his albumin were low, we would try to determine whether he had decreased synthesis of proteins, for example, as might occur in liver disease or in malnutrition. Alternatively, he might have lost albumin; the two sources of albumin loss would be his kidney and his gastrointestinal tract. Third, he could have increased vascular permeability secondary to inflammatory disease or some kind of injury, although I admit that a localized inflammatory process could not explain this much weight gain. Finally, drainage from the interstitial space could be reduced if he had lymphatic occlusion or lymphatic disease.

So the main concern is why his vessels leak fluid.

> The patient was short of breath when he climbed stairs but not on ordinary exertion. He denied orthopnea, paroxysmal nocturnal dyspnea, and chest pain. He was eating well and taking no medications, and he had no gastrointestinal complaints. He did have nocturia, four to five times a night, but no other genitourinary symptoms.

The shortness of breath does not seem impressive and could simply be related to the need to carry an extra 30 pounds of weight. It is hard to tell: He may well have minor chronic lung disease, but those findings are not consistent with pulmonary disease severe enough to account for this degree of fluid retention. The shortness of breath suggests the possibility that he may have volume overload rather than retention of fluid secondary to a low oncotic pressure. Of course, he could also have pleural effusions or ascites secondary to hypoalbuminemia, and either of those could make his respiratory function a little poorer in response to exercise, but there is nothing at the moment to suggest that possibility.

Frequent nocturia suggests prostatic obstruction. I would be interested to know whether he urinates frequently during the day as well. Obstructive uropathy could explain salt and water retention and could produce a volume-overloaded state. Mild congestive heart failure might also explain the nocturia. Patients with congestive heart failure may be operating at their peak cardiac output most of the time and may fail to concentrate their urine at night. That disturbance can produce some degree of nocturia, though four to five times is more than I would anticipate from urinary tract obstruction. Of course, he could have some disor-

der of concentrating ability, but I do not see any reason to consider any of those yet. This much nocturia suggests either that his bladder is not holding the volume or that he is excreting larger than normal amounts of urine.

> The patient had a 150-pack-year smoking history and a history of heavy drinking, but he had not smoked or used alcohol in 2 years. Stage D cancer of the prostate had been treated 2 years earlier by orchiectomy; he had neither symptoms nor signs of active disease since, and his prostate-specific antigen (PSA) was not elevated. He had no history of hypertension. His family history was unrevealing.

With that smoking history he could well have chronic obstructive lung disease, but he does not have much dyspnea, cough, or sputum production, which still leads me to believe that he does not have severe enough pulmonary disease to produce cor pulmonale.

He did use alcohol until 2 years ago. Could he have cirrhosis with hypoalbuminemia? Could a low albumin account for the fluid in his legs? We certainly have to keep that in mind. He stopped drinking 2 years ago, and assuming that he eats well and has no other stigmata of cirrhosis, we will put the diagnosis of cirrhosis on hold.

We do have to concern ourselves with the possibility of obstructive uropathy. It could explain his nocturia; in addition, the early phase of obstructive uropathy is associated with retention of sodium and volume overload.

We must concern ourselves with his smoking history of 150 pack-years, which suggests the possibility of some tobacco-related malignancy, particularly a pulmonary malignancy. Could such a malignancy explain some or all of his clinical manifestations? The answer is yes, on two counts. First, he might have nephrotic syndrome associated with a pulmonary malignancy. Histologically, such lesions are either membranous glomerulonephritis or membranoproliferative glomerulonephritis, which can produce the classic picture of nephrotic syndrome with proteinuria, low serum albumin, and peripheral edema. Second, he might have salt retention secondary to a pulmonary lesion; he could have a tumor that is producing ACTH (adrenocorticotropic hormone), which in turn would lead to a mineralocorticoid effect with sodium retention and potassium loss. The sodium retention could explain the edema, and potassium depletion (rather than nephrotic syndrome) might explain the polyuria because we would expect a somewhat reduced urine output in nephrotic syndrome.

> His blood pressure was 190/92 mm Hg, and his pulse was 84 per minute. He was obese and not jaundiced. Neck veins were not distended. A few early expiratory wheezes were heard in both lungs; cardiac examination revealed an S_4 gallop but no S_3 gallop and no murmurs. The abdomen was obese, with no palpable organs or masses and no evident ascites. Liver size was apparently normal. The prostate was hard and nodular. There was 4+ pitting edema up to the knees and none elsewhere.

Given that he did not have a history of hypertension and now has a slightly elevated diastolic and mildly elevated systolic pressure, I suspect that he may, in fact, be slightly volume overloaded. The presence of an S_4 gallop with no S_3 gallop might be consistent with a recent rise in blood pressure, but it also might mean that his left ventricle is less distensible than normal. Clearly, he has no evidence of cardiac failure, and I am now willing to exclude this disorder as a cause of the edema. His abdomen is obese, but he has neither hepatomegaly nor ascites, and I think that we also can eliminate liver disease as a cause. We know that he has 4+ pitting edema only in the legs. The edema could be the nonspecific consequence of renal salt and water retention and thus be dependent edema, or it could be the result of a mechanical obstruction that limits it to his lower extremities. Although he had cancer of the prostate, careful examination disclosed no lateral extension of a mass along the pelvic floor that might have obstructed either lymphatic or venous return, and his PSA was not elevated.

> Laboratory findings at this time were as follows: hemoglobin 14.9 g/dL, hematocrit 50%, white cell count 11,900 with 83% segs, 5% bands, 5% lymphs, and 7% monos, BUN 23 mg/dL, creatinine 1.2 mg /dL, fasting glucose 133 mg/dL, albumin 3.2 g/dL, calcium 9.3 mg/dL, biliru-

> bin 0.4 mg/dL, alkaline phosphatase 64 IU/L, lactate dehydrogenase 487 IU/L, and aspartate transaminase 55 IU/L. International Normalized Ratio was 1.0, and partial thromboplastin time was 22 seconds. Urinalysis: specific gravity 1.015; trace amounts of protein and glucose. Urine sediment was unremarkable. The electrocardiogram showed sinus arrhythmia, left axis deviation, and nonspecific anterolateral T-wave changes.

The patient's serum albumin is slightly low, but it is not in the nephrotic range, and his urine protein is negligible. I am now satisfied to exclude the diagnoses of nephrotic syndrome and cirrhosis. His hemoglobin is at the upper limit of normal for a man his age. If he does have pulmonary disease, it is probably not severe. The hemoglobin suggests one of three things: (1) he is more hypoxic than I thought; (2) he has a lesion that is causing his hematocrit and hemoglobin to be elevated (the lesion could be a malignancy that is producing either erythropoietin or cortisol excess); or (3) he has hemoconcentration, which does not sound likely. His white count is slightly elevated, and he has a significant left shift. His blood sugar is mildly elevated. These findings also go along with excess cortisol.

> Routine admission electrolytes: sodium 150 mEq/L, potassium 2.1 mEq/L, chloride 93 mEq/L, total CO_2 45 mEq/L. Blood gases (patient breathing room air): pH 7.62, PCO_2 46 mm Hg, PO_2 57 mm Hg. Calculated plasma bicarbonate 47 mEq/L.

Aha! These data give us the answer! Given this serum sodium, the finding of sodium retention, hypertension, and the other features suggesting volume overload, a pattern of primary sodium retention emerges. This, in combination with severe hypokalemia and metabolic alkalosis, implies an acceleration of sodium exchange with potassium and hydrogen ion that is typically seen in hypercorticism. Because the patient had been a heavy smoker, the first diagnosis that comes to mind is a neoplasm stimulating cortisol production directly through ACTH secretion. He could have an adrenal lesion, but I think that is a less likely possibility. You could also get edema with cathartic abuse. There is no doubt that this is a picture of corticoid excess, and the only question is whether we are dealing with a primary adrenal lesion or with another neoplasm that is stimulating the adrenals through the production of ACTH. The 150-pack-year history of smoking suggests that the latter is more likely.

> **Urinary electrolytes (spot specimen): sodium 77 mEq/L, potassium 48 mEq/L, chloride 58 mEq/L.**

Given the serum potassium of 2.1, a urinary potassium of 48 represents overt potassium wasting and is most consistent with hyperadrenocorticism. The urinary chloride concentration of 58 is even more interesting from a diagnostic standpoint. Most patients with hypokalemic metabolic alkalosis of this severity have virtually no chloride in their urine, and the absence of chloride is a good indicator that they have lost chloride as a consequence of vomiting or the use of diuretics. Such patients are chloride dependent; you can treat them with either sodium or potassium chloride and readily correct their alkalosis. But there is a subset of patients who are sodium chloride resistant—that is, their alkalosis does not correct with sodium chloride administration. These individuals have significant amounts of chloride in their urine, as this patient did, and many of them have adrenocortical hyperfunction.

> **The chest x-ray revealed bilateral interstitial changes and nodular densities in the right lower lobe consistent with malignancy.**

This finding supports the suspicion that a tumor is causing the hyperadrenalism. All we need are the hormonal data.

> **His plasma cortisols were as follows: random morning value 46 μg/dL; evening value 56 μg/dL. After dexamethasone suppression (1 mg, overnight): morning cortisol 46 μg/dL. After 0.5 mg, every 6 hours, for 2 days: morning cortisol 48 μg/dL. After 2 mg, every 6 hours, for 2 days: morning cortisol: 50 μg/dL. ACTH 500–922 pg/mL (normal <130 pg/mL). Plasma renin and aldosterone normal.**

This is an obvious ACTH-producing lesion, and the high level of ACTH production is almost

certainly caused by the pulmonary neoplasm. The patient has a neoplasm that is producing ACTH, which in turn stimulates the adrenals to produce cortisol at an unremitting rate. The high cortisol levels lead to salt retention, potassium wasting, and salt-resistant alkalosis. Most people would "escape" from the sodium-retaining effect of cortisol, but if he has mild cardiac dysfunction, he might not escape. The other possibility that might explain the edema is severe potassium depletion. The mechanism of salt retention in potassium-depleted patients is not known, but in some patients, potassium replacement leads to a striking diuresis.

> **Outcome: Bronchoscopy revealed multiple lesions in the right-upper- and lower-lobe bronchi. Biopsy of the lesions revealed small-cell anaplastic carcinoma; prostate-specific antigen stain was negative. Large quantities of potassium chloride were given to treat hypokalemia and metabolic alkalosis, and spironolactone was added later. Normal plasma potassium and bicarbonate values were not achieved. The patient was given a course of chemotherapy, but he died at home several weeks later.**

Analysis

This patient suffered a tragic outcome, but we offer the discussion of his case as an excellent example of causal, or physiologic, reasoning. We have much to learn about the kinds of reasoning that physicians use to build a diagnosis from the clues they abstract from the environment. Elsewhere, we describe Bayesian (or probabilistic) reasoning, a diagnostic approach that relies exclusively on the statistical relations between clinical findings and ignores a pathophysiologic explanation (see cases 23 and 27). For example, in the Bayesian framework, hypertension might be viewed as correlated with renal artery stenosis without acknowledgment that the stenosis was the proximate cause of renin release, which in turn produced the elevation of blood pressure. Pulmonary edema might be viewed simply as a likely finding in patients with cardiac failure, without any acknowledgment that the high pulmonary venous pressure produced the capillary leak in the lungs. This probabilistic approach is valuable, especially when causal relations between clinical variables are uncertain or unproved, but in our everyday lives, our commonsense reasoning probably is not characterized largely by statistical associations. Indeed, it seems quite likely that causality dominates much of our routine problem solving. We are quite accustomed to causal connections that describe the real world: What goes up must come down; black clouds and thunder portend rain; the faster we drive, the worse the crash. Causal reasoning is important in medicine; witness the amount of time devoted to physiology and biochemistry in medical schools. Despite the emphasis on physiologic principles at the undergraduate level, causal reasoning has received little attention as an approach to medical diagnosis.

The transcript presented here provides a superb example of how probabilistic relations take a back seat to physiologic reasoning in solving some diagnostic dilemmas. Although the case we selected is ideally suited to this kind of approach, the discussant's bent toward physiologic reasoning is evident early in the exercise. In this case, the etiology of edema was an uncommon disorder; after taking a brief stab at the possibility that edema was cardiac or pulmonary in origin, the discussant reverted to a consideration of the possible physiologic causes of salt and water retention (e.g., increased hydrostatic pressure, low oncotic pressure, increased vascular permeability, obstruction to lymphatic or venous outflow). He then considered and rejected many of those possible causes. Later, when he learned that the patient's blood pressure was high and he had no previous history of hypertension, he considered the possibility that the patient was volume overloaded. With a volume-expanded state in mind, he used the high hematocrit, the left shift, and the mild hyperglycemia to support the possibility that hyperadrenalism produced the volume expansion. Finally, he pounced on the serum and urinary electrolyte abnormalities as convincing evidence that a hyperadrenal state existed and correctly proposed lung cancer as the cause.

There is little evidence that he was thinking probabilistically; rather, he seemed to follow causal (physiologic) paths throughout. Though he was not explicit about it, he knew that cortisol stimulates erythropoiesis and produces leukocytosis and hyperglycemia. He correctly identified the alkalosis as the chloride-resistant variety and appreciated that this acid-base disturbance can be caused by hy-

peradrenocorticism. Finally, he made the correct causal connection between excessive production of ACTH and certain cancers and concluded that the patient must have a lung cancer that was causing the hyperadrenal state.

He did not explain why he selected lung cancer as the likely cause, and we can only guess at the reason: Perhaps he used the observation that lung cancer is highly correlated with heavy smoking (a statistical correlation); perhaps he used the observation that most extraadrenal ACTH-producing cancers are in the lung (another statistical correlation), or perhaps he used the observation that some lung tumors actually secrete ACTH (a causal relation). No matter how he made the connection between hypercorticism and lung cancer, he appeared to employ causal reasoning as a diagnostic tool and as a means to justify his approach.

This transcript aptly illustrates the value of causal reasoning in diagnostic problem solving. We have yet to identify which kinds of problems are best approached with causal reasoning, which kinds should be approached with Bayes' rule, and which should be approached with other techniques (e.g., flow charts or algorithms). Because causal reasoning is based not on associations that must be committed to memory but on physiologic relations and concepts, users always can return to first principles to solve the problem by a commonsense or logical process.

In another discussion, we quote the master of deductive reasoning, Sherlock Holmes (see case 54). Not unexpectedly, Holmes had great regard for causal reasoning. In "The Five Orange Pips," Holmes explained to Dr. Watson,

> The ideal reasoner would, when he had once been shown a single fact in all its bearings, deduce from it not only all the chain of events which led up to it but also all the results which would follow from it. As Cuvier could correctly describe a whole animal by the contemplation of a single bone, so the observer who has thoroughly understood one link in a series of incidents should be able to accurately state all the other ones, both before and after.[213]

Yet Conan Doyle appreciated that to solve complex problems by causal reasoning, an individual required command of a certain body of facts. Holmes continued,

> To carry the art, however, to its highest pitch, it is necessary that the reasoner should be able to utilize all the facts which have come to his knowledge; and this in itself implies, as you

will readily see, a possession of all knowledge, which, even in these days of free education and encyclopedias, is a somewhat rare accomplishment. It is not so impossible, however, that a man should possess all knowledge that is likely to be useful to him in his work, and this I have endeavored in my case to do.[213]

Although these comments were made by a not-so-successful physician reflecting on detective work, the scientific basis for causal reasoning and the place of knowledge in human problem solving is well described.[46,47,137,214]

The lesson from this transcript is a simple one: When possible, use physiologic principles and causal relations to solve diagnostic problems. Not only is such reasoning sound, but also the diagnostic process one follows can be justified readily on the basis of these principles. The lesson from Conan Doyle for students is equally clear: Causal reasoning is an ideal aid in the deductive process that underlies medical diagnosis, but you have to know pathophysiology to use it.

CASE 35. THE TRICKY TASK OF ATTRIBUTING CAUSATION

> A 44-year-old man was transferred to the hospital for recurrent episodes of fever, malaise, headache and confusion.

This could be a serious situation. In anyone with fevers, headaches and confusion, I would be concerned about central nervous system infection. Since he was transferred from another institution, I would wonder if he has already been studied, and if no cause was found, he might have an unusual central nervous system infection. If he has had these symptoms for some time, then bacterial infections such as meningococcus infection is unlikely.

> The patient was in good health until 6 weeks prior to admission, when he was admitted to a local hospital with gastrointestinal bleeding from gastritis that was attributed to aspirin and nonsteroidal antiinflammatory drugs that he had been taking for chronic back pain. He also had a long history of depression.

It is hard to know if this history is relevant to his current symptoms. Certainly if he were continuing to take nonsteroidal anti-inflammatory drugs, then aseptic meningitis due to these medicines would be a possibility. The combination of gastrointestinal bleeding and back pain raises the possibility of some type of inflammatory bowel disease and a concomitant spondyloarthropathy. Possibly while in the hospital, he acquired a nosocomial infection, perhaps related to the endoscopic procedure, and the complication is only now becoming clinically apparent.

> His current symptoms began 1 month later when over the course of 2 days he became increasingly lethargic, confused, and ataxic. At work, he was found sitting at his computer not knowing what to do. His temperature was 39°C, and he was taken to the hospital.

If the current symptoms were related to his hospitalization a month earlier, then we are dealing with an indolent process. On the other hand, it may be totally unrelated. The confusion raises the question of some type of encephalopathy. The ataxia makes me think of something going on in his cerebellum or perhaps a peripheral neuropathy or perhaps some type of ear infection that has led to a brain abscess. I am thinking about the possibility that some drug could have caused these symptoms. I do not think that proton pump inhibitors could be responsible. If he were achlorhydric from the proton pump inhibitor, he might be more susceptible to an infection like tuberculosis. My main concern at this time is some type of basilar meningitis.

> He was very lethargic but awake. He had difficulty saying "Methodist Episcopal." There was mild left–right confusion and difficulty in repeating. He was diffusely weak with no other focal findings. The remainder of his physical examination was not revealing. Complete blood count, blood glucose, electrolytes, and serum calcium were normal. Lumbar puncture was normal, and a toxic screen was negative. The neurologist was concerned about encephalitis and initiated acyclovir therapy.

He appears to have a diffuse encephalopathy with signs of bilateral cortical dysfunction. He could have a vocal apraxia or something more serious like a loss of language itself. The diffuse weakness makes me think of some type of toxin with systemic effects. Could he have one of the viral encephalopathies? Does he live in an endemic area? Is it the right time of year? He does not appear to have any metabolic abnormalities. Given the potential seriousness of herpes encephalitis, the initiation of acyclovir seems reasonable since the potential benefits outweigh the risks at this point. Finally, could he have some type of a paraneoplastic syndrome?

> Head CT, magnetic resonance imaging (MRI), and electroencephalogram (EEG) were unremarkable. Chest X-ray showed a possible right basilar infiltrate. Blood and cerebrospinal fluid (CSF) cultures were negative. Acyclovir was stopped, and ceftriaxone therapy was initiated. His symptoms gradually improved, and he was discharged. The final diagnosis was probable viral syndrome and depression.

The presence of a possible pulmonary infiltrate and neurologic dysfunction makes me wonder about the possibility of a *Legionella* infection, although the ataxia would be unusual. The improvement of his symptoms in the hospital could be related to the antibiotics or could just be coincidental.

> He returned one week later with similar symptoms. Blood and urine cultures were negative. Mono spot and thyroid-stimulating hormone were normal. Lyme titers and a purified protein derivative (PPD) test were negative. Other routine lab studies were unremarkable. Chest CT raised the question of a right-middle-lobe consolidation, and he was given clarithromycin. By the third hospital day he had improved remarkably, and he was discharged.

Does he have some type of relapsing disease, or could he have a partially treated infection? Could he have some type of occult abscess that is causing intermittent symptoms? Is he being exposed to some kind of toxin? Still disease could be associated with intermittent fevers and back pains, but not central nervous system symptoms, and vasculitis must always be on the differential of intermittent febrile illnesses; it can involve the central nervous system.

> Two days later he returned with the same symptom complex, including slurred speech, ataxia, and confusion. Meanwhile he had been given paroxetine 30 mg daily for depression and pantoprazole 40 mg daily for his stomach symptoms.

I am still wondering about undiagnosed basilar meningitis, central nervous system tuberculosis, and fungal infections. Prior to HIV disease, cryptococcal disease often occurred in immunocompetent hosts. Is the patient taking any illicit drugs?

> The patient lived with his wife and worked as a sewer inspector. He had a distant history of cigarette smoking. He denied recent travel, sick contacts, or pets. He had abused alcohol in the past but had been sober for 6 years. He exercised regularly before his recent illness.

Given his work as a sewage inspector, leptospirosis immediately comes to mind. This can be a relapsing illness associated with confusion but also hepatic and renal disease.

Has he been bitten by a rat and acquired rat bite fever? I doubt it. The regular exercise makes one wonder if he were using performance-enhancing drugs such as anabolic steroids or the like.

> He was in no distress. His blood pressure was 100/65 mm Hg, and his heart rate was 54 per minute with no orthostatic changes. He was afebrile. General examination was unremarkable. He was oriented but slow to respond. He could not remember his phone number. He was ataxic and unsteady on his feet. The rest of the neurologic examination was normal.

His ataxia appears to be central in origin. Central nervous system infection still is on my list, but could he have one of the avitaminoses, such as thiamine deficiency, or another nutritionally related illness?

> The following laboratory studies were normal: electrolytes, glucose, liver function tests, serum calcium, serum magnesium, and creatine kinase. White cell count was 7,400 with a normal differential. Complete blood count was unchanged. Sedimentation rate was 53 mm/hr.

Hepatitis serologies and HIV test were negative. *Brucella* titers were negative.

If his outside studies have been reviewed and
are normal, then repeat imaging studies are unlikely to be very helpful. Is he taking any health
foods of any kind?

On further questioning, the patient's wife said
that 2 months previously the patient had started
taking kava kava and valerian root for his depression. Each time he was admitted to the hospital, he stopped the herbal medications and his
symptoms subsided. No further tests were performed, and except for drugs for depression, no
other medications were given. As before, within
2 days the neurologic findings disappeared. He
was advised not to take the herbal products. The
patient subsequently had no recurrence of his
symptoms.

Analysis

Inferences about causality have long been known
to be essential to every-day experiences. In the great
novel *War and Peace*, Tolstoy wrote, "The totality
of causes of phenomena is inaccessible to the human mind, and without grasping in their count-
less complexity the conditions of phenomena, of
which each separately may appear as a cause, takes
hold of the first, most comprehensive approximation and says: here is the cause."[215] This caution-
ary note applies in medicine as well. From minute
to minute, we make inferences: Which medicine
caused a patient's blood pressure to fall; which test
caused acute kidney damage; why did a patient
on a steady dose of warfarin start to bleed? The
patient described here provides an unusual opportunity to consider causal relations. Three times the
patient presented with confusion and ataxia, and
twice he improved during a short hospital stay, yet
the physicians caring for him did not recognize
the nature of his illness until the third time he recovered. The discussant seemed wiser; even after
she heard the information from the patient's first
admission, she raised the possibility of "some type
of toxin," and she repeated this concern when she
heard about the information from the second and
third admissions. Rapid improvement in symptoms during hospitalization on repeated occasions

is a signal to invoke a classic causal hypothesis,
namely "*post hoc, ergo propter hoc*" (after this, therefore because of this). There are not many disorders
that fit a relapsing and recovering pattern, but exposure to a toxin (and subsequent elimination of
the toxin) is one. Examination of the literature on
the toxicity of these herbal substances is frustrating principally because so little research has been
done on the side effects of these materials. Most
sites list no side effects of valerian root and only
liver toxicity for kava kava. Yet the case for kava
kava and/or valerian root as the toxin in this case
is quite convincing, based on the return of symptoms after exposure and improvement after cessation of the herbals. In essence, this is the nature
of the "challenge–dechallenge–rechallenge" concept, the idea that the strength of a causal attribution increases if the response disappears when a
stimulus is removed and reappears when the stimulus is reapplied.[216] In this patient, dechallenge
and rechallenge occurred twice after the initial
event, providing convincing evidence of a cause-
and-effect relationship between the herbals and the
patient's illness.

Given the multiple recurrent episodes, it is
safe to make the causal connection here, but it is
critically important not to become overly enam-
ored with the "*post hoc, ergo propter hoc*" notion,
simply because an inference between a single stimulus and a single effect could well be coincidental,
and because of such random effects, invoking the
causal connection is frequently a logical fallacy.
Thus, it is generally hazardous to attribute causality solely based on the order in time in which events
occur. Other factors must always be taken into account in making causal attributions.

What are these factors?[44,45,47] A useful framework for considering causality has the following
components: a causal field, cues to a causal relation, and factors that influence causal strength. A
causal field is a context in which judgments about
probable cause are made. The causal field is analogous to or possibly even the same as the context
or problem space in which probabilistic reasoning takes place (see case 7). A context is thought
to be triggered by unusual, unlikely, or abnormal
findings or events that produce recognizable differences in background, violate expectations, and
thus arouse an interest in causality. In the case presented here, repeated relapse and recovery sets up

a cause-and-effect hypothesis, a causal field, or the context, which then demanded satisfaction and explanation. The causal field in this instance could be construed as a chain consisting of a simple explanation, namely, could a toxin at home be the cause of symptoms? The causal field also is important in setting the number of alternative explanations for an event or finding. For example, in the case we are considering, numerous possible diagnoses were raised, from serious infections to vasculitis.

Cues to causality are probabilistic indicators of causal relations. Factors frequently considered cues of a relation between an observed effect and a putative cause include a comparison between the intensity of a cause and the extent and severity of an effect, the contiguity between cause and effect in time, and the contiguity between cause and effect in space. In the case considered here, the intensity of the stimulus and the result are probably concordant even though data on the toxicity of the herbals was difficult to come by. Necessarily, this relation is a probabilistic one: On the basis of the cues alone, we would be justified only in being suspicious that the herbals caused the central nervous system manifestations. Nonetheless, as with most judgments about the state of the world, our assessment of this cause-and-effect relation yields only a probability that an effect is linked to some cause.

Several measures make it possible to test the *strength* of the link between a cause and an effect, the third component of the framework for assessing causality. The credibility of the entire causal chain, as well as that of the each link in the chain, is one such measure. The covariation between two phenomena is another: When a change in a response correlates closely with a change in a stimulus, the stimulus can be construed as a more probable cause of the response. Similarly, if there is substantial congruity of duration and magnitude between a response and a suspected stimulus, the strength of the cause and effect is enhanced. Many of these measures were satisfied in our patient, but the relation in time and space between the putative stimulus and the response was the most potent. Of course, these relationships are only correlations. As noted, care must be taken to avoid using spurious correlations to enhance causal strength.

Finally, the strength of a given causal hypothesis must stand the test of alternative possible explanations. The fact that a single causal explanation appears to account for all the observed findings does not ensure that this causal chain is the correct one. Alternative constructions of the chain must be sought deliberately and tested for their strengths. In the patient presented here, other explanations gained little credibility.

Detailed rules for causal attribution in medicine are not available, yet physicians assiduously delve for causal explanations of the clinical phenomena they observe. Such searches for a cause not only are the basis for understanding the pathogenesis of clinical manifestations in individual patients, but, in some cases, also may be the modality by which new hypotheses about the mechanisms of disease are first identified.

CASE 36. THE RIGHT ANSWER FOR THE WRONG REASON

> **A 36-year-old man with a history of multiple hospital admissions for drug overdose was admitted with lethargy and incomprehensible speech. He had taken excessive amounts of a drug or drugs, otherwise not identified.**

We are given a lot of information in this first sentence, mainly that this patient has a long history of drug overdoses and that his physical and mental states are consistent with a drug overdose.

> **The patient had a history of drug abuse, depression, and suicide attempts. He had had a cholecystectomy followed by a hepatojejunostomy for a common bile duct stricture. His recent medications included thioridazine (50 mg three times a day) and alprazolam (as required). He had taken lithium at some time in the past.**

The questions we would have to raise are these: Does he still have access to the lithium, and has he in fact ingested any of the medications that he has on his person? The history of common bile duct stricture is the only other thing of note here. Occasionally, stricture recurs, and this can be a source of infection. But our index of suspicion for biliary disease is not terribly high right now, given the patient's history.

Examination showed the following: blood pressure 110/80 mm Hg, pulse 64 per minute, respirations 20 per minute, temperature 36.6°C. He was lethargic but arousable and was mildly agitated. Deep tendon reflexes were slightly depressed, but the remainder of the neurologic examination was unremarkable. The neck was supple. Skin turgor was normal. There were no abnormal physical findings.

The physical examination, other than showing some depression of consciousness and depressed deep tendon reflexes, does not yield any localizing findings. He is not febrile, and again the major concern is that the change in this patient's mental status can be explained by a drug overdose. I think we should find out if he has anything in his stomach and get some blood studies.

Laboratory findings were as follows: complete blood count normal, BUN 8 mg/dL, creatinine 0.8 mg/dL, blood glucose 103 mg/dL. Sodium was 142 mEq/L, potassium 4.3 mEq/L, chloride 110 mEq/L, total CO_2 29 mEq/L. Blood gases: pH 7.32, arterial PCO_2 46 mm Hg. The chest x-ray was normal, as was the electrocardiogram, except for a Q-T$_c$ interval of 0.46. Toxic screen on serum, urine, and gastric contents showed no identifiable agent. A serum lithium level, not part of the toxic screen, was requested. A blood sample for alprazolam was sent out for analysis.

The only thing of note in the laboratory data is that he has a slight respiratory acidosis, with a pH of 7.32 and a PCO_2 of 46. We are not given the PO_2. His anion gap is 3, a low value, and the prolonged Q-T interval is of interest. These findings make me wonder what is contributing to the serum sodium. Is this an artificial elevation as recorded by the autoanalyzer? I will be most interested in this patient's lithium level.

The patient was treated with charcoal, sorbitol, magnesium citrate, naloxone, thiamine, and intravenous fluids, and he became less lethargic over the next 2 hours. At that time, the serum lithium level was reported to be 11.9 mEq/L. The patient denied taking lithium, but he was not fully alert.

So, clearly, lithium was found. Presuming that this was a reliable assay, he appears to be a victim of lithium intoxication.

Because of a gross discrepancy between the patient's clinical status and the lethal lithium blood level, a resident questioned the diagnosis of lithium overdose. After some investigation, the resident found that the heparinized tube in which the patient's sample was sent for blood-gas analysis had also been sent for analysis of blood lithium. The anticoagulant in the tube was lithium heparin. Another lithium level from a properly collected specimen of clotted blood was less than 0.2 mEq/L.

So this error was the consequence of faulty blood collection—not of laboratory measurement!

The patient's mental status improved over the next 12 hours. He said that he had ingested 50 alprazolam tablets in a suicide attempt. The alprazolam blood level at admission was 280 ng/mL (therapeutic range 19–55 ng/mL). Serum electrolytes at follow-up were sodium 142 mEq/L, potassium 4.3 mEq/L, chloride 109 mEq/L, total CO_2 22 mEq/L. The calculated anion gap was now normal (11 mEq/L). The patient was transferred to an inpatient psychiatric unit for further therapy.

An interesting lesson.

Analysis

There are several interesting aspects of clinical problem solving here. The discussant, an able clinician, immediately discovered that the patient had an abnormally low anion gap, a finding that few other clinicians not working in the domain of fluid and electrolyte metabolism would have appreciated. The discussant promptly raised the possibility that lithium in the patient's plasma accounted for the low anion gap: a rational and appropriate hypothesis, given the information at hand. However, later, when the lithium level was reported, the same discussant failed to comprehend the significance of the result. Instead of appreciating the discrepancy between the patient's clinical manifestations (quite mild reduction in consciousness) and the remarkably elevated plasma lithium level, his initial reaction was to attribute the central nervous system manifestations to lithium overdose. A superb performance followed by a missed clue!

Why the error? Here we have an opportunity of seeing the interaction between knowledge, the generation of diagnostic hypotheses, and the evocation of clues to a causal connection. An accepted model of the process of hypothesis generation requires that some prior knowledge be imbedded in long-term memory and that plausible candidates be evoked and activated into working memory by a process that involves checking against incoming data.[105] On the other hand, causal hypotheses, which tentatively attribute a given effect to some specific cause, may be evoked by a somewhat different mechanism. A causal hypothesis, it appears, is evoked when expectations are violated. To fit these seemingly diverse concepts together in the context of the foregoing exercise, we offer the following construct:

1. The discussant knew about lithium intoxication, had the ability to recognize when abnormal amounts of lithium are in the bloodstream (via the low anion gap), and knew that plasma levels of lithium were useful in identifying patients with a lithium overdose.
2. The discussant did not have an accurate working model of the relation between lithium blood levels and a patient's clinical state.
3. As a consequence, the discussant failed to appreciate an essential clue that the resident identified: namely, the discrepancy between the lithium level and the patient's status.
4. This essential piece of knowledge, when missing, failed to evoke a clue to a causal relation (or, in, this case, the lack of a causal relation).

In other cases, we have discussed some of the theories that explain how such knowledge is stored. In this case, such knowledge might be in the form of a condition–action pair, such as: **If** a patient is still conscious (or alive), **and** plasma lithium concentration is greater than 6 mEq/L, **then** the lithium level must be a laboratory error. Or, it might be in the form: **If** a patient is still conscious (or alive), **and** the plasma lithium level is greater than 10 mEq/L, **then** search for some laboratory error.

The knowledge could, of course, be in a quite different form, such as some algebraic relation between lithium levels and a patient's status. Other forms are also possible.

Should the discussant be faulted for failing to appreciate the discrepancy between the lithium level and the patient's clinical state and thus failing to appreciate that an expectation had been violated? Should such knowledge be stored rather than merely accessible in books? To answer this question, we should explain again how these protocols are collected. We present clinical material, organized in "chunks," to clinicians who have no advance preparation, and we ask them to think aloud as they try to solve the clinical problem. We record their comments, transcribe the tape verbatim, and edit the remarks only slightly; we are careful not to change the content.

Most of the discussants are academic clinicians, who are accustomed to making their thought processes explicit as part of their didactic role. Given the spontaneous nature of their comments and their inability to use their usual sources of information when they perceive their knowledge in a certain area to be insufficient, we cannot know whether the clue missed in this format would be missed in the clinician's natural setting. Only a detailed audit of an individual physician's practice would identify such errors. We are not aware of such a peer-reviewed analysis of an individual physician's practices over a prolonged period.

The discussant, a distinguished internist, was in the right church but the wrong pew. He posited immediately that lithium must be present in the plasma, but the lack of a single piece of information led him to believe that it got there from the patient's intestinal tract rather than from the tube in which his blood was collected. This unusual error provides an important lesson. No matter how accurate any laboratory test is, a mishandled specimen can produce just as confusing a false-positive or a false-negative result. Even the most sensitive tests (e.g., polymerase chain reaction) are susceptible to such errors.

CASE 37. A POINT-BY-POINT DISSECTION OF CLINICAL REASONING

NOTE We depart here from our usual framework of first presenting sequential case information and accompanying discussant's remarks with analysis tacked on at the end. Instead, the analysis of the discussant's remarks is presented directly in the text of her remarks. The comments in bold italics represent an analysis of her reasoning in "real time."

> **A 77-year-old man with asymptomatic mitral regurgitation secondary to mitral valve prolapse was seen in clinic with insomnia and shortness of breath for 5 days.**

My first thought in this setting would be congestive heart failure. [*Here, with no more than the patient's age, sex, one historical fact, two symptoms, and the time course of symptoms, she offers her first diagnostic hypothesis—cardiac failure.*] Why he would go into CHF (congestive heart failure) is less clear with this limited information. He could have progressive mitral regurgitation leading to pressure buildup in the lungs and even pulmonary edema. If so, we would also have to figure out why his mitral regurgitation would be getting worse. [*Here she is apparently reasoning causally, trying to understand why the condition in her first hypothesis might have occurred.*]

> **He denied chest pain, orthopnea, cough, fever, edema, or history of similar symptoms. He was short of breath when walking across the room. The murmur of mitral regurgitation had first been noted 9 years earlier. He also had benign prostatic hyperplasia. He had not smoked in 40 years and did not drink alcohol. He was not taking any medications. He was a former tile cutter.**

The absence of orthopnea makes left-sided CHF less likely. The lack of cough is nonspecific but with the absence of fever makes a pulmonary infection less likely. [*Here she examines her second hypothesis, namely pulmonary infection, and considers it probabilistically, arguing that certain features (lack of fever) reduce its likelihood.*] The lack of peripheral edema does not affect my thinking about left-sided failure since not all patients with left heart failure, especially when more acute, have pedal edema due to right-sided heart failure. [*Here she returns to her first, temporarily favored hypothesis, pointing out that the lack of a common finding (pedal edema) does not dissuade her from a diagnosis of heart failure.*] Signs of right heart failure due to left heart failure usually occur in more chronic settings. The shortness of breath on exertion makes me think more strongly about a pulmonary process in addition to a cardiac one. Interstitial lung disease or pulmonary hypertension comes to mind. [*Here she posits that more than two conditions (cardiac failure and lung disease) might coexist, presumably because she believes that the symptoms are too extreme for one condition alone. She has also replaced the hypothesis "a pulmonary process" with two more specific disorders, interstitial lung disease and pulmonary hypertension.*] If his mitral regurgitation was due to rheumatic heart disease, he could have some mitral stenosis as well, but he denied symptoms of orthopnea. His being a former tile cutter brings entities like asbestosis or silicosis to mind if he had the proper exposure. These could result in pulmonary pathology that could present with dyspnea on exertion. [*Here she offers evidence that might argue in favor of interstitial lung disease. Note that so far her differential diagnostic list contains only three hypotheses.*]

> **On examination, he was in no distress. Blood pressure was 144/84 mm Hg. Pulse was 100 per minute and regular. Respiratory rate was 28 per minute. He was afebrile. There was no jugular venous distension. Lungs were clear. Cardiac exam revealed a regular tachycardia. A 4/6 holosystolic murmur was present at the apex and radiated to the axilla. There was no peripheral edema. The remainder of the examination was unremarkable. Complete blood count, electrolytes, blood urea nitrogen (BUN), and creatinine were normal. Stool was guaiac negative. Electrocardiogram (ECG) showed sinus tachycardia. Left atrial enlargement and**

possible left ventricular hypertrophy were noted. There were no acute changes. Chest x-ray showed a tortuous aorta, left ventricular hypertrophy, and no evidence of heart failure. The physician wondered if his symptoms were due to progressive mitral valve disease and ordered a stat echocardiogram (EKG).

The vital signs are noteworthy for the mild tachycardia and increased respiratory rate. He appears to be in mild respiratory distress. The described murmur sounds like his known mitral regurgitation and, given its loudness, makes me think his mitral regurgitation is fairly severe. I am trying to reconcile the lack of orthopnea with his severe regurgitation. [*Another use of causal reasoning to explain an apparent discrepancy.*] The exertional nature of his symptoms makes me wonder if an exertion induced tachycardia makes his mitral regurgitation transiently worse. The lab results are not really surprising. The EKG is what I would have expected. The lack of CHF on x-ray could be consistent with pulmonary hypertension. [*Here she cites a negative finding to support her latest, most-favored diagnostic hypothesis.*] I would like to see an ambulatory oxygen saturation in a patient like this to see how much hypoxia he has with exertion. The high respiratory rate makes me think he has a significant degree of hypoxia. [*Here she uses her model of the disease entity—pulmonary hypertension—to predict expected clinical findings.*]

Echocardiogram revealed a normal left ventricular ejection fraction, 3–4+ mitral regurgitation and 3+ tricuspid regurgitation. The estimated peak pulmonary pressure was 64 mm Hg. Because the pulmonary hypertension was the only new finding compared to an echocardiogram done 1 year previously, the echocardiographer thought that the pulmonary hypertension was unlikely to be due to the mitral valve disease.

As I mentioned, in a patient like this, we need to consider pulmonary hypertension. Why he has the new pulmonary hypertension is the next question we have to answer. [*Her suspicion of pulmonary hypertension now confirmed, she looks for a causal explanation.*] I would be interested in

a blood gas for starters. [*She asks for this test, perhaps suspecting that the result will help confirm her suspicion of disorders that cause pulmonary hypertension.*]

Blood gases on room air were pH 7.41, partial pressure of oxygen (PO_2) 61 mm Hg, partial pressure of carbon dioxide (PCO_2) 34 mm Hg.

This blood gas implies some sort of ventilation/perfusion (V/Q) mismatch. The differential is long here, but the possibility of pulmonary embolism is high on that list. This would present with a widened A-a (alveolar–arterial) gradient and a significant degree of hypocapnia. In addition, severe pulmonary disease from many causes can result in this type of gradient. [*Cardiac failure has disappeared from her differential diagnosis; now the list contains disorders that cause pulmonary hypertension and interstitial lung disease.*]

A V/Q scan revealed multiple perfusion defects with a normal ventilation scan; high probability for pulmonary emboli.

It appears that this patient has suffered from multiple pulmonary emboli. I suspect that this process has been going on for more than a day or two. At this point, the patient should be started on heparin. His previously noted guaiac-negative stool makes the risk of anticoagulation reasonable. He should have an overlap of heparin and warfarin therapy for approximately 5 days. [*Satisfied that the scan clinches the diagnosis of pulmonary embolism, she recommends standard treatment, but first assesses the risk (possibly because the patient is elderly and thus is at greater risk of anticoagulation?).*] The question now is what is the cause of his pulmonary emboli? In an elderly patient, we need to think about the possibility of an underlying cancer. Adenocarcinomas are the classic cancers associated with a hypercoagulable state. Other causes of a hypercoagulable state would be less likely in this setting. [*Once again, she reasons in a causal framework beyond the unifying diagnosis of pulmonary embolism to consider why the patient developed the disorder.*]

The patient was admitted and treated with intravenous heparin. A Doppler study revealed a deep venous thrombosis extending from the left mid thigh to the level of the groin.

I am not sure I would have proceeded with the Doppler studies. Since we knew the patient has had pulmonary emboli, the results of the Doppler study were unlikely to change my therapy. [*She makes a relevant point here: unless the result of a diagnostic test changes the approach to therapy, what is the point of doing it?*] I do not think this patient needs to be considered for an IVC (inferior vena cava) filter at this point. I would only consider that intervention if the patient does not respond to our therapy or developed a contraindication to anticoagulation. [*Again, she is reasoning prospectively, weighing the benefits and risks of this therapeutic intervention.*]

On the second hospital day the partial thromboplastin time (PTT) was greater than 2 minutes and the patient's stool became guaiac positive. The combination of a deep venous thrombosis and gastrointestinal bleeding provoked by anticoagulants raised the possibility that an occult gastrointestinal neoplasm had induced a hypercoagulable state. Studies of the gastrointestinal tract were initiated.

Once again, adenocarcinomas, especially from the gastrointestinal tract, can be associated with a hypercoagulable state. The bleeding, even in the context of a prolonged PTT, raises the possibility of a colon cancer or a gastric cancer. I would proceed with endoscopic evaluation of the GI (gastrointestinal) tract. [*A set of findings triggered the hypothesis of pulmonary embolism. This diagnosis in turn triggered the hypothesis of a hypercoagulable state. The diagnosis of a hypercoagulable state triggered a diagnosis of possible cancer, which in turn led to diagnostic testing.*]

Colonoscopy revealed a large polypoid tumor at the splenic flexure. Biopsy showed adenocarcinoma. Abdominal computed tomography (CT) scan showed no definite evidence of metastatic disease. A Greenfield filter was inserted because of the risks of continued anticoagulation. He then underwent a left hemicolectomy. Liver metastases were found at the time of surgery. The postoperative course was un-

complicated, and he was referred for follow-up chemotherapy.

The insertion of an IVC filter at this point is certainly appropriate, given the problems and risks with anticoagulation in this patient. The whole presenting picture of this patient now makes sense. [*Finally, she asserts that all the linkages are coherent: all the positive findings and negative findings are consistent with the working diagnosis, and the diagnosis is parsimonious, that is, it is a simple explanation of all the findings. Unfortunately for the patient, a rapid and correct diagnostic approach in this instance provided little benefit.*]

CASE 38. LEAVING NO STONE UNTURNED

A 66-year-old woman with schizophrenia was brought to the Emergency Department from a psychiatric day hospital because of increasing paranoia, confusion, and disorientation.

When a patient is transferred from a psychiatric day center because her clinical state has deteriorated, I think about the possibility of physical and organic causes along with psychiatric disorders, but that is as far as I would be willing to go at this point.

She had had a mitral commissurotomy and aortic valve replacement 8 years earlier and was receiving diltiazem and warfarin. She had had adult-onset diabetes mellitus for 3 years, which was controlled with oral hypoglycemic agents.

So we know that she has heart disease with previous valve surgery, has diabetes, and has been receiving certain drugs. Adult-onset diabetes mellitus is not likely to get out of control suddenly, although it certainly can. Also, oral hypoglycemic agents can produce complications, so high or low blood sugars can be a possible explanation. I doubt that she has diabetic ketoacidosis. Diltiazem and warfarin typically do not cause paranoia, confusion, and disorientation. Other cardiac changes leading to increasing paranoia would be possible but not too likely.

> She was well dressed and cooperative, but she was drowsy, had slurred speech, looseness of associations, and delusional thinking. Her affect was inappropriately elated. The artificial valve sounds were heard on physical examination, which was otherwise normal.

The physical disorders that might lead to deterioration of her psychiatric condition are not likely to have manifestations that would be easily found on physical examination. I am afraid this information provides no particular clues.

> Arrangements were made to admit the patient to the psychiatry service, but before she was admitted, a battery of tests was ordered.

What type of tests would one want to get in a person like this? I would be interested, of course, in her diabetes, so a blood glucose would be important. I would certainly want to see an INR (International Normalized Ratio). Checking her serum electrolytes and renal function makes a certain amount of sense. Except for studies of thyroid function and a drug screen, I cannot think of other laboratory tests that might be used to ascertain psychological abnormalities.

> Laboratory findings: Serum electrolytes were sodium 121 mEq/L, potassium 4.9 mEq/L, chloride 84 mEq/L, total CO_2 23 mEq/L. Blood glucose 180 mg/dL, BUN 8 mg/dL, creatinine 0.6 mg/dL. She was admitted to the medical service.

I presume that the leading diagnosis was inappropriate antidiuretic hormone (ADH) secretion of some sort. For the hyponatremia to explain her worsening confusion and disorientation, one might guess that the sodium level had fallen abruptly, because most people can tolerate a serum sodium of 121 or so without too much psychological malfunction if hyponatremia develops slowly. However, she did have schizophrenia, so maybe it took only a small additional stress to make her worse.

To sort out different kinds of hyponatremia, we would first want to know whether the patient actually had hyponatremia with respect to plasma water or whether the low serum sodium was just an artifact. In other words, could there be something occupying space in the plasma—such as lipids or proteins? That does not seem likely, but a plasma osmolality would settle the question. If the osmolality corresponded to the serum sodium concentration, it would rule out hyperlipidemia or other kinds of artifactual hyponatremia. Assuming that there were no signs of hyperlipidemia, the osmolality would be approximately 240 to 260. Could hyperglycemia be the cause? No, because the blood glucose is not high enough to cause any transient shift of water out of the cells to dilute the sodium in the serum. So if we exclude these pseudohyponatremias, we are left only with hyponatremias that result from elevated antidiuretic hormone levels. Then it is our job to decide whether the elevation of antidiuretic hormone was appropriate or inappropriate.

Appropriate elevations might be found in patients with circulatory insufficiency such as might result from dehydration or heart failure, perhaps a circulatory abnormality, liver disease, or nephrotic syndrome. Except for her heart history, we do not have clues that any of those is present; her kidneys seem fine, given a serum creatinine of 0.6 and a BUN of 8. We will keep in mind the possibility that she has some cardiac or circulatory abnormality and consider especially dehydration. We are not told anything that would help us decide whether or not she is dehydrated. If she had been given a diuretic for her heart disease, the drug could produce enough volume contraction to give her a circulatory abnormality, which in turn could produce an appropriate ADH release, but we have no such information. However, she has serious psychiatric illness, and she could be taking diuretics at home. If at the same time she had been drinking a fair amount of water, she could certainly have induced this clinical and chemical picture.

> A call to the psychiatric facility disclosed that the patient was receiving the following medications: trifluoperazine 25 mg daily, lithium 600 mg daily, trihexyphenidyl 2 mg daily, diltiazem 120 mg daily, warfarin 5 mg daily, and chlorpropamide 250 mg daily.

Now we have other possible causes of inappropriate antidiuretic hormone. Of these multiple drugs, trifluoperazine in ordinary doses, as well as diltiazem, warfarin, and trihexyphenidyl, have little effect on the kidneys' excretion of water. Chlorpropamide and lithium do, but they have opposite effects. Lithium causes an inability to concentrate the urine and to retain water. Toxic amounts of this drug would lead to dehydration, which ordinarily would lead to hypernatremia rather than hyponatremia. If lithium were at fault, she would be expected to have a large urine volume and accompanying thirst. It is thought that a primary effect of lithium is stimulation of thirst, as well as impairment of the ability to concentrate the urine, but I doubt it.

Chlorpropamide has the opposite effect. It may enhance the effect of antidiuretic hormone, so that even with small circulating amounts of the hormone, the kidneys do an extra good job of concentrating and thus retaining water. With continued habitual intake of water, the syndrome of inappropriate antidiuretic hormone is produced, even though the absolute amount of the hormone released may not be unusually large. In other words, the effect of small amounts may be amplified by the chlorpropamide.

Schizophrenia itself may have some effect on her fluid intake, and it would be interesting to know whether she habitually drinks a lot of water. Not uncommonly, patients who are habitually big water drinkers do not have any difficulty excreting the water until somebody gives them a diuretic (which produces a modest degree of dehydration and circulatory impairment) or chlorpropamide (which enhances the effect of the tiny amount of antidiuretic hormone that may be normally released). At that point, hyponatremia may be precipitated, and sometimes it is quite severe.

So I would guess that the patient is a habitual water drinker and that in the presence of the chlorpropamide she is retaining water—probably with no relationship to her lithium therapy.

> Fluid restriction was initiated. Four hours after admission the laboratory results were as follows: sodium 141 mEq/L, potassium 4.9 mEq/L, chloride 106 mEq/L, total CO_2 24 mEq/L. Blood glucose 142 mg/dL, BUN 6 mg/dL. Creatinine 0.7 mg/dL. Because the electrolytes had changed so rapidly, the intern wondered whether the initial laboratory results had been incorrect.

So do I. If I had been the intern, I would have first called the laboratory and asked them to save all the blood for repeat testing. I would also go back and look at her intake and output. I would inquire whether this sudden change occurred in relation to a seizure. Serum sodium concentration can rise abruptly after a seizure; that would suggest that the muscles have become permeable to water, which consequently has entered the muscle compartment.

Another explanation for the rapid change might be a sudden reduction in the volume of her extracellular fluid compartment. In other words, if water did not leave her body, water might have left the extracellular fluid and thus raised the concentration of sodium in the plasma. The most common cause of such a shift is glucose. In her case, blood glucose fell only from 180 to 142—not nearly enough to account for the change in sodium concentration. But before invoking internal shifts, we should try to find out whether she excreted the water.

> The intern assumed that he had identified the cause of the patient's hypo-osmolar state and its rapid correction when he discovered that the admission urinalysis showed specific gravity 1.001, osmolality 52, pH 7, no glucose or protein, and no sediment abnormalities.

I do not think he did discover it. Presumably, her urine output during the 4 hours was very large, but we would have to measure it and calculate whether the loss of water was sufficient to raise the sodium concentration from 121 to 141. Even if the change in the external water balance was consistent with the rise in sodium concentration, it does not explain why she got so hyponatremic to start with. It only means that whatever was wrong has gone away, and we have the same speculations as before.

> The psychiatric resident later reported that the patient had had a long-standing relationship at the day hospital with a male patient who had psychogenic polydipsia. The patient had apparently mimicked his habit of drinking large quantities of water.

It is hard to believe that she could have become this hyponatremic from polydipsia alone.

The findings are more consistent with some concomitant impairment in her ability to excrete water, though she did not have much impairment during the 4 hours in the emergency ward. I would guess that she did have a slight impairment of water excretion before she came in. Ordinarily, this defect is the result of mild volume depletion. It could even be caused by the chlorpropamide, except that the half-life of the drug is so long that the effect would not wear off as quickly. I suppose it also could have been related to psychological factors that cause release of antidiuretic hormone, but I do not know how that disorder would be suddenly turned off.

> **Hyponatremia did not recur during the remainder of her hospitalization. The patient returned to the day hospital.**

The final possibility is that the entire syndrome was caused by an enormous water intake. Her urine osmolality was 52, an extremely low value. If she was excreting urine with an osmolality of 52 all the time and was eating a normal amount of food (which produces 800 to 900 mOsm/day), she would be able to excrete 600 to 700 mL of fluid per hour with no problem. But if she drank more over a short period, would she get into trouble? I guess she could. Certainly, that possibility would explain all the facts.

NOTE Chlorpropamide, the drug that was putatively partly responsible for the patient's inability to excrete the large volume of water she had ingested, is rarely used today, yet the example of a patient receiving a drug and later developing water intoxication is so common, and the cognitive aspects so compelling, that we opted to preserve the case. Currently used drugs that have the same effect as chlorpropamide on water excretion include tricyclic antidepressants, phenothiazines, serotonin reuptake inhibitors, carbamazepine, and cyclophosphamide.

Analysis

This case illustrates several problem-solving tactics, including diagnostic discrimination, diagnostic coherence, and diagnostic adequacy. Early in his responses, the discussant "fishes around" and tries to fix on a cause of the patient's disordered mental state. Not surprisingly, given the enormous number of disorders that could explain these nonspecific symptoms, he mentions several heterogeneous disorders, including hypo- and hyperglycemia, heart disease, and thyroid disease. After the plasma electrolytes are presented, however, he focuses on the hyponatremia. He decides (1) that hyponatremia could and probably does cause the new central nervous system dysfunction, (2) that the hyponatremia is real, and (3) that his job is to determine how hyponatremia developed. In the last task, he adeptly displays the discrimination tactic and the concepts of coherence and adequacy.

A discrimination strategy is a technique that narrows down diagnostic possibilities from many to a few and then (when possible) a single one.[19] The literature on discrimination strategies is rather incomplete. The discussant does not use a statistical method that we have discussed earlier, namely Bayesian analysis, to discriminate among diagnostic options. Instead, he relies exclusively on his knowledge of the pathophysiology of water balance. First, he excludes kidney and liver disease; he considers diuretic therapy as a cause and comes back to it later. Then he concentrates on various drugs the patient has been receiving. At one point, when the serum sodium quickly returns to normal, he even begins to question his earlier judgment that the hyponatremia is real. However, he soon gets back on the track; after he learns about the rapid spontaneous correction of hyponatremia, he again accepts that the hyponatremia was real and tries to explain its pathogenesis. Because he understands what is required to produce the combination of rapid and spontaneous correction of hyponatremia and a dilute urine, he further narrows the diagnostic possibilities to three: mild volume contraction, resolving syndrome of inappropriate ADH (SIADH), and extreme water loading. Finally, he ends up with only the last two hypotheses, and at the very end, he appears to concede that massive water loading alone may have been the unique explanation. This discrimination strategy appeared to be based exclusively on the physiology of water balance and its aberrations.

The discrimination approach is one of several "case-building" strategies—tactics used by physicians to evaluate and refine hypotheses, incorporate new data into existing hypotheses, and modify or eliminate hypotheses. Concomitantly, physicians seek to evaluate diagnostic hypotheses for their coherence and adequacy, and these attributes of diagnostic problem solving are well illustrated by this session. A diagnosis can be considered coherent when the links between the clinical findings are appropriate—when physiologic links are satisfactory and when predisposing factors or complications are sensible and acceptable. A diagnosis can be considered adequate when it encompasses all the surviving elementary hypotheses and when it explains all the abnormal and normal clinical findings and test results. Indeed, one of the important judgments one can make of a diagnosis is whether it meets the rigorous criteria of coherence and adequacy.

We use the transcript presented here as an example of these diagnostic attributes because the discussant is so dogged in his zeal to satisfy these criteria. Though he probably does not appreciate that he is doing so, he satisfies the concept of diagnostic coherence by carefully exploring the links between water intake and water-excretion defects and by considering the factors that might predispose to each. He satisfies the concept of diagnostic adequacy by his tenacious attempt to account, in a single "package," for all the findings and all the hypotheses he offered earlier. Indeed, he persists long after many would have given up trying to explain how the patient became hyponatremic. At first, he holds fast to his belief that some defect in water excretion must have been responsible, even after he learns that the metabolic disorder corrected itself rapidly after admission. When the patient's psychosocial history was consistent with a huge water intake, the discussant conceded that massive water intake alone could be responsible for all the findings, although he explains that a preexisting water-excretion defect cannot be excluded. His unwillingness to accept the simple answer of excessive water intake as the cause of the hyponatremia was justified by his accurate comprehension of the physiology of water balance.

CASE 39. VERIFICATION

A 54-year-old man was admitted to the hospital because of slurred speech and difficulty walking.

I have limited amount of information at this point. I would like to know whether these signs developed over 20 minutes or whether they had been increasing in severity over the past 2 to 3 weeks. If they had come on only 20 minutes ago, I would be more concerned about an acute ischemic event. If they had been developing over a long period of time, I would be more concerned about a toxic problem such as alcohol or a more serious problem such as a brain tumor. I cannot go any further than that, but I am obviously focusing on a neurologic process as the immediate cause of the patient's problems.

The patient had felt well until several weeks before admission, when he began to have transitory difficulty in walking and slurring of speech. Over the 3 days preceding admission, he noticed dizziness, nausea, and vomiting. He denied headaches.

It appears that the problem is more of a chronic one. That makes an acute ischemic event much less likely and a space-occupying lesion more likely. I would still be interested in knowing more about his history. Specifically, I would question the patient about drug ingestion and obtain a cardiac history. The presence or absence of headaches is not impressive to me. Ultimately, I shall need the results of a physical examination.

The patient had been told he had severe hypertension 5 years earlier. He was on therapy for 2 years but was lost to follow-up thereafter. He had a family history of hypertension and had smoked one pack of cigarettes a day for several years. He was taking no medications. He drank half a pint of whiskey per day.

We now have a history of high blood pressure, although I do not think that is directly related to what is going on. If he had an intracranial hemorrhage secondary to hypertension, I suspect the symptoms would have been much more acute in onset. The history of cigarette use simply would increase the likelihood of cerebrovascular or cardiac disease. He was taking no medications, so I do not have anything to point to, such as phenytoin intoxication. The consumption of a half pint of whiskey a day certainly raises the possibility of alcohol intoxication. That, however, would also be much more acute in nature, and thus I would be worrying about some chronic neurologic problem related to alcohol, such as cerebellar degeneration. Even so, I would still be concerned about a space-occupying lesion. On physical examination, in addition to knowing his blood pressure, I would be particularly interested in the appearance of his optic disks. I have not yet homed in on anything specific beyond a relatively chronic neurologic problem.

> On examination he was in no distress, but his speech was slurred. Blood pressure was 255/176 mm Hg, and pulse was 116 per minute and regular. He had bilateral hemorrhages in the fundi and papilledema, right greater than left. Visual fields were intact, and lungs were clear. There was a 2/6 systolic ejection murmur. No abdominal masses, tenderness, or bruits were noted. There was no peripheral edema. Pulses were intact. Neurologic exam revealed normal orientation. He was ataxic on the left side and mildly hyperreflexive.

He has extraordinarily marked hypertension with hypertensive retinopathy. This complicates matters a bit diagnostically, but I do not believe it does therapeutically. By this I mean that papilledema in a nonhypertensive patient might strongly suggest a space-occupying lesion. In this patient, it probably is part of his hypertensive process. At any rate, his blood pressure needs to be brought down rapidly to respectable ranges by intravenous antihypertensive medications. The rest of the examination is not as markedly abnormal as I would have suspected. He has minimally focal neurologic signs with left-sided ataxia. Can one have focal abnormalities with hypertensive encephalopathy? The answer is yes. So we have at least one very good diagnosis. The only question: Are we still missing something? I would bring this patient's blood pressure under control, and I would still be concerned about a space-occupying lesion. I need to know what his renal function is before doing anything, such as contrast studies.

> Laboratory data were as follows: sodium 138 mEq/L, potassium 2.9 mEq/L, chloride 102 mEq/L, bicarbonate 30 mEq/L, BUN 28 mg/

dL, creatinine 2.2 mg/dL, and cholesterol 266 mg/dL. Urinalysis: specific gravity 1.015, pH 7.0, 4+ protein, and 1+ blood. The sediment had 20 to 30 red blood cells (RBCs) and 5 to 10 oval fat bodies per high-power field, free fat globules, and no RBC casts. Hematocrit was 50%, and white cell count was 8,000. The ECG showed left ventricular hypertrophy with strain, and echocardiogram revealed concentric left ventricular hypertrophy with a normal ejection fraction. Chest x-ray showed moderate cardiomegaly. Head CT scan revealed a lacunar infarct in the left internal capsule and a possible hypodense area in the left cerebellum.

The cerebellar abnormality would accord with the patient's clinical findings. I would have to discuss the significance of that with the radiologist to see whether it is likely to be a tumor or whether this is consistent with alcoholic cerebellar degeneration. The patient clearly has evidence of end-organ damage from hypertension. He has hypertensive retinopathy. His kidneys are damaged, as reflected by hematuria and an elevated BUN and creatinine. The data are consistent with both primary and secondary causes of hypertension, and a more thorough history is required. In addition, the patient clearly has cardiac hypertrophy according to ECG, echocardiogram, and chest x-ray. I would bring his blood pressure down while I continued his evaluation. I need to learn more about the significance of this "possible hypodense area" in the left cerebellum.

> The patient's blood pressure was aggressively lowered and eventually controlled on several antihypertensive drugs. Renal ultrasound demonstrated normal kidney size bilaterally with no obstruction; 24-hour urine protein excretion was 4.2 g; serum albumin was 2.8 g/dL. The patient was considered to have malignant hypertension superimposed on essential hypertension and was followed as an outpatient.

His allegedly normal kidney size is consistent with an acute deterioration in renal function secondary to relatively acute elevation of his blood pressure; by "acute," I mean present for no more than 2 to 3 months or so. The protein excretion is a little high, but with malignant hypertension, you can get a glomerular pattern of proteinuria. If the malignant hypertension were the cause of his proteinuria, I would expect that the protein excretion would resolve over the next month or two. If it went up to 10 to 12 g as his blood pressure was controlled, I would get suspicious that I was missing some primary renal disease. Following him as an outpatient is reasonable. I have no further information regarding the interpretation of the CT scan finding in the left cerebellum.

> **Three months later all neurologic symptoms and findings had resolved. On the same medications his blood pressure was 130/80 mm Hg, but 3 to 4+ peripheral edema had developed. Creatinine was 3.1 mg/dL, and serum albumin was 3.3 g/dL. Urinalysis now showed specific gravity 1.020, pH 5.5, 4+ protein, 0 to 1 white blood cell, and 0 to 1 RBC per high-power field, many oval fat bodies, 2 to 5 fatty casts per high-power field, and free fat. The 24-hour urine protein excretion was 5.6 g.**

There are several key observations here: His blood pressure is well controlled, and I shall assume that it has been well controlled since the first week or two of his hospitalization. Despite that control, however, his kidney function has deteriorated and his 24-hour protein excretion may have risen a bit, or at least it has not fallen. I would be willing to follow the 24-hour protein excretion for another 3 months, but the rising creatinine bothers me. In patients with malignant hypertension whose blood pressure is promptly reduced, it would not be surprising to see the creatinine increase from about 2, where it had been on admission, to 3 or 4. However, I would expect to see some improvement in renal function over a period of time. I would be interested in seeing a series of serum creatinines. That would tell me if the creatinine had gone up right after his blood pressure became more normal or if it has been sneaking up over 3 months. The latter would be a bit unusual for malignant hypertension and would make me think that I might be missing something. At that point, the question of renal biopsy would come up. At this time, I would probably not do a biopsy, but if the serum creatinine reached 3.5 to 4.0, I would step in and be more aggressive. In fact, one could argue that his hypertension got so bad initially because he had

some acute renal process that triggered the acute episode.

> **A renal biopsy revealed advanced membranous glomerulopathy and moderate to severe nephrosclerosis. The revised diagnosis was membranous glomerulopathy with secondary malignant hypertension. He was treated with prednisone, 120 mg every other day. Five months later, when his prednisone dose had been decreased to 20 mg every other day, his serum creatinine was 1.8 mg/dL and his 24-hour urinary protein excretion was 2.66 g.**

Analysis

In this discussion we deal with the process of diagnostic verification and failures in the process, a notion sometimes described as "premature closure."[217] The physicians caring for this patient failed to keep an open mind about the cause of the patient's hypertension and simply assumed that he had primary malignant hypertension. The discussant, however, was far more cautious. At the time of the patient's discharge, he was willing to accept the provisional diagnosis of malignant hypertension superimposed on chronic essential hypertension, and he pointed out that the available data (including presenting symptoms, history, and laboratory data) were consistent with that diagnosis. Nonetheless, he made the point that the working diagnosis would have to be confirmed or reevaluated depending on the patient's subsequent course. He stated that if the protein excretion did not decrease as the blood pressure control was maintained, he would be concerned that he "might be missing something." Here is a careful clinician. Although he missed the significance of fat in the urine (it probably was a clue that the patient had primary renal disease), he was not willing to accept his provisional diagnosis as verified; he certainly was not guilty of premature closure.

Verification is the concept that has thwarted international attempts to control the proliferation of nuclear weapons. It also is, we shall argue, a concept that embraces both the deepest reaches of science and the humblest diagnostic efforts. We also point out that the frustration with this concept in foreign affairs, science, and medicine is an inevitable consequence of a fundamental notion:

namely, that absolute verification of hypotheses is unattainable.

Because our concern is problem solving in medicine, let us first focus on the problem of confirming—or verifying—a diagnosis. To state the issue explicitly, at what point in the diagnostic process should we be satisfied that we have arrived at the correct answer? How early should we close our mind to collecting more data? Is it appropriate to accept a diagnosis before we have examined *all* the collectible data? How about all the risk-free and low-cost data? Do physicians keep an open mind—do they even try to do so—when they are involved in the diagnostic process? Is premature closure a real issue in diagnosis, and, if so, what are the risks of jumping to premature conclusions? When are we justified in concluding that we need to go no further?

Concepts of diagnostic "adequacy" and "coherence" are useful in thinking about verifying diagnostic hypotheses. "Adequacy" is a test of whether all the clinical findings are explained by specific diagnostic hypothesis. "Coherence" examines whether a diagnostic hypothesis is pathophysiologically consistent with all the clinical findings. Once a causal relation is established, for example, between some effect and its putative stimulus, coherence testing should ascertain whether any causal relation other than the currently accepted one can explain the same findings.

What constitutes "proof" that a diagnosis is correct? Before we elaborate on medical efforts to grasp this problem, it will be fruitful to explore the most sophisticated approach to this problem—the one used in scientific discovery.[111] Once an induction is made and a theory is "discovered," scientists take on the task of confirming the theory. Because a universal generalization can never be verified unequivocally by a finite set of observations, verification usually is considered in a framework in which the weight of evidence favors the theory or opposes it. Attempts to verify a theory are usually based both on probabilistic and statistical approaches. In the Bayesian model, evidence accumulates and progressively increases the probability that a given hypothesis is correct.[218] In the statistical approach, according to the null hypothesis, the harder it is to explain a set of observations by random processes, the more credible the hypothesis becomes. Of course, neither a high probability nor

a highly significant "p" value truly confirms a scientific hypothesis. Sometimes theories can be disproven, however, if strong evidence is adduced to show that the hypothesis is false.[161] This approach is useful, of course, only if convincing evidence opposing a theory appears; until it does, one is justified in retaining a theory derived by induction from a set of observations. [111] So, here is the bad news: Even in hard science, there are no absolutes. We can identify theories that are parsimonious, that are quite consistent with the observable data within some criteria of accuracy, that are highly probable, and for which no detracting data exist. However, no matter how convincing at the time, we should not delude ourselves into believing that we have an ironclad answer. Despite two centuries of vigorous debate, philosophers of science have not achieved consensus either on what constitutes a verified induction or on whether verification is even possible.[111]

What have we done in medicine to explore when to accept or reject a diagnostic hypothesis? Not much. Although some physicians have argued that we should refrain from making even diagnostic hypotheses before a complete list of problems has been formulated,[219] others have shown that clinicians instinctively do not behave in that way. Instead, they generate diagnostic hypotheses with only minimal data and revise them as they collect additional clinical information.[18,19] Confirmation of diagnostic hypotheses has received only passing notice.[19] Despite the ambiguity and arbitrariness in the process of verification, physicians must come to a conclusion about how to proceed and thus how to define a "working diagnosis," which, although perhaps incomplete and imprecise, forms the basis for needed action (usually therapy).

Failing to find a vigorous approach to verification of a diagnostic hypothesis, how can we test whether a given diagnosis is sufficiently verified to be useful clinically? Here are some useful criteria: (1) Is the working diagnostic hypothesis highly likely? (2) Is it the most parsimonious explanation? (3) Are there other hypotheses that cannot be easily dismissed? (4) Does the working diagnosis explain all the principal clinical findings—positive, negative, and normal findings? (5) Within this diagnosis, are all the clinical features pathophysiologically consistent? (6) Do causal links fit, or are there other causal explanations that are equally convincing?

(7) Do predictions based on the hypothesis come to pass? (For example, does it correctly predict test results and prognosis?)

If a given diagnostic hypothesis passes all these tests, we gain confidence in it and accept it as a working diagnosis. However, we must be cautious not to hold on too avidly to a diagnosis, even if it seems quite attractive. As the distinguished author Primo Levi explained, "There is trouble in store for anyone who surrenders to the temptation of mistaking an elegant hypothesis for a certainty."[220]

We must appreciate that, no matter what we would like to believe about the accuracy of our verification methods, accepting a diagnosis as confirmed remains an act of faith. No matter what methods we use or promises we receive, we could say the same, of course, about the verification that certain countries have suspended their plans to produce nuclear weapons. In medicine, such uncertainty must not, however, paralyze our will to act.

CASE 40. A METICULOUS APPROACH

A 55-year-old woman who had immigrated to the United States from Hong Kong 3 months earlier presented in the Emergency Department with anorexia, nausea, and light-headedness. She spoke very little English. Before a translator arrived, the house officer did a cursory examination and found that the patient appeared to be dehydrated and had postural hypotension. The physician ordered several laboratory tests and observed the patient closely.

The woman appears to be moderately ill. We have two areas of concern: First, what is the nature of the acute illness, and what therapeutic measures should be initiated before we arrive at a diagnosis? Second, how should we proceed to determine the cause of the underlying problem? I would start an intravenous infusion after blood is drawn for initial laboratory tests and begin to hydrate the patient. I need more of her history and a more detailed physical examination. On the basis of the available data, I do not know whether the patient has a cardiovascular problem, an infection, a metabolic abnormality, or some other disorder.

The following laboratory results became available before the translator arrived: hemoglobin 9.6 gm/dL, hematocrit 27%, white cell count 4,100 with 42 polys, 3 bands, 17 lymphs, 2 atypical lymphs, 5 monos, and 31 eosinophils.

The patient is moderately anemic and has a mild neutropenia and a striking eosinophilia. If she is both dehydrated and moderately anemic, we will have to follow her hematocrit closely during rehydration because it may fall even more. Eosinophilia of this magnitude in a woman from Hong Kong raises the possibility of parasitic infection. If she does have a parasitic infection, the workup can be done at a somewhat leisurely pace. Adrenal insufficiency is also a possibility. As a rule, Addisonian patients are salt depleted, and therefore there is a real danger of circulatory collapse, which is unpredictable; it can happen even over a period of minutes and can be fatal. Salt alone helps prevent the circulatory collapse that occurs in patients with Addison's disease. Therefore, for hydration, I would use normal saline, with or without glucose.

In the initial blood studies, I would obtain a plasma cortisol assay and an ACTH (adrenocorticotropic hormone) level. If I were concerned about circulatory collapse from Addison disease, I would also give dexamethasone—approximately three times the physiologic replacement dose. Because dexamethasone does not interfere with the cortisol assay, that intervention would allow me to treat the patient, and, at the same time, it would not confuse my diagnostic evaluation, which would probably include an ACTH-stimulation test. The ACTH test would help me to determine whether there is glucocorticoid deficiency and, if so, whether it is a primary adrenal disease or ACTH deficiency. One administers cosyntropin, a synthetic analog of ACTH, 0.25 mg intravenously, and measures plasma cortisol and aldosterone at the time of injection and again 30 and 60 minutes postinjection. If there is primary adrenal damage (mainly Addison disease or destruction of the gland by tuberculosis, histoplasmosis, or tumor), neither the cortisol nor the aldosterone will rise. ACTH deficiency will blunt the normal rise in plasma cortisol. Because aldosterone secretion is primarily under the control of the renin–angiotensin system, plasma aldosterone would respond normally to ACTH. I would therefore pursue both diagnostic and therapeutic approaches, specifically considering Addison disease. I still need to know more about the history and the general physical examination because we certainly cannot exclude parasitic disease or other causes of marked eosinophilia.

> **The house officer was not surprised to learn that the patient was hyponatremic (serum sodium, 122 mEq/L), but she was confused when she learned that the BUN was 3 mg/dL and the creatinine was 0.4 mg/dL; she had expected both values to be increased.**

The house officer presumably thought that if the patient was dehydrated, she would exhibit prerenal azotemia. These findings, however, are consistent with glucocorticoid deficiency, in which hyponatremia results from a disturbance in free water excretion. In Addison disease, muscle mass tends to be decreased, so a low BUN and a normal creatinine are not unexpected. I must admit, however, that if the patient is really severely dehydrated, I would expect both the BUN and the serum creatinine to be higher. If we are considering adrenal insufficiency, we also should be alert to the possibility of hyperkalemia, which can itself be dangerous.

Now that we know that the patient is hyponatremic, we should consider other possible causes of this metabolic abnormality. Included would be the syndrome of inappropriate ADH secretion and the tumors associated with it, as well as the many medications that can cause defects in free water excretion, especially diuretics.

> **The history disclosed that 16 months earlier, the patient had a nasopharyngeal squamous cell carcinoma and was treated with radiation over a 3-week period. In the last 6 months, she had experienced diplopia, nausea, anorexia, fatigue, and weakness. She had not taken diuretics or other drugs.**

Now we have considerably more history. Although it used to be thought that the anterior pituitary gland was relatively resistant to radiation, we now know that patients who receive several thousand rads to areas near the sella turcica for treatment of tumors either in the nasopharynx or in the brain can acquire anterior pituitary deficiency.

Rarely, posterior pituitary deficiency can occur as well. It is not possible to predict which of the anterior pituitary hormones will be deficient; almost any combination can occur. We now have a reason to suspect ACTH deficiency and consequent glucocorticoid deficiency in our patient. We also have to consider the possibility that some of her symptoms are due either to effects of radiation on the brain or to metastatic carcinoma. The anorexia may reflect a radiation effect on taste sensation. The fact that she had not taken diuretics or other drugs leads us to believe that the hyponatremia is not drug related and that it probably reflects hormonal deficiency.

If she had deficiency of multiple pituitary hormones, the one that should be treated immediately is the ACTH deficiency. In this setting, thyroid-stimulating-hormone deficiency is usually not so severe that patients are at any considerable risk of myxedema coma. Therefore, if she is hypothyroid, it may be contributing to the symptoms but does not need to be treated immediately. One certainly would want to evaluate that, however. I might add that severe hypothyroidism also can be associated with a water-excreting defect.

> **Examination disclosed a thin woman with dry skin and dry oral mucosa. Vital signs were (supine) blood pressure 108/60 mm Hg, pulse 100 per minute; (standing) blood pressure 60/0 mm Hg, pulse 112 per minute. Bilateral 6th nerve palsies and right 12th nerve palsy were present.**

This confirms the previous observation of orthostatic hypotension. The supine pulse was rapid to begin with and rose when the patient stood up, although not as much as I would have expected, given the drop in blood pressure. The bilateral 6th nerve palsies and the right 12th nerve palsy are consistent with the history of diplopia. A rapidly growing pituitary tumor can cause 6th nerve palsies, but I do not believe that would ever cause a 12th nerve palsy. Therefore, I think that finding reflects either metastatic disease from her nasopharyngeal carcinoma or radiation effects.

I presume there was no hyperpigmentation. If there is ACTH deficiency, one would not expect hyperpigmentation. If there is glucocorticoid deficiency from adrenal damage, one would expect ACTH to rise and its melanocyte-stimulating activity to be expressed as hyperpigmentation. Certainly, we have no reason to suspect that primary hypoadrenalism is present.

> Further laboratory data were as follows: sodium 120 mEq/L, potassium 3.4 mEq/L, chloride 85 mEq/L, total CO_2 24 mEq/L. Urine specific gravity 1.016. Urine sodium (random specimen) 35 mEq/L, potassium 14 mEq/L.

The serum and urinary electrolytes are informative. The normal serum potassium suggests that neither aldosterone deficiency nor primary adrenal damage is present. Typically, with adrenal insufficiency secondary to pituitary disease, there is enough aldosterone to enable the kidneys to excrete potassium. Given that the patient was not taking diuretics and did not have renal disease, the high urinary sodium excretion argues against volume depletion because sodium excretion is close to zero in the volume-depleted state. The combination of hyponatremia, renal sodium wasting, and a urine more concentrated than it should be strongly suggests that the patient has SIADH. In this disorder, sodium excretion reflects sodium intake in the steady state.

> Additional studies: reticulocyte count 1.6%, mean corpuscular volume (MCV) 56.8, serum iron 45 μg/dL, iron-binding capacity 165 μg/dL, serum folate 8 μg/dL. Serum ferritin 245 μg/dL. Hemoglobin electrophoresis: normal. Lactate dehydrogenase 197 IU/L. Total bilirubin 1.7 mg/dL. Random blood sugar 67 mg/dL.

The patient's anemia is accompanied by a low reticulocyte count. Patients with hypopituitarism can have significant anemia. With an MCV of 56.8, I also wonder if the patient has thalassemia trait, which is not uncommon in Asians. The blood sugar is low, but not dangerously so. One occasionally sees severe hypoglycemia in Addison disease or in hypopituitarism, and if the patient had been severely ill and comatose, I would have given her glucose immediately.

> Additional blood studies: plasma cortisol (morning value) 3.0 μg/dL. After cosyntropin stimulation, 10.2 μg/dL. Plasma thyroxine

> 3.5 μg/dL (normal, 4.2–12.0) Thyroid-hormone binding ratio 0.94 (normal, 0.82–1.2) Free thyroxine index 4.1 (normal, 5.5–11.5).

The rise in plasma cortisol is subnormal. I consider a normal response of the plasma cortisol to be at least a doubling, with the stimulated value being greater than 18 at 1 hour after cosyntropin administration. I assume this test was done with a bolus injection of the ACTH analog. A more prolonged infusion would give a better indication of the state of adrenal responsiveness. The data are most consistent, however, with secondary adrenal insufficiency. A normal aldosterone response to cosyntropin would be even stronger evidence of pituitary disease. The low free thyroxine index also points to pituitary damage.

The data imply that this patient will need both glucocorticoid and thyroxine replacement. When such replacement is to be used, one should give the glucocorticoid first since there are reports that giving thyroxine first can occasionally precipitate Addisonian crisis. Those reports are from the older literature, made at a time when thyroid hormone replacement was given in higher doses than we use today, but there is every reason to be prudent and no particular reason to be aggressive with thyroxine therapy, especially if one considers the mild nature of the thyroid defect. A TSH (thyroid-stimulating hormone) level would be of interest. If the patient has secondary hypothyroidism, the value should be low.

> CT scan of the head showed a mass lesion in the sella turcica that had invaded the sphenoidal sinus and the clivus and extended anteriorly into the pterygoid region and posteriorly along the foramen magnum. Sinus biopsy disclosed a malignant tumor suggestive of a poorly differentiated carcinoma. Lumbar puncture showed the following cerebrospinal fluid values: protein 125 mg/dL, glucose 45 mg/dL, 22 white blood cells (84 lymphs, 16 monos), and 287 RBCs.

Here we have anatomic evidence of a tumor, which could certainly cause damage to the anterior pituitary and explain the biochemical findings. The histology of a poorly differentiated carcinoma and the location and extent of the tumor are consistent with my earlier remarks about a 12th nerve palsy being unusual for a typical pituitary adenoma. The histologic finding of poorly differentiated carcinoma is compatible with the nasopharyngeal carcinoma that was diagnosed before. We need to keep in mind the possibility of a pituitary carcinoma, although those are very rare. When present, they can be very aggressive and can present with a nasopharyngeal mass, but statistically, one would certainly more readily suspect a primary nasopharyngeal lesion, especially in an Asian.

> **The patient's fluid intake was restricted, she was treated with levothyroxine sodium and prednisone (in "replacement" doses), and radiation was directed at the tumor. Within days, plasma electrolytes returned to normal, postural hypotension disappeared, and the cranial nerve palsies partially resolved.**

The response to glucocorticoid replacement occurs within minutes. The response to thyroxine replacement occurs more slowly, over a period of weeks. I think the patient's presenting findings are due to hypopituitarism secondary to her tumor. She had evidence of SIADH, which responded to hormone replacement and treatment of the tumor.

Analysis

The discussant who solved this clinical problem did a superb job of systematically working through its complexities. She quickly appreciated that the patient had adrenal insufficiency, identified its cause as disordered pituitary function, and then discovered other, related hormonal disorders. She accomplished this task despite conflicting clinical data. On the one hand, some data—hyponatremia, postural hypotension, and dry mucosa—suggested that the patient was volume depleted. On the other hand, the metabolic data argued strongly against volume contraction; the patient's lower-than-normal BUN and serum creatinine indicated a supernormal glomerular filtration rate, and her urine sodium concentration was moderately high. Although there is room for argument, we are inclined to believe that this postural hypotension was caused not by a volume deficit but by a deficit of adrenal hormones and that the patient did have SIADH with volume expansion. If that physiologic construct is valid, the patient had a water-excreting defect secondary to hypopituitarism and

became volume expanded with the syndrome of inappropriate ADH secretion. In this context, the dry mucosa must be viewed as a misleading finding.

The synthetic approach used by the discussant in this case deserves comment. As she assembles a diagnosis of hypopituitarism, she takes great pains to be sure that the diagnosis is both adequate and coherent.[19] A diagnosis can be considered adequate when it encompasses all of the elementary hypotheses and accounts for all (or at least nearly all) of the normal and abnormal findings. In this instance, we have one diagnosis that accounts for virtually all of the findings: an invasive nasopharyngeal carcinoma. A diagnosis is considered coherent when physiologic links are appropriate (e.g., high urine sodium is related to volume expansion; normal response to cosyntropin is consistent with primary pituitary, not primary adrenal insufficiency). A diagnosis is also considered coherent when predispositions or complications associated with the disease entity are appropriate. In this instance, the patient's race is an appropriate predisposing (risk) factor for the carcinoma, and the pituitary dysfunction is an appropriate complication of the cancer.

Apparent also in this problem-solving session is the care with which the discussant seeks to explain *every* finding according to her proposed hypothesis. The major findings—including the electrolyte abnormalities, the hormone results, and the anemia—either are used to solidify her hypothesis or are explained by it. This meticulous interpretation of all of the data is the hallmark of an excellent clinician.

CASE 41. A DIAGNOSTIC QUANDARY

> **A 52-year-old machine shop owner was evaluated for recurrent fever, chills, and sweats for 6 years.**

Six years of illness seems to me a very long time for an infectious disease, unless it is something like tuberculosis. It also seems too long for the usual malignant process, so I tend to think of something like a connective tissue disorder or perhaps some type of occupational exposure to fumes or other organic substance. Those are the things that occur to me off the top. I would like to have more data before I really try to guess what has been going on.

> He was well until 7 years ago, when he was admitted to a hospital for chest pain. On the basis of electrocardiographic findings, he was said to have sustained a myocardial infarction. Six years ago, he reported the first of several episodes of fever and pleuritic chest pain, diagnosed each time as pneumonia and treated with antibiotics. Sometimes the fevers were associated with pain in his calves, thighs, and arms, and on other occasions with pain in his wrists, knees, and ankles. This set of symptoms usually resolved in 5 to 10 days.

Some ideas come to mind. If we assume this is all part of one problem and the myocardial infarction set off periodic episodes of fever, we could consider the post–myocardial infarction, or Dressler, syndrome. That disorder is probably some type of allergic response to myocardial tissue. The patients usually get pleuritic pain and fever and sometimes a pulmonary infiltrate. I must admit that I have never seen one that went on for 6 years, but that would be a possibility. Another thought is that maybe they were wrong the first time around and what he had instead of a myocardial infarction was pericarditis. Conceivably, he could be having recurrent episodes of pleuropericardial disease. With the arthralgias and other symptoms, I think of something in the lupus family. There is a remote possibility that he had a vasculitis that somehow affected the myocardial vessels and now he is having other kinds of problems related to vasculitis, but I think that is highly unlikely.

> Three years ago, he began to experience almost daily fevers as high as 40°C with chills, drenching sweats, and migratory polyarthralgias. During at least one febrile episode, he complained of exquisite pain above the right shoulder and right hip, but x-rays of those regions were normal. He recalled a fleeting red rash on his trunk during some episodes of fever.

I must admit that I have never seen anybody with lupus or polyarteritis who had been sick with daily fevers for 3 years, but I suspect that may reflect my limited experience. I am still most interested in that possibility. I am still concerned about occu-

pational exposure, and I would like to know if he ever took time away from his usual environment and noticed any change in his fever during the past 3 years. The rash does not help me much; I think it would be compatible with lupus or vasculitis. People with Dressler syndrome do not usually get cutaneous manifestations, so that disorder becomes less likely.

> Extensive tests both in and out of the hospital failed to disclose the cause of his complaints, and the patient was treated with a variety of medications. Colchicine and dapsone had no effect. Prednisone (up to 25 mg daily) and indomethacin (up to 125 mg daily) relieved the joint pains but offered only slight relief from fever; steroid therapy induced muscle weakness and diabetes mellitus.

Some patients with connective tissue disease or vasculitis might not respond to the prednisone dose that was given. I need some serologic data or some tissue. I would like a biopsy of the rash or of an organ if I can get some indication that the organ is worth looking at. I want to see if his alkaline phosphatase is elevated to give me some idea if something may be going on in his liver. I would want to know whether he has hematuria or something else that would make me want to look at his kidneys or some chronic cutaneous lesions that I could perhaps biopsy. I have a sense that I am dealing with something in the polyarteritis or lupus family and that I will need either serologic or pathologic information before I can make a diagnosis.

> His only foreign travel in recent years was to Aruba 8 years ago. He had not been camping, and he lived in a city. He had a history consistent with Raynaud phenomenon. His family history was unremarkable.

The rest of the information does not help me very much. The foreign travel makes me think that whoever summarized the history was thinking about an infectious problem, but I think the answer is elsewhere. Raynaud phenomenon would certainly fit in with a presumed connective tissue disease.

> Physical examination was unremarkable. White cell count was 12,000 to 14,000; on two

occasions, there were 51% polys and 24% bands. Hematocrit was 36 to 38%. Platelet count was 350,000 to 430,000. Sedimentation rate was 70 to 90 mm/hr; α_1- and α_2-globulins, C-reactive protein, and antinuclear antibodies were elevated when measured during one of his hospitalizations.

It surprises me that he had such a high percentage of bands. That suggests more acute inflammation, but his low hematocrit is consistent with a chronic illness, as are the elevated α-globulins and sedimentation rate. None of this really changes my mind, and I am still looking for information about a connective tissue disease or a vasculitis. Nothing here so far makes me want to look for an infectious or malignant cause.

All of the following studies were normal or negative: urinalyses, serum albumin and electrolytes, renal function studies, liver function studies, thyroid function studies, pulmonary function studies, angiotensin-converting-enzyme level, rheumatoid factor and antinuclear antibodies, urine for light chains, serum iron and iron-binding capacity, rectal biopsy for amyloid, hemoglobin electrophoresis, multiple blood, urine, and stool cultures, stools for ova and parasites, hepatitis antigen, and antibodies, multiple chest x-rays, hip x-ray, upper GI series, CT scan of abdomen and pelvis, electrocardiogram, echocardiogram, bone marrow biopsy, febrile agglutinins, *Brucella* titers, *Blastomyces* antibodies, antimalarial antibodies.

This is a rather extensive workup. One test strikes my eye. The antinuclear antibodies are negative, which means that either he has one of the mixed connective tissue diseases or he has an unusual form of lupus. There is nothing here that helps me rule out polyarteritis. I suspect that we are going to have to get some tissue. One of the things one could do to investigate polyarteritis is perform a renal arteriogram. Another possibility, which I should have mentioned earlier, is a factitious fever. There was no documentation of the fever anywhere in the data. I am still leaning toward something like a vasculitis, however.

Abnormal studies included low titer antimicrosomal antibody (one occasion). Abdominal CT scan 8 months earlier disclosed normal-appearing liver, but the spleen was enlarged. Liver biopsy 8 months earlier yielded two different interpretations: (1) chronic inflammatory changes secondary to systemic inflammation; (2) acute and chronic changes suggesting a "primary hepatic process." (Neither acid-fast bacilli nor granulomas were seen.)

I do not get any more thoughts from these additional data. I am slightly concerned that this could be a lymphoma, but I still think I would probably proceed with a renal arteriogram. It might be useful to take another look at the spleen to see if it is indeed enlarged, but the CT scan of the abdomen and pelvis should have revealed that, and I suspect it is probably not enlarged.

On the basis of the fever, leukocytosis, anemia, evanescent rash, polyarthralgias, and evidence of chronic inflammation in the liver biopsy, adult-onset Still disease was diagnosed. High-dose salicylate therapy was recommended.

This impresses me as a long time for Still disease to be going on without the development of more joint symptoms. In most of the patients I have seen with Still disease who present with a fever of undetermined origin, the rheumatic illness usually becomes a little more prominent after a year or two.

On 15 aspirins per day, the patient's fever and arthralgias disappeared. He remained somewhat weak but returned to work 2 weeks after starting salicylate therapy.

This is an interesting case—clearly not one that I would have diagnosed on the basis of the long history and the rather minimal rheumatic complaints. The response to salicylates is gratifying, and I would be very interested in seeing what happens to the patient over time. Should he become ill again, I would still be interested in looking at his renal arteries to see whether there might be evidence of a vasculitis.

Analysis

Even after all the history, physical findings, and extensive laboratory findings were available, we still are not confident that we know what is wrong with this patient. We chose such a patient for presentation because, from time to time, we do find ourselves in just such a diagnostic quandary, and we wished to explore how we deal with it.

When a physician begins to explore the cause of a patient's complaints, he or she does not start with a "blank page." Instead, a patient's age, sex, principal complaints, and physical appearance, as well as a myriad of other subtle (and frequently not explicit) clues, suggest certain diagnostic possibilities. Complaints such as dysuria narrow the possibilities greatly, but other presenting manifestations, such as weakness or fatigue, are far less directive. No matter what the starting position or methods that are used to gather additional data, we usually wind up with enough information to formulate a working diagnosis, one that allows us to take the next step—that is, to treat the patient or perhaps to proceed with a risky, invasive diagnostic test. But what if no clear diagnosis emerges? How does such a quandary occur, and when it does occur, what can we do about it?

First, we will develop two models that explain how we end up with an uncertain diagnosis. To do so, we must assume that at any given point in such an exercise, an intermediate or tentative diagnosis can be represented as an array of possible diseases, each associated with some probability, and that the sum of all such probabilities is 1.0.[156,221] In such a scheme, we devise two models, each of which consists arbitrarily of three possible diseases. In the first model, the probabilities of the three diseases at a given point during the collection and interpretation of clinical data are disease 1, 0.8; disease 2, 0.1; and disease 3, 0.1. In this first model, any clinical finding with a likelihood ratio that favors diseases 2 and 3 will lower the probability of disease 1.

If, for example, one is inclined to believe that a patient has idiopathic nephrotic syndrome and serum complement is found to be low, the diagnosis of lipid nephrosis becomes much less likely and that of membranoproliferative glomerulonephritis much more likely. It is easy to imagine in this model how a set of clinical findings more highly correlated with the other two diseases (specifically, findings whose conditional probabilities are far higher for diseases 2 and 3 than for disease 1) could reduce the probability of disease 1 and raise the probability of diseases 2 and 3, such that the probabilities of all three diseases end up the same or nearly the same. This situation—equal probability of all diagnostic possibilities—describes maximum diagnostic uncertainty, or a quandary like the one we are considering.

In our second model, the probability of each of the three diseases at a given point in time is the same, namely 0.33. If the conditional probabilities of some clinical findings identified thereafter are higher for one of the possible diseases (say, disease 3), that disease becomes more likely and the other two diseases less likely. If additional data emerge later in which the conditional probabilities of the findings favor one or both of the other two diseases, the probabilities of all three diseases may end up equal or nearly equal again.

If, for example, a patient is considered to have an equal likelihood of hepatitis, cholestatic jaundice, and extrahepatic biliary obstruction, an elevated alkaline phosphatase would reduce the chance of hepatitis and increase the chance of obstruction (either type), but the subsequent finding of a very high alanine transaminase (ALT) might reduce all three diagnostic possibilities to equivalent values. Clearly, these models are merely two examples of how a diagnostic quandary can be reached.

What should be done, then, when we do not have a definitive diagnosis? Many have been puzzled, in such situations, to observe senior clinicians who have no difficulty with such quandaries: They declare the patient to have a certain disease (usually one that cannot be either proved or disproved) and recommend treatment based on the diagnosis they have designated. This practice is analogous to the apocryphal reply of a baseball umpire: When asked how he decided whether a pitch was a strike or a ball, he declared, "They ain't nothing until I calls them."

Clearly, just giving a patient a diagnostic label does not necessarily make it so, and although some seasoned clinicians seem to have a way of intuitively sensing the correct diagnosis, such an approach does not readily lend itself to objective examination. Another of the interesting approaches in such a situation is to wait it out—that is, to continue to observe the patient until findings emerge that clarify the picture. This practice often is referred to as using "tincture of time." A third approach, closely allied to the second, is typified by a one-liner attributed to the distinguished clinician Robert F. Loeb: "If you don't know what to do, don't do anything."[222]

When all is said and done, what should we do when we do not have a definite diagnosis? Some expert clinicians who often deal with such patients (e.g., those with fever of undetermined origin) advocate taking a fresh approach and "starting from scratch"—namely, taking the history over again, repeating a complete physical examination, and reordering selected laboratory tests. Its occasional success is explained by several possibilities. First, the fresh look may be more extensive than the initial evaluation and may uncover previously overlooked historical features (e.g., an exposure to a certain infectious agent) or physical findings (e.g., a patch of chorioretinitis). Second, some tests that were either positive or negative earlier may give different results because the initial results were either falsely positive or negative. Third, the patient's disease may still be in evolution, and new, diagnostically helpful findings may have developed.

The advice not to do anything when the diagnosis is in doubt clearly was never meant to be universally applicable. In fact, almost everyone appreciates that not making a decision is tantamount to making a decision, namely, not to change the existing or current approach. When the patient's welfare does not hinge on an immediate change in therapy, tincture of time is certainly appropriate, and reassessing the patient repeatedly for new findings is warranted.

Unfortunately, we are not always afforded the luxury of extra time. Both acute and chronic situations that demand immediate action despite uncertain diagnosis readily come to mind. We must choose a therapeutic approach immediately for a patient who is unable to provide a coherent history and presents with shock from an unknown cause. In such cases, we treat all the manifestations of shock and often resort to treating all the likely causes until we are able to get more data. We may be forced to treat a cancer patient blindly with radiation therapy if a lesion threatens to compress the spinal cord, even though the lesion has not been identified by biopsy as metastatic.

In some cases, we may be forced to accelerate the diagnostic workup, using risky, invasive tests sooner than we would have liked. In a patient with progressive, severe weight loss, for example, delaying those tests may compromise the patient's chance of recovery even more than immediate exposure to the risky procedures. Many of these decisions can be aided by decision analysis. If a full set of the diseases that could be affecting the patient can be identified; if the therapeutic approaches, their efficacies, and complications can be ascertained; and if the values (utilities) of all outcomes can be specified, then the optimal approach will be the one with the highest expected utility. Even the value of combined therapeutic approaches—that is, using more than one treatment—can be assessed with this tool.

Fortunately, the incidence of frustrating diagnostic quandaries that stop clinicians in their tracks and lead to paralysis of therapeutic decision making is small and getting smaller with the advent of noninvasive scans and minimally invasive biopsies. Nonetheless, we know little about how to proceed in such circumstances. We do not even have a means of identifying them when they occur, and we do not have a classification for them. Clearly, we need to learn more about this interesting and potentially important dilemma. Folklore is no longer a sufficient basis for medical decision making.

CASE 42. DIAGNOSIS BY FIAT

A 39-year-old woman with a history of hypertension, asymptomatic proteinuria, β-thalassemia trait, and hypothyroidism presented with a 3-week history of shortness of breath. She was found to be in congestive heart failure.

My first thought is that the β-thalassemia trait probably has nothing to do with the development of the congestive heart failure. Second, the congestive heart failure presumably could be related to the hypertension, although I have no history of the severity or duration of the hypertension, and I do not know whether it has been treated and whether she was on medication. Similarly, hypothyroidism could be important, but then again I do not know how long she has had it and whether it has been properly managed with replacement therapy. Congestive heart failure could be due to many things, and it may be unrelated to the history that is available at this point.

> Blood pressure was 164/110 mm Hg. Rales were present over both lung fields. Cardiac examination revealed an S_3 gallop with no rubs or murmurs. The spleen tip was felt. Slight pedal edema was present. Initial laboratory data were as follows: white cell count 10,400, hemoglobin 13.6 g/dL, hematocrit 35%, MCV 77, and platelets 91,000. Electrolytes were normal, BUN 19 mg/dL, creatinine 1.6 mg/dL, creatine kinase (CK) 863 IU/L, MB 10.3%. Urinalysis: specific gravity 1.020, pH 6.0, protein >100 mg/dL. Sediment examination revealed a few white blood cells. ECG showed sinus tachycardia. T-wave changes consistent with inferior and lateral ischemia were present.

The low MCV is consistent with the thalassemia trait. The low platelet count suggests an additional process and may be related to the palpable spleen. The high CK might indicate myocardial damage, especially with the elevated MB percentage, or it might be related to inadequately treated hypothyroidism. The proteinuria suggests that the patient has some kind of renal disease, but we do not know whether it is secondary to hypertension or whether the hypertension is secondary to the renal disease. The palpable spleen and the low platelet count could go together, but I cannot relate these findings to any of the other information.

> Cardiac failure and hypertension were aggressively treated with diuretics and vasodilators. An echocardiogram revealed a moderate-sized circumferential pericardial effusion. Concentric left ventricular hypertrophy was present, with a hypokinetic inferoposterior wall. Ejection fraction was 65%. Viral titers were negative. Cardiac catheterization disclosed normal coronary arteries. Free thyroxine index was 0.8, TSH 227 μU/mL, antithyroglobulin antibody 1:25,600. Thyroid replacement therapy was initiated. Her 24-hour urine protein excretion was 2.5 to 4.2 g. Serum albumin was 3.4 g/dL, and

> cholesterol was 206 mg/dL. Antinuclear antibody was 1:5,120 in a nucleolar pattern.

The low thyroxine index, elevated TSH, and positive antithyroglobulin antibody suggest thyroiditis or some type of autoimmune disorder. There appears to be a renal lesion causing protein loss in the nephrotic range, but I would like to know what the protein is. The patient is a young woman, and the question of lupus comes up, but the nucleolar pattern of the antinuclear antibody is not the pattern typically seen with lupus. The nucleolar pattern could be seen in a variety of other diseases.

> The following studies yielded negative or normal results: CH_{50}, C4, C3, C2, C1q, rheumatoid factor, hepatitis B antigen, anti-dsDNA (antibody to double-stranded DNA), anti-ss (single-stranded) DNA, anti-Ro, anti-La, anti-Scl-70, anti-Sm, anti-RNP.

These results argue against mixed connective tissue disease, against systemic lupus, and against scleroderma. What do they suggest? It is still possible that she has an autoimmune thyroiditis, but that does not account for the protein loss in urine or explain the whole picture.

> A consulting clinician felt that a definitive diagnosis of systemic lupus erythematosus (SLE) could not be made because the patient did not fulfill the American College of Rheumatology's (ACR) criteria for the diagnosis of SLE. A renal biopsy was recommended to help clarify the diagnosis.

I guess the main purpose of the renal biopsy would be to clarify the nature of the renal disease that is causing a lot of protein loss but not really impairing renal function that much. It is possible that a renal biopsy is not going to be of much help in the management of the patient. I do not remember all of the ACR criteria, but I believe they include skin involvement, joint involvement, and probably some specification of the type of autoantibody that is seen. It typically should be anti-dsDNA in an abnormal titer. With active disease, I would think that CH_{50} and the C3 should be down, but I do not remember if they are in the ACR criteria for lupus.

A renal biopsy revealed diffuse thickening of capillary loops consistent with membranous nephropathy. Subepithelial, subendothelial, and mesangial deposits were found. The patient was thought to have the membranous glomerulopathy of lupus. Therapy with corticosteroids and immunosuppressive agents was recommended.

I think the rheumatologist was correct—that the whole picture does not meet the criteria.

The patient refused treatment. Two months later, she presented with vasculitis that produced ischemia in several fingertips. She was treated with plasmapheresis, prednisone, and cyclophosphamide, with a good response. Over the next several months, she had intermittent exacerbations of her disease, characterized by recurrent vasculitis of her fingers, decreases in her serum complement activity, and increased proteinuria. Her anti-dsDNA levels remained normal. Nine months after her initial presentation, she was in remission on prednisone. Her antinuclear antibody titer was 1:640 with a nucleolar speckled pattern. Her creatinine was stable at 1.1 mg/dL with a 24-hour urinary protein excretion of 2.1 g.

In this case, I would be more comfortable using a broader term than systemic lupus and say that the patient had an autoimmune disorder that certainly affected her thyroid and her kidneys and possibly affected her heart. She did not have a number of features that most people recognize as components of the diagnostic entity systemic lupus erythematosus.

Analysis

This patient presented with proteinuria and declining renal function secondary to an immune complex glomerulonephritis, which a renal pathologist identified as consistent with lupus nephritis. Her antinuclear antibody titer was markedly elevated, but no other clinical manifestations or laboratory evidence of SLE were identified despite an extensive search. A consultant recommended that the patient be treated aggressively for lupus nephritis, even though she failed to satisfy widely accepted criteria for the diagnosis of SLE. Should the consultant be criticized for making an inappropriate judgment with flimsy evidence? Retrospectively, of course, it seems quite obvious that his recommendations were appropriate; indeed, he appears almost prescient, because within 2 months the patient manifested flagrant vasculitis.

Here is the issue raised by this case: How appropriate is it to require that a diagnosis fits the fixed criteria of some defined recipe? How critical are the conditions for setting up such criteria? When such criteria have been established for a given disease and a given patient fails to meet all the criteria, should we not diagnose that disease? Should we simply keep the diagnosis "on hold" until more data appear?

The practice of making diagnoses by adhering to set criteria has been applied in several settings.[223,224] Some of the purposes of establishing fixed diagnostic criteria are as follows:

1. *To make a diagnosis* that will be a guide to therapy. Criteria have been fashioned to diagnose a number of diseases, including acute rheumatic fever (the venerable Jones criteria),[225] allergic bronchopulmonary aspergillosis,[226] Behçet disease,[227] rheumatoid arthritis,[228] and systemic lupus erythematosus.[229]
2. *For clinical research.* For this application, criteria usually are used to identify a homogeneous patient population for study.
3. *For reimbursement purposes.* Coding into categories by set diagnostic criteria provides an unambiguous approach to identification of patients who are eligible for insurance coverage.[230]

The second purpose is essential to proper clinical research; the third purpose also seems rational, especially when done carefully and thoughtfully. However, the first approach—namely, setting criteria solely for the purpose of fitting a patient into a diagnostic pigeonhole—deserves comment.

A fundamental concept in the definition of a disease is the notion of a gold standard. This standard is often based on histologic features and less frequently on specific radiologic features or even on a particular response to therapy. Once the gold standard is established, the clinical and laboratory features of the disease can be identified. Because not all features are invariably associated with the disease in a given patient and because some manifestations occur in one stage of the disease and not in another, it is convenient to describe the occurrence of clinical features and laboratory manifestations in probabilistic terms.

Among patients with lung cancer, for example, how many have Horner syndrome? How does the frequency of this feature vary with the location, duration, or type of tumor? How often is Horner syndrome associated with other tumors? With other, non–tumor-related disease? Once we know these probabilistic associations, we are in a position not only to interpret clinical signs and laboratory abnormalities, but also to engage in differential diagnosis—the process of differentiating among the many diseases that can produce similar clinical and laboratory manifestations.

The process of interpreting such clinical data and integrating them into a coherent working diagnosis (i.e., a diagnosis that is a guide to further testing or therapy) is often performed implicitly and without calculation but can be conducted formally by means of Bayesian analysis, as described earlier.[156,176] The Bayesian approach has special value as a model of the diagnostic process because it identifies many of the traps behind the integration of clinical and laboratory data. It requires, for example, that the diagnostic possibilities form an inclusive and complete set and that manifestations included in any calculation be mutually exclusive of each other.[103] The latter requirement avoids "double counting" for the strength of two or more different manifestations that are fundamentally part of the same physiologic disturbance. The benefit of the Bayesian framework is that it focuses on the interplay among all the diagnostic possibilities: Once a complete set is assembled, evidence favoring one diagnosis over another must, *pari passu*, yield a reduction in the likelihood of one or more alternative diagnostic possibilities.

Against this Bayesian model, let us consider diagnosis according to fixed criteria—in particular, the diagnosis of systemic lupus erythematosus by the ACR criteria. Compared with the Bayesian model, the ACR criteria appear flawed. First, they were not originally based on a gold standard. Second, they stand in isolation rather than in relation to other diagnostic possibilities. They thus fail to ask the important questions: If this is not systemic

lupus, what else could it be? What are the other competing diagnoses? Third, the criteria are simply additive: If the patient has fewer than a given number of criteria, the diagnosis of lupus should not be made, whereas if the patient has more than the sufficient number of present criteria, the diagnosis of lupus can be made with confidence.

Yet the Bayesian model shows quite clearly that unless likelihood ratios for all clinical findings are the same (a distinctly unusual phenomenon), a simple arithmetic combination of individual criteria (whether clinical or laboratory) does not adequately describe how a feature affects a given diagnostic possibility. In fact, it is the strength of the correlation between a given feature and a given disease that determines how a single feature should be weighted. The presence of a feature that occurs in 99% of patients with lupus and 0.001% of patients with another disease (such as high levels of double-stranded DNA) is a far more powerful argument in favor of a diagnosis of lupus than is the presence of a feature that occurs in 80% of patients with SLE and in 6% of patients with diseases that often are confused with lupus.

Given these shortcomings of diagnosis by fiat, what can we offer in its place? Careful Bayesian analysis is one approach. Discriminant analysis is another because it combines the gold standard with careful studies of the frequency of manifestations and thus gives appropriate weight to findings that are either present or absent. Short of using these quantitative approaches, the best guidelines are the following: Consider all relevant diagnostic possibilities, weight each manifestation according to the frequency with which it occurs in all the competing disorders, avoid double-counting physiologically related manifestations, and remember that features derived from the history and physical examination may be as discriminating as those derived from the chemistry laboratory or imaging unit.

Whether the patient described here has lupus or some yet unnamed disorder is uncertain. If it is not lupus, as our discussant argues, it is a close relative. No matter whether we diagnose by fiat or by combining probabilistic variables, it may not be prudent to sit and wait for new manifestations to appear before treating. Even though our confidence in a given diagnosis may be enhanced by watching and waiting, the golden opportunity for intervening in a potentially lethal disease may sometimes pass us by.

CASE 43. IRON PYRITE AND DIAGNOSTIC CONFIRMATION

Example 1

A 28-year-old woman was admitted to the hospital with a 10-week history of nausea, vomiting, and abdominal bloating. Six years before admission she had undergone laparoscopy for abdominal bloating; no abnormalities were found. Two years before admission she had had another laparoscopy for a right tubal pregnancy. She had been well otherwise. On admission, her abdomen was distended. A fluid wave and mild diffuse tenderness were detected. Abdominal CT scan confirmed the ascites and disclosed a 5 × 3.5-cm right adnexal mass. A CA 125 level was 800 (normal, 0 to 35).

Exploratory laparotomy disclosed a right corpus luteum cyst and multiple white implants on the parietal and visceral peritoneum. A frozen section of one of the implants in the cul-de-sac was reported as "consistent with adenocarcinoma of unknown primary; cannot rule out acute inflammation." On the basis of this finding, a total abdominal hysterectomy and bilateral salpingo-oophorectomy were performed. The postoperative diagnosis was adenocarcinoma.

Review of the permanent sections revealed only multiple noncaseating granulomas involving the fallopian tubes. There was no malignancy. The patient was treated for granulomatous peritonitis with antituberculous medications and adrenal corticosteroids.

Example 2

A 44-year-old man presented with right flank pain of 3 months' duration. Abdominal ultrasound and CT scan revealed a solid 11-cm right adrenal mass. His history was unremarkable. Plasma cortisol levels and urinary excretion of catecholamines, vanillylmandelic acid, and metanephrines were all normal. A right adrenalectomy was performed. The pathologic diagnosis was pheochromocytoma.

Six weeks later the patient had an episode of intraabdominal bleeding, which necessitated a repeat laparotomy. No bleeding site was found. Another biopsy specimen was thought to be consistent with pheochromocytoma. Because of recurrent bleeding, an oncologist was consulted. This physician thought that the clinical course was inconsistent with a pheochromocytoma and requested that special histologic studies be done on the original tissue specimens. The special stains disclosed that the tumor was an angiosarcoma, not a pheochromocytoma. (Note: An extensive discussion of this patient can be found in case 66.)

Example 3

A 52-year-old man had a laparotomy for acute appendicitis. The specimen showed acute inflammation and a tiny perforation, but it also contained a tumor. The pathologist described the lesion as a carcinoma of the appendix that originated in a villous adenoma, and he recommended further surgery. Postoperatively, the surgeon recommended that the patient undergo a right hemicolectomy.

The patient's gastroenterologist was skeptical of the diagnosis of cancer of the appendix because this disease is extremely rare. He reviewed the histologic sections and concluded that the findings thought to be consistent with cancer, namely glandular structures in the adventitia, resulted not from metastatic spread of the tumor but from an artifact attributable to the technique by which the specimen was sectioned. The gastroenterologist recommended observation only. The patient has been entirely well in the 25 years since.

Analysis

These three examples raise a problem rarely discussed and for which we have few data: the clinical situation in which a usually impeccable and reliable "gold standard" turns out to be simply wrong and the patient suffers because of the error. All three cases illustrate the same fundamental principle of clinical decision making, yet in each the outcome was determined by whether the physician responsible for the patient's care recognized that the standard was not gold but only looked like gold.

The patient with the granulomatous lesions on her peritoneal membrane lost her uterus and fallopian tubes unnecessarily; the histologic interpretation on the frozen section was not definitive (adenocarcinoma *or* inflammation), yet the subsequent surgery was done for cancer. A definitive reading of the biopsy as inflammation came only after the fact.

The patient with the abdominal angiosarcoma was subjected to a delay in the administration of chemotherapy. The correct diagnosis was made only after a consultant recognized that pheochromocytoma was not a plausible explanation for all of the patient's clinical findings.

The man with an appendiceal adenoma endured the anxiety of thinking that he had cancer and that he would require another laparotomy. In this case, the unlikelihood of cancer of the appendix led the gastroenterologist to search for a more plausible diagnostic hypothesis. The gastroenterologist was confident that the histologic findings were far more consistent with a benign villous adenoma.

We have argued that a diagnosis is a belief in the state of a patient and that certainty in diagnosis is difficult, if not impossible, to attain. We have also laid out ground rules for the verification of diagnostic hypotheses (see case 39). Here we offer three specific examples in which tissue histology, putatively our most reliable confirmatory diagnostic aid, yielded an incorrect initial diagnosis. Even the final arbiter—the pathologist—does not always have the right answer. We see from these examples that it can make a difference: In one case, a patient had an unnecessary hysterectomy and salpingo-oophorectomy; another patient nearly had a partial colectomy. What signals should we look for in identifying such problems?

Some clues can be found in the three case histories. In the patient with the granulomatous peritoneal lesions, an equivocal histologic interpretation should have been a signal to study the tissue further before proceeding with more surgery. In the patient with the abdominal angiosarcoma, atypical clinical features should have suggested the possibility that the tumor was not a pheochromocytoma. In the man with suspected appendiceal cancer, the rarity of the lesion should have raised more questions about the validity of its designation as malignant.

In all three cases, therefore, some feature that was not fully consistent with the suspected diagnosis might have been the essential signal that a new diagnostic hypothesis should be entertained. Finally, all three examples of erroneous interpretation involved rare diseases: granulomatous peritonitis, abdominal angiosarcoma, and appendiceal villous adenoma.

One of the problems encountered here is a special case of a concept we have considered before, namely the notion of adequacy of diagnosis[19] (see cases 38, 39, and 40). Adequacy is a criterion that asks the following question: Are all the findings in the patient explained by the working diagnosis? Clearly, in one of the cases we described (the angiosarcoma), all findings were not adequately explained by the working diagnosis. In another case (the appendiceal lesion), both cancer and adenoma would have explained all the findings, but the gravity of the cancer diagnosis led to a search for a different, equally plausible explanation.

Here are some lessons from the tarnished gold standard: (1) Beware if the criterion of adequacy is not satisfied. If it is not, seriously question the working diagnosis and search for a more plausible diagnostic hypothesis.[26,134] (2) Exercise special caution when making a diagnosis of a rare disease, particularly when the prognosis for that disease is poor. (3) Beware of positive findings in tests ordered for the wrong reason: As we noted before, positive results often turn out to be false positives (see case 23). (4) If you are not certain whether your findings match a given diagnosis, consult your colleagues, the experts, or the literature. It may be dangerous simply to assume that discrepant or unexplained findings just represent variations on a theme of disease.

CHAPTER 18

Therapeutic Decision Making

CASE 44. THE SURGEON OPTS TO OPERATE: WHY?

> A 38-year-old man with a 12-year history of ulcerative colitis was admitted to a community hospital with bloody diarrhea and abdominal pain. *Campylobacter* was found in his stool, and he was treated with a macrolide antibiotic for 10 days, but the diarrhea worsened. Sigmoidoscopy showed a diffuse, erythematous, friable mucosa, and mucosal biopsy was consistent with ulcerative colitis. Treatment with steroids was begun. Abdominal pain and diarrhea persisted, and an abdominal plain film showed distention of the transverse colon with air–fluid levels. The white cell count was 14,600 with 58 polys and 6 bands.

Any time a patient with ulcerative colitis presents with exacerbation of symptoms, regardless of whether the disease has been active or inactive, several things should come to mind. For starters, it could be just an exacerbation of the disease, which will respond quickly to medical management with steroids and bowel rest. These patients must be closely followed in the hospital because of the potential for complications, such as toxic megacolon and perforation. It is probably not appropriate to attribute the worsening of symptoms in such patients to infectious causes without clear-cut documentation that their ulcerative colitis is quiescent. I think, therefore, that the *Campylobacter* here probably is just a red herring. The distention of the transverse colon associated with the elevated white cell count is an ominous sign: The evolution of toxic megacolon in this setting can be rapid and life threatening, especially in patients on steroids, which might mask the clinical progression of the disease. It is important that the patient be followed closely with serial abdominal films.

At this point, I would not manipulate the colon any further and would not use any antidiarrheal agents, especially any anticholinergic agents that might further depress motor function of the bowel. Probably, broad-spectrum antibiotics and complete bowel rest should be prescribed and the patient followed closely for a period to see if the abdominal findings will resolve. Otherwise, it is probably important to have a surgical consultation early to make sure that if symptoms and signs progress despite optimum medical management, preparation has been made for surgery.

> Parenteral nutrition was instituted, and the patient was allowed nothing by mouth. Sharp left-upper-quadrant pain with shoulder radiation was treated with meperidine.

Parenteral nutrition is important in these patients, although it is a little unclear how acute the need for parenteral nutrition was in this case. If the patient was otherwise healthy and he was in good nutritional shape, that probably would not have been my top priority. The emergence of sharp left-upper-quadrant pain in this setting is strongly indicative of perforation. The shoulder pain is related to diaphragmatic irritation from an inflammatory process in the left upper quadrant, and in this setting, it is almost certainly related to perforation of the colon. I think treating with meperidine is not going to do anything but mask the symptoms. I would get a repeat plain film of the abdomen and prepare the patient to go to the operating room.

> Repeat plain film was said to be consistent with toxic megacolon, and the patient was transferred to Tufts Medical Center. On admission, he was afebrile, and his vital signs were normal. His abdomen was distended, with diffuse tenderness but no rebound tenderness. No bowel sounds were heard. Rectal examination disclosed liquid brown stool that was guaiac positive. Flexible sigmoidoscopy was unchanged from before.

The patient clearly has toxic megacolon. I would not be misled by the fact that he is afebrile and has normal vital signs. The patient is probably on fairly high doses of steroids, so the vital signs and temperature can be deceiving. The abdomen is distended, with diffuse tenderness. I believe the patient probably already has a perforated bowel, so I do not think it was necessary to do a sigmoidoscopy. Assuming he has had a good physical examination and if his abdomen appears to be that tender and distended, I think that perforation has to be the leading diagnosis. If the colon has perforated, the surgical mortality increases to 50% to 70%, compared with a fairly acceptable rate of probably 12%, maybe 18%, for nonperforated toxic megacolon. I think it is important that the patient be evaluated for surgery on a relatively urgent basis.

> After admission another abdominal plain film showed a dilated ascending colon and transverse colon and a very large aneurysmal dilation of the splenic flexure with air–fluid levels throughout. Blood pressure was 115/75 mm Hg, pulse rate 100 per minute, and temperature 38°C. White cell count was 7,200 with 60 polys and 19 bands.

I think that this patient is in serious trouble and should be operated on without delay.

> Because the patient had been treated with antibiotics 2 weeks earlier, the possibility of *Clostridium difficile* enteritis was entertained. The *C. difficile* stool assay obtained on admission was reported to be positive. The patient was treated with oral vancomycin (500 mg four times a day) and followed closely. After 2 days of therapy, abdominal pain began to subside, the patient remained afebrile, and there was a decrease in the degree of the left shift. After 1 week the diarrhea began to diminish, the plain film showed fewer abnormalities, and the stools became guaiac negative. The patient was discharged after a 3-week hospitalization.

I think you were lucky. It is nice that the patient was able to keep his colon, but I suspect he is going to lose it in the not too distant future. He is 38 years old and has had chronic ulcerative colitis for 12 years. His risk of colon cancer now is probably in the 10% range, and by the time the patient is 50 years old, it will be close to 40%. Thus, he is probably going to lose his colon some time in the next 10 to 15 years.

Analysis

Internists sometimes consider a surgeon's clinical judgment that differs from theirs a consequence of an undefined but widely acknowledged "surgical mentality." Likewise, surgeons invoke a "medical mentality" when they judge that an internist has used medical therapy too long before referring the patient for possible surgery. Some surgeons even acquire a reputation of being "medically oriented" and some internists are considered "surgically oriented." Indeed, these designations sometimes even evoke pejorative connotations. Perhaps we should not be surprised that strong opinions sometimes exist when the alternative choices—typically medical therapy versus surgical therapy—imply such different approaches and potential outcomes.

Applying quantitative approaches to clinical decisions has made it possible to assess some of the factors responsible for these differing judgments,[231] but here we use another approach, namely analyzing the "thinking aloud" behavior of physicians engaged in the decision-making process.[61] The patient described in this transcript was managed by an expert gastroenterologist, and the surgeon to whom we presented the clinical material is an expert gastrointestinal surgeon. Of course, the internist had the advantage of a direct patient encounter, whereas the surgeon's encounter was in the form of a "paper exercise." Nonetheless, the surgeon's explanations of his opinions reveal differences from the internist's judgments. The discussant appears to have a lower threshold for intervening and clearly would have recommended surgery earlier than the internist.

Several factors appear to account for this approach. First, the surgeon viewed the chance of perforation (or incipient perforation) as being quite high and based this view largely on the location and radiation of the patient's abdominal pain. By contrast, we know from the hospital record that the gastroenterologist was impressed that the patient was afebrile, that vital signs were normal, that no rebound tenderness was present, and that the white cell count was normal. He judged the chance of perforation to be low. Second, the surgeon considered unlikely the possibility that a treatable and reversible infectious cause of toxic megacolon could be responsible for the acute clinical manifestations. Third, the surgeon raised serious concern that a delay in surgery would be associated with an increasingly high, unacceptable surgical mortality.

In fact, after the surgeon learned that the patient had recovered from toxic megacolon with medical management alone, he expressed the view that both the gastroenterologist and the patient were lucky. The implication of this remark is that the outcome would have been adverse more often than favorable in comparable circumstances. Finally, the surgeon, after learning the outcome (perhaps guided by retrospective bias[143,144]) opines that the patient will eventually require colon resection to avoid colon cancer. Thus, he implies that even if the colon had been unnecessarily removed on this occasion, it would have been justifiable for other reasons.

Of course, a transcript such as this fails to uncover much of the reasoning of both the internist and the surgeon. We do not know whether either of the physicians considered other relevant factors: the morbidity of surgery, the impact of colectomy on the quality of the patient's life, and the risk of recurrent episodes of toxic megacolon. It is quite likely that these factors were considered, albeit not explicitly. These issues may well have had an important impact on the therapeutic choices of both the gastroenterologist and the surgeon.

Clearly, this level of analysis merely scratches the surface in analyzing differences between medical and surgical approaches. Nonetheless, it points up the fact that such analyses are feasible. In our view, they are also desirable. We believe that it is intrinsically important for physicians to identify and explain differences in clinical judgment. Moreover, because the "territories," or domains, of the internist and the surgeon intersect in many common clinical problems (e.g., acute pancreatitis, upper gastrointestinal bleeding, and acute abdominal pain), such an elaboration of judgment should serve the patient's best interest.

Any parent of a growing child knows that he or she can no longer sing "the dog chased the cat; the cat chased the rat" when the child reaches age 5 or 6 years without explaining why. We look forward to detailed studies of clinical judgment that probe the explanations of physician behavior.

CASE 45. TREAT OR KEEP TESTING?

A 64-year-old woman was admitted to the hospital with knifelike anterior chest pain accentuated by moving, coughing, and deep breathing. The pain was accompanied by shortness of breath, and, the night before admission, the cough was productive of white, pink-tinged sputum.

When evaluating patients with pleuritic chest pain, I think about illnesses that cause inflammation of the pleura—either directly or indirectly by a process that involves the underlying lung. When a patient presents with shortness of breath, pleuritic pain, and pink-tinged sputum, one would be most concerned about pulmonary embolism. Another strong possibility would be pneumonia, especially if the patient is febrile and her sputum is purulent.

Three weeks before admission, while attempting to board a train, the patient fell and sustained a subcapital fracture of the left hip and a left Colles fracture. She underwent a closed-reduction internal fixation with a two-hole side plate. She was in Buck traction for 2 days, was ambulating with the aid of a walker on postoperative day 7, and left the hospital on hospital day 13. In the period between discharge and readmission, she had been walking on crutches.

Because the patient has just suffered a major trauma, namely, a hip fracture, I am even more concerned about pulmonary embolic disease. At this point, I would want to see just how sick she is so I could get some idea of the urgency of her problem. In terms of diagnosis, our options include D-dimer, ventilation-perfusion scan, or computed tomography (CT) pulmonary angiogram. In the meantime, I would empirically treat her with heparin, assuming there were no obvious contraindications, because another pulmonary embolus could prove fatal.

At the time of admission, chest pain had been present for 3 days. She had not had calf or leg pain, fever, chills, weight loss, edema, nocturnal dyspnea, or orthopnea. Her vital signs were normal. Examination of the chest revealed decreased excursion on the right side, decreased

breath sounds at the right base, and a localized right anterior pleural friction rub in the midclavicular line just below the breast. Cardiac examination was normal. Her legs were normal, and Homans' sign was not present. The remainder of the examination, including a pelvic exam, was normal.

The first thing that occurs to me is that no one actually measured the respiratory rate. With major embolic disease, it is unusual for a patient not to have tachypnea and a respiratory rate greater than 20. Most such patients also have tachycardia, although less consistently. Occasionally, patients with massive pulmonary embolic disease have a right ventricular heave and accentuated P_2 due to pulmonary hypertension. Neither is described, but I would wish to confirm their absence personally rather than accept that observation from another observer. The fact that the examination of the legs was not informative does not dissuade me from considering pulmonary embolic disease the most likely diagnosis, since examination of the extremities is notoriously unreliable in thromboembolic disease. Because the patient was afebrile, pneumonia is less likely.

Hemoglobin was 12 g/dL, hematocrit 36%, and white cell count 12,400 with 67 polys, 1 band, 28 lymphs, 2 monos, and 2 eos. Blood urea nitrogen (BUN), creatinine, electrolytes, and blood glucose were normal. Sedimentation rate was 70 mm/hr. Sputum examination revealed scarce white blood cells, scarce red cells, and no bacteria.

I do not find these data very helpful. The diagnosis we are concerned about here is pulmonary embolism, and one therefore has to either obtain a lung scan or a CT pulmonary angiogram or treat with anticoagulants on the clinical suspicion alone. I think a chest x-ray might be useful, but most of the other tests that are often ordered reflexively in patients with similar presenting symptoms are much less helpful in pursuing what seems to be by far the most likely diagnosis in this patient.

Chest x-ray: The right pulmonary artery is a little prominent but probably within nor-

mal limits. The azygous vein is not distended. The main-stem bronchi are not especially splayed. The heart is normal in size. The right costophrenic angle is blunted. A pleural effusion that layers out in the right lateral decubitus position is new since the previous admission. An electrocardiogram (ECG) shows normal sinus rhythm, rate 72, axis 0 degrees, no S_1, Q_3, T_3 pattern, and no other abnormalities.

The chest x-ray is helpful because it excludes the possibility of pneumonia. It is a little surprising that her pulse rate is only 72 because sinus tachycardia is so common in pulmonary embolic disease. Occasionally, especially with overwhelming pulmonary hypertension and multiple emboli, one will see a pattern of right ventricular strain. Axis deviation occurs in 10% to 15% of patients. Actually, left-axis deviation is about as common as right-axis deviation. The classic S_1, Q_3, T_3 pattern probably occurs in no more than 5% to 10% of patients, and therefore its absence is not often useful. The ECG findings are not particularly helpful in this patient; I am still eagerly waiting for the results of a lung scan or a CT scan. I suspect, given the sequence in which the data have been presented, however, that I will next be given the results of arterial blood gases.

Blood gases (on room air): pH 7.51, arterial partial pressure of carbon dioxide (PCO_2) 32 mm Hg, arterial partial pressure of oxygen (PO_2) 65 mm Hg.

The patient has moderate hypoxemia and mild respiratory alkalosis. It used to be thought that patients with pulmonary embolic disease always had an arterial PO_2 of less than 80. When we examined patients who presented in our emergency room with lung scans positive for pulmonary embolic disease, 10% to 15% had a PO_2 greater than 80. The patient's blood gases are consistent with a diagnosis of pulmonary embolism. The increase in her alveolar–arterial oxygen gradient, however, could also be caused by underlying lung disease.

A lung scan was carried out (Figure 18.1).

There seem to be major defects in the left upper lobe, probably at the right base, and at the

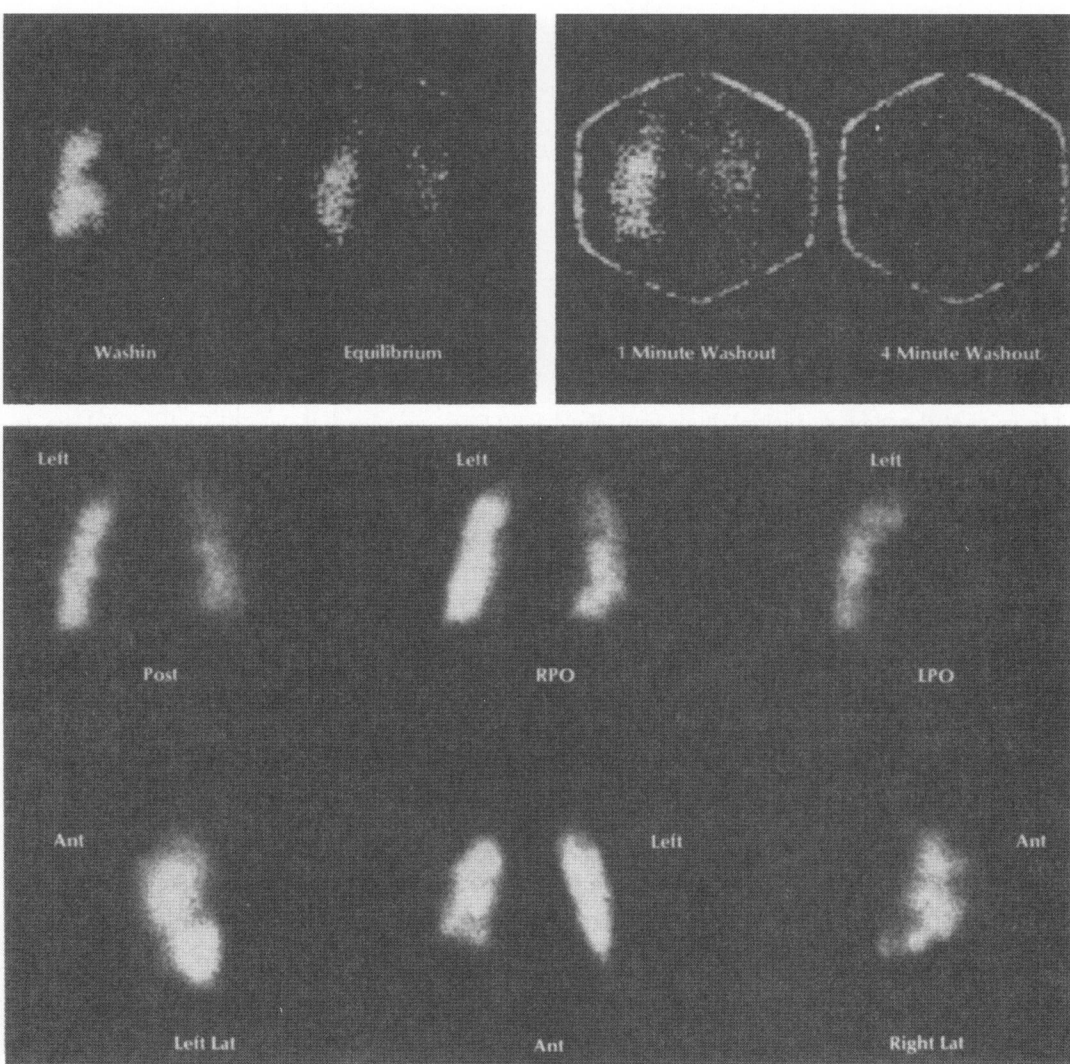

Figure 18.1 • Ventilation-perfusion lung scan; case 45.

right apex. The right basilar defects are difficult to interpret since we know that she has an effusion in that location, but clearly the left side is very abnormal. I would be quite willing to treat her for pulmonary embolic disease on the basis of her history and these findings. An interesting question would be whether to use thrombolytic therapy as opposed to conventional heparin treatment. In view of her recent hip trauma and surgery, I would tend to use heparin, although I am not sure whether there is an absolute contraindication to thrombolytic therapy, given that her surgical procedure was done 3 weeks ago.

The official reading of the scan was as follows: "Decreased ventilation to the entire right lung, possibly compatible with reduced volume secondary to atelectasis. Perfusion scan showed bilateral multiple small defects that were indeterminate in appearance. In conclusion, low suspicion for pulmonary embolus."

I have reservations about this interpretation. I think the scan is more suggestive of pulmonary embolism than did the radiologist. If I had read the scan myself, I would have treated the patient with anticoagulants on the basis of that scan. Given this different interpretation, however, I would review the study with the radiologist. If he or she was convinced that the suspicion of pulmonary embolism on the scan was quite low, I would do the definitive study—a CT pulmonary angiogram—because of my strong clinical suspicion that the patient has a pulmonary embolus.

> In spite of the "low-suspicion" lung scan, the clinicians taking care of the patient felt that the likelihood of a pulmonary embolus was so high that they initiated heparin therapy without performing a CT scan. The patient had an uneventful recovery.

Analysis

The solution to this patient's clinical problem illustrates multiple aspects of the clinical problem-solving process, including (1) the overt violation by an expert of the data-gathering rules we teach our students, (2) the willingness of an expert clinician to rely on clinical convictions rather than on laboratory tests, (3) the folly of trying to separate diagnostic reasoning from therapeutic decision making, and (4) the concept of the "threshold" approach to therapy.

Even before the discussant learned that the patient had undergone an orthopedic procedure 3 weeks preceding the onset of dyspnea, hemoptysis, and pleuritic chest pain, a diagnosis of pulmonary embolism was uppermost in his mind. His concern about this diagnosis increased on learning her history, and before he learned the remainder of the history, the data from the physical examination, or the laboratory findings, he asked to see the lung scan. However, the sequence in which the clinical data on the patient were obtained did not match this request, so the discussant waded through the other data, willingly interpreting the usual sequential findings obtained in the workup of such a patient. In doing so, he displayed impatience at not being given what he apparently perceived to be the critical data, namely the results of the scan. He was clearly violating the standard, sys-

tematized approach that we teach our students: Obtain a complete history, do a complete physical examination, order all the "simple" laboratory tests, and only then order the expensive and risky ones.

Should we be dismayed at the discussant's desire to bypass this orderly process, or can we learn something from it? It is our view that the "shunting" process he used is one that characterizes the expert clinician and that we should acknowledge that this process is not only valid but also often desirable. In this instance, we have notable clues to the rationale for requesting data "out of step." The many negative physical findings did not dissuade the discussant from his conviction that the patient had sustained a pulmonary embolus, the ECG findings were not helpful, and the blood gas analyses did not alter his opinion. Apparently, at this point, he implicitly used a valuable clinical rule: Choose a safe test with the highest possible information content, that is, a test that is most likely to confirm or exclude a highly probable diagnosis with the least possible harm to the patient. Although the ECG and the blood gases were risk-free tests, their interpretation was not likely to convince him that he was right or wrong, and thus he was not particularly interested in the results. This kind of experience suggests that we should begin to teach students how we actually solve problems, not what the traditions dictate. We might paraphrase a famous expression as follows: "Do what I do, not what I say you should do."

The second feature of this clinical problem-solving session is the strong reliance by the discussant on his clinical judgment when it came to initiating lifesaving therapy. He announced his desire to initiate heparin therapy when the only information he had was that the patient suddenly developed dyspnea, pleuritic chest pain, and slight hemoptysis 3 weeks after orthopedic surgery. When the official interpretation of the scan was less confirmatory than his, he remained convinced that the patient had a pulmonary embolus, and he wished to explore the official interpretations in more detail. He was even willing to recommend a CT pulmonary angiogram despite a low-suspicion scan because he was so confident of the diagnosis of pulmonary embolism.

Was he simply being stubborn? We think not. His assessment of the probability of pulmonary embolism, principally on the basis of the history, was so high that even a low-suspicion scan failed to dissuade him of the diagnosis. In Bayesian terms (in which the prevalence of the disorder is taken into account in interpretation of laboratory results), the low-suspicion scan did not importantly lower the probability of pulmonary embolism from its extremely high a priori value. It is equally interesting that the clinicians who were taking care of the patient were so convinced that she had a pulmonary embolism that they did not feel obliged to carry out a CT angiogram, even when their own radiologist interpreted the lung scan as "low suspicion for pulmonary embolism."

The emphasis here should be placed on the necessity to interpret test results in the context of the clinical situation. Although the scan was considered "low suspicion," the pretest clinical context was a high prior probability of pulmonary embolism. In the Prospective Investigation of Pulmonary Embolism Diagnosis (PIOPED) study, 40% of patients strongly suspected of having pulmonary embolism who had low-probability scans had pulmonary embolism.[232] Only a completely normal scan in such circumstances would be sufficiently sensitive to "rule out" pulmonary embolism.

Another interesting feature of this problem-solving session is the tightly integrated consideration of both the diagnostic and the therapeutic decision-making tasks. In an effort to be explicit about both of these tasks, we often arbitrarily separate them. For years, students in their first clinical rotations have been told to ignore therapeutic issues and concentrate on diagnosis. The protocol presented here, as well as other experience, suggests that expert physicians do not make that distinction when they solve clinical problems.[19] If that is true, why continue to teach these practices as separate and distinct? With little more than a few symptoms and the history of the recent hospitalization, the clinician announced that he was ready to give the patient anticoagulants, at least until he was more certain that the patient either had or did not have a pulmonary embolus. He was willing to treat (assuming there were no contraindications to the use of anticoagulants) because even without proof of the diagnosis, the net benefit of treatment would be greater than that of not treating. Later, his interpretation of the scan enhanced his suspicion of

pulmonary embolism, and he announced his intention to continue the anticoagulants. He did not first make a firm diagnosis and then decide how to treat; he made a preliminary diagnosis, recommended treatment, added further support to his diagnosis, and then would have continued treatment. In fact, he never made an unequivocal diagnosis, yet he made several therapeutic decisions.

The relation between the certainty of diagnosis and the characteristics of a treatment that governs therapeutic decision making is aptly illustrated by the problem of pulmonary embolism and by the case presented here in particular. For a given disease for which there exists treatment with defined efficacy and risk, clinicians should be willing to give the treatment if they are certain that a patient has the disease. And, of course, they should not use the treatment if they are sure that the patient does not have the disease. When the disease is neither definitely present nor definitely absent, the decision to give or withhold treatment should depend on the degree of certainty of the diagnosis and the efficacy and risk of treatment.

If a treatment is not very effective and is also risky (e.g., some forms of chemotherapy), one should treat only if one is highly confident of the diagnosis. If a treatment is highly effective and is also quite safe (e.g., penicillin for streptococcal pharyngitis), one need not be highly confident that the throat infection is streptococcal before prescribing penicillin. The higher the benefit-to-risk ratio of a treatment, the lower must the probability of disease be before one recommends therapy. When no tests are available, those characteristics of the treatment will define the threshold probability of disease—above which, treatment is the more appropriate choice, and below which, withholding it is more appropriate.[58]

In circumstances in which a lung scan, spiral CT scan, ultrasonography, or D-dimer test are available, the decision making is only slightly different. Do not use heparin when you are quite sure the patient has not experienced a thromboembolic event; use it when you are quite sure he or she has; and use the test when your assessment of the probability of thromboembolism falls somewhere between "quite sure it's present" and "quite sure it's not." The test result merely increases or decreases your suspicion of embolism. If it increases your suspicion, you treat; if it decreases your suspicion, you do not. Thus, when a test is available, there are two thresholds: one that represents a probability of disease below which you withhold treatment and above which you perform the test, and another that represents a higher probability of disease below which you would test and above which you would treat.[59]

Those thresholds are illustrated here, even though the discussant never mentioned the concept and used no formal analytic methods. He was quite sure that the patient had pulmonary emboli but not so sure that he was willing to commit her to a full course of therapy. He used the lung scan to alter his view of the probability of embolism; his interpretation of the scan enhanced his suspicion of embolism, and he recommended treatment. When this high suspicion was questioned by the official scan interpretation, the discussant wanted another test done, that is, a CT pulmonary angiogram, to confirm his high suspicion and thus his decision to treat. The interaction of the effectiveness and the risks of treatment is also apparent in the decision he made regarding thrombolytic therapy. Although thrombolytic therapy may lyse clots more quickly than heparin for pulmonary embolism, the discussant believed that it was riskier, given the patient's recent surgery. This threshold approach can be applied explicitly, with numerical values for benefits, risks, and disease probabilities, as well as in the manner considered here.

This exercise in thresholds is relevant also to the issue of certainty in the diagnosis of pulmonary embolism. As in this case, many clinicians do not feel compelled to order a CT angiogram in every patient suspected of having a pulmonary embolus. When the suspicion on clinical grounds combined with noninvasive tests is sufficiently high, they treat. After all, it is the overall outcome that a clinician seeks to optimize, not the diagnostic certainty.

Finally, in this case we must be impressed with the discussant's confidence in his diagnostic acumen. He dismissed the normal respiratory rate, arguing that it probably was never actually measured (he was probably right), and he was ready to do battle with the radiologist about the scan interpretation. We presume that this behavior, enhanced by years of experience, is the essence of good clinical judgment.

CASE 46. WATCH AND WAIT, OR OPERATE?

> A 71-year-old woman was seen in consultation for hypercalcemia, which was initially discovered when routine chemistries were ordered during her first evaluation 1 year earlier. Since then, her serum calcium concentration had varied between 10.6 and 11.9 mg/dL (normal range, 8.8–10.4 mg/dL) and her serum phosphate concentration had varied from 2.6 to 3.7 mg/dL (normal range, 3.0–4.5 mg/dL). The history disclosed only untreated labile hypertension and fibrocystic disease of the breasts. She had no history of kidney stones or peptic ulcer disease. Although she reported no bone pain, she did complain of stiffness and pain in her knees, hips, elbows, and shoulders. She was taking no medications other than a nonsteroidal anti-inflammatory drug on an as-needed basis. Her blood pressure was 140/88 mm Hg. Joint findings were consistent with osteoarthritis. Other findings were normal.

We have here a fairly common situation of apparently asymptomatic hypercalcemia discovered during a routine evaluation. This biochemical abnormality had been present for a year in an elderly woman whose only complaints were joint stiffness and pain and whose only physical findings were consistent with osteoarthritis. Her serum phosphate varied between normal and slightly low values. In a woman this age, one of the common elements of the differential diagnosis would be use of a thiazide diuretic. I raise that possibility particularly because of the history of labile hypertension; however, we are told that she was not receiving such medication. Of course high on the list of causes of hypercalcemia would be primary hyperparathyroidism and malignancy-induced hypercalcemia; less likely would be sarcoidosis or other granulomatous disease, hyperthyroidism, hypervitaminosis D, and chronic lithium therapy. The negative history helps to differentiate among these disorders. The longer the hypercalcemia has been stable, the less likely it is to be malignancy induced. By contrast, stable hypercalcemia is common in patients with primary hyperparathyroidism. The constellation of the joint findings and the slightly high serum calcium concentrations would make one wonder about pseudogout, which may also occurs in patients with primary hyperparathyroidism. Without further information, however, I would guess that the joint manifestations and the hypercalcemia are unrelated. The key test in this patient is measurement of serum parathyroid hormone. The results of serum protein electrophoresis and measurements of serum 25-(OH)-vitamin D and alkaline phosphatase would also be of interest.

> **Laboratory findings: hemoglobin and white cell count, normal. Urinalysis: specific gravity 1.013, no protein, rare granular cast. Serum calcium 10.6 mg/dL, phosphate 3.2 mg/dL, alkaline phosphatase 119 IU/L (normal range, 40–100 IU/L), parathyroid hormone 72 pg/mL (normal range 10–65 pg/mL), creatinine 0.8 mg/dL, electrolytes normal. Serum and urine electrophoresis, normal. ECG, normal. Repeat serum calcium 11.3 mg/dL, phosphate 3.5 mg/dL, parathyroid hormone 74 pg/mL. Her urinary calcium excretion was 365 mg/day (normal range, 100–300 mg/day). Bone densitometry reveals T scores of –0.5 to –0.9 in the spine and several regions of the hip; the score for the total hip is –0.7.**

These biochemical findings establish the diagnosis of primary hyperparathyroidism to my satisfaction. In favor of this diagnosis are her mild chronic hypercalcemia, intermittent hypophosphatemia, and slightly high serum parathyroid hormone concentrations. Keep in mind that patients with hypercalcemia of any other cause have low serum parathyroid hormone concentrations. But first, I want to digress to consider—principally, to exclude—a diagnosis of malignancy-induced hypercalcemia. The malignancy that most regularly causes hypercalcemia is multiple myeloma, and the normal serum and urinary electrophoreses exclude that diagnosis. Other tumors, such as non–small-cell lung cancers and breast cancers, secrete parathyroid hormone–related protein, which has similarities to parathyroid hormone but is not measured in parathyroid hormone assays. Parathyroid hormone–related protein can be measured, but I see no reason to do that in this case.

Given the long history and the other negative findings, I believe that the case for primary hyperparathyroidism in this woman is convincing. It is, of course, usually caused by a parathyroid adenoma. In passing, one should consider whether she might be a member of a family with multiple endocrine neoplasia type 1 because patients with hyperparathyroidism in these families tend to have parathyroid hyperplasia rather than a parathyroid adenoma.

To decide whether she should be referred for parathyroid exploration, two issues must be considered: Does she have any complications of the primary hyperparathyroidism? We already know that she does not have kidney stones or compromised renal function as a consequence of nephrocalcinosis or chronic hypercalcemia. Her urinary excretion of calcium is consistent with hyperparathyroidism, and her bone density study is unremarkable. So what should be done with an asymptomatic patient with primary hyperparathyroidism and with mild hypercalcemia? Clear indications for surgery are bone disease (which she does not have), renal impairment (for which there is no evidence), and moderate or severe hypercalcemia, usually defined as serum calcium concentrations greater than 1.0 to 1.6 mg/dL above the upper limit of the normal range.[233] She does not have this either. Among patients with lesser elevations, progression in any way—more severe hypercalcemia, onset of nephrolithiasis, decrease in bone density—is unusual.[234]

What to do in this situation is controversial. Administration of estrogen or raloxifene can lower serum calcium concentrations by about 0.5 mg/dL. Cinacalcet, which directly inhibits parathyroid hormone secretion, lowers serum calcium concentrations by about 1.0 mg/dL, has side effects, and is not approved for treatment of primary hyperparathyroidism. Treatment with bisphosphonates raises bone density in patients with primary hyperparathyroidism, as it does in other patients, but has little effect on hypercalcemia. Whether one should recommend parathyroid surgery at this stage is debatable. There is controversy about whether patients with so-called nonspecific symptoms of hypercalcemia such as fatigue, weakness, and depression improve in response to restoration of normocalcemia. I suppose her joint and muscle aches might improve, but that outcome seems unlikely, and she will probably remain stable and never have any complications. On the other hand, she is basically healthy now, but if in 5 years she develops symptomatic hypercalcemia, she may then have other medical problems that would make her a poor surgical candidate. For now, I would not recommend surgery. I would urge her to maintain a high fluid intake because the most frequent serious threat is dehydration, but I would not restrict dietary calcium.

> **Follow-up: The patient was followed for 6 years. At age 77 years, when last seen, she continued to be in good health. She had a cystocele, which was repaired uneventfully 1 year earlier. Her serum calcium has varied between 10.7 and 11.6 mg/dL, and her renal function is normal. Repeat bone densitometry on two occasion during follow-up revealed very small decreases in T score; she does not yet have osteopenia, much less osteoporosis.**

I am not surprised and am a little relieved, and I would continue to follow her.

Analysis

This case illustrates the didactic value of assessing clinical material prospectively, and it underscores the problem of trying to be objective about the process of clinical decision making when the outcome is already known. The discussant evaluating the clinical data in this case quickly made a diagnosis and then struggled with the principal dilemma: whether to recommend parathyroid exploration for what is almost certainly a parathyroid adenoma. Before he knew that the patient did well for the next 6 years, the choice was not an easy one. If the follow-up data had been available before he expressed his opinion, there is some chance that the favorable outcome might have biased his viewpoint.[144] The problem of retrospective bias affects discussants at clinicopathologic conferences in which the patient's entire clinical course is presented before the discussion is held. The advantage of the format in this exercise is that the discussant has no advance information.

Why is the decision so difficult in this case? Primarily because there are competing risks. The discussant reasons that because the patient was 71 years old when the initial recommendation for or against surgery was required, she might never have complications of hyperparathyroidism and would

probably die of some unrelated disorder. If that course is the most likely one, why put her through unnecessary surgery? He is not explicit about the negative aspects of such surgery, but he is undoubtedly aware that they include short- or long-term hypocalcemia, vocal cord paralysis, and cardiovascular complications—not to mention the morbidity associated with neck surgery. Against those factors, he weighs the risks the patient will face if either the hyperparathyroidism or the hypercalcemia does cause serious complications such as severe hypercalcemia, nephrolithiasis, osteoporosis, and fracture at a time when the operative risk may be prohibitive.

The decision is difficult for two reasons: First, each choice may have negative sequelae, some of them quite onerous. Yet the probability of each is very small. Second, the value (in decision-analysis terminology, the expected utility) of the two choices is nearly the same. In other words, there may be no difference in average overall outcome; the choice may be a toss-up.[60]

The uneasiness with which the discussant made this choice is well illustrated by his expression of relief when he learns that the outcome was good. It should be emphasized that the favorable outcome in this case does not prove that the decision to follow the patient was a good one. Such a conclusion can be drawn only after careful analysis of data from studies of large groups of comparable patients. Few such studies are available, but those that are available do not reveal much benefit of surgery in patients with mild primary hyperparathyroidism, and little progression in those who are not operated on. The choice in this exercise was, however, a thoughtful one, and its rationale was carefully explicated.

CASE 47. AN APPLE OR AN ORANGE?

> **A 50-year-old woman with insulin-dependent diabetes mellitus of 16 years' duration was admitted for repair of a displaced right ankle fracture. Because of this admission electrocardiogram (Figure 18.2) a medical consultant was asked for "preoperative clearance."**

The fact that this patient is diabetic puts her at increased risk of a variety of problems,

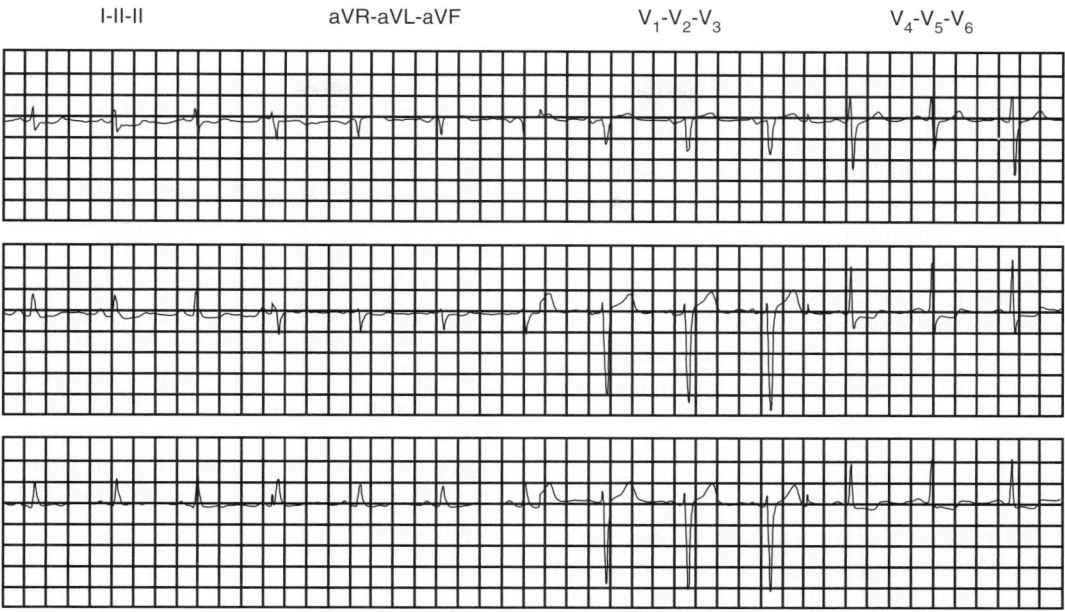

I-II-II   aVR-aVL-aVF   V₁-V₂-V₃   V₄-V₅-V₆

Figure 18.2 • Electrocardiogram; case 47.

including coronary artery disease. The electrocardiogram demonstrates normal sinus rhythm. Some repolarization changes represent the most striking abnormality. There is ST-segment and J-point depression in leads V_5 and V_6. I do not think these electrocardiographic changes are "nonspecific." Rather, they may well be consistent with ischemic changes. The fact that the T waves are still upright and the ST segment is both depressed and downsloping is worrisome. A preoperative electrocardiogram is done to screen for cardiac disease. We must say that the screening test is positive in this case, and now we have to look at the patient in more detail and see what is going on.

The patient had fractured her ankle 1 month earlier. Since then she had put weight on her foot and had subluxed her talus. In the last month, the patient had no cardiac symptoms. The ST- and T-wave changes on her current electrocardiogram were more pronounced than those on an electrocardiogram 1 month earlier. The patient had an episode of pulmonary edema in 1982, thought to be secondary to a non–Q-wave myocardial infarction. She had no previous history of angina. Six months be-

fore admission an echocardiogram revealed a 48% ejection fraction with inferoposterior hypokinesis and mild mitral regurgitation. The patient was obese and had a history of mild hypertension.

We now know that this obese, hypertensive, insulin-dependent diabetic woman has a previous history of ischemic heart disease. A recent cardiac evaluation revealed mild ventricular dysfunction and mitral regurgitation, perhaps secondary to papillary muscle dysfunction. The fact that her ST-segment abnormalities were more marked than in her previous tracing raises the question of an acute event, whether it is an infarct or only active ischemia. I do not think she had a non–Q-wave infarction because in that circumstance I would expect to see persistent T-wave inversions or changes. The current electrocardiogram is more consistent with ongoing ischemia, with the persistent J-point and ST-segment depression. Because the patient is diabetic, she could have an autonomic or sensory neuropathy and may be having silent ischemia, which is a difficult problem to manage.

We need to weigh the urgency of surgery versus further workup and evaluation of the patient's cardiac stability. I would play a waiting game. As far as I can see, there is little urgency for immediate ankle surgery. First, I would measure some cardiac enzymes and obtain serial electrocardiograms to see if any further cardiac problems were developing—although clearly, if an event happened during the last month, it is unlikely that we would catch anything by measuring enzymes. The likelihood that we would find evolving electrocardiographic changes is also small. The decision would be easy if we did because that would convince me that the risk of proceeding with surgery was too high. I am stalling because I am not quite sure what to do. I do know that the more I stall, the safer it is for the patient, from a cardiac point of view.

> The possibility of a silent non–Q-wave myocardial infarction sustained over the preceding month was raised, and the patient was transferred to the medical service for further evaluation. The orthopedic surgeon stressed the importance of early surgical repair of her ankle if she was to regain adequate function.

I would discuss the timing of surgery with the orthopedic surgeon. I need to know quantitatively the likelihood that her leg function will decline as a result of delaying surgery. Just saying that it will decrease is not enough. The question is: If we delay surgery 2 or 3 weeks, does the chance of a good functional result in this patient fall from 90% to 10%? If I am going to give an optimal preoperative evaluation, the orthopedist and I will have to balance the risk of a bad functional result in the leg against the chance that she will get into significant trouble. What trouble could she get into? If she has had a myocardial infarction recently or if she has active ischemia, there is a markedly increased risk that she will have another infarction or ischemic event during an operation. The more recently an infarct has occurred, the greater is the risk. If surgery is needed, how can we minimize the operative risk? I would explore whether surgery can be done under local as opposed to general anesthesia. I would try to do the least-risky operation.

I also would ask the patient how she felt about the possible functional loss in the face of an increased operative risk. She is not going to lose her foot. How important is some stiffness in her ankle, when compared with taking what might be substantial cardiac risks? If she were my patient, I certainly would include her in the decision-making process.

> Cardiac enzyme determinations revealed no evidence of acute infarction. The ST and T waves returned to their original configuration. Repair of the foot under regional anesthesia was accomplished uneventfully. The patient's internist, concerned about the possibility of silent myocardial ischemia, ordered a dipyridamole nuclear scan. The scan revealed a fixed inferolateral wall defect, mild left ventricular dilation, and partial redistribution of flow to the lateral wall. Consultation regarding cardiac catheterization was requested.

I did not think she had a recent infarction, and I still do not. She most likely had active ischemia, which quieted down after admission. The possibility of silent ischemia is a real one in this diabetic woman, as I mentioned before. A dipyridamole thallium scan really is no different from an exercise stress test. The patient cannot exercise, so instead of using the stress of exercise, one uses dipyridamole to maximize blood flow and reveal ischemic areas. The scan revealed a fixed inferoposterior wall defect that corresponded to the area of hypokinesis on the echocardiogram. The important finding is the partial redistribution of flow to the lateral wall. The lateral wall matches the area of the changes on the electrocardiogram, so now our suspicion of ischemia appears confirmed.

The question is whether cardiac catheterization should be performed. I think so. She is a relatively young diabetic with known coronary artery disease. I am concerned about the possibility of multivessel disease and would want to look into it further.

> A consultant felt that it was highly unlikely that the patient had a life-threatening (i.e., left main) lesion and recommended medical management. The patient was transferred to a rehabilitation facility.

I am not sure I totally agree with the consultant. The consultant seems to be satisfied with medical treatment because the patient has no angina. But this woman is a diabetic who may have a defective warning system and thus may be experiencing silent ischemia. I get a little nervous with such patients because I cannot use their symptoms to monitor disease activity.

Although the defect on the thallium scan was on the lateral wall, I do not think that excluded a problem with the anterior wall circulation, as would be seen with a left main lesion. I do not think that the sensitivity and specificity of the dipyridamole thallium scan are sufficiently high to confidently exclude left main disease.

Furthermore, this patient has at least two-vessel disease. The old inferior myocardial infarction probably represents disease in the right coronary artery, and the lateral wall defect seen on the thallium scan implies disease in the circumflex artery. If we factor in her diminished ejection fraction and mitral regurgitation, I am not sure that I would not consider surgery or angioplasty. I would need to look very closely at the data. My approach would be influenced by my opinion that coronary surgery is an extraordinarily good operation, and as much as I hate to admit it in light of the economics, I tend to be very aggressive in my approach to patients like this.

Analysis

There is an old adage that one cannot compare apples and oranges. Where this notion originated we do not know, but in our view, it is a fatuous concept. In everyday life, we frequently find it necessary to make difficult choices between disparate items. So, too, in medicine, and the problem presented by the patient here is a classic example. Her ankle requires surgical repair to prevent a significant long-term disability. The orthopedist would have proceeded immediately to fix the ankle, but on admission, she was found to have an abnormal electrocardiogram, which probably represented at least acute ischemic heart disease and at most an acute myocardial infarction. If we wait to fix her ankle, there is some chance that she will not regain full function. If we operate immediately, there is some chance that she will have some serious complication of ischemic heart disease. Here we *must* compare apples and oranges. We must balance long-term disability in one foot against the short-term risk of a life-threatening cardiac complication. The choice

is complicated principally because we do not have all the facts, but from the remarks of the discussant, we can identify the facts that we would need to make an informed recommendation.

First, we need to know several things about the disability. How severe is it likely to be? What is the effect of waiting? Will the disability increase as a result of the delay in surgery? If so, will the disability be severe or only minor? That information would be obtained from an expert—the orthopedist. Finally, how does the patient feel about having a permanent disability? After all, it is she who must live with it. How much is she willing to risk for a good ankle?

Second, several issues have to be weighed with respect to the cardiac risk. Has she had an acute myocardial infarction or only an acute ischemic event? Does it matter which she has had in terms of the cardiac risk? How high is that risk, and what exactly are the serious consequences? If one of the serious consequences does ensue, how likely is the patient to die? Is there any risk of permanent disability from cardiac disease if she sustains a perioperative acute myocardial infarction? Is she prepared to accept possible lameness for the rest of her life to avoid a one-time, short-term risk even if the risk is small?

Clearly, we would have to ask those questions if we were to carry out a formal analysis of the problem by means of a quantitative method, such as decision analysis. Each event would have to be described in terms of its probability and its utility (value). The short-term events would be rather easy to define because the principal worry is death, an anchor point in many decision analyses. Long-term disability can also be expressed in numerical terms as an adjustment to the quality of a patient's life, with input from the patient.[235] The principal issues are as follows: on the one hand, an uncertain chance of chronic disability with an uncertain severity of disability; on the other, an uncertain chance of a serious cardiac event with an uncertain severity of a complication. How both the physician and the patient view the risks and consequences of each of the outcomes should determine which choice is made. In the patient discussed here, the procedure ultimately was carried out under local anesthesia, and we can assume that the physicians responsible for her care thought that the risk could be minimized by doing so. Thus, they found a way of avoiding the more difficult choice between a long-term quality-of-life issue and a short-term disastrous consequence.

Finally, we appreciate that we have avoided discussing the issue of cardiac catheterization. The omission was not accidental. We did not have a full explanation of the consultant's opinion to withhold catheterization, so we were unable to compare the arguments pro and con. Even if we had all the facts, we may have come to an impasse. Experienced cardiologists have vastly differing views about how to proceed in the same patient. We explored some of the reasons for this disagreement in another discussion (see case 25).

CASE 48. A DIFFICULT TRADEOFF

After spending more than 8 hours on an airplane, a 75-year-old physician with a passion for rock climbing had a pulmonary embolism. He did well with anticoagulation, although he noted some residual shortness of breath with exertion. His evaluation for possible clotting abnormalities was negative. His physician recommended that he continue to take anticoagulants indefinitely. Because of his rock-climbing avocation, however, the patient preferred not to. An analysis of the data defining the benefits and risks of long-term anticoagulants was made.

Analysis

The analysis of the seemingly simple choice—long-term anticoagulation or not—is not so simple. It involves assessing whether the pulmonary embolism can be attributed to a prolonged flight, determining the optimal anticoagulation regimen for such an embolism, finding data on the risks of long-term anticoagulation, adding in the patient's preferences for possible outcomes, and, finally, making a recommendation after weighing all of these factors.

First, we examine pulmonary embolism related to air travel. Whether prolonged travel increases the risk of venous thromboembolism remains controversial.[236] Some studies suggest that the risk is increased, others found no increase, and one review found increased risk only when travel exceeded 10 hours. In eight prospective studies of flights exceeding 4 hours, asymptomatic deep venous thrombosis was found in 2.2% of 3,051 fliers. The rate was 1.4% in the 2,056 travelers with no risk factors and 4.0% in 995 fliers with predispositions such as prior thromboembolism, recent surgery or trauma, cancer, estrogen use, older age, obesity, and thrombophilia.[236] The World Health Organization Research Into Global Hazards of Travel (WRIGHT) project on air travel and venous thromboembolism confirmed this finding from eight prospective trials: For healthy travelers, the risk of venous thromboembolism for flights greater than 4 hours was 1 in 6,000, but it increased with longer travel duration and multiple

flights within a short period.[237] The WRIGHT findings are based on epidemiologic studies including a population-based case–control study, a retrospective cohort study among employees of international organizations, and a retrospective cohort study among professional pilots.

More data are available. In a systematic review of 25 randomized, controlled trials and cohort studies, the risk of symptomatic venous thromboembolism was 27 per 1 million travelers.[238] Logistic regression analysis identified the following risk factors: mean duration of air travel less than 6 hours (odds ratio [OR] 0.01) or greater than 8 hours (OR 2.3), prior deep venous thrombosis, hereditary hypercoagulable disorder, body weight less than 90 kg, limited mobility, and cancer or large varicose vein (OR 3.6). From these data, it is reasonable to conclude that even normal people can develop thromboembolism after plane flights, but usually after long flights, and that the patient's age, multiple consecutive flights, and flight duration may have enhanced his chance of developing one.

Next, we examine the evidence of efficacy of long-term anticoagulation after pulmonary embolism. First, here are recommendations from guidelines. The Seventh American College of Chest Physicians Conference on Antithrombotic and Thrombolytic Therapy recommended that all patients with a first episode of pulmonary embolism from a transient or reversible risk factor should receive anticoagulants, specifically a vitamin K antagonist, for at least 3 months.[239] However, if the cause cannot be identified, then long-term anticoagulation should be considered for those with achievable monitoring and no risk factors for bleeding. Both of these are strong recommendations based on clear benefit from randomized, controlled trials that did not have important design limitations. This guideline also states "that patients with first-episode idiopathic pulmonary embolism be considered for indefinite anticoagulant therapy." This recommendation was an "intermediate strength" recommendation, in which the best action may depend on circumstances or patient or societal values. In a 2008 guideline, "intermediate strength" was eliminated.[240]

There are few randomized, controlled trials of long-term anticoagulation of only patients with pulmonary embolism. The first task is to categorize our patient's embolism so we can compare his condition to those in published studies. In one trial of extended anticoagulation beyond 3 months after the first episode of venous thromboembolism, venous thromboembolism was defined as idiopathic in the absence of a lower limb fracture, bed confinement for more than 3 days, general anesthesia, and a hereditary hypercoagulable condition or malignancy.[241] In another study of extended anticoagulation after a first pulmonary embolus, a risk factor was defined as immobilization for more than 7 days.[242] Thus, because exclusion criteria in these studies would have required immobilization for 3 to 7 days as opposed to a long plane ride, this patient's pulmonary embolus could be classified as idiopathic. (Note, however, that these studies were not limited to only patients with pulmonary embolus.) Nonetheless, if we accept an "idiopathic" classification for our patient, then based on these randomized trials, the likelihood of recurrent venous thromboembolism would be 4% to 27% per patient-year untreated versus 1% to 3% per patient-year among those treated with a vitamin K antagonist.[241–243] Among patients with untreated proximal deep venous thrombosis, about 50% experience clinically detected pulmonary embolism. Finally, the death rate from pulmonary embolism is high: In the only randomized trial comparing anticoagulation with no treatment, mortality without treatment was 26%,[244] with no embolism-related mortality in the treated group. We conclude from this analysis that the patient does not fit the profile of patients in these studies precisely, but it is safe to conclude that anticoagulants, if taken long term, have a good chance of protecting the patient against recurrent embolism.

Of course, the analysis is incomplete without an assessment of the risks of the proposed therapy itself. Two studies show that physicians have difficulty estimating the long-term risk of bleeding during outpatient anticoagulant therapy.[236] Estimates of long-term bleeding risk typically arise from observational studies in cohorts of patients on anticoagulants. These patients differ from patients fulfilling enrollment criteria in randomized trials, which typically restrict inclusion to those at low risk for bleeding.

Mathematical models based on preliminary studies have identified risk factors that are associated with an increased risk of bleeding. In one such study, risk factors were increasing age, gastrointestinal bleeding, a serious comorbid condition, and past or present stroke or transient ischemic attack. Based on this one model, the patient would have a 3.6% annual bleeding risk.[245] Another preliminary study identified hypertension, cerebrovascular disease, ischemic stroke, heart disease, and renal insufficiency as risks for bleeding. At present, these studies cannot be used for solid predictions, at least not until validated, that is, until they are applied to other patient populations and found to yield accurate predictions. However, two validated models have identified risk factors for anticoagulant-related bleeding as age greater than or equal to 65 years, female sex, a history of gastrointestinal bleeding, a history of stroke, and recent myocardial infarction, renal insufficiency, severe anemia, diabetes mellitus, and coexisting malignancy. The likelihood and consequences of a major bleeding episode vary among studies and depend in part on the indication for the anticoagulation (whether for prosthetic heart valve, atrial fibrillation, ischemic heart disease, or venous thromboembolism). In a systematic review of 33 studies, major bleeding had a fatality rate of 13%. The death rate was 46% for those with intracranial bleeding and 10% for those with extracranial bleeding.[246] In another study, the mortality from intracranial bleeding was 26% in patients who were not anticoagulated versus 52% in those who were.[247] From these data, we conclude (mostly based on our patient's age) that he faces an increased risk of bleeding from anticoagulant therapy, and if a major bleeding episode occurred, it could lead to an extremely serious outcome.

Given the patient's high level of intellectual and physical function, he said he equated anticoagulation-related intracranial bleeding leading to a long-term disability as being equivalent to being dead.

A final task is to incorporate this information into a recommendation, making certain not only that the patient's preferences are taken into account, but also that the patient understands the elements of the decision and makes his own choice. First, the guideline recommendation for indefinite anticoagulation after idiopathic pulmonary embolism was of intermediate strength, according to which the optimal choice depends on circumstances, patient values, or societal values. The guideline recommendation explicitly states that it is based on placing a relatively high value on preventing recurrent thromboembolic events and a relatively low value on bleeding and cost. Any decision, however, must consider a substantial element of personal choice or values.[193,248,249] Hence, the patient's preference to avoid disability and death from intracranial hemorrhage and his passion for rock climbing must be weighed in the clinical decision on whether to continue anticoagulation for a prolonged period. Finally, the patient must make that choice in partnership with the physician, ideally through shared decision making.[250-253]

As in case 30, a formal decision analysis was performed at the Tufts Medical Center to help the patient make the difficult choice of taking long-term anticoagulants or not (the analysis is not shown here). In addition to the intermediate-strength recommendation from the guideline and the significance of patient preferences, the analysis extrapolated the randomized, controlled trial data that had at most 4 years of follow-up to a lifetime. The analysis also allowed for switching from no therapy to anticoagulation (and vice versa), depending on the therapeutic strategy selected in the event of a thromboembolic or serious bleeding event.

By quantifying the patient's preferences and explicitly incorporating the probabilities of harms and benefits as described previously, the result supported lifelong anticoagulation as the optimal choice. Based on the decision analysis, the patient opted for long-term anticoagulation. His comment on his involvement in the decision analysis was, "For me, it helped greatly in accepting a major life long (hopefully long lifelong) therapeutic decision." In follow-up 1 year later, he had had no more embolic events and no bleeding and was planning to participate soon in slab climbing rather than face climbing.

CASE 49. MAKING JUDGMENTS WHEN THE EVIDENCE IS NOT DEFINITIVE

A 57-year-old white man presented with a 6- to 12-month history of progressive lower urinary tract symptoms with poor force of stream and nocturia. He had a history of angioplasty and stent placement of his left anterior descending (LAD) artery. His prostate was large (40 g), smooth, and symmetric with no nodules. His prostate-specific antigen (PSA) was 5.7 ng/mL (previous PSA readings had been between 4.1 and 5.1 ng/mL). A prostate biopsy was recommended, although the urologist thought his mildly elevated PSA could be secondary to benign prostatic hypertrophy (BPH).

His biopsy revealed a small amount of carcinoma. One of 14 cores contained carcinoma with a Gleason score of 6. The therapeutic options were discussed with the patient. Given his relatively young age and good health, the urologist recommended a radical prostatectomy. The urologist was concerned that the sensitivity of the biopsies might be limited by the patient's large prostate. He also felt that in view of the patient's prostate enlargement, a seed implant would not be feasible. The urologist acknowledged that surveillance was an option, but he did not have hard data to make that recommendation.

The patient and his wife discussed the options and did their own research. The patient decided that he wanted to wait and not undergo surgery. A big factor in his decision was his concern about the risk of loss of sexual function with surgery. The urologist accepted the patient's preference. The plan was to check his PSA every 4 to 6 months and repeat a biopsy in a year or so to reevaluate the histology. He was treated medically for his symptoms of BPH.

Over the next 3 years, his PSA stayed in the 4 to 6 range. He had two subsequent biopsies, both of which were identical to the original, with a small focus of carcinoma in 1 of 14 samples with a Gleason score of 6. The patient opted for continued surveillance.

This patient faced a challenging decision about management of clinically localized prostate cancer, diagnosed as a result of PSA testing. He was not alone; in the United States, widespread PSA testing has almost doubled the risk a man will have to deal with a prostate cancer diagnosis over his lifetime.[254]

Favorable prognostic factors known at baseline included a relatively low PSA level of 5.7 ng/mL; an apparently slow PSA rate of rise based on the previous values; a nonsuspicious digital rectal examination, making the clinical stage T1c; only 1 of 14 cores positive on the initial biopsy; and a Gleason sum of 6, for practical purposes the lowest value assigned by modern pathologists. On the other hand, at age 57 years, even with coronary artery disease status post revascularization, the patient probably still has a life expectancy of up to 20 years, over which even an indolent cancer might cause trouble.

It is ironic this man's prostate cancer was probably diagnosed through serendipity.[255] In all likelihood, the PSA was elevated not because of the cancer, but because of coexisting BPH, judging from his lower urinary tract symptoms and the enlarged prostate. In fact, his "PSA density," derived by dividing the PSA level by the prostate volume, was just under 0.15 ng/mL/g, more consistent with BPH than cancer.[256] However, as the prevalence of underlying histologic prostate cancer is at least 30% among men in their 50s, a biopsy done for a PSA elevation driven by BPH has a good chance of diagnosing a prostate cancer too small to be responsible for the PSA elevation.

Men with clinically localized prostate cancer like this one face a bewildering choice of management options, including radical prostatectomy (using an open, laparoscopic, or robot-assisted technique), radiation therapy (external beam radiotherapy using a 3D [three-dimensional] conformal or intensity-modulated technique, brachytherapy, or proton beam therapy), and cryoablation.[257] Another option to consider, particularly for men with a favorable prognosis, is a strategy of expectant management referred to as "active surveillance."[258] With active surveillance, attempted curative therapy (and the possible side effects of these therapies) is deferred unless and until there is evidence that the cancer is progressing or less favorable prognostic features become evident. Unfortunately, there are no randomized trials comparing these management strategies among men with cancers detected through PSA screening. As the relative effectiveness of these strategies is uncertain and the side effect profiles vary, informed patients can reasonably make different decisions about their preferred option; that is, the optimal decision for a given patient is "preference sensitive."

Given this man's relatively long life expectancy, his urologist raised the concern that his cancer might be "a wolf in sheep's clothing." That is, since even modern extended-patterned biopsies only sample a small percentage of prostate tissue, perhaps he might have had more extensive or higher-grade cancer missed by the initial biopsy. In fact, up to half of Gleason 6 cancers may be upgraded when the entire specimen is examined after surgery.[259] For these reasons, active surveillance strategies include careful monitoring by digital rectal examinations and PSA measurements, as well as periodic repeated biopsies. The stable PSA level and similar results from two follow-up biopsies over the next 3 years provide reassurance that active surveillance remains a reasonable strategy for him.

What is the prognosis for men diagnosed with clinically localized prostate cancer who elect active surveillance? What is the likelihood their cancers will "escape from cure" despite close monitoring? Most prognostic data available for men with clinically localized cancers not initially treated come from the pre-PSA era. Even with these older data, the likelihood of dying of a Gleason 6 prostate cancer left untreated has been estimated at about 15% over 15 years.[260] However, when the effects of lead time and overdiagnosis attributable to PSA testing, as well as the upward "creep" in assignment of Gleason grades over time, are considered,[261,262] current models predict few if any prostate cancer deaths would occur among such men over 15 years.[263] However, predictive models cannot substitute for prospective outcome studies.

While many academic medical centers are now reporting series of prostate cancer patients on active surveillance,[264] few have adequate follow-up. In one of the most mature series from the University of Toronto, initiated in 1995, criteria for active surveillance (for men under 70 years old) included a PSA less than 10 ng/mL, Gleason sum of 6 or less, and stage T1c or T2a cancer. Criteria for delayed treatment have evolved to a PSA doubling time less than 3 years, progression to Gleason 7, or patient preference. PSA and DRE (digital rectal exam) are monitored every 3 months for 2 years and then every 6 months; repeat biopsies are performed at 1 year and then every 3 years. After a median follow-up of 5 years, about one third of patients have opted for active treatment; the 8-year actuarial prostate-cancer specific survival is estimated at 99.2%.[265]

This patient's urologist is to be congratulated for both respecting and actively supporting his choice of management.

> **Six years after his original diagnosis, he underwent a transurethral prostatic resection for progressive obstructive symptoms. All of the specimens from the operation were negative for tumor. His PSA levels fell below 1.0 ng/mL. Eight years from the original diagnosis, he continued to do well. His latest PSA was 0.67 ng/mL.**

Analysis: The dramatic response of the patient's PSA level to transurethral prostatectomy confirms the suspicion that BPH, rather than prostate cancer, was driving the PSA elevation. BPH starts in the peri-urethral transition zone of the prostate, and as the benign prostatic tissue coalesces and expands, it compresses the peripheral zones of the prostate, which are preferentially affected by prostate cancer, outwards against the prostate capsule. In this case, a small volume prostate cancer was probably left behind when the central benign prostatic tissue was resected; thus, the negative pathology report. The PSA value following transurethral resection can now serve as a baseline for further active surveillance of this man's prostate cancer, which certainly still seems like the preferred management strategy.

CASE 50. USING AND CITING PUBLISHED EVIDENCE

> **A 67-year-old woman was seen for a general medical evaluation. She had hypertension and non–insulin-dependent diabetes mellitus and was a smoker. Her review of systems was negative, with no neurologic symptoms. On physical examination, bilateral carotid bruits were heard and neurologic examination was normal.**

The approach to the patient with asymptomatic carotid bruits should be individualized. Certainly, this patient has many risk factors for atherosclerosis, including hypertension, diabetes, and cigarette smoking. Her carotid bruits are both a marker for generalized atherosclerosis and a specific indicator of stroke risk. The presence of the carotid bruits gives evidence of generalized involvement of her vascular system with atherosclerotic disease and should prompt an investigation to prevent the complications of that process. The most important investigations should focus on her coronaries and her carotids, but she may also have lower-extremity arterial disease and an aortic aneurysm.

Initial management includes risk factor analysis and control. Her diabetes, hypertension, and smoking should be assessed. In addition, a lipid profile should be obtained. Careful control of her hypertension, diabetes, cholesterol, and triglycerides is essential. If she is on oral hypoglycemic agents, some thought should be given to switching her to insulin to optimize control. Statin therapy will almost always be started, and, especially in diabetics, therapy targeted at reducing triglyceride levels is also important. She should be urged to quit smoking immediately, and adjunctive smoking cessation treatments should be offered. An electrocardiogram should be performed to look for evidence of prior myocardial infarction or ischemia or any myocardial conduction system damage. If she is not already on aspirin, it should be started, although the optimal dose is not clearly defined.

The specific qualities of the bruit may provide some clue as to its significance. The pitch of carotid bruits is important. Low-pitched bruits tend to be associated with less significant disease, while high-pitched bruits tend to be associated with more significant disease. The duration of the bruit is also important. Short bruits may represent transmitted heart sounds or external carotid lesions, while holosystolic bruits and bruits extending into diastole are often associated with more severe carotid disease. Also, the location of the bruit is important. Bruits that are loudest low in the neck often result from subclavian or common carotid origin pathology, whereas bruits loudest at the angle of the mandible tend to be associated with disease in the carotid bifurcation. A high-pitched bruit that extends throughout systole into diastole and is loudest at the angle of the mandible is generally associated with about 80% stenosis.

TABLE 19.1

Duplex Velocity and Waveform Criteria for Carotid Stenosis Determination

Stenosis (%)	PSV (cm/sec)	EDV (cm/sec)	Turbulence
<30	<120	Any	Minimal
30–50	<120	Any	Present
50–79	>120	<140	Present
80–99	>120	>140	Present

EDV, end diastolic velocity; PSV, peak systolic velocity.

The optimal study for evaluation of asymptomatic carotid disease is duplex ultrasound, performed in an accredited vascular laboratory. Duplex is noninvasive, readily available, and, when performed by experienced technicians, highly accurate and reproducible. There are standardized criteria for determining the severity of the carotid stenosis based on duplex-derived velocities and waveforms (Table 19.1).[266,267] In addition, duplex images yield important information regarding plaque morphology.

> **Noninvasive studies were performed. There was a 30% to 50% right internal carotid artery stenosis with ulceration and greater than 80% left internal carotid artery stenosis with ulceration and/or hemorrhage. The patient remained asymptomatic.**

Two large-scale prospective, randomized trials permit evidence-based decision making in this case.[268,269] Both the Asymptomatic Carotid Atherosclerosis Study (ACAS) and the Asymptomatic Carotid Surgery Trial (ACST) compared the results of medical management alone and medical management plus carotid endarterectomy (CEA) in patients with 60% or greater carotid stenosis. In both trials, surgery was shown to be beneficial, with approximately 50% relative stroke risk reduction at 5 years follow-up. In the ACAS, 834 medically managed patients had a 5-year stroke risk of 11%, while 825 patients undergoing surgery had a 5-year stroke risk of 5.1% ($P = .004$).[269] Similarly, in the ACST, 3,120 asymptomatic patients with 60% or greater carotid stenosis were randomized to medical management versus medical management plus CEA. After 5 years of follow-up, stroke or perioperative death had occurred in 6.42% (±0.70) of the CEA group and 11.78% (±1.0) of the medical management-alone group (absolute difference = 5.35%, 95% confidence interval [CI] = 2.96%–7.75%, $P < .0001$).[268] Based on these data, left carotid endarterectomy can be recommended to this patient with confidence.

The presence of ulceration and/or hemorrhage noted on duplex in the left carotid plaque is significant. In general, echo-dense or calcified plaques are more likely to remain stable and are less likely to be associated with symptoms. Echolucent plaques are those with intraplaque hemorrhage or large, lipid-debris-filled cores, and these tend to rupture with embolization, resulting in transient ischemic attacks or overt stroke. Plaque ulceration may result from prior plaque rupture, so such a finding in an asymptomatic patient is of uncertain significance. Still, the presence of plaque ulceration should be considered as an indicator of prior and potential future plaque instability and would be another factor favoring surgery in this patient.

Of course, the patient's operative risk must be taken into account prior to making a recommendation for surgery. Exclusion criteria in both the ACAS and the ACST included age greater than 79 years, significant heart, lung, kidney, or liver failure, any disease process anticipated to cause death within 5 years, or excessive operative risk (usually related to coronary disease). When considering the risk-to-benefit analysis for patients with asymptomatic carotid disease, the magnitude of the benefit associated with surgery should be considered. Even though the benefit is statistically significant in both ACAS and ACST, it is not large. In ACAS for example, the absolute risk reduction is 6%; the number treated to prevent a single stroke is, therefore, 16. Thus, patients should be selected carefully for surgery. In this patient population, especially in the presence of diabetes, preoperative risk stratification with radionuclide stress imaging seems prudent. Perioperative beta-blocker, aspirin, and statin therapy should be routine. Surgeon-related factors should also be considered. Surgeons in the ACAS and the ACST were selected for participation based on their past performance of carotid endarterectomy with very low (<2%) stroke and mortality rates. In current practice, combined perioperative stroke morbidity and all-cause mortality for endarterectomy in asymptomatic patients should be less than 3%.

More recently, carotid stenting has been suggested as an alternative to carotid endarterectomy, especially in patients at high surgical risk. One randomized trial comparing carotid endarterectomy and carotid stenting in patients at high risk for endarterectomy due to anatomic factors or medical comorbidities found that stenting was associated with a statistically significant reduction in the incidence of periprocedural stroke, MI (myocardial infarction), or death as a combined endpoint.[270] The differences in the incidences of individual endpoints failed to reach statistical significance. More than 70% of the high-risk patients in this trial were asymptomatic. The lack of a medical-treatment-only arm in this and other similar stenting trials makes their results difficult to interpret since many high-risk patients are probably best treated with medical therapy alone. At present, there are insufficient data to permit definition of a role for carotid stenting in asymptomatic carotid disease.

> She underwent an uncomplicated left carotid endarterectomy. Three years later, she has continued to do well with no neurologic events.

The long-term stroke risk in patients who have undergone carotid endarterectomy, that is, the stroke risk in the ipsilateral hemisphere, is approximately 1% per year. With current surgical techniques, the incidence of clinically relevant recurrent carotid stenosis should be less than 5%. The natural history of her right-sided carotid lesion is most often benign. In a patient with less than 50% contralateral stenosis, as in this case, the annual incidence of contralateral carotid-related symptoms is less than 5%, and the probability of progression to 75% stenosis (or more) over 5 years is 14%.[271,272] There is significant controversy as to the most appropriate follow-up for this patient. In our practice, we would get a follow-up duplex at 6 months and then every 2 years unless the disease progressed.

Analysis

In this instance, we departed from our usual practice of presenting the clinical material to a clinician, recording the discussant's "thinking aloud" utterances, and then transcribing and editing the discussant's remarks. Instead, we gave the material to an expert in carotid artery disease (a surgeon) and asked him to analyze the material as he would if he were the patient's physician. What emerges is an exercise in evidence-based medicine, as described in Chapter 8. The discussant begins his analysis by noting that he is undoubtedly not dealing with isolated carotid disease and notes that attention must be paid to other arteries, including efforts to stop the progression of disease with therapeutic interventions (cessation of smoking, use of statins). Then he launches into a detailed analysis of diagnostic issues, bringing evidence to bear on the patient's disorder.

His analysis, with data and references provided, examines data on the outcomes of two major clinical trials, and he compares the patient to the cohorts of patients in these trials. His decision includes a thoughtful risk/benefit analysis and a consideration of alternate approaches.

We suspect that he has internalized all the evidence to which he refers, and that on a day-to-day basis, he does not need to go through this detailed exercise. Nonetheless, having his decision process made explicit shows how even someone with lesser degrees of expertise could approach a similar problem.

CASE 51. A LITTLE MATH MAKES THE MEDICINE GO DOWN*

> A 44-year-old previously healthy man presented with a 3-week history of fatigue and temperatures as high as 38.2°C (100.8°F). The man was a medical resident at a municipal hospital.

Despite the long list of causes of fever and fatigue, I would be most worried about occupationally related illnesses, such as primary human immunodeficiency virus (HIV) infection and hepatitis in its prodromal phase.

*Originally published by Kopelman RI, Wong JB, Pauker SG. N Engl J Med 1999;341:435–439. For references see http://content.nejm.org/cgi/content/extract/341/6/435. Reprinted with permission of the Massachusetts Medical Society.

The fevers usually occurred at the end of the day and were associated with myalgias and chills. The patient began to take acetaminophen. He was seen at a local emergency room for epigastric pain, where a physical examination, a complete blood count, electrolyte levels, and radiographs of the kidneys, ureter, and bladder were all normal. In the previous week, he had noticed some shortness of breath when he was climbing stairs, a dry cough, and a single episode of night sweats. He had lost 2.7 kg in weight in the preceding 6 months. A review of organ systems was otherwise unremarkable.

At what time of year did this occur? Normally, body temperature peaks in the evening and is lowest in the early morning. Swings in body temperature tend to be a little wider in febrile states. Dyspnea suggests the possibility of viral pneumonia, but I am still focused on the occupational risk factors.

The patient grew up in India, where he had received bacille Calmette–Guérin (BCG) vaccine as a teenager. Twenty years earlier, he had had a positive skin test for tuberculosis with purified protein derivative (PPD). He had lived in Barbados, Jamaica, and the Bahamas before coming to the United States 3 years earlier. He had no recent history of travel or needle sticks. His clinical rotations over the last 9 months had been in municipal and Veterans Affairs hospitals. He did not recall caring for any patients with active tuberculosis, but had been exposed to varicella in the previous month. He smoked a half pack of cigarettes daily and was taking no medications other than acetaminophen.

Exposure to BCG vaccine can permanently affect the results of the PPD skin test, so a skin test might be useful at this point to determine whether the patient is anergic. Schistosomiasis and strongyloidiasis are endemic in the Caribbean. It is inconceivable to me that this man has not been exposed to tuberculosis, given his personal and professional history.

The patient appeared to be in good health. His vital signs and temperature were normal. Physical examination was unremarkable. Serum electrolyte, creatinine, and calcium levels were normal, as were liver function results and a complete blood count.

I continue to be concerned about the possibility of acute HIV infection and tuberculosis. Varicella is possible but unlikely in the absence of skin lesions. I would obtain a chest film, especially given the patient's occupational history. Varicella can cause a severe pneumonia, often associated with hemoptysis. In its wake, the findings on the chest film are almost pathognomonic, with very tiny (2 to 3 mm), densely calcified, perfectly round lesions that are too small to be anything but varicella.

A chest film showed numerous small nodules bilaterally in a miliary pattern. The right hilum, right paratracheal region, and aorticopulmonary window appeared slightly larger than they had 1 year earlier and were thought to reflect the presence of enlarged lymph nodes. An infectious disease consultant thought that the likelihood of tuberculosis was high.

I would test the patient for tuberculosis while the workup proceeds. The diagnostic yield of a sputum specimen from a patient with miliary tuberculosis is not as good as in patients with cavitary lesions. I would like to recheck the results of this patient's skin tests because a negative result could mean that anergy has developed. The PPD test is usually positive in patients with miliary tuberculosis, but in this patient, it could also be positive because of the BCG immunization. At this point, the likelihood of tuberculosis is roughly 70%. If this patient were in California, fungal diseases, such as coccidioidomycosis, would be higher on my list. I would dilate his pupils and search his optic fundi for granulomas, which, if present, would rule out the possibility of varicella.

The results of the PPD skin test were negative, with a positive reaction to control antigens. Bronchoscopy revealed mild to moderate bronchial inflammation; examination of bronchoalveolar-lavage fluid was negative for cancer. A transbronchial biopsy revealed compact, noncaseating granulomas with occasional giant cells, consistent with the presence of sarcoidosis. Staining for acid-fast bacilli and methenamine staining for fungi were negative.

Although noncaseating granulomas are compatible with the presence of sarcoidosis, they are also compatible with the presence of many other things. The negative acid-fast stain does not rule out tuberculosis. This man does not have anergy, and I would have expected his PPD skin test to be positive because he had received BCG vaccine. Tuberculosis can occur in people who have received BCG vaccine. I would still treat him for tuberculosis until the results of the culture become available. I would also seek additional evidence of sarcoidosis, such as skin lesions or abnormalities on slit-lamp examination of his eyes. A finding of noncaseating granulomas at another site would be helpful. Whether to begin treatment with corticosteroids is problematic without a more definitive diagnosis.

The angiotensin-converting-enzyme level was normal. Treatment with isoniazid, rifampin, pyrazinamide, and ethambutol was begun. The patient was advised not to return to work for 2 weeks. His wife was asked to undergo a PPD skin test and chest radiography.

The angiotensin-converting-enzyme level is neither specific nor sensitive enough to rule out sarcoidosis because it can be abnormal in any patient with a granulomatous process. I would still seek further evidence of sarcoidosis: I would check the patient's alkaline phosphatase level and examine his lacrimal and parotid glands. If his wife's chest film is also abnormal, the likelihood of tuberculosis would increase.

The patient continued to have fevers, and 2 weeks later, his shortness of breath became more severe. Cultures for mycobacteria remained negative. Treatment with 60 mg of prednisone per day was begun because of the possibility of sarcoidosis. Because the patient was not anergic and had potentially been exposed to tuberculosis in the past as a physician and in India, antituberculosis therapy was continued pending final culture results.

I am in thorough agreement with this approach. What does alarm me, however, is the patient's increasing dyspnea. He appears to be re-

ceiving adequate antituberculosis therapy, so the progressive symptoms could indicate a resistant strain of *Mycobacterium*. I would obtain another chest film.

The patient's symptoms improved markedly after 3 days of treatment with prednisone. After 6 weeks, the cultures for mycobacteria were still negative and the antituberculosis medications were discontinued. The working diagnosis was sarcoidosis.

The problem we often have when considering a diagnosis of sarcoidosis is how much evidence is enough. Is a finding of granulomatous tissue at only one site in a patient with a somewhat atypical clinical story enough? The patient clearly seems to have had a good response to the corticosteroid therapy. Fortunately, tuberculosis seems to be highly unlikely.

Analysis

Distinguishing between pulmonary sarcoidosis and pulmonary tuberculosis can be a challenge, even for experienced clinicians. The main effects of both diseases typically are in the lungs, in association with predominant symptoms of fever, malaise, anorexia, weight loss, and, depending on the degree of pulmonary involvement, dyspnea or cough. Both diseases can involve the same organ systems; both can produce granulomas, which may reveal neither caseation nor organisms on histological examination. Both can mimic a variety of diseases [1–4] (the reference numbers refer to those in the paper cited in the footnote giving the source of this case).

Although ordinarily a specific diagnosis is made before a treatment is chosen, we must often make therapeutic choices before the diagnosis has been established. As evidence becomes available, we interpret it, decide whether to gather more information, and choose whether or not to initiate treatment. As the clinical picture evolves, we constantly balance the benefits and risks of additional tests against those of immediate therapy. Some decisions involve determining whether one disease is sufficiently likely that the potential benefits of treatment outweigh the potential side effects and complications [5]. As was true in the case under discussion, other therapeutic decisions may be required when there are several diagnostic alternatives, when each has its own risks, and when the treatment used for one possibility could pose an additional risk to the patient if one of the other diagnoses is correct.

Both the clinicians caring for this physician and the discussant were strongly attracted to a diagnosis of tuberculosis. The basis for that belief may have been the possibility of an occupational exposure or the patient's history of travel, in conjunction with his symptoms and findings on the chest film. When the PPD skin test was found to be nonreactive, the angiotensin-converting-enzyme level was found to be normal, and noncaseating granulomas were identified on transbronchial lung biopsy, should the clinicians have abandoned the diagnosis of tuberculosis?

A simple Bayesian analysis offers some assistance. Let us assume that the patient had either tuberculosis or sarcoidosis. Table 19.2 summarizes the probability of each finding in the presence of tuberculosis and sarcoidosis, both individually and in combination. A Bayesian calculation (Table 19.3) shows that if the probability of tuberculosis on clinical grounds is 70% before the three results are known (a value suggested by the discussant), the revised, or posterior, probability of tuberculosis, which includes the information on the joint probability of all three findings, would still be quite high: 37%.

What does a posterior probability of tuberculosis of approximately 40% tell us about the advisability of treatment with antituberculosis agents or corticosteroids? Because neither tuberculosis nor sarcoidosis was an established diagnosis, the decision hinged on the tradeoffs with respect to the benefits and risks of both proposed treatments. The fact that miliary tuberculosis is life threatening argues strongly for the use of antituberculosis therapy, at least until the diagnosis can be ruled

---

TABLE 19.2

Probabilities of Various Findings in the Presence of Miliary Tuberculosis and Sarcoidosis

Finding	Probability of Finding with Miliary Tuberculosis (%)	Probability of Finding with Sarcoidosis (%)
Nonreactive PPD skin test[a]	25	95
Noncaseating granulomas[b]	20	100
Normal angiotensin-converting-enzyme level[c]	95	20
All three findings[d]	4.75	19

[a] The likelihood of a negative purified protein derivative (PPD) skin test in patients with miliary tuberculosis ranges from 10% to 62%, with an average of 25% [6–10]. About 10% of patients who receive bacille Calmette-Guérin vaccine become nonreactive to PPD after 10 years, and nearly all are nonreactive after 25 years [11]. Because sarcoidosis does not result in a positive reaction to PPD and because the patient in question had been vaccinated 30 years earlier, the likelihood of his being nonreactive to PPD is 95% if he has sarcoidosis.
[b] Approximately 20% of patients with miliary tuberculosis will have noncaseating granulomas without identifiable acid-fast bacilli [12]. Virtually all patients with sarcoidosis will have noncaseating granulomas on biopsy.
[c] Angiotensin-converting-enzyme levels are normal in 20% of patients with sarcoidosis, whereas the levels are normal in 95% of patients with tuberculosis [13].
[d] Each value is the product of three individual probabilities, assuming that each one is independent of the others.
From Kopelman RI, Wong JB, Pauker SG. A little math helps the medicine go down. *N Engl J Med* 1999;341:435–439. For references see http://content.nejm.org/cgi/content/extract/341/6/435. Reprinted with permission of the Massachusetts Medical Society.

TABLE 19.3

Calculation of Revised Probability of Tuberculosis in the Presence of Various Findings

Diagnosis	Initial Estimate of Probability Based on Clinical Grounds (%)	Joint Probability of All Three Findings for Each Diagnosis[a] (%)	Product of the Initial Estimate and the Joint Probability of All Three Findings	Revised Probability[b] (%)
Tuberculosis	70	4.75	332.5	37
Sarcoidosis	30	19	570	63
Total			902.5	

[a] Each value is the product of three individual probabilities, assuming that each one is independent of the others.
[b] The revised probability was calculated by dividing the product of the initial estimate and the joint probability of all three findings by the total.
From Kopelman RI, Wong JB, Pauker SG. A little math helps the medicine go down. *N Engl J Med* 1999;341:435–439. Reprinted with permission of the Massachusetts Medical Society.

out [1,6–10]. Although isoniazid-related hepatitis is not infrequent, in a young man who would be closely followed, there would only be a tiny chance of a fatal reaction within the relatively short period before culture results became available [14–16]. If the patient had tuberculosis, the balance between the benefits and risks would clearly favor the use of antituberculosis therapy; if the patient had sarcoidosis, treatment with isoniazid would expose him to unnecessary risks.

Somewhere between these two diagnostic certainties, there must be a probability of tuberculosis at which the benefits of treatment equal the risks. This level is called the therapeutic threshold [5]. For values above that threshold, antituberculosis treatment should be given, and for lower probabilities, treatment should be withheld. The threshold value depends on the benefit-to-risk ratio (B:R) for the treatment and, in fact, equals the quotient of the following expression [5]: $1 \div (B:R + 1)$.

How can one estimate the benefits and risks in order to determine the therapeutic threshold? Once again, we will assume that the patient has either tuberculosis or sarcoidosis. If we also assume that treated miliary tuberculosis has a mortality rate of 20%, as compared with a rate of 50% without treatment [1,6–10], then treatment is associated with an absolute benefit of 30% in terms of survival if a patient does have tuberculosis and receives appropriate treatment. Isoniazid-related hepatitis is the main risk of treatment. Although the risk of this complication is typically 1%, it is somewhat

higher in Asian men, perhaps 2%. Each patient in whom isoniazid-related hepatitis develops has a 7.6% risk of dying from that complication. Thus, the overall mortality rate among all Asian men who take isoniazid is 2% × 7.6%, or approximately 0.15% [15–17]. Patients who are treated for miliary tuberculosis but who actually have sarcoidosis would be exposed to this risk without any benefit. The benefit-to-risk ratio for treatment is therefore roughly 200 (30% ÷ 0.15%). Thus, the therapeutic threshold for antituberculosis therapy is 0.5%, or $1 \div (200 + 1)$. Working backward, we can see that as long as the clinical probability of tuberculosis (the probability before the findings of the nonreactive PPD skin test, the normal angiotensin-converting-enzyme level, and the noncaseating granulomas on biopsy have become known) exceeds 2%, administering antituberculosis therapy is appropriate.

The discussant estimated that the clinical probability of tuberculosis was 70%. Certainly, that value far exceeds the therapeutic threshold and is at a level at which therapy should provide a substantial benefit. Even after the results of the PPD skin test, the serum angiotensin-converting-enzyme level, and the bronchial biopsy became known, the probability of tuberculosis was almost 40%, a value that was still well above the very low therapeutic threshold. Viewed another way, if the probability of tuberculosis is 40%, a cohort of 10,000 similar men would include 4,000 with tuberculosis and 6,000 with sarcoidosis. Without antituberculosis therapy, only 2,000 of those with tuberculosis (50%) would survive. With antituberculosis therapy, 3,200 would survive (80%) but 5 would die of isoniazid-related hepatitis. On the other hand, among the 6,000 men with sarcoidosis, 9 would die of isoniazid-related hepatitis. For the cohort of 10,000 men as a whole, the use of antituberculosis therapy would improve survival by 1,186 men (1200−5−9). Of course, if there were additional benefits of antituberculosis therapy (e.g., if treatment also prevented the transmission of infection to others), the net benefit of therapy would be even greater, the benefit-to-risk ratio would be higher, and the therapeutic threshold would be even lower.

If the patient had tuberculosis but was treated with corticosteroids for presumed sarcoidosis in addition to antituberculosis drugs, what would have been the risk of disseminated tuberculosis? The risk of corticosteroid therapy in patients with pulmonary tuberculosis, especially miliary tuberculosis, is far lower than is generally believed. Studies extending over four decades emphasize the safety, if not the benefit, of corticosteroid therapy, as long as antituberculosis therapy is given concomitantly [17–20]. On the other hand, if the patient had sarcoidosis, would initially withholding corticosteroids have posed a risk as long as his condition remained stable? Aggressive treatment of patients with pulmonary sarcoidosis who have progressive respiratory symptoms decreases the extent of permanent end-organ damage [3,21]. The benefit-to-risk ratio for the use of corticosteroids in the presence of progressive dyspnea, such as occurred in the patient under discussion, would be high, and the therapeutic threshold would be rather low. On this basis, we might conclude that once progressive dyspnea developed and the probability of sarcoidosis exceeded 60% (Table 19.3), the clinicians did select a superior management strategy: They added corticosteroids to the antituberculosis-drug regimen until the results of mycobacterial cultures became known and the diagnosis of tuberculosis could be ruled out.

The key to approaching patients who are acutely ill and in whom the diagnosis remains uncertain is to think probabilistically. First, use the available information to estimate the likelihood of each disease. Once that is done, assess the potential benefits and risks of each proposed therapy quantitatively. Sometimes, rather than choose between two therapies, the best strategy may be to give both treatments and wait for more information, as was done in the case under discussion.

CASE 52. A REWARDING PURSUIT OF CERTAINTY*

A 53-year-old, previously healthy college professor was brought to the emergency room in status epilepticus. He had no history of seizures.

After giving intravenous medication to stop the seizures, I would obtain some medical and social history. Does the patient have hypertension or underlying vascular disease? Is he a drinker or a user of recreational drugs? These days we must always keep the possibility of human immunodeficiency virus (HIV) infection in mind.

Three weeks earlier he had seen his physician for new bifrontal headaches that were relieved with aspirin. His physical examination was normal at that time. On the day before his seizure, he awoke at 4 a.m. with a diffuse, piercing headache that was relieved with aspirin. He then felt well enough to work that day. In the emergency room, the patient's wife said that he had had neither constitutional symptoms nor difficulties with his gait, vision, or speech. He had no history of head trauma but had played touch football a few weeks earlier. Twenty years ago, he had undergone orchiectomy for what was said to be a benign lesion. He smoked one pack of cigarettes a day and had done so for 30 years; he drank socially. He took no medications. He had three children.

I would want to know whether the orchiectomy was performed because of an undescended testicle or a lesion in a descended testicle. If it was for an undescended testicle, the risk of cancer in the contralateral testicle is increased. Even at the patient's age, germ-cell tumors can present with

*Originally published by Pauker SG, Kopelman RI. *N Engl J Med* 1993;329:1103–1107. For references, see http://content.nejm.org/cgi/content/extract/329/15/1103. Reprinted with permission of the Massachusetts Medical Society.

central nervous system metastases. The fact that he has three children is of interest because 15% to 20% of men with testicular lesions are infertile before their diagnosis.

Aspirin helped his headache but could also cause an occult lesion to bleed, although there is no history of a stiff neck. He has had no symptoms suggesting a systemic illness, but the subacute history of headaches suggests a mass lesion, perhaps from an infectious or neoplastic process. Chronic meningitis due to an organism such as *Cryptococcus* seems less likely.

> **The seizures were controlled with diazepam, phenytoin, and phenobarbital. After they stopped, the patient's blood pressure was 140/70 mm Hg, his pulse rate was 70 per minute, and his respiratory rate was 12 per minute. He was afebrile. Physical examination was unremarkable except for a blurred nasal portion of the left optic disk, an absent left testicle, and moderate prostatic enlargement with no nodules. He was drowsy and had a decreased attention span. He responded to questions with one-word answers and did poorly on tests of comprehension, ability to name objects, and ability to repeat a list of items. He did not follow commands. The remainder of the neurologic examination showed no focal findings. The complete blood count, differential count, blood glucose and blood urea nitrogen (BUN) levels, and serum electrolyte, creatinine, calcium, magnesium, and alkaline phosphatase levels were all normal. The erythrocyte sedimentation rate, chest x-ray film, and results of urinalysis were normal. A stool guaiac test for occult blood was negative.**

At this point, the patient's altered mental state does not help me distinguish between a mass lesion and meningitis. His normal temperature argues against many infections, although a patient with a suppurative brain abscess could be afebrile, as could a patient with toxoplasmosis. The blurred optic disk raises the possibility of increased intracranial pressure. The rest of his physical findings are not helpful. His impaired sensorium could just represent a postictal state.

From an oncologic viewpoint, it would be unusual for a patient with disseminated cancer, especially one originating below the neck, to have all these normal laboratory values. Melanoma could present with a metastatic brain lesion without obvious evidence of a primary lesion. If he has a metastatic germ-cell tumor, the chest film should not be normal. Certainly, a primary tumor of the central nervous system is possible.

Because of the possibility of increased intracranial pressure, I would order a computed tomographic (CT) scan of his head before attempting a lumbar puncture.

> **CT scan of the head with contrast showed a well-defined 2-by 2-cm lesion in the left parietooccipital region. There was ring enhancement around a large area of attenuation (Figure 19.1). An additional 1-cm area of low attenuation without ring enhancement was seen in the left temporal lobe.**

He appears to have multifocal disease. The differential diagnosis includes a brain abscess

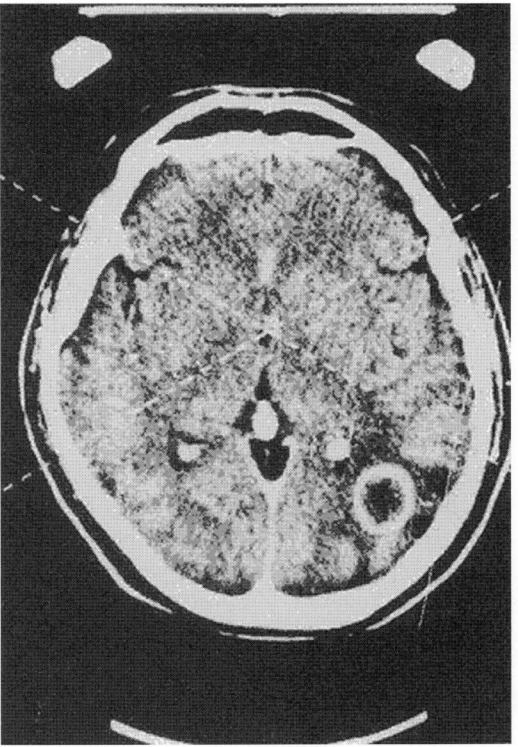

Figure 19.1 • Contrast-Enhanced CT Scan Demonstrating a 2-by-2-cm Lesion in the Left Parieto-Occipital Region. Case 52.

(either bacterial or perhaps resulting from *Toxoplasma* infection), lymphoma, and a glioma, which can be microscopically if not grossly multifocal. Ring enhancement suggests that there is an inflammatory component and excludes the possibility of causes such as a bland infarct. Even though the patient is afebrile, septic emboli are possible, but the normal blood count and sedimentation rate argue against that.

> **The patient was treated with dexamethasone. Over the next 24 hours, his mental status cleared and his neurologic results returned to normal. Magnetic resonance imaging (MRI) of the head was interpreted as strongly suggestive of a metastatic lesion in the left parietooccipital region and an old infarct in the left temporal region.**

The MRI suggests that he may not have multifocal disease. A search for a primary tumor may not be productive. I would draw an analogy to patients who have adenocarcinomas of unknown primary origin; there, the yield of such searches has been low. Because it would be nice to find a site other than the patient's brain to biopsy, I would look elsewhere for possible infectious or neoplastic causes, even though the yield is likely to be low.

I am uncertain why the MRI scan was interpreted as suggesting a neoplastic as opposed to an infectious cause. Although we have to be careful not to overinterpret radiologic studies, my experience has been that MRI is fairly good at distinguishing tumor from infection.

> **A chest CT scan was normal. An abdominal CT scan revealed a 1-cm cystic structure in the right lobe of the liver and a 1-cm cystic structure in the superior pole of the right kidney. A pelvic CT scan was normal. A bone scan showed mild uptake in the lower lumbar spine but no discrete abnormalities. The prostate-specific antigen level was 6 μg/L (normal range for men older than 40 years old is 0.5–4.0 μg/L).**

The prostate-specific antigen result is irrelevant. In the absence of bony lesions, the chance that a patient with prostate cancer has an isolated brain lesion is extremely low. I am still reluctant to label an isolated brain lesion as neoplastic without further proof. We still have to look for occult infection.

> **The patient felt well. A repeated CT scan showed resolution of the edema. Blood cultures were negative. Plans were made for a brain biopsy before beginning radiation therapy for the presumptive diagnosis of metastatic cancer from an unknown primary site.**

A tissue diagnosis is obviously necessary before radiation therapy is even considered in this man. However, infection has not been excluded. I would still like to know whether he has any risk factors for HIV infection and whether he has traveled recently. I neglected to ask earlier whether the patient had any dental work done before the onset of his recent symptoms. I raise this question because brain abscesses can originate from infections around the teeth.

> **Brain biopsy showed necrotic material but no tumor. Staining revealed long, filamentous branching rods that were gram positive. Until culture results became available, the patient was treated with penicillin and a sulfonamide.**

The results of Gram's staining raise the possibility of actinomycosis or nocardiosis. The initial antibiotic coverage seems appropriate.

> **Cultures were positive for *Actinomyces odontolyticus*. On further questioning, the patient recalled that he had had a tooth capped 3 months earlier. Although the patient had no pain in this tooth, the cap was removed and an apical abscess was found and drained. Those cultures were also positive for *A. odontolyticus*.**

A large percentage of primary brain abscesses are of dental origin. In retrospect, it is unclear whether the workup of this patient should have been different. Some clinicians might have proceeded to brain biopsy sooner and thereby reduced the duration of anguish of the patient and his family over the clinical assumption that the mass was cancer.

> **The patient received penicillin for 6 months. He had no further seizures and no residual neurologic deficits. Anticonvulsant medications were**

discontinued. At the end of his course of therapy, a CT scan showed only a small glial scar.

Analysis

Brain abscesses are uniformly fatal if not diagnosed [1,2] (the reference numbers refer to those in the paper cited in the footnote giving the source of this case). Over most of the last half century, the case fatality rate of brain abscess was fairly constant, approximately 30% to 50% [1–5], but in the last decade it has dropped sharply, to the range of 10% to 15% [2,3,5–10]. That improvement has been ascribed to the early diagnosis made possible by modern imaging studies, to early surgical intervention, and to improved antibiotic therapy [3,8]. The chief risk of brain abscess is that of an expanding intracranial mass, not of infection [1,2,4,6].

As was the case with this patient, most patients with brain abscesses have headache or lethargy [2,3,6], but fewer than half have fever, focal neurologic signs, signs of increased intracranial pressure, or altered mental status [2,3,6,9,11]. One third have seizures [2,3,6]. Ten percent of brain abscesses are caused by penetrating trauma to the skull, and 20% are cryptogenic, but fully half arise by contiguous spread from the sinuses, the mastoids, and the middle ear [1,3,7,10–12]. Of interest, the 20% that arise by hematogenous spread from a remote site are more insidious in their onset, and patients with such abscesses often present with seizures or status epilepticus [7]. A common source is dental infection, but lung abscesses, abdominal or pelvic infections, osteomyelitis, and occasionally endocarditis can also be the source [1,3,8,10–12]. Patients with right-to-left shunts caused by pulmonary arteriovenous fistulae or cyanotic congenital heart defects are particularly prone to brain abscesses, especially if the shunt is large enough to cause polycythemia [3,7,10,11]. Hematogenous abscesses often fall within the distribution of the middle cerebral artery and occur at the junction between the brain's white and gray matter, where capillary flow is slowest [3,7,13].

Streptococci, *Bacteroides*, and gram-negative species, such as *Proteus*, *Klebsiella*, and *Pseudomonas*, are most commonly cultured from brain abscesses, although staphylococci predominate when penetrating trauma is the cause [3,6–11].

One fifth of brain abscesses are sterile [3,6,7]. *Toxoplasma* is becoming a more common agent as the incidence of acquired immunodeficiency syndrome increases [6]. Actinomyces is an unusual cause of brain abscess but a common inhabitant of the oral cavity and a common cause of dental and craniofacial infections [14,15]. Actinomycotic brain abscesses can arise from either contiguous structures or hematogenous spread from remote sites [16–18], as was presumably the case here. Although craniofacial actinomycosis has been reported in association with HIV infection [19], its incidence does not appear to be consistently increased among immunocompromised patients [14].

The first priority in a patient with status epilepticus is to control the seizures [20], but the next order of business is to identify the cause. In adults, the majority of grand mal seizures are in patients with preexisting epilepsy [21,22]; the underlying cause is found in only one fourth of adults with new seizures [23,24]. The majority of the causes are relatively evenly distributed among vascular disease, trauma, tumors, and alcoholism [22]. Only a minority are caused by degenerative disease or infection [21,22]. The causes of a new seizure disorder depend strongly on the patient's age [23,24]. Among neonates, birth trauma and infections are common, but in early childhood, head trauma and idiopathic epilepsy are more likely. Among young adults, brain tumors and alcohol withdrawal are the predominant causes, only to be overshadowed by cerebrovascular disease in middle age and beyond.

Given the history of headache and a blurred optic disk but the absence of fever, meningismus, and laboratory signs of infection, the clinicians worried about the risk of herniation as a complication of lumbar puncture and first obtained a CT scan [1,4,8,12]. As shown in Figure 19.1, the scan revealed a parietal occipital lesion with radiologic signs of inflammation and edema. Brain abscesses commonly demonstrate a thin ring of enhanced uptake of contrast on CT scan, but thicker, more irregular rings can also be seen in patients with brain tumors [13,25], especially if an area of central necrosis is present. MRI is said to distinguish more clearly between abscesses and tumors, demonstrating a thin capsule pointing toward the ventricles in the latter [13], but findings can overlap. In one study that applied Bayes' rule to distinguishing among brain abscess, tumor, and vascular disease, the finding that discriminated best was the uniformity of thickness of the ring-enhancing capsule caused by brain abscesses [26]. In this patient, when the MRI scan was interpreted as strongly suggestive of metastatic disease, the clinicians at first appeared to foreclose other diagnostic possibilities. However, after a cursory search for bacteremia, they planned a brain biopsy. Their assumption was that they would find metastatic cancer and then proceed with radiation therapy.

Although the identification of *Actinomyces* on the brain biopsy was a surprise, the discussant had persisted in his concern about central nervous system infection all along. It is not clear why, because the history is certainly consistent with the possibility of another intracranial mass lesion, such as a tumor. Had this been a brain tumor presenting as status epilepticus, the prognosis would have been quite grim. With the possible exception of a germ-cell tumor [27], a cancer with two intracerebral metastases but no established primary lesion relegates almost any therapy to the realm of palliation. Perhaps that knowledge led the discussant to focus on the patient's orchiectomy. However, with his long history of tobacco use, the lung would certainly be the leading source of cancer in a man of this age.

In any case, before the clinicians abandoned further diagnostic studies and resigned themselves to treating a disease with as poor a prognosis as that of metastatic cancer, they wanted to be quite certain of their diagnosis. Foreclosing consideration of some diagnoses too soon is a common cognitive error known as premature closure [28]. In effect, clinicians are probably guided by what we might call a threshold of diagnostic abandonment. Only when the likelihood of the untreatable and presumably rapidly fatal disease is above that threshold do they feel comfortable resorting to palliative therapy. The threshold of diagnostic abandonment is analogous to a probability of disease known as the test-treatment threshold, above which empirical treatment is indicated [29]. If the benefit of identifying a treatable disease is large (as in the case of patients with a brain abscess), then the threshold of abandonment should be high, unless the risk of performing the test or the risk of delaying palliative therapy in the event of a false-positive result is very high. In most cases, these risks are small because a patient with a rapidly fatal disease has little to lose as compared with what a patient with a treatable disease has to gain.

A rough approximation can be made by comparing the potential net benefits and risks. This patient stood to gain roughly 20 years of survival with treatment if he had a brain abscess. (This net benefit of therapy is calculated by multiplying his normal life expectancy [24 years] by the likelihood of his surviving a brain biopsy [99%] and by the likelihood of his surviving with a treated brain abscess [85%].) His net risk is the loss of only 0.005 year if he has metastatic cancer. (This value is calculated by multiplying the average life expectancy for such patients [6 months] by the chance of dying from a brain biopsy [1%].) If brain biopsy can accurately identify a brain abscess, then the test-treatment threshold [29] can be calculated as $1 - (0.005/20)$, which means that if the chance of brain abscess is greater than 0.005/20, or 1/4,000, a brain biopsy should be performed. Even if brain biopsy could identify only three fourths of brain abscesses, the threshold probability of brain abscess would only rise to $1/(4,000 \times 3/4)$, or 1/3,000. Because the clinicians could certainly not deny that the probability of brain abscess was higher than these extraordinarily low values, they were obliged to carry on the search until they were quite sure of the nature of the brain lesion.

It is not always reasonable to pursue every diagnostic possibility. At some point, we abandon the chase and turn our attention to providing comfort. However, in a patient with no evidence of cancer elsewhere, even fairly characteristic imaging studies do not raise the chance of a brain tumor to sufficiently high levels of certainty. In this patient, it was necessary to establish a tissue diagnosis, but was a brain biopsy the best diagnostic test? Should a less invasive course have been followed? Perhaps a detailed history could have revealed the recent dental procedure; perhaps a "shotgun" series of imaging studies would have discovered the apical abscess. Even if the dental infection had been identified, should the clinicians have assumed that the patient had a brain abscess? Would it still have been necessary to get a tissue specimen from the brain? The infamous bank robber Willy Sutton, when asked why he robbed banks, answered, "Because that's where the money is!" When tissue is needed to confirm a diagnosis, the patient is often best served when the doctor follows Sutton's law. Brain biopsy involves some risk [30–32], but the risk is quite low when the procedure is guided by modern imaging studies [33–35], especially relative to the information the biopsy provides.

Except for small brain abscesses, multiple lesions, and abscesses located deep in the brain, surgical drainage is the treatment of choice [3,7], followed by an intense and prolonged course of appropriate antibiotics directed at the organism identified. In this instance, knowledge of the causative agent led to additional focused questions about recent dental work, to the appropriate choice of antibiotics, and to a cure for the patient. In many instances, the quixotic quest for diagnostic certainty leads us to perform many more tests than necessary; most of the time we learn little from these superfluous studies [35]. In this case, however, the clinicians' persistence until the cause was uncapped was the key to a successful outcome.

CASE 53 TREATING BEFORE KNOWING*

A 52-year-old man with a history of mild hypertension and nephrolithiasis presented with progressive dyspnea, productive cough, and fever for 3 days.

The first thing that comes to mind is pneumonia. An upper respiratory tract infection does not usually cause dyspnea unless there is underlying cardiac or pulmonary disease. Hypertensive cardiomyopathy can produce congestive heart failure, but this man has only mild hypertension. Nephrolithiasis can cause advanced renal disease and hypertension but may also be an incidental finding.

Two weeks before admission the patient had fatigue, myalgias, and nasal congestion. Four days before admission he noticed shortness of breath and a cough, productive initially of greenish sputum, which became brownish red the next day. At a local clinic, a chest film

*Originally published by Pauker SG, Kopelman RI. *N Engl J Med* 1992;327:1366–1369. Reprinted with permission of the Massachusetts Medical Society.

showed bilateral infiltrates. The patient refused admission and was given a prescription for cephalexin. Respiratory distress developed overnight, and he was hospitalized.

Greenish sputum bespeaks an infection; in a bacterial infection, brownish-red sputum can be associated with hemorrhage into the infected alveolar spaces. Although his condition deteriorated, the patient had not been taking the antibiotic very long. In a previously healthy man with bilateral pulmonary infiltrates and brownish-red sputum, pulmonary hemorrhage comes to mind even without frank hemoptysis. Diseases associated with pulmonary infiltrates and hemorrhage include Wegener granulomatosis and Goodpasture syndrome. But bacterial pneumonia is highest on my list.

The patient's hypertension had resolved 5 years ago after he lost weight. His last kidney stone developed 13 years earlier. Recently, his creatinine level had been 1.3 mg/dl, and urinalyses had not shown any hematuria. He worked as a clothing shipper. He did not drink and had not smoked for 10 years. There was no history of drug abuse, and he had not had sex with men.

The history is consistent with mild essential hypertension. The serum creatinine may be normal if he is a large man. I would dismiss chronic renal stone disease as a cause of renal failure and volume overload. Patients with anti–glomerular basement membrane (GBM) antibodies are more likely to have pulmonary hemorrhage if they have an underlying pulmonary injury, such as that caused by tobacco abuse. He does not appear to have risk factors for human immunodeficiency virus infection, which would predispose him to opportunistic infections.

In the emergency room, the patient was markedly dyspneic. His blood pressure was 174/101 mm Hg, his pulse was 98 per minute, his respiratory rate was 30 per minute, and his rectal temperature was 37.3°C. His skin was warm, and he had no rashes. Diffuse rales were present bilaterally. The rest of the physical examination was unremarkable. Other laboratory data were as follows: hemoglobin 11.3 g/dL; hematocrit 34%; and white cell count

17,100 with 78% polys, 12% lymphocytes, 1% atypical lymphocytes, 7% monocytes, and 2% eosinophils. The platelet count was normal. The electrolytes were normal. The BUN was 34 mg/dL, and the creatinine was 2.0 mg/dL. The chest film showed diffuse bilateral infiltrates consistent with pulmonary edema. The electrocardiogram showed no acute changes. On room air, the arterial blood gases were as follows: pH 7.42, partial pressure of oxygen 27 mm Hg, and partial pressure of carbon dioxide 39 mm Hg.

I do not think the infiltrates would be so diffuse with bacterial pneumonia, but viral pneumonia could give this picture. The patient is a little old for *Mycoplasma* pneumonia, but *Legionella* pneumonia is possible. I would try to distinguish between noncardiac and cardiac pulmonary edema. Despite severe hypoxemia, he is not hyperventilating, which suggests inadequate alveolar ventilation. Some patients with cardiogenic pulmonary edema are unable to hyperventilate, and respiratory acidosis develops. I would expect more focal findings if this were pulmonary hemorrhage. I am eager to see his urinalysis. If the elevated serum creatinine is a manifestation of rapidly progressive glomerulonephritis associated with Goodpasture syndrome, therapy needs to be begun immediately.

With supplemental oxygen, the partial pressure of oxygen increased to 100 mm Hg. Erythromycin and ceftriaxone were begun. His respiratory status deteriorated shortly thereafter, and he was intubated. The sputum was brown with streaks of blood. Gram staining revealed moderate numbers of polymorphonuclear neutrophils with gram-positive cocci and gram-negative rods, but no predominant organisms were seen. Dipstick examination of the urine showed 4+ blood and 3+ protein. The urine sediment contained 10 to 15 white cells per high-power field and 15 to 20 red cells per high-power field. Numerous coarse granular and white-cell casts were seen. There were clumps of red cells but no red-cell casts.

I would continue broad-spectrum antibiotics. Acute renal failure has been associated with *Legionella* and viral pneumonias, but granular and white-cell casts reflect renal parenchymal injury. With glomerular disease, the sediment typically contains more red cells than white cells, and one would expect to see red-cell casts. With inflammatory tubulointerstitial disease, there are more white cells than red cells, and one would anticipate seeing white-cell casts or renal tubular epithelial casts. White-cell casts can be seen both in interstitial diseases, such as interstitial nephritis or pyelonephritis, and glomerulonephritis, but in the latter case usually when there are red-cell casts as well.

With so much hematuria and this pulmonary picture, I suspect that this patient does indeed have a glomerulonephritis, although the absence of the red-cell casts is worrisome. If no red-cell casts are seen on repeated urinalyses, these urinary findings would suggest hemolytic uremic syndrome, but neither the childhood nor the adult form of hemolytic uremic syndrome, which may resemble thrombotic thrombocytopenic purpura, fits the pulmonary picture. The only thing I can think of that explains the whole picture would be rapidly progressive glomerulonephritis with pulmonary hemorrhage.

I would order serologic tests for the various forms of glomerulonephritis, but I would not rush to do a kidney biopsy if the patient remains stable.

Serologic studies were ordered of antinuclear antibodies (ANAs), C3, C4, total complement (CH$_{50}$), anti-DNA antibodies, anti-GBM antibodies, and antineutrophil cytoplasmic antibodies (C-ANCAs). Immunosuppressive therapy was considered for a "pulmonary-renal" syndrome.

In Goodpasture syndrome, prednisone and cyclophosphamide can suppress antibody formation and plasmapheresis can remove pathogenic anti-GBM antibodies. But this therapy needs to be started early. If we wait until the patient's creatinine level is greater than 4 mg/dL, until he is oliguric, or until crescents occupy more than 80% of his glomeruli, then renal function will be lost, perhaps forever. With Wegener granulomatosis we have more time because the prognosis for recovery of renal function is good even if therapy is delayed until renal failure develops.

If the patient had a negative C-ANCA test and a negative anti-GBM titer, then the remaining immune-complex diseases might be managed with prednisone alone, so these serologic tests might keep us from resorting to kidney biopsy, if we could get the results back quickly. If his creatinine continues to rise, I would opt for the biopsy.

> On the second hospital day, the pulmonary-capillary wedge pressure was 31 mm Hg. An echocardiogram revealed normal valves and normal ventricular function. Vigorous diuresis was begun. An indirect immunofluorescence assay for anti-GBM antibodies was negative, but repeat urinalyses showed definite red-cell casts. Pending a specific diagnosis, plasmapheresis and immunosuppressive therapy with cyclophosphamide and prednisone were initiated. Plans for a renal biopsy were made.

A Swan-Ganz catheter can be useful in separating cardiogenic from noncardiogenic pulmonary edema. The echocardiogram implies that this is not primarily cardiac disease, but rather fluid overload due to the kidney disease. The red-cell casts validate the diagnosis of glomerulonephritis. If a patient has anti-GBM antibodies, there is a 60% chance of detecting them with indirect immunofluorescence. The negative result does not reduce the probability of glomerulonephritis sufficiently to warrant withholding therapy.

> The results of serologic studies of samples drawn on admission were reported on the third hospital day: CH_{50} 156 (normal 150–250); C4 0.33 (normal 0.15–0.54); and C3 0.42 (normal 0.87–2.20). The assays for ANA, C-ANCA, and cold agglutinins were all negative. A percutaneous renal biopsy was performed, and the preliminary findings were negative for anti-GBM antibodies. Staining for immunoglobulin A (IgG) and IgA was negative. Antistreptolysin O and streptozyme assays were positive. A culture of sputum obtained at the local clinic on the day before admission was reported as growing moderate amounts of group A beta-hemolytic streptococci and a few gram-negative bacilli. Immunosuppressive therapy was discontinued.

The negative C-ANCA assay argues strongly against a diagnosis of Wegener granulomatosis.

The kidney biopsy is the gold standard for determining whether a patient has a disease caused by anti-GBM antibodies, and a negative result suggests that he does not have rapidly progressive glomerulonephritis associated with Goodpasture syndrome. There is no evidence of lupus, endocarditis, or cryoglobulinemia. The normal serum C4 level in the face of the low C3 suggests activation of the complement system by the alternative pathway. The anti–streptolysin O and streptozyme tests indicate that the patient was truly infected with streptococci and not just colonized. I suspect that light microscopy of the kidney-biopsy specimen will show a diffuse proliferative glomerulonephritis. Electron microscopy of the specimen will clinch the diagnosis of poststreptococcal glomerulonephritis if it shows subepithelial deposits, although I would have expected the staining for IgG to have been positive.

In children, hypertension and pulmonary edema are classic findings in poststreptococcal glomerulonephritis, a diagnosis that brings the whole clinical picture together.

> The renal biopsy showed exudative glomerulonephritis with subendothelial, subepithelial, and mesangial electron-dense deposits. Granular deposits of C3 were noted along glomerular basement membranes. The findings were consistent with postinfectious (poststreptococcal) glomerulonephritis. The patient's antibiotic was changed to penicillin, and immunosuppressive therapy was discontinued. His pulmonary infiltrates cleared. At discharge on the 13th day, his creatinine was 1.4 mg/dL.

Analysis

Out of context, even the most familiar friend can be difficult to recognize. Presented with the picture of glomerulonephritis in a child with hypertension and edema, few physicians would fail to place acute poststreptococcal glomerulonephritis near the top of their list of suspected diagnoses.[273,274] Even in a patient older than 50 years of age, acute glomerulonephritis presents primarily with acute renal failure, hypertension, and edema.[275] However, an acutely ill, middle-aged man with pulmonary edema evoked other, quite appropriate diagnostic hypotheses. Once it was clear that the patient had glomerulonephritis, the discussant maintained a narrow focus because he perceived a need to identify rapidly progressive glomerulonephritis associated with Goodpasture syndrome quickly and to begin therapy before irreversible renal damage occurred.[276–278] Although he weighed the possibility of other "pulmonary-renal" syndromes, such as Wegener granulomatosis, and argued for the continuation of antibiotics to cover his most likely diagnosis of pneumonia, he appears not to have considered poststreptococcal nephritis until the rather specific complement and positive streptococcal titers became available.

Of interest, the discussant raised the specter of Goodpasture syndrome before any clinical findings suggested renal involvement; the case presentation included only respiratory distress, hemoptysis, and bilateral pulmonary infiltrates. Although this cut to the chase was a surprising anticipation of the patient's renal involvement, it is perhaps understandable that pulmonary hemorrhage would suggest a pulmonary-renal syndrome to a nephrologist. By the same token, however, a specialist in renal disease would be intimately familiar with acute poststreptococcal glomerulonephritis, so it is surprising that that possibility was initially ignored. Perhaps concern about a rapidly progressive disease with potentially irreversible consequences was too great for other possibilities to be considered. Perhaps the clinical picture of a middle-aged patient with respiratory distress was too disparate; not many patients with acute poststreptococcal glomerulonephritis present as this patient did, and extremely few middle-aged adults with these clinical manifestations have acute poststreptococcal glomerulonephritis.

Selecting a management strategy when the spectrum of diagnosis remains broad is a complex task. At one extreme, the clinician can defer therapy and gather more information, either performing diagnostic tests or observing the evolution of the disease process, as might be done when a patient presents with acute abdominal pain but has no localizing findings. At the other extreme, the clinician can begin therapy empirically, either to use the patient's response to therapy as a diagnostic marker or because the likelihood of disease exceeds some therapeutic threshold at which the benefits of therapy exceed its risks or costs. Sometimes the clinician settles on a mixed strategy, treating one possible disease empirically while ordering diagnostic studies to confirm or exclude alternative diagnoses. Occasionally, the physician can begin several empirical therapies at once to cover several diagnostic possibilities. Perhaps the most common reason for this latter strategy is the selection of antibiotics in a patient in whom sepsis is suspected before bacteriologic confirmation of sepsis is available.

In the simplest case, choosing whether or not to begin therapy depends on the likelihood of disease and the benefits, risks, and costs of therapy. When a diagnostic study might be performed, the optimal solution depends on the costs and risks of the test and the diagnostic information it might provide. When the delay engendered by performing a diagnostic test can diminish the benefits of therapy, the decision also depends on the duration of such delays and their effect on the patient's prognosis with and without the use of empirical therapy.

This patient's initial presentation led his doctors to perform two invasive procedures and to administer potentially dangerous immunosuppressive therapy. Neither the doctors caring for this patient nor the discussant had foreclosed possibilities other than Goodpasture syndrome, even as they pursued that diagnosis and administered appropriately aggressive and timely therapies. They continued giving antibiotics to treat bacterial pneumonia; they inserted a pulmonary-artery catheter and performed an echocardiogram to evaluate the possibility of intrinsic cardiac disease.

The rationale for both renal biopsy and empirical immunosuppressive therapy turns on the likelihood that the patient had the rapidly progressive glomerulonephritis of Goodpasture syndrome. Although he was intubated, the patient appeared clinically stable, allowing the doctors time to obtain the results of serologic studies. Although immunosuppressive therapy and plasmapheresis might be begun without histologic confirmation of Goodpasture syndrome if anti-GBM antibodies were present on indirect immunofluorescence assay, renal biopsy can be helpful in treating a patient who has acute glomerulonephritis of unknown cause.[279] The discussant mentioned that the indirect immunofluorescence assay had a sensitivity of 60%. If the specificity of the test were 100%, a negative result would reduce the odds of anti-GBM disease to roughly half their previous level. (If the test were less specific, it would have less effect on the probability of anti-GBM disease.) Since the negative indirect immunofluorescence studies lowered the likelihood of disease and since there was no evidence of progressive renal failure, it is interesting that both the clinicians and the discussant still opted for empirical treatment with cyclophosphamide and prednisone. It is not clear why.

As the patient's clinical course evolved, the first suggestion that he had postinfectious glomerulonephritis arose when serologic studies revealed a normal C4 level while C3 levels were low—evidence for activation of the alternative complement pathway. That pattern suggests acute poststreptococcal or membranoproliferative glomerulonephritis.[273,280,281] With that evidence in hand, the clinicians ordered serologic tests for streptococci and discovered elevated titers. The results of the culture of sputum obtained some 5 days earlier confirmed the presence of infection with group A beta-hemolytic streptococci.

In retrospect, the patient's history of hypertension may have obscured the nature of his new disease. Nondependent edema is less frequent in older patients with acute glomerulonephritis than in children and young adults.[275] Had the positive sputum-culture results been available in a timely fashion (within 1 to 2 days of admission), the correct diagnosis probably would have been obvious far sooner, and the patient might well have avoided the risks entailed by renal biopsy, plasmapheresis, and even brief immunosuppressive therapy.

CASE 54. A DEFECTIVE DETECTIVE

Here we present two independently recorded discussions of a renal diagnostic problem, one by a medical intern and the other by an experienced nephrologist. Although we know little about the phylogeny of diagnostic acumen, it is instructive to compare the consecutive responses to the same clinical data of two individuals with widely different training and experience.

> A 40-year-old man who was known to abuse alcohol and various other drugs was seen in the emergency room for excruciating back pain. The orthopedic resident asked the medical resident for help when he found a creatinine of 3.7 mg/dL, a blood urea nitrogen (BUN) of 47 mg/dL, and no evidence of bone or joint disease.

Intern: We are called to see a patient with back pain, a BUN of 47, and a creatinine of 3.7. I would certainly want to know where the back pain is because if it is in the flank, that may suggest a renal etiology. One of the first things I would want to know is whether the elevated BUN and creatinine are new findings or if they have been a chronic problem. First, I would want to find out how long he has had the back pain and whether he has had fever. I would also want to know if he has had any urinary symptoms. All those features would favor an acute renal etiology, although I recognize that he may have chronic renal disease. The location of the back pain may be useful information. He could have prerenal azotemia or pyelonephritis. I would want to examine the patient and order several other laboratory tests, particularly a CBC (complete blood count) and differential count, chemistries, and urinalysis.

Nephrologist: Excruciating back pain with dysfunction of the kidneys makes one wonder whether it is the kidneys that are hurting. I would be interested to know the location of the back pain, whether there is radiation, and what factors exacerbate or relieve the pain. I would want to know if there is accompanying tenderness. If I found that the pain is localized to the costovertebral angles and that there is tenderness in the kidneys, those findings would guide a lot of the history taking

that I would do. I probably would try to elicit tenderness in the back before spending a lot of time taking the history. Then I would want to know when all the manifestations started. I would want to know whether he has a history of back trouble or any similar episodes, and I would explore the course, the pace, and the nature of the pain.

> The patient had felt well until the night of admission, when he consumed large quantities of alcohol and used cocaine. Twenty to 30 minutes after his first cocaine injection (with a dirty needle), he experienced severe, persistent, bilateral flank pain, which increased on motion. His urine was described as cola colored, and pain did not increase on urination. He continued to drink alcohol and shoot cocaine and also took tranquilizers and an antibiotic. The severe pain persisted, and he came to the emergency room.

Intern: I assume that his urine previously was not cola colored. This sounds like an acute event characterized by dark urine and acute flank pain. In a patient who abuses intravenous drugs, the findings suggest the possibility of impurities in the material he was injecting, although I cannot make a connection immediately between such impurities and the bilateral flank pain and dark urine. Dark urine could contain bilirubin or blood. I still would like to know his white count and whether he is febrile. I continue to worry that he has bilateral pyelonephritis, although I admit that the diagnosis is not terribly likely. Another thing I continue to wonder is whether he has some sort of an acute reaction to an injected impurity.

Nephrologist: So the pain was increased by motion. And the new information answers the question about the duration. He had not had it more than an hour or so, and it came on while he was consuming large quantities of alcohol and using cocaine. We know that he is taking many other drugs and that he used a dirty needle. He certainly could be infected with a variety of organisms.

The cola-colored urine is perhaps the most specific finding and suggests that he is passing either blood or bile. We are not told whether he is jaundiced. Barring a few rare disorders, the cola-colored urine probably represents hematuria. So my initial concern would turn toward solving a problem consisting of bilateral severe renal pain accompanied by renal insufficiency and gross hematuria. We do not know whether the hematuria preceded this episode or not. I will not speculate about what it means if it did go back in time, because the history suggests that he took one injection, got severe pain, and then passed dark urine. I am a little worried about this assumption, however, because the serum creatinine of 3.7 and the BUN of 47 suggest that something has been going on for a long time.

> On physical examination, he was extremely anxious. Pulse was 100 per minute; other vital signs, including temperature, were normal. There were no murmurs. Moderate paraspinal and costovertebral angle tenderness was elicited. The remainder of the examination was normal.

Intern: Again, the observations are nonspecific. If he has an infection, I would expect him to be febrile, but he is neither febrile nor hypothermic. His vital signs are normal. Most likely he is not septic. I am now less concerned that he has an infectious process, but I would not be willing to exclude one. I would still want to see the white count and more laboratory data.

Nephrologist: So, he is not jaundiced. We have to assume that some asymptomatic disorder of his kidneys predated this recent illness in order to explain the serum creatinine of 3.7. I would have to conclude that he had some preexisting renal failure, and that he had either a subacute illness or an acute illness that occurred over the past few days. He could have glomerular disease, obstruction from stones, or embolic renal disease. It is probably not an infection. Glomerular disease would include disorders caused by intravascular infections such as endocarditis. Infection also could play a role in the genesis of glomerular disease if he had hepatitis, but we have little evidence to support this possibility. Renal impairment could be the result of ingestion of a nephrotoxin. We should keep in mind that drug users and alcoholics are more likely than the general population to be exposed to a variety of toxins. None of these diagnoses, however, accounts for the sudden bilateral renal pain

that he had shortly after his intravenous cocaine injection.

> In the preceding 15 years, he had had the following illnesses: an abdominal stab wound, hepatitis B, an abscess in the arm, syphilis, and gonorrhea. He had no history of kidney disease.

Intern: Neither the history of an abscess in the arm nor the history of syphilis and gonorrhea is particularly helpful. It could be important to know when and where the abdominal stab wound occurred and whether he had any damage to his kidneys. With respect to hepatitis, if he had chronic hepatitis with an exacerbation, he could have bilirubinemia and bilirubin in his urine. However, I do not think this history tells me a whole lot.

Nephrologist: The history of an abscess in the arm, the syphilis, and the gonorrhea is probably not relevant to the current problem. Some of these findings do raise the possibility of a sexually transmitted disease and the possibility of HIV infection. We have not been told about HIV risk factors.

> Laboratory findings were as follows: white cell count 10,900 with 84% polys, 10% lymphs, 6% monos; hemoglobin 15.4 g/dL; hematocrit 45%. Electrolytes were sodium 133 mEq/L, potassium 4.8 mEq/L, chloride 100 mEq/L, total CO_2 20 mEq/L. Urinalysis: specific gravity 1.012, protein 2+, blood 3+, negative glucose, 2 to 5 white blood cells (WBCs) and 5 to 10 red blood cells (RBCs) per high-power field, numerous granular casts, and a few cellular casts. Chest x-ray and electrocardiogram (ECG) were normal. Abdominal plain film showed kidneys of normal size and no abnormalities.

Intern: I am unimpressed with the white count and the electrolytes. His urine contains 2 to 5 white blood cells, but there is no mention of bacteria. It concerns me that his urine tests 3+ for blood and contains 5 to 10 red cells. Bilirubin is not mentioned, so I suspect it is not the cause of his dark urine. I think the dark urine is caused by blood. I am puzzled about the cause of his problem. One thing we have to think about in an intravenous drug user is endocarditis. But he has no murmurs, he has a normal white count, and he is afebrile. This is not a diagnosis that I would entertain seriously. At this point, the question is what we should do to evaluate his bilateral flank pain and hematuria. I would have to consider other tests to assess the anatomy of his urinary tract.

Nephrologist: Now here is the first startling item. I assume the cola-colored urine does contain a fair amount of blood. Although if tests only 3 out of 4+, which is not the strongest reaction, this finding is far beyond what I would expect from 5 to 10 red blood cells per high-power field. These findings suggest that some substance other than the few red cells is contributing to the color of the urine and the positivity of the dipstick reaction. The principal candidates are either hemoglobin or myoglobin. Of course, lysed red cells could produce the same findings, but because the specific gravity of the urine is 1.012—that is, approximately isotonic—there is no particular reason for lysis of red cells. I would try to find out whether there is evidence of hemolysis or release of myoglobin into the blood. At this point, the most helpful information would include a plasma haptoglobin and a serum free hemoglobin. I suspect we will find a normal haptoglobin and negative serum free hemoglobin because hemolysis is not very likely, given the hematocrit of 45.

The pigment in the urine probably is myoglobin. The electrolytes are not remarkably abnormal. They give us little information about the duration of the renal disorder. The fact that the kidneys are normal in size argues that this is an acute problem. It would be interesting to know if they were larger or smaller than they were the day before.

Serum findings a few hours later were creatinine 4.8 mg/dL, BUN 56 mg/dL, potassium 5.4 mEq/L, uric acid 14 mg/dL, calcium 8.4 mg/dL, and phosphorus 7.5 mg/dL.

Intern: He has a rapidly rising BUN, creatinine, and serum potassium. We do not know what his uric acid was previously, but this value is quite high. Serum phosphorus also is very high. He clearly is in acute renal failure.

There are some things I should have checked earlier. I assume he did not have postural hypotension because his vital signs were normal, but one of the things that I should have looked at first was his state of hydration. At this point, he has rapidly progressive renal failure, and I think that renal studies clearly are warranted. The first thing that we should be sure of is that he does not have urinary tract obstruction as a cause of renal failure. The first study that I would order at this point is an abdominal ultrasound, which would also give us an indication of kidney size.

Nephrologist: Things are changing rather rapidly, thus confirming that this is an acute event. If his illness had been evolving for a few weeks or even for a few days, one would not expect such a rapid rise in BUN and creatinine over a matter of a few hours. The combination of a high serum phosphorus, slightly low serum calcium, rapidly rising serum potassium, and high uric acid is consistent with the dumping into the blood of potassium, purine metabolites, and phosphate from some compartment. The slightly low serum calcium probably is the consequence of hyperphosphatemia. The rate of rise of the creatinine and BUN suggests that he has essentially no renal function. Even with no renal function, the rate of rise of the serum creatinine is a little rapid, which suggests that there is rapid delivery of intramuscular creatinine pools into the blood. Again, this finding is consistent with myoglobinuria.

Other results were aspartate transaminase (AST) 1,160 IU/L, alanine transaminase (ALT) 369 IU/L, lactate dehydrogenase (LDH) 1,900 IU/L, and creatine kinase (CK) 42,000 IU/L. On repeat urinalysis, there was 3+ blood, zero to two RBCs per high-power field, and numerous reddish-brown casts.

Intern: We do not know what his bilirubin is, but most likely, he has acute hepatitis. A CK of 42,000 in somebody who has been drinking heavily could be caused by rhabdomyolysis. Excessive alcohol intake is a common cause of rhabdomyolysis. The CK cannot be elevated on a cardiac basis because a CK of this magnitude would imply such severe muscle necrosis that a patient would not survive such a cardiac event. Rhabdomyolysis also occurs in elderly people who lie in one position and in patients with sepsis and hypotension. Because he is an alcoholic, there is a good chance that he fell and sustained trauma. Such an event would explain the CK of 42,000. I would still want to know his bilirubin, and given that his repeat urinalysis showed red cells and reddish-brown casts, I am suspicious that he has acute glomerulonephritis. I would still want to see a renal ultrasound study.

Nephrologist: All of this argues for tissue destruction, probably muscle destruction and probably causing release of myoglobin into the blood and hence into the urine. It would still be nice to know the serum hemoglobin, haptoglobin, and aldolase, although I doubt that the results would contribute much. I think it would be useful to try to figure out whether the source of back pain is his kidneys or his muscles.

> The patient's peak creatinine and BUN reached 9.2 and 83 mg/dL, respectively. He was not oliguric, and he did not require dialysis. He did not develop hypercalcemia in the recovery period. Back pain resolved slowly over a 2-week period. Follow-up values for creatinine and BUN 1 week after discharge were 1.6 and 23 mg/dL, respectively. The patient was followed jointly by psychiatry and social service in the substance abuse clinic.

Intern: I am afraid I have not managed to arrive at a totally satisfactory diagnosis. One of the first things that I would have done in a patient like this is to send off liver function tests. His AST is very high, and other enzymes also are abnormal. I still wonder what is wrong with his liver.

[At this point, the intern was told that the correct diagnosis was acute renal failure secondary to rhabdomyolysis.]

Oh, of course, I should have gotten the diagnosis much earlier! We should have alkalinized his urine early on. We would have had the CK result in an hour, seen that it was 42,000, and at that point alkalinized the urine immediately. This treatment might have helped deter the development of renal failure.

Nephrologist: Now that the diagnosis is clear, it would be interesting to try to wrap up the loose ends. I wonder if the whole thing could have dated from the injection. The sudden back pain was said to have begun 20 to 30 minutes after the first cocaine injection, but he continued after that to drink alcohol and shoot more cocaine. The entire clinical course seems to have evolved over a period of a few hours. It is difficult to imagine that the serum creatinine increased to 3.7 in a period of a few hours. This rate of rise is quite fast, but it is possible.

So what caused the back pain? It could be the kidneys' response to damage by myoglobin. Sometimes such damaged kidneys do produce pain because they become swollen. But pain also could emanate from damaged muscles. A CK of 42,000 implies substantial damage of muscle mass, and if the necrosis was widespread in his back, severe back pain could occur. It seems likely that some combination of the alcohol he was drinking and the shot he gave himself caused sudden and nonspecific muscle damage.

Analysis

Clinicians and detectives have much in common. Both deal with problems that may have subtle and well-hidden solutions. Both take detailed histories, examine physical details, and apply diagnostic tests. Throughout our comments about the comparative problem-solving capacities of the intern and the nephrologist, we will interject some comments by the most famous fictional sleuth of all, Sherlock Holmes. That Holmes's words should be directly applicable to medical problem solving should be no surprise to Sir Arthur Conan Doyle's readers; terms common to medical diagnosis and criminology, such as "facts," "deduction," "inference," "clues," "hypothesis," and "discrepancies," are sprinkled liberally throughout his writings. Of more than passing interest is the fact that Conan Doyle was a physician.

With regard to the case at hand, we would be unwise to generalize about the comparative problem-solving approaches of interns and subspecialists on the basis of this limited sample, but certain patterns of their remarks are worthy of comment. Clearly, the nephrologist was quicker, more accurate, more efficient, and more complete than the intern. The patient's initial diagnostic findings were confusing: The high creatinine led away from a diagnosis of acute renal failure, and back pain (never fully explained even later) is a nonspecific symptom. Nonetheless, the nephrologist summarized the problem as one consisting of back pain, renal insufficiency, and gross hematuria. The intern at this stage had only a poorly formulated hypothesis ("some sort of acute reaction to an injected impurity") and was considering the rather improbable diagnosis of bilateral pyelonephritis. Considering the fact that problem formulation is an essential component of the problem-solving process, it is not surprising that subsequently the nephrologist was better prepared than the intern to receive and evaluate new data.

Indeed, the next remarkable difference was their interpretation of the urinary findings. The nephrologist recognized promptly that there was a discrepancy between the 3+ test for blood and the finding of 5 to 10 red blood cells per high-power field; the intern thought that the urine contained blood but failed on two occasions to recognize the discrepancy between the occult blood test and the microscopic findings in the urine. In fact, he posited a diagnosis of rhabdomyolysis only after the remarkable CK results became available, and even then, he never connected the rhabdomyolysis with the acute renal failure.

Holmes would never have missed this important clue. In *A Study in Scarlet*, he remarked to Inspector Lestrade of Scotland Yard (as the nephrologist might have explained to the intern)

All this seems strange to you because you failed at the beginning of the inquiry to grasp the importance of the single real clue that was presented to you. I had the good fortune to seize upon that, and everything that has occurred since then has seemed to confirm my original supposition, and indeed, was the logical sequence of it. Hence, things that have perplexed you and made the case more obscure have served to enlighten me and to strengthen my conclusions.[282]

The nephrologist's approach probably would have seemed impressive to the intern. In *The Crooked Man*, Holmes explains to Dr. Watson, "It is one of those instances where the reasoner can produce an effect which seems remarkable to his neighbor, because the latter has missed the one little point which is the basis of the deduction."[283]

By the close of the diagnostic session, the intern still was puzzling about the enzyme abnormalities and persevered on the presence or absence of jaundice. By this time, the nephrologist had "wrapped up" the diagnosis and was attempting to explain many of the previously obscure findings.

This exercise should not be used to denigrate the intellectual capacities of house officers. We selected the transcript from several we had recorded with interns specifically because it illustrated faulty problem solving. In any given case, an intern might be a far more effective problem solver than a highly trained and experienced subspecialist. Even experts make mistakes; nonetheless, in this case the intern performed poorly and the nephrologist admirably.

What factors account for the superior performance of the expert? The extent of knowledge must be one factor, pattern recognition (positive occult blood test with few red cells in the urine) probably is another, and experience with similar cases (the availability heuristic) is still another.[27,28] Other factors undoubtedly are involved. Holmes would have had no difficulty explaining the less-than-perfect performance of the intern. In *The Sign of Four*, commenting on the capabilities of the prominent French detective François le Villard, Holmes said, "He possesses two out of the three qualities necessary for the ideal detective. He had the power of observation and that of deduction. He is only wanting in knowledge, and that may come in time."[284]

CASE 55. REMEDIES FOR FAULTY HYPOTHESIS GENERATION

A 61-year-old woman was being evaluated for mild anemia and an elevated sedimentation rate.

The connection between the abnormalities is vague. If I assume they are related and do not represent an acute process, many diagnostic possibilities come to mind. Treatable disorders with these abnormal findings include polymyalgia rheumatica, temporal arteritis, connective tissue disorders such as vasculitis, and chronic infections such as tuberculosis and osteomyelitis. Of course, we would have to think of malignancies, especially lymphoma or multiple myeloma, when the sedimentation rate is very high. I obviously need much more data.

Nine months earlier her hematocrit was 35%, and 5 months previously, when her doctor saw her for upper respiratory tract symptoms and weakness, it was 32%. Treatment with iron seemed to relieve her weakness somewhat. Two months ago, her major complaints were tinnitus and anxiety. She was still receiving iron, and her hematocrit was 38%. The mean corpuscular volume (MCV) was 78, reticulocyte count 2%, platelets 400,000, and white cell count 12,000

with a normal differential. The sedimentation rate, first measured at that time, was 83 mm/hr.

There are two pieces of information that I find intriguing. The most striking number is the MCV of 78, which implies some problem with hemoglobin formation. If she had iron-deficiency anemia with an MCV of 78, I would have expected the hematocrit to be lower. She could have thalassemia minor, but there the MCV typically is even lower. Other causes of microcytic anemia include pyridoxine deficiency, lead poisoning, and chronic disease. I would want to look at a peripheral blood smear for more information.

The sedimentation rate is obviously abnormal, and my earlier differential diagnosis still holds. I am not sure what to make of her tinnitus. That symptom can be seen with quinidine or salicylate use but not with iron therapy, to the best of my knowledge. There is no information regarding headache or hearing loss that would make me look for cranial nerve pathology. I still need more information in order to decide on the extent of my workup.

She was admitted to the hospital. On admission, she complained only of anxiety and tinnitus. She was postmenopausal. She did not use alcohol or other drugs. A detailed review of systems revealed only that she had sustained two episodes of near-syncope in the previous 6 months. She did not think that she hyperventilated prior to the attacks. Her appetite was good, and her weight was stable. On examination, she appeared anxious. Blood pressure was 150/88 mm Hg, pulse 92 per minute and regular, and respirations 18 per minute. Head, eyes, ears, nose, and throat were normal. The thyroid was not palpable. Lungs were clear. Cardiac exam revealed no murmurs. Abdominal exam was unremarkable. Neurologic exam disclosed no focal findings.

Given the new data, I am concerned principally about the two episodes of near-syncope. There is no doubt that people with syncope due to a cardiovascular cause have an increase in mortality over the subsequent 1 to 2 years, whereas syncope due to other causes tends to carry a fairly benign prognosis. Given that she has tinnitus, I wonder whether she has experienced vertigo, which may produce a vagal response and near-syncope. At a minimum, I think she needs to have an evaluation for a cardiac arrhythmia, with long-term monitoring. Additional history would be useful in evaluating the possibilities of hypoglycemia and orthostatic hypotension.

The hematocrit was 40%, MCV 79.7, WBC 11,200 with a normal differential, and sedimentation rate 49 mm/hr. Urinalysis: 1+ blood and zero to three red blood cells per high-power field. Serum calcium, electrolytes, uric acid, and glucose were normal. Liver function and thyroid function tests were normal. The stool was guaiac negative. Radiologic studies of her gastrointestinal and urinary tracts were normal. Cystoscopy disclosed only chronic cystitis. Chest x-ray was normal, and purified protein derivative (PPD) test was negative. The ECG showed normal sinus rhythm, nonspecific ST and T-wave changes, and right ventricular conduction delay (incomplete right-bundle-branch block [RBBB]). The ANA titer was 1:16, with a diffuse pattern. Serum protein electrophoresis showed no spike and high levels of alpha- and gamma-globulins.

I am struck most by the enormous amount of effort that is going into evaluating a woman who does not seem to be terribly ill. From what I know, it is not clear that hospitalization was necessary at this point—unless her doctors were concerned about her syncopal symptoms and felt she required long-term monitoring. The reason for the GI (gastrointestinal) workup is not clear to me either. It is possible that the iron therapy corrected a preexisting iron-deficiency anemia, and the physicians wanted to rule out an occult source of blood loss. The guaiac-negative stools, however, decrease the likelihood of finding significant pathology.

I am not sure what to make of the microscopic hematuria. I suspect that given her age, the physicians involved in her care were concerned enough that they felt it was important to look for upper tract disease and do cystoscopy to rule out a bladder tumor, which, although more common in men than in women, clearly becomes a problem at her age. I would have predicted, however, that those tests would have a low yield.

The low titer of antinuclear antibodies is non-specific, and I doubt that it is of any significance. The sedimentation rate has fallen, and I probably would not pursue it further at present.

Nothing here really helps me evaluate her episodes of near-syncope. There is no evidence on electrocardiogram of a major conduction problem. An incomplete right-bundle-branch block is a common variant, especially in women. I still feel that more evaluation for the syncope is needed. If the tinnitus is significant, the possibility of an acoustic neuroma might be considered. In that case, an audiogram or a CT (computed tomography) scan might be indicated.

The patient was discharged without a definitive diagnosis and followed as an outpatient. Over the next month, she complained about an occipital buzzing ("like a bee in my head"). She was seen by a neurologist, who found no abnormalities and felt that some of her symptoms were related to anxiety. Audiometry showed a mild bilateral high-frequency hearing loss. The etiology of her symptoms and high sedimentation rate remained uncertain.

The audiogram described is consistent with her age. There is no evidence of a lateralizing problem. The mildly elevated sedimentation rate is still unexplained. The possibility of polymyalgia rheumatica or temporal arteritis still exists. Individual cranial nerves can be affected in temporal arteritis, which is sort of a cousin of polymyalgia rheumatica, and I wonder if her occipital buzzing, which I suspect is just severe tinnitus, could be related to this kind of neuropathy. I think any decision about proceeding with a temporal artery biopsy would be conditioned a great deal by talking to the patient and finding out whether she has the other symptoms that you would expect to find in that illness, such as shoulder aches and pains, chronic fatigue, headaches, or irregularity of the temporal arteries on palpation. Finally, I am still concerned that the syncope, which could be a very significant symptom in a 61-year-old person, seems to be left unexplained.

One month after discharge she came to the emergency room complaining of palpitations and increasing anxiety and was readmitted. She

was found to have a paroxysmal supraventricular tachycardia, which responded promptly to therapy with antiarrhythmic agents. Physical examination was unchanged. Hematocrit was 39%, and sedimentation rate was 52 mm/hr.

I still think we are probably dealing with two problems. In series of patients with arrhythmia and syncope, tachyarrhythmias are about twice as common as bradyarrhythmias, and many patients with supraventricular or ventricular tachycardias present with syncope without other obvious cardiovascular symptoms. Rhythm disturbances can also present as near-syncope, although loss of consciousness typically is rather precipitous in onset in patients with arrhythmias.

Paroxysmal supraventricular tachycardia is not usually associated with any medical problems and does not usually lead me to do an extensive workup. To decide whether the patient had a supraventricular tachycardia that was due to atrioventricular nodal reentry or perhaps due to conduction through an accessory pathway, both the rate of the supraventricular tachycardia and its morphology may be helpful. Distinguishing between these mechanisms might affect my choice of therapy. I still think that the elevated sedimentation rate is a separate problem, and my thoughts about it are unchanged.

An echocardiogram (Figure 20.1), performed to evaluate the new rhythm disturbance, revealed a minimally enlarged left atrium that contained a large pedunculated, freely moving mass originating from the atrial septum. The mass had the characteristics of a myxoma.

Aha! This finding explains all. Patients with an atrial myxoma can present with various characteristics, including those manifested by this patient. They may have low-grade fever, chronic elevation of the sedimentation rate, and sometimes arthralgias. I am not sure that the arrhythmia was due to the myxoma, but I guess the tumor could create the conditions conductive to a reentry pathway. I am not aware of any association between tinnitus and myxoma.

The left atrial myxoma was removed without complications. Five months later the patient's

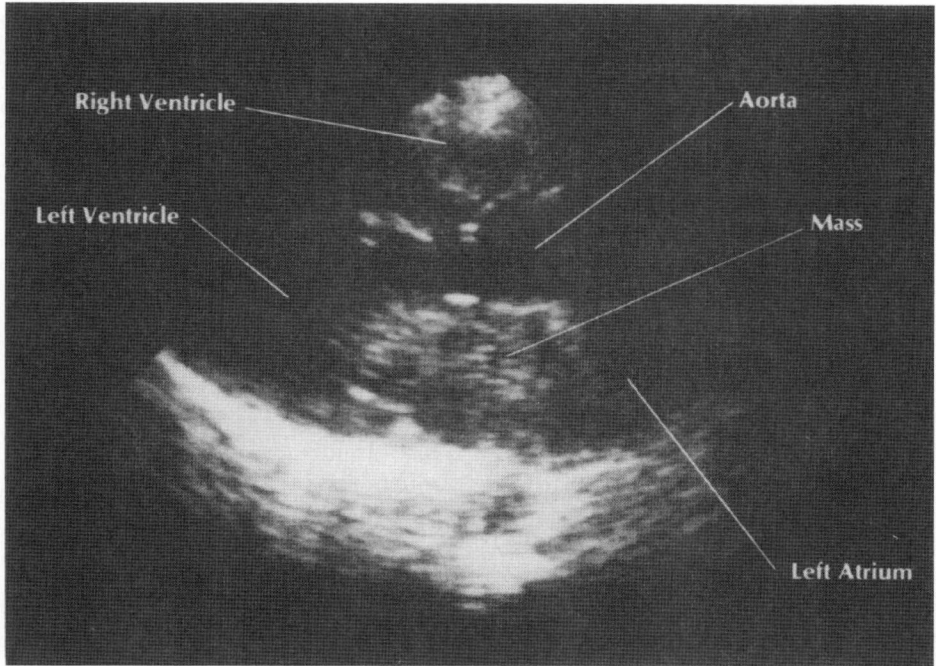

Figure 20.1 • Echocardiogram; Case 55.

> hematocrit was 43%, MCV 89, and sedimentation rate 13 mm/hr. Anxiety and tinnitus persisted.

Except for the persistence of some symptoms, this is a nice outcome for the patient because she suffered no serious complications from the myxoma. The hematocrit, MCV, and sedimentation rate are now normal. I must admit that in my clinical practice I have had very little luck in finding an etiology for tinnitus or in treating it. Hence, I am not surprised that her symptoms persisted. Finally, I feel that since the etiology of her near-syncope is not clearly due to the tumor, a valid argument could be made for further evaluation with Holter monitoring.

Analysis

The diagnosis of atrial myxoma was missed both by the clinician who discussed this patient and for some time by the physicians taking care of her. The patient's doctors stumbled on the diagnosis only after they ordered an echocardiogram as part of a "routine" workup of a new rhythm disturbance,

not because they suspected an atrial myxoma. What defect in diagnostic reasoning was responsible for this failure? We speculate that this defect is a "triggering" error. At the inception of the diagnostic process, certain findings (historical data, physical findings, laboratory results) produce important diagnostic clues that trigger one or more diagnostic hypotheses. Those hypotheses serve in turn as the framework for further diagnostic inquiry. A combination of weight loss and anxiety might trigger "hyperthyroidism"; diarrhea without a nocturnal component might trigger "functional bowel disease"; and sudden severe muscle weakness in a heavy smoker might trigger "Eaton-Lambert syndrome." Throughout the diagnostic investigation of this patient and throughout the discussion by the consultant, the possibility of atrial myxoma did not surface. In retrospect, every good clinician can identify the telltale findings: mild anemia, near-syncope, and persistently elevated sedimentation rate.

If the defect lies in faulty triggering, how can it be avoided? Certainly, atrial myxoma cannot be considered in every patient for whom there is no evident explanation for a high sedimentation rate.

Neither should the evaluation of a patient with a high sedimentation rate include routine echocardiography or chest CT scan. How, then, can the physician become more alert to this diagnosis? Although atrial myxomas are rare, they are extremely dangerous, and they are curable; thus, the premium for thinking of the diagnosis is great. Perhaps the diagnosis would be triggered more readily if texts and training programs emphasized the constellation of clinical findings that should do so— for example, pulmonary emboli without an obvious source, a right atrial lesion (tumor or thrombus), systemic emboli or acute pulmonary edema without an obvious source, or a left atrial lesion. Atypical presentations of vasculitis, endocarditis, rheumatic fever, and cardiomyopathy and unexplained central nervous system manifestations in a patient with a high sedimentation rate are other likely constellations.

Once the diagnosis is suspected, the stumbling blocks are not passed. Although noninvasive cardiac studies have enormously enhanced our ability to confirm a suspected diagnosis of atrial myxoma, they are, like all tests, imperfect. In some instances, thrombi, mitral valve vegetations, and even metastatic tumors can mimic a myxoma on the echocardiogram.

Atrial myxomas were once a medical curiosity: a challenge to diagnose and a hopeless prognosis once discovered. Because of the success of surgery and the high accuracy of noninvasive tests, the triggering mechanism is the essential step in their diagnosis. Unless the disorder is considered, appropriate tests will be delayed or even not done; the consequences of delay in diagnosis are grave. The patient under discussion was fortunate that a rhythm disturbance, perhaps not even related to the tumor, led to the diagnosis and to the prompt and uncomplicated removal of the lesion before life-threatening consequences supervened.

CASE 56. A DISASTER AVERTED

A 31-year-old Hispanic man with a history of cirrhosis was admitted for possible liver transplantation.

My first question relates to what is meant by Hispanic. Depending on the country of origin of this patient, certain causes of chronic liver disease would come to mind. Does this person come from an area where hepatitis C is endemic? Or does this person come from a place like the Caribbean or South America where schistosomiasis is endemic? I like to view the patient in the context of his cultural background, native diet, cultural exposures, and belief systems. I would wonder whether the man might have a genetic predisposition to certain types of diseases.

Seven years ago he developed fatigue and jaundice while in his native Puerto Rico. He was diagnosed with hepatitis A and B. His jaundice resolved, but his fatigue persisted and he has been disabled ever since. Five years ago, he developed abdominal distention and edema, for which he was given diuretics. There was no history of gastrointestinal bleeding or encephalopathy.

Given that he comes from Puerto Rico, it makes me think more strongly of schistosomiasis. It is somewhat unusual to be diagnosed with both hepatitis A and B. Hepatitis A is usually an acute disease and does not usually progress to chronic liver disease. Hepatitis B can certainly lead to cirrhosis, as well as to complications such as portal hypertension and hepatomas. Maybe this man had chronic hepatitis B and then got superimposed acute hepatitis A. Hepatitis C is still a possibility, given the information we have at hand. He has abdominal distention and edema, which imply portal hypertension with ascites, but at least so far, he has not had variceal bleeding. The absence of encephalopathy is interesting to me because usually by the time someone gets severe ascites from typical cirrhosis, encephalopathy often occurs as well. By contrast, in cirrhosis caused by toxins or schistosomiasis, or in the entity known as cryptogenic cirrhosis, there tends to be much more scarring and less parenchymal dysfunction.

Two years ago, endoscopy showed no evidence of varices. A liver biopsy 18 months ago showed inactive cirrhosis in a mixed macro-micronodular pattern. At that time, CBC was normal and the platelet count was 284,000. Serum creatinine and urinalysis were normal. Bilirubin was 2.2 mg/dL (mostly indirect),

> alkaline phosphatase 89 IU/L, ALT 42 IU/L (normal 0–25), AST 55 IU/L (normal 0–25), and serum albumin 2.0 g/dL.

The biopsy is disappointing because a competent histopathologist should be able to at least see schistosomiasis. He or she should be able to distinguish the different architectural disarray that occurs in the liver in these different disorders. Maybe the patient has combined disease, or maybe he has chronic hepatitis B or undiagnosed hepatitis C or E. I still would like more history, including exposure to exogenous toxins, medications, herbal remedies, and alcohol.

> Paracentesis showed that the ascitic fluid was a transudate. Alpha-1 antitrypsin level was normal. Hepatitis C antibody was negative. The Fe/total iron-binding capacity (TIBC) was 64/265. Copper level was 67 mcg/dL (normal, 70–158). Antimitochondrial and antinuclear antibodies were negative. Over the next 18 months, the edema, ascites, and fatigue persisted, and he was referred for possible liver transplantation.

Can I assume that this man was not found to have a history suggesting exposure to benzene or hydrocarbons of any kind and he was not a big drinker? Based on the laboratory tests ordered, it appears that his physicians are looking for possible causes of cirrhosis including, alpha-1 antitrypsin deficiency, hemachromatosis, Wilson disease and immunopathic liver disease.

> His past medical history was unremarkable. His only other hospitalization was 8 years previously for a stab wound to the chest. He had never had a blood transfusion and he did not drink alcohol excessively. He did not smoke or use illicit drugs. He had no family history of liver disease. He worked making wooden chairs in a factory and was exposed to a number of unknown chemicals. His only medications were bumetanide and triamterene.

In the course of the stabbing, could he have been exposed to the blood of the attacker? The absence of blood transfusions is important. If we can believe the history about no drug use or alcohol abuse, those are important pertinent nega-

tives. The lack of family history of liver disease is against disorders such as Wilson disease, alpha-1 antitrypsin disease, and hemochromatosis. The occupation history is intriguing, and I would need to do more exploring about exposures to glues or hydrocarbons, some of which are hepatotoxic.

> On examination, he appeared chronically ill. Blood pressure was 110/76 mm Hg, pulse 76 per minute and regular. The skin was nonicteric. No spider angiomata or palmar erythema were noted. Lungs were clear. Cardiac exam was normal. The abdomen was soft, nontender, and mildly distended. Shifting dullness was present. No organomegaly was appreciated. There was mild proximal muscle wasting and 2 to 3+ pedal edema. Neurologic exam was unremarkable.

Interesting, he does not have the kind of angiogenic findings we would expect in chronic liver disease such as palmar erythema and spider angiomata, both of which are thought to be caused by an increase in estrogenic substances that the diseased liver fails to break down. In addition, he is not icteric, which I find surprising. He certainly is not a typical patient with end-stage liver disease. I might have expected to see splenomegaly from portal hypertension, although sometimes it is hard to feel the spleen in the presence of ascites. The mild proximal muscle wasting goes along with a chronic disease of any sort. I am missing something here.

> Laboratory data: WBC 4,700 with a normal differential. Hemoglobin was 14.6 g/dL, and hematocrit was 42%. Platelet count was 227,000. International Normalized Ratio (INR) was 1.2. Electrolytes were normal. BUN was 19 mg/dL, and creatinine was 1.2 mg/dL. Bilirubin was 1.9 mg/dL (all indirect). Alkaline phosphatase was 84 IU/L, ALT was 19 IU/L, and AST was 33 IU/L. Serum albumin was 3.2 g/L.

He still has an elevated bilirubin. I am surprised that this chronically ill man has a hematocrit of 42. I wonder if he has a hepatoma that is producing erythropoietin. The platelets are not terribly elevated, but they are not terribly depressed either. If he had splenomegaly from portal hypertension, I would have expected thrombocytopenia. Something is not working for me here.

> Hepatitis B surface antibody was reactive. Hepatitis B surface antigen and hepatitis C antibody were negative. Herpes simplex and varicella zoster antibodies were positive. Toxoplasmosis titer was positive, and cytomegalovirus (CMV) titer was negative. Alpha-fetoprotein level was 4.8 (normal 0–9). Serum ceruloplasmin was 51.4 mg/dL (normal 23–44). HIV antibody was negative.

He apparently can mount an antibody response, as noted by the positive herpes antibodies. He does not appear to have HIV disease. Toxoplasmosis is fairly common, so the positive titer may not mean anything. The normal alpha-fetoprotein makes a hepatoma unlikely. I do not really suspect Wilson disease, although I do not know the prevalence of Wilson disease in patients from Puerto Rico.

> Pulmonary function tests showed a mild restrictive defect and a moderate reduction in diffusing capacity. Echocardiogram showed the right atrium to be mildly enlarged with findings consistent with elevated right-sided pressures. Systolic function was normal, as was valvular function.

The pulmonary function tests could be important. Does he have a form of pulmonary hypertension that could lead to congestive hepatopathy, which could lead to hepatic cirrhosis? Usually the alkaline phosphatase is a little higher. On the other hand, pulmonary hypertension can be seen in patients with underlying cirrhosis due perhaps to inadequate breakdown of vasoactive substances.

> The gastroenterologist to whom the patient was referred did not think that the patient's findings were consistent with the admitting diagnosis—cirrhosis. He pointed out that the patient's hepatic synthetic function was not seriously impaired, and his platelet count was normal.

We have been putting a lot of emphasis on the findings in one liver biopsy. Do we have confidence in the reading of that biopsy? Was it read by an experienced hepatopathologist? Was it read by someone who is familiar with diseases that may be seen more frequently in Puerto Rico? The prevalence of diseases obviously may vary among geographic regions, and we constantly need to remind ourselves of that.

> Given the echocardiographic findings, a cardiologist was consulted. The cardiologist found the cardiac examination was normal. She specifically noted that the patient's jugular venous pressure did not appear to be increased. A chest CT showed pericardial thickening and calcification. On cardiac catheterization, mean right atrial pressure was 24 mm Hg with a prominent x and y descent. Pulmonary artery (PA) pressure was 42/24 mm Hg, wedge pressure was 24 mm Hg, and left ventricular pressure was 115/26. The findings were consistent with pericardial constriction.

Now it is starting to make some sense. The patient does have a picture consistent with some type of pulmonary hypertension. Pericardial constriction could be idiopathic or postviral. We must consider tuberculosis as well, especially in a man from the Caribbean. Finally, this could be due to the stabbing he received in the chest.

> The findings were consistent with cardiac cirrhosis. The patient underwent an uncomplicated pericardiectomy. He did well clinically and said he "felt great." All of his symptoms resolved.

Analysis

Imagine how tragic the outcome would have been if the diagnosis of the referring physician had not been overturned at the referral hospital. The patient might have had a liver transplant that he did not need and would not have had the surgical procedure he actually did need. It is always important to step back in instances such as this and analyze how something as dangerous as this misdiagnosis occurred, as well as how it was corrected.

There certainly was logic behind the original diagnosis of cirrhosis. The patient had had hepatitis B with jaundice, followed 2 years later by edema and ascites, and a liver biopsy at that time showed a picture of "inactive cirrhosis." Looking at the diagnosis of cirrhosis retrospectively, it is certainly appropriate to ask whether the histologic diagnosis was correct or whether the original biopsy might have shown the telltale characteristics of passive congestion and thereby might have signaled a closer look at an alternative diagnosis of cardiac cirrhosis. The previous histologic diagnosis of cirrhosis and the same admitting diagnosis raise an important issue for any physician taking a "hand-off" of a patient from another source. The problem is that once a specific diagnosis is made, it can easily be perpetuated unless someone is alert to the possibility that the existing diagnosis is wrong. How to avoid such errors is rarely considered, but some rules might be as follows: Keep an open mind; approach a new patient de novo as much as possible; examine old records, not just hearsay; reexamine biopsy material and scans with experts. It is always wise to recall one of President Ronald Reagan's favorite caveats, namely, "It's still trust but verify. It's still play, but cut the cards. It's still watch closely. And don't be afraid to see what you see."[285] Although he applied these warnings to United States–Soviet relations, they are just as relevant as diagnostic principles.

In this particular instance, as the patient's fluid retention became refractory to treatment, he was initially considered to be in the late stages of cirrhosis, yet more and more inconsistencies and discrepancies in the diagnosis of end-stage liver disease became evident. More than the clinical manifestations and laboratory findings that the patient *had*, it is the disease attributes that the patient *did not have* that should have alerted his physician that he was barking up the wrong tree. What are these negative attributes? They are the absence of palmar erythema and spider angiomas, the normal or near-normal liver function tests, the normal INR and platelet count, the lack of esophageal varices, and the lack of hepatic encephalopathy. Any one of these features could be missing in a patient with advanced cirrhosis, but surely not all. Although it took some time for our discussant to mention the correct diagnosis, namely constrictive pericarditis, she was skeptical all along that cirrhosis could explain the entire clinical picture. On two occasions she expressed his frustration by saying, "I'm missing something here" and "Something is not working for me here."

This kind of response should always alert the clinician to look skeptically at the current diagnostic hypothesis, question it, and look for another di-

agnosis that could explain all the findings instead. When the clinicians finally did so, even then not all the findings were consistent with constrictive pericarditis, an often-neglected cause of peripheral edema and ascites. The liver biopsy failed to show passive congestion (was it overlooked by the pathologist?), and the patient had minimal neck vein distention, one of the hallmarks of pericardial constriction. As noted, not all of the "classic" findings need be present, and one missing physical finding certainly would not exclude a diagnosis when all other manifestations fit.

We pay a lot of attention to positive findings as we wend our way through the diagnostic process, but we should pay just as much attention to negative test results, normal findings, and lack of certain clinical manifestations.[188] Such a comprehensive approach to diagnosis should help us avoid the kind of potentially disastrous error that characterized this patient's course.

CASE 57. DERAILED BY THE AVAILABILITY HEURISTIC

> **A 78-year-old man sought medical attention because of intermittent nausea, shivering sensations during the day, drenching night sweats, and weight loss.**

The first piece of information leads me to focus my attention toward a disease affecting a particular age group, the elderly. A constellation of symptoms, rather than any one particular symptom, is offered, and they are fairly nebulous. Intermittent nausea, shivering sensations during the day, drenching night sweats, and weight loss imply subacute or chronic duration and make me think of things that haven't been going on just for hours. The combination of shivering sensations (which I interpret as chills) and drenching night sweats often is associated with an inflammatory process. Weight loss would certainly go along with that, and I wonder if he is having fevers.

I would like to know quite a bit more history. Was the man well until these symptoms developed? Is this his first encounter with medical disease? I would like some more information about the duration of the symptoms and some objective data to convince me that he has something serious.

> He was a heavy cigarette smoker for 45 years. Fourteen years ago, a routine chest x-ray disclosed a coin lesion in the left lower lobe, and a localized small-cell carcinoma was removed by lobectomy. He stopped smoking at that time. Except for mild dyspnea, he had no complaints in the interim period.

He had a lung cancer that was resected 14 years ago, and I think for all intents and purposes that he was cured of that disease. He stopped smoking at that time. There is evidence that his risk from smoking has abated to that of the general population. I am going to assume the symptoms developed in an otherwise healthy person.

When elderly persons present as this patient did, many of the inflammatory conditions that come to mind, such as tuberculosis, can be subacute. It is important to know whether he has an abnormal chest x-ray to start because one of the things that I suspect will come up in the evaluation will be a chest x-ray, and I need to keep in mind that he had a resected lung cancer.

> Two weeks before the sweats and weight loss began, his previously healthy wife was hospitalized with a stroke that left her aphasic and hemiparetic. The patient was concerned about his wife but claimed not to be depressed; except when he awoke with night sweats, he slept well. He thought his appetite was unaffected, but he had lost 5 pounds.

I am getting a better feeling about the subacute nature of this illness. I know that there has been a course of several weeks' duration. I also have a feel for the patient's social setting. He must be upset by his wife's illness. Elderly patients with depression may not always present with classic early-morning awakening, loss of appetite, and some of the other symptoms but just with weight loss. The patient denies depression, however.

One of the things that run through my mind is whether there is any association between his wife's illness and what happened to him. It appears that she had a fairly straightforward vascular event, and I cannot easily connect what happened to her with her husband's current symptoms. However, we should always think of what is going on in the patient's environment.

I would like to focus for a moment on his weight loss. The patient notes no difference in his appetite but has lost 5 pounds. I do not have an impression of a person who is clearly losing more material than he is taking in—from diarrhea or malabsorption, for example. It bothers me that the weight loss appears not to be related to decreased caloric intake. I would add that a 78-year-old man whose wife is not able to cook may in fact be eating less despite the fact that his appetite is unchanged. Otherwise, I would be concerned that he was in a hypermetabolic state, which would be consistent with his original presentation. Thyroid disease comes to mind, but again, it does not usually present with drenching night sweats. I am thinking he has an inflammatory disease with secondary hypermetabolism, but I need to keep in the back of my mind there may be some noninflammatory cause of his manifestations.

> He had no other complaints (including abdominal pain, diarrhea, anxiety, heat intolerance, and fever), and he had no respiratory or genitourinary complaints. Physical examination was normal. He was not febrile. Laboratory tests, including complete blood count, urinalysis, electrolytes, BUN, creatinine, and chest x-ray, were normal. Sedimentation rate was 10 mm/hr. An antibiotic was prescribed, but it did not affect the symptoms, and weight loss continued.

This additional history addresses many of my concerns. Diarrhea was not present. The absence of heat intolerance seems to rule out hyperthyroidism, but in the elderly, that disorder can present in an apathetic state. Also, I am told that he did not have fever. So, many of my original ideas about trying to categorize this illness have not been further developed by additional history. I am forced to turn to the laboratory data, and I am given a variety of important negatives. If indeed he has a serious inflammatory disease, I would have expected some additional clues: a low-grade fever, an elevated white count and sedimentation rate, and an abnormal chest x-ray.

Despite this array of negatives, his physician gave him a therapeutic trial—something I would not have done at this point. In any event, it had no effect on the symptoms. I would keep going back and focus on the magnitude of his weight loss and on some of the environmental issues that I asked about. When I am facing a weight loss question, I always wonder about caloric intake, and since I know that there are complicating social factors, I suspect that that is not normal.

> **Six weeks after the onset of night sweats, the patient had lost 15 pounds, and he consulted another physician. The same laboratory tests were again normal, as were thyroid tests; no evidence of malabsorption was found.**

The second doctor was similarly focused on the combination of night sweats and weight loss but could not find anything either. This is a fairly generic description of thyroid tests, and I would want to make sure a T_3 level was drawn because elderly patients with thyrotoxicosis occasionally have normal T_4 levels. Similarly, the physician focused on the question of a balance between intake and output as a cause of the weight loss. I imagine a D-xylose test or something like that was done here, and perhaps an examination for stool fat. So again, we are faced with someone still having a lot of sweats and who now has lost 15 pounds. I am back to wanting to know more about caloric intake, but in the back of my mind I am still quite concerned about all those sweats.

> **A physician observed the patient on two occasions during one of his "spells." The first, during the day, occurred in an air-conditioned environment. The patient was shivering and appeared cyanotic and vasoconstricted; he wore a towel around his neck to soak up the sweat. Vital signs were normal. The second observed episode occurred when the patient awoke in the morning. He was covered with a large number of blankets, and he and the bedclothes were drenched with sweat. He had no fever, and vital signs were again normal.**

I am now quite concerned about the magnitude of these sweating episodes. I do not think that something as simple as poor dietary intake from depression and a change in social situation can totally explain his illness. In the sequence of events described, he shivers, becomes vasoconstricted, and sweats. There is no fever and no change in blood pressure. It almost sounds as if intermittent dis-

charges of some substance into his bloodstream may be occurring. However, when I think of the things that make people either suddenly flush and sweat or suddenly vasoconstrict and sweat, I think of things that also affect the blood pressure—pheochromocytoma or tumors that liberate histamine or an adrenergic substance.

Despite the absence of vital sign changes, I am becoming increasingly concerned that this man has a mass lesion releasing a vasoactive substance that is causing the weight loss and other symptoms.

> **The patient continued to lose weight. After he had lost 20 pounds, more tests were done. Multiple cultures of blood and urine were sterile, CT scans of the chest and abdomen were negative, and CBC remained normal. Bone films showed a small lesion in the pelvis that was attributed to Paget disease.**

We are not making a tremendous amount of progress with this man. He has lost more weight and is continuing to go downhill. I agree with his physician's concern. Multiple blood cultures were done for evidence of some kind of subacute infectious process, such as endocarditis or salmonellosis. Those cultures were negative, as I would have expected in the presence of normal CBCs and sedimentation rates. It is quite surprising that this apparent degree of severe illness is not reflected in the patient's blood count or sedimentation rate. Despite a negative chest film on two separate occasions, the physicians continued to look for something in his chest, for reasons that are not clear.

Now we know that he has a lesion in the pelvis that is attributed to Paget disease. There are other lesions that are called Paget disease on bone films but that turn out not to be Paget disease after biopsy. I have had experience with some such cases. Certainly, one would want to pursue the abnormal bone film a little bit more. A bone scan should pick up both an inflammatory process and a Paget disease lesion, but perhaps not in the same way as if this was some kind of metastatic disease. We are told the lesion is in the pelvis, but it is not more specifically localized. The pelvis is a common site of Paget disease, as well as metastatic lesions, but it is not a usual site of infectious lesions.

Where could this man be hiding a tumor or an infectious process that might give him this combination of symptoms? The gastrointestinal tract comes to mind and has not yet been studied. I am moving further and further away from an inflammatory process and more and more toward a neoplasm that is consuming him metabolically, is releasing a vasoactive substance, and is related to the pelvic lesion. I will need to pursue that.

> The patient continued to have severe sweating spells and lost more weight. Total weight loss was 30 pounds. He was referred to a consultant in infectious diseases, who repeated many tests and still could find no explanation for the spells or weight loss.

The only additional information I am given here is that this subacute to chronic disease is not going away spontaneously but is continuing unabated. Again, there is less and less indication that he has an infectious or inflammatory disease.

> Concerned about the continued weight loss during the next 2 months and having no better idea what to do, the patient's physician prescribed amitriptyline, 50 mg daily.

This brings us back to some of the earlier discussion concerning the possible role of depression as a cause of the patient's weight loss. The physician has now made a second attempt at a therapeutic trial. However, I would not really be happy with a therapeutic trial until I knew more about his gastrointestinal tract and the lesion in his bone. I am disturbed by the sweats and the observed cyanosis. I would like to know more about the alkaline phosphatase and a couple of other blood chemistries, although I am told that all of his chemistries were normal. While I subscribe to therapeutic trials in patients who are not terribly ill, I think that this patient is continuing to do badly enough to contraindicate such action. But I can understand the physician's frustration in not being able to make a diagnosis. I would have pursued further testing before this therapeutic trial.

> Within 2 weeks the patient's sweats began to abate, and within 3 weeks his weight stabilized. One month later the patient's wife returned home, still paralyzed but less aphasic. The patient took over the responsibility for her total care. During the next 6 months, the pa-

> tient had few sweating episodes, and he began to regain his lost weight. He continued to take amitriptyline.

He appears now to be on the way back to good health. Two things have happened. One of them was a therapeutic trial of an antidepressant, and the other was an important change in his social situation. His wife is back home, and he now has some responsibility and reason for his existence. We need to remind ourselves that the psychosocial situation is of concern in patients of all ages but particularly so in adolescence and older age. This man went through an elaborate workup for an illness that appears to have turned out to be depression. I must say I am still a little bit concerned about what those "spells" were, but in view of the long-term follow-up, the other diagnostic possibilities seem increasingly less likely. If he did have a metastatic illness or an inflammatory process, one would not expect that this intervention would have gotten him better.

> His wife died. The patient continued to take amitriptyline for an additional 6 months and then discontinued it. He had regained all the weight he had lost. In the subsequent 10 years, he continued to be well. Neither the sweats nor the weight loss recurred.

I think that one of the major concerns of a physician is not to miss a diagnosis. One should constantly review the situation when pieces of data do not fit together terrifically well. In this case, I am reassured because the initial symptom complex did not recur and he continued to be well. The fact that his symptoms did not recur when he stopped taking amitriptyline after his wife's death implies that over time he adjusted to the social situation created when his wife had her stroke and that he was able to cope with her death.

Analysis

The symptoms manifested by this elderly gentleman usually are associated with organic disease, but in this case, they were caused by depression. Our discussant was increasingly suspicious that depression was the cause but was thrown off track by the striking description by a physician who observed the patient during two sweating episodes.

To make it possible for the reader to analyze this interesting derailment in clinical reasoning, we present our analysis of two elements of the problem-solving process: the hypotheses under consideration, and the discussant's assertions (i.e., his tentative conclusions) about each of those hypotheses.

The discussant weighed three major hypotheses: (1) an inflammatory process, (2) the combination of depression and decreased caloric intake, and (3) other serious, noninflammatory disorders, such as hyperthyroidism and tumors. We did not include every hypothesis raised by the discussant in these categories; we believe that such omissions are minor and do not contribute to the understanding of the diagnostic reasoning. Figure 20.2 shows both the hypotheses under consideration and the discussant's assertions about those hypotheses as he is given data. It is easy to follow the discussant's impression about each principal hypothesis from this array of assertions. The correlated curves represent the approximate strength of the discussant's conviction in each of the three diagnoses as those impressions changed with the information provided.

The discussant views the possibility that the patient has an inflammatory process as rather slight at first ("come to mind"), but after the third chunk of data it gains strength ("I'm thinking he has"). However, after the review of systems and laboratory tests are found to be unrevealing, an inflammatory process fades in interest ("would have expected some additional clues"), and it never regains prominence.

The discussant's tenacity with respect to the hypothesis that the patient was depressed and had been eating less undergoes far more striking changes. Initially he is only mildly interested in the hypothesis ("may in fact be"), but after he learns that routine studies, thyroid tests, and absorption studies are unrevealing, his interest in this hypothesis heightens ("wanting to know more about"). The next fragment of information, however, changes his opinion completely about depression and inadequate caloric intake. After the stark description of the patient's appearance during a sweating episode, the discussant declares that the psychosocial factors could not "totally explain his illness." Even after the antidepressant has had a salutary effect, the discussant is not totally convinced. He says that

it "appears to have turned out to be" depression. He becomes convinced that his diagnosis is correct only when the patient's recovery is sustained.

By contrast, the discussant's acceptance of the diagnosis of a noninflammatory, serious organic disorder is modest to begin with ("need to keep in the back of my mind," "concerned that he was in a hypermetabolic state"), and it increases dramatically after the striking description of the sweating episode ("I'm becoming increasingly concerned that this man has a mass lesion"). Later, when depression and poor diet become a more likely explanation, his acceptance of the hypothesis of a serious organic disease falls off. Although he "would have pursued further testing" and although he asserts that he remained "still a little bit concerned" about the possibility of an organic cause, he finally admits that such disorders are "increasingly less likely." Thus, a careful inspection of the transcript strongly suggests that the discussant was shunted from an on-target hypothesis to an incorrect (albeit plausible) one by a vivid description of the patient.

Why did the discussant err? We suspect that he, as well as the physicians caring for the patient, was tripped up by the availability heuristic. The concept of heuristic methods in problem solving is a valuable by-product of research in artificial intelligence. To solve a complex, ill-defined problem, as exemplified by diagnostic problems in medicine, methods must be used that limit the number of questions we need to ask and the number of tests we need to carry out. Those methods, called heuristics, use information about the nature and the structure of the problem domain (in our case, the specific diseases under consideration) to limit the search.

Heuristics have been defined variously as rules of thumb, strategies, tricks, or simplifications. Heuristic methods generally improve the efficiency of the problem-solving process, and they offer solutions that are "good enough most of the time."[27,28] Indeed, the occasional lapse in efficiency and accuracy of our clinical heuristics, which in turn produces cognitive errors, is the focus of our concern in the case presented here. Cognitive errors have been studied extensively by cognitive psychologists, but there are few descriptions in medicine.[28,56,109,286] Several heuristics have been identified, including those termed availability, representativeness, and anchoring: In another case we

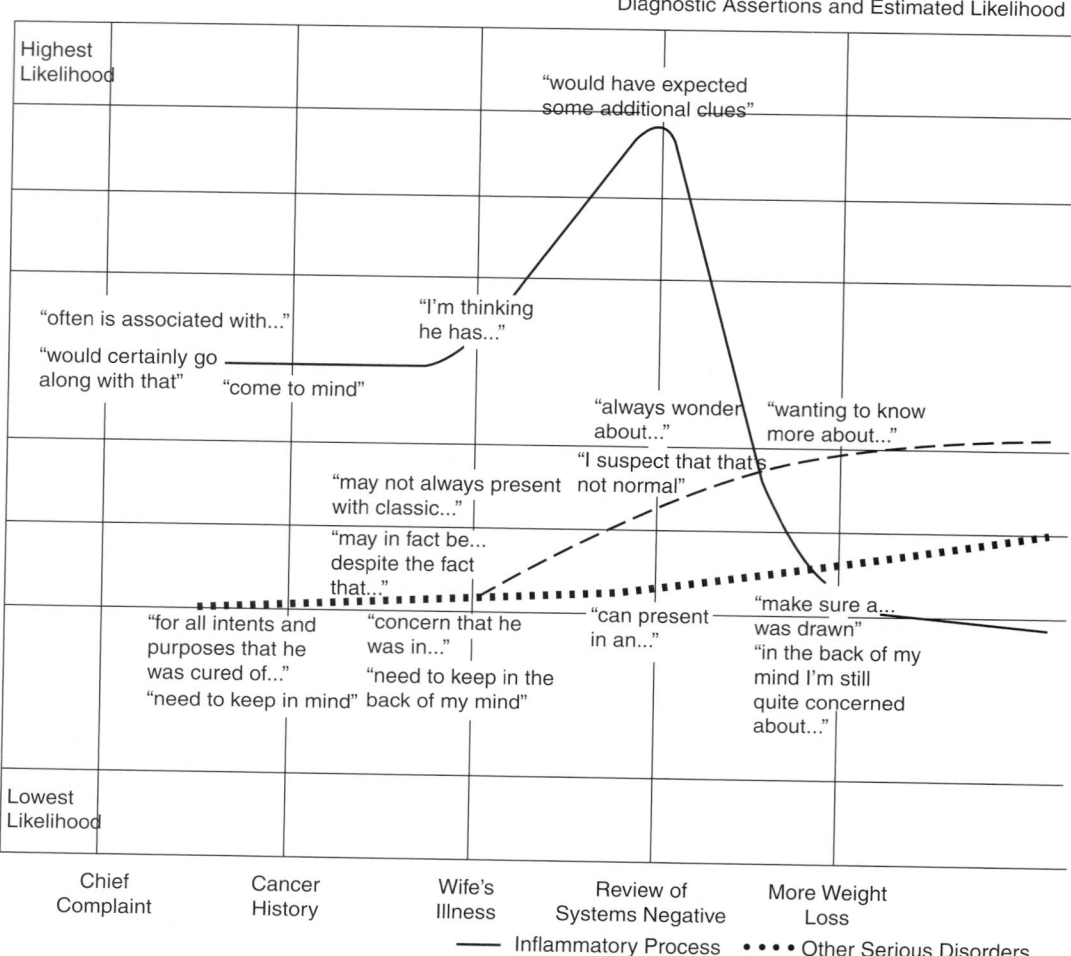

Figure 20.2 • An example of hypothesis revision in the case of an elderly man with weight loss and spells of sweating and shivering. The hypotheses under consideration were an inflammatory process (*solid line*), depression (*dashed line*), and other serious disorders such as a secreting tumor (*dotted line*). The figure shows sequential revision of these hypotheses as new information became available to a physician discussant. The ordinate describes the approximate likelihood of each of the three hypotheses. The sequential attributes of the patient's illness made available to the discussant are plotted on the abscissa. The assertions by the clinician/discussant are given in quotes. Note that initially depression was not even considered, but by the time all the information had been provided, it was the most likely diagnostic hypothesis. Note also the striking effect on the discussant's view of the likelihood of a secreting tumor after he learned about the striking character of the patient's "spells." Case 57. (*continued*)

describe a diagnostic error accountable to the representativeness heuristic (see case 23).

In the patient described here, we believe that the cognitive error can be accounted for primarily by the availability heuristic, which, used to judge frequency and probability, relies on the ease with which instances or occurrences can be brought to mind.[27,28,287] Because, as a general rule, frequent events are easier to recall or imagine than infrequent ones, availability is a valid approach for judging frequency.[27,28,287] But it is not infallible. In a classic illustration of an error attributed to the availability heuristic, subjects presented with a list containing equal numbers of males and

as Affected by Sequential Data Provided

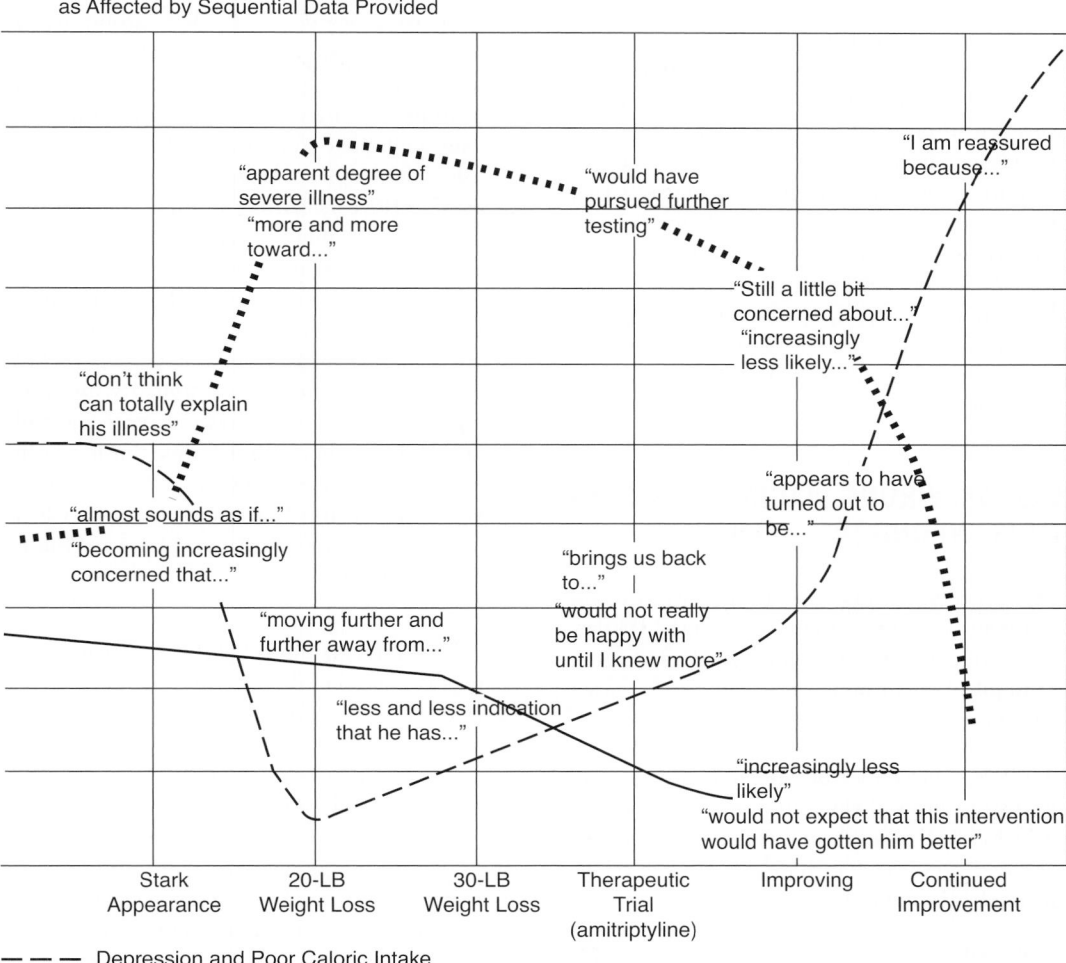

Figure 20.2 • (*Continued*)

females guessed that the list contained more of one sex when it contained a disproportionate number of famous persons of that sex.[27,28] In the case presented here, we believe that the ease with which a secretory tumor was brought to mind by a physician's vivid description of the patient produced the cognitive error.

Clearly, we must strive to avoid errors in judgment that delay or impair our capacity to make an accurate diagnosis. Observations suggest that it may be possible to minimize such errors if alternative outcomes are considered actively and if we pay increased attention to certain types of usually ignored data.[288] How can we make these recommendations in clinical practice?

Imagine first how a psychiatrist might have evaluated the patient presented here. Psychiatrists, of course, would be expected to establish an emotional disorder as the predominant hypothesis. Given that orientation, it seems quite likely that psychiatrists would have weighed far more heavily the recent history of a remarkable change in the patient's life and related it to depression. In addition, they would have delved more deeply into the patient's symptoms to assess whether additional manifestations were consistent with depression. How they would have accounted for the striking sweating episodes is uncertain. Nevertheless, they would have embarked, we suspect, on a far more directed, efficient diagnostic process.

We must learn from our mistakes. Perhaps next time we will enhance our sensitivity to the elderly patient who develops an unexplained illness after a traumatic personal experience, and we will consider the possibility of depression sooner when what seems to be a physical ailment fails to conform to a clear, well-recognized pattern. Perhaps next time we will dig deeper for signs of depression when we suspect it. Perhaps the courage of our convictions will be sufficient so that a single description of the patient will not be weighed inappropriately and throw us off the track.

Perhaps this process hones our expertise. Perhaps that is what is meant by "practice."

CASE 58. WRONG DIAGNOSIS, WRONG TESTS, WRONG TREATMENT

A nephrologist was asked to see a 61-year-old woman on her 13th hospital day. She had hematuria, impaired renal function, fever, confusion, and purple spots on her toes, which are shown in Figure 20.3.

This constellation of signs and symptoms suggests a diagnosis of vasculitis. Since the nephrologist was asked to see the patient on her 13th hospital day, I presume that those problems developed during her hospital stay.

The patient had been admitted to the hospital for increasing angina. On admission, her blood pressure was 150/90 mm Hg and her pulse was 72 per minute. She was obese, and

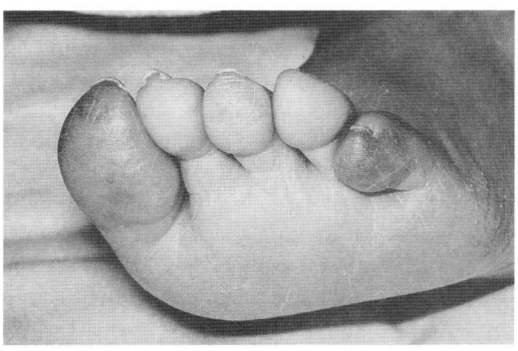

Figure 20.3 • Discoloration of toes; case 58.

bruits were heard over the left carotid artery and the mid-abdomen. Laboratory values were hemoglobin 11.8 g/dL, white cell count 12,200, creatinine 1.5 mg/dL, and BUN 7 mg/dL. The urine contained no protein, red cells, or white cells. The history disclosed that she had had a stroke 10 years earlier, multiple transient ischemic attacks thereafter, and a left carotid endarterectomy 1 year before this hospitalization. Five years after the stroke she had had a coronary artery bypass graft, and she had had persistent angina since. She was hypertensive, but her blood pressure was controlled with antihypertensive drugs. For several years, she had had headaches; her sedimentation rate had been persistently elevated, but temporal artery biopsy was not revealing. Members of her family had coronary and cerebrovascular disease and lupus erythematosus.

This information is helpful. The patient has extensive vascular disease. She has already experienced many complications of coronary and cerebrovascular disease, and the diffuse bruits on physical examination are evidence that vascular involvement is widespread.

The initial serum creatinine of 1.5 represents a modest decline in glomerular filtration rate for a woman of her age. On admission, however, her urinary sediment examination showed no evidence of an active process. I think we can infer that she started out with modest renal damage, possibly related to nephrosclerosis.

The history of headaches and a persistently elevated sedimentation rate and a family history of lupus suggest the possibility of an inflammatory vasculitis. Temporal arteritis was an appropriate diagnosis to consider, but temporal artery biopsy was negative. Although a negative result makes the diagnosis of temporal arteritis less likely, one should remember that biopsies can be negative in this disorder because of the "skip nature" of the pathologic findings. In other words, even in patients with documented temporal arteritis, some segments of the temporal arteries fail to show the classic findings on biopsy. The results of antinuclear antibody (ANA) and complement studies may be of interest. However, I would have difficulty integrating the appearance of hematuria and purple toes with temporal arteritis into a coherent diagnosis with inflammatory vasculitis as the underlying theme.

If I had to choose a dominant diagnostic theme now, it would be cholesterol embolization. The manifestations of atheroembolism can be protean; they depend on the distribution of the atherosclerotic lesions and the nature of any invasive procedures performed on the patient. If there is significant carotid disease with ulcerated plaques, cholesterol emboli can travel to the eyes and produce transient visual changes. Examination of the fundus in such patients can be diagnostic: Bright orange collections of cholesterol crystals sometimes are seen, frequently lodged at the bifurcations of arterioles. If you tap on the eye, you can often knock the embolus loose. Cholesterol emboli also can cause transient ischemic episodes. Occasionally, atheroembolism causes pancreatitis or ischemic disease of the bowel with guaiac-positive stools. Emboli also can lodge in the arms, legs, or skin. It is worth noting that on occasion the process of cholesterol embolization can be precipitated by anticoagulation.

Renal insufficiency frequently occurs, sometimes accompanied by flank pain and hematuria. The renal manifestations probably are a function of the size of the emboli. If the emboli are large enough to occlude major branches of the renal artery, segmental renal infarction with flank pain and hematuria result. If the emboli consist only of cholesterol crystals that partially occlude renal arterioles, renal ischemia results. In such patients, hypertension and renal insufficiency are the predominant manifestations; hematuria often is absent. If the emboli reach the small vessels, kidney biopsy will show characteristic clefts: The cholesterol that previously inhabited the clefts is dissolved out in the fixation process.

Although atheroembolism is the most attractive diagnosis, we should keep an open mind. Hypersensitivity vasculitis remains a possibility. Other disorders, such as urinary tract obstruction and drug-induced renal disease, can produce both hematuria and decreased renal function.

> On the patient's second hospital day, cardiac catheterization was carried out. During the procedure, the patient became hysterical and was found to have a blood pressure of 250/130 mm Hg and a pulse of 200 per minute. Her blood pressure was quickly brought under control and her pulse fell, but the patient remained confused and agitated. There were no focal neurologic signs. On the third hospital day, the patient's level of alertness was variable. Her left hand was noted to be cyanotic. Her temperature was 38.8°C; her white cell count was 36,600 with 12% bands. Sedimentation rate was 129 mm/hr. The urine was grossly bloody; it contained 2+ protein and many RBCs and WBCs per high-power field. Creatinine was 1.4 mg/dL; BUN was 17 mg/dL.

A severe hypertensive response during cardiac catheterization is a rare event. It can result from dissection of the aorta or renal artery by the catheter. It also can result from renal atheroembolism: The emboli partially obstruct flow to the juxtaglomerular apparatus and activate the renin–angiotensin system. All of the findings are consistent with atheroembolism, including the central nervous system manifestations, cyanosis of the hand, and hypertension. Leukocytosis is probably indicative of segmental renal infarction, and the blood in the urine is consistent with that interpretation. It is surprising that kidney function was not impaired.

> On the fourth hospital day, her mental status remained unchanged. A neurologist found no focal signs and made a diagnosis of "acute encephalopathy" but appended a long differential diagnosis. The left hand remained blue. A rheumatologist suggested ordering the following tests: assays for C_3, C_4, CH_{50}, anti-DNA antibodies, hepatitis B surface antigen (HBsAg), and cryoglobulins. The treatment he recommended—methylprednisolone (100 mg per day) and cyclophosphamide (100 mg per day)—was initiated.

The rheumatologist obviously was willing to treat empirically for vasculitis with immunosuppressive and anti-inflammatory agents. I would not have given those drugs without stronger evidence for an inflammatory process because the treatment has substantial potential risk. I suspect that too much weight was given to the sedimentation

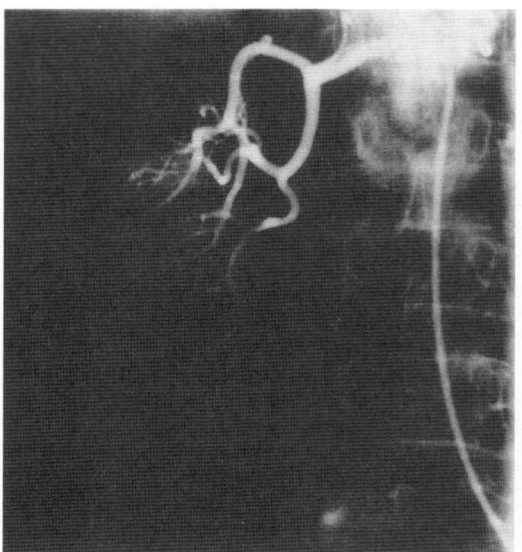

Figure 20.4 • Renal arteriogram; case 58.

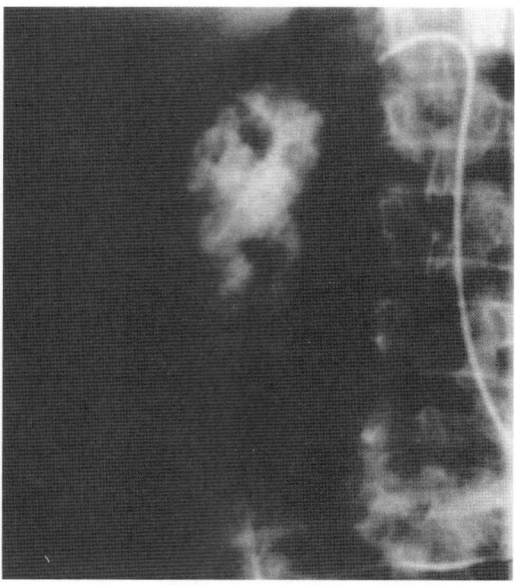

Figure 20.5 • Renal arteriogram, postinjection phase; case 58.

rate. I still think the patient has cholesterol embolism to the brain and kidneys and probably has extensive but asymptomatic embolism in other organs as well.

> On day 5 the creatinine was 2.1 mg/dL, BUN was 56 mg/dL, and the urinary sediment continued to show red cells, too numerous to count. A renal arteriogram was performed for diagnostic purposes. The arterial and parenchymal phases are shown in Figures 20.4 and 20.5.

I assume that the arteriogram was done in the expectation of finding renal arterial aneurysms, thereby hoping to confirm a diagnosis of polyarteritis nodosa. Obviously, I would not have done that test—first, because I think that diagnosis is unlikely; and second, because I believe the patient had atheroembolism. The strong possibility of atheroembolism is a particularly compelling reason not to do further arterial studies. Her aorta must be full of friable, loose, ulcerated atheromas that can be fragmented by stiff catheters, thus risking acceleration of the embolic process.

The study shows patchy ischemia of both kidneys with marked attenuation of distal renal arteries. Given this patchy cortical filling, my suspicion of atheroembolism is further enhanced.

> On day 6, both legs and feet appeared mottled, and the toes took on their purple appearance. CT scan of the brain showed a left occipital infarction. Between days 7 and 13, the encephalopathy persisted, and the mottled appearance of the left hand and both feet remained unchanged. Hematuria also persisted; creatinine ranged between 1.9 and 2.1 mg/dL.

I am even more confident that the patient has widespread atheroembolism now that we know that the vessels of both her brain and legs are affected. I am less clear about whether she had a single shower of emboli initiated by the cardiac catheterization, a second shower of emboli from the renal arteriogram, or multiple episodes of embolism. The history strongly suggests two independent episodes. It is reasonable to assume that the confusion and hypertension resulted from cerebral and renal emboli secondary to the cardiac catheterization because both manifestations followed shortly after this procedure and both the CT scan of the head and the renal arteriogram showed evidence of blocked arteries. The legs were not apparently involved before the renal arteriography, but afterward the classic picture of livedo

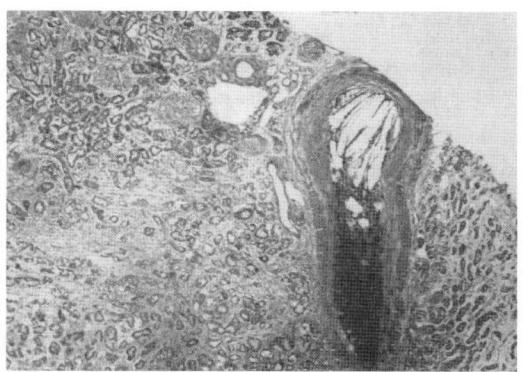

Figure 20.6 • Renal biopsy; case 58.

reticularis evolved, and the toes became blue. The kidneys appear to have suffered from both procedures. Serum creatinine increased only after the renal arteriogram—but because progressive decline of renal function can occur after even a single shower of emboli, the deterioration in renal function could have resulted from the first procedure, the second one, or both.

> A kidney biopsy, shown in Figure 20.6, was carried out.

I do not think a biopsy was needed, because the case is such a classic. Nonetheless, what we see here are cholesterol emboli. The vessels are nearly or totally occluded by crystals, debris, and a reactive endothelial proliferation. This is a case in which a serious error was made at the beginning. When I heard the initial constellation of symptoms, I also thought of vasculitis. When I heard more history, however, I reconsidered my initial presumption. Although vasculitis was still a possibility, in a patient with angina, a stroke at the age of 51 years, diffuse bruits, and a family history of vascular disease, cholesterol embolization immediately came to mind.

> Outcome: Methylprednisolone and cyclophosphamide were discontinued. One month later the patient remained confused. Her skin lesions were slowly resolving. Creatinine was 1.8 mg/dL. The patient's mental function declined progressively, and she died 3 months after discharge.

Analysis

This problem-solving exercise provides a rare opportunity to trace the evolution of an inappropriate diagnostic and therapeutic course that had a fatal outcome. Simultaneously, we can observe the reasoning of our discussant, not only as he proceeds correctly but also as he criticizes the actions of those who took the wrong path.

As the discussant asserts, an important error was made at the start. Although the physicians involved in the patient's care correctly identified the system involved (arteries and arterioles), they mistakenly assumed that the vascular involvement was an inflammatory one. That assumption led them to treat the patient with a drug regimen that had no potential benefit and was, at the same time, potentially harmful. It also led them to perform renal arteriography, which our discussant correctly assumed was done in an effort to identify renal aneurysms. Given the final diagnosis, the test was of no value and almost certainly contributed to later morbidity.

Although some of the early findings (multisystem involvement and a high sedimentation rate) were consistent with vasculitis, other manifestations were not explained by this diagnosis. In particular, it was not reasonable to attribute the sudden change in clinical manifestations after cardiac catheterization to vasculitis; at that point, the correct diagnosis should have surfaced. Indeed, it is an excellent general principle that any sudden, unexplained change in the clinical course of a hospitalized patient should raise the possibility of an iatrogenic complication.[289] Drugs and diagnostic procedures are most frequently at fault.

Why the striking discrepancy between the incorrect approach that contributed to the patient's death and the skillful approach of our discussant? Our discussant is a nephrologist who is intimately familiar with the syndrome of catheter-induced atheroembolism. Although vasculitis was his first diagnostic choice, he quickly abandoned that hypothesis when the history disclosed extensive vascular involvement by atherosclerosis and posited the correct interpretation. Familiarity with the features of diagnostic entities clearly is an essential ingredient of the diagnostic process. Those clinical features serve not only to trigger a diagnostic hypothesis, but also are essential to the confirmation of such hypotheses. Clinicians presumably remember complex patterns of diseases and syndromes against which they match the findings in an individual patient.[162] In the patient discussed here, every subsequent manifestation in her clinical course apparently matched the pattern of atheroembolic disease conceptualized by the discussant, and he became convinced that his diagnosis was correct—so convinced, in fact, that he considered the final proof (kidney biopsy) unnecessary.

This discussion provides an example of how the quality of medical care can be assessed by a prospective approach. Most attempts to determine the quality of care have centered on measuring the number of tests or treatments given to a patient or on medical outcomes in patient populations. In this instance, our discussant judged the quality of the medical decisions prospectively and repeatedly. He first disagreed with the diagnosis of vasculitis (the most serious error because it led to multiple errors) and criticized the decision to treat with steroids and cyclophosphamide. Later, he criticized the decision to do renal arteriography and the renal biopsy. Here, an expert is reviewing the quality of decisions as they were made rather than after the fact. The value of that approach as a tool for assessing the quality of medical decision making is clearly evident. Indeed, the discussant could have commented on other decisions but did not. For example: Was coronary arteriography indicated? Was a renal arteriogram an appropriate test, given that polyarteritis nodosa was strongly suspected? This format deserves study not only as a tool for determining the quality of clinical decisions, but also for teaching decision making to students and house officers.

CASE 59. RECONSIDERING FAILURES OF THERAPY

A 59-year-old woman office manager was seen by a gastroenterologist in his office for severe abdominal pain (9/10) and a 60-pound weight loss. She had a history of hypertension and migraine headaches, and had a coronary angioplasty 22 months ago. She was known to have bilateral carotid bruits. She had smoked 1/2 pack of cigarettes per day for many years but did not use alcohol. Fifteen months ago, she was treated for abdominal pain and severe regurgitation with H_2-blockers, but these drugs failed to relieve the symptoms. She began losing weight. One of her sons and one of his sons have celiac disease, and though the patient complained of constipation and no diarrhea, celiac disease was suspected. After a duodenal biopsy done 12 months ago showed "mild villous blunting and nonspecific chronic inflammation," she began following a gluten-free diet, but her weight loss continued.

Six months ago, she was subjected to a fundoplication procedure for her regurgitation. It also failed to relieve her symptoms, and her weight loss continued. She began having upper abdominal pain and flank pain. Several observers noted that the abdominal pain was particularly prominent after eating. When seen, she was complaining of diffuse abdominal pain that was aggravated by eating, moving, and lying down. She had been anorexic and had associated nausea and constipation. She appeared emaciated and pale.

Blood pressure was 138/78 mm Hg; pulse was 68 per minute. Bilateral carotid bruits were present, left louder than right. Radial and pedal pulses were diminished. The digits appeared normal. The remainder of the examination was unremarkable. Except for a BUN of 31 mg/dL, the rest of her laboratory studies were within normal limits. A CT angiogram demonstrated severe stenosis of the superior and inferior mesenteric arteries and moderate to severe stenosis of the celiac trunk.

After a period of hydration and total parenteral nutrition, a bypass graft was inserted between the left iliac artery and the superior mesenteric artery. She recovered uneventfully from surgery and gradually lost her abdominal pain. On follow-up 6 months postoperatively, she was eating normally, had no abdominal pain or reflux symptoms, and had gained 25 pounds.

Analysis

In retrospect, the diagnosis of mesenteric ischemia seems so obvious. The patient not only had classic symptoms, namely pain after eating (a form of abdominal angina), but also readily available evidence of severe vascular disease, including a history of coronary disease, carotid bruits, and reduced peripheral pulses. We might speculate why this obvious diagnosis was missed for two years (did her physicians fail to examine her pulses? did they forget about her coronary disease and bruits?), but instead we will focus on two other examples of diagnostic errors, namely failure of a therapeutic trial.

Once a tentative diagnosis is established, it should be subjected to a simple evaluation: Are all the patient's manifestations explained by the diagnosis? Are all the positive and negative findings consistent with the diagnosis? That is, is the diagnosis sufficient to explain the patient's illness? Often these questions are supplemented by a test of treatment. If a specific treatment is available for a condition and the treatment improves the patient's symptoms, this response provides further support that the diagnosis is correct. If, however, such a treatment is applied and fails to improve symptoms, the diagnosis should come under suspicion. In essence, the test of therapy becomes just another diagnostic test.

In the instance, we have two such tests of therapy: H_2-blockers and fundoplication for gastroesophageal reflux disease (GERD), and a gluten-free diet for celiac disease. Both failed. GERD was an appropriate diagnosis, given the patient's initial symptoms, but failure of treatment should have triggered the suspicion that some other condition was at play. Despite the family history, celiac disease seemed an unlikely cause of the patient's manifestations, especially because it is usually accompanied by diarrhea, not constipation. When the diet failed to improve the patient, it too should have been a sign that the physicians were barking up the wrong tree.

What should a physician do when a tentative diagnosis no longer becomes tenable and the patient continues to suffer? Needless to say, the answer is: Look for one or more diagnoses that might be. In the case of this patient, a thorough look at the patient's record might have revealed the history of vascular disease, a carefully taken history would have turned up the classical pain pattern, and a careful examination would have demonstrated diminished pulses. Fortunately, one observer did put all this information together, made the correct diagnosis, and probably saved the patient's life.

It goes without saying that optimal diagnosis requires getting all the relevant information and a careful physical examination, but when tests of treatment fail, it is time to go back to the drawing board. Start from scratch. Scour the old records, talk to the patient, check her pulses.

CASE 60: THE CHEETAH AND THE SNAIL

A 35-year-old, previously healthy male presented with an 8-month history of vague abdominal discomfort, fatigue, malaise and a 40-pound weight loss.

In a patient with these kinds of constitutional symptoms, the differential diagnosis is quite broad, but in a 35-year-old, a malignancy would be less likely, although it cannot be excluded. Given the longstanding presentation, I think more of chronic diseases such as collagen vascular disorders and endocrine disorders. The history raises the question of adrenal insufficiency, which can present with vague abdominal discomfort with fatigue and malaise. The degree of weight loss strikes me as a little extreme but could be seen with severe adrenal insufficiency. There are no specific collagen vascular disorders that jump to mind, although I guess polyarteritis nodosa among the vasculitides should be considered. Rare disorders such as familial Mediterranean fever can cause chronic, hard-to-diagnosis abdominal discomfort. Chronic infections could also be possible but are less likely. I still think that given his age, malignancy should be further down the list.

Eight months prior to admission the patient noticed vague periumbilical discomfort, worse in the morning and sometimes associated with halitosis. He also had mild fatigue, dizziness, lack of appetite, and mild nausea with motion. At that time, his physical examination was unremarkable. Laboratory studies showed a low white cell count and mild transaminitis. He was not anemic, and his T_4 level was 5.3 pmol/L (normal 4–12 pmol/L). He was given a diagnosis of functional dyspepsia and was prescribed an H_2-blocker with relief of his abdominal discomfort.

The additional history is still relatively nonspecific. The vague periumbilical discomfort and other symptoms do not point me in any one direction. The dizziness makes me wonder if the patient had some mild orthostasis. I am not surprised that the physical examination is normal, given the presenting symptoms. The low white count is interesting. HIV-related disease must always be considered in situations like this. I would be interested in his CD 4 count to see if he is at risk for opportunistic infections. The mild transaminitis is not helpful to me since it is so nonspecific. He does not appear to have hypothyroidism, although I would like to see a TSH (thyroid-stimulating hormone) to be sure of that. At this point, the treatment with an H_2-blocker seems reasonable, and I see no need for further aggressive workup at this time.

> The malaise, fatigue, anorexia, and excessive eructation persisted, and 4 months before admission his gastrointestinal discomfort recurred. Additional negative studies included HIV, CMV, and Epstein-Barr virus (EBV) antibody titers. After recurrence of symptoms despite the H_2-blocker, switching to a proton-pump inhibitor had no effect. He began to notice weight loss.

If he had longstanding HIV infection, the HIV antibody test should have been positive. Since I did not think he had acute HIV infection, the negative test should allow us to eliminate HIV from the differential. The negative CMV and EBV titers are helpful in this patient, who could have had a mononucleosis-like syndrome that can be associated with mild transaminitis. I am not surprised that the omeprazole did not help. The weight loss raises the concern for significant underlying pathology. With the vague abdominal discomfort, we should consider things like inflammatory bowel disease, more likely Crohn disease than ulcerative colitis since the latter is more likely to have diarrhea and bloody stools. I do not think he has chronic pancreatitis. The weight loss makes irritable bowel syndrome much less likely. The eructation makes me think of something like gastroparesis, but I have not heard about things like early satiety, which could go along with it. I would be interested in more laboratory data, especially a cortisol level since adrenal insufficiency is my leading diagnosis at present. CT imaging of the

abdomen is unlikely to be helpful unless he has an underlying malignancy or some process such as lymphoma, which would be associated with lymphadenopathy.

> Seven weeks before admission he saw another physician, who obtained the same history. The patient had begun to notice some tingling of his legs and arms, especially when in bed. He had always preferred warm weather but began to notice an extreme sensitivity to cold. He denied fevers. He stated he had no interest in eating and felt his memory was slipping. He was taking no medications. He did not smoke and denied alcohol excess. The patient had begun to lose time at work and was unable to perform his normal leisure time activities. He denied marital problems or depression. In fact, he had seen a psychologist for an opinion as to whether the symptoms were psychological in origin. He just wanted his problem "to be fixed." Family history was positive for a father with hypothyroidism and a sister with a congenital heart lesion.

The additional history is interesting. The tingling makes me think of a peripheral neuropathy. I would like to know more about the distribution of these symptoms. Were they stocking glove in distribution? Diabetes does not seem likely to me, given the rest of the picture. New-onset diabetes should not be associated with a neuropathy. Could he have B_{12} deficiency, which can be associated with Crohn disease due to involvement of the terminal ileum? Could he have some cervical spine process leading to a myelopathy of some sort since he appears to have a bilateral process involving both the arms and the legs? I have a hard time tying that idea with his abdominal symptoms. The sensitivity to cold raises the question of hypothyroidism again. Could he have cryoglobulinemia presenting with some neuropathic manifestations? The memory problems are consistent with B_{12} deficiency. This illness appears to be having a major impact on the patient's life, including his job, which makes a functional disorder much less likely. The father's hypothyroidism may indicate that the patient is at greater risk for some autoimmune conditions.

> His physical examination at that time was described as normal. His abdominal examination

was benign, with no organomegaly or tenderness. The physician was not sure of the cause of this chronic illness. He postulated a metabolic illness, a depressed cardiac output from a cardiomyopathy of some sort, an internal malignancy of the abdomen, or a lymphoma.

At this point, my top considerations would be inflammatory bowel disease or adrenal insufficiency. One rare disorder that can present with abdominal symptoms is acute intermittent porphyria. We really do not have a history suggestive of episodic symptoms. I still think malignancy is less likely because of the age. Hypothyroidism is not usually associated with weight loss. Apathetic hyperthyroidism can present with fatigue and weight loss, but that is usually a disease of the elderly.

Laboratory studies were as follows: WBC 4,700 with 62 polys, 28 lymphs, 4 monos and, 2 eos; hematocrit 48% with an MCV of 88. Sedimentation rate 5 mm/hr. Sodium 133 mEq/L, potassium 4.7 mEq/L, chloride 91 mEq/L, and total CO_2 26 mEq/L. Serum glucose 78 mg/dL. BUN 15 mg/dL, creatinine 2.0 mg/dL. Bilirubin 1.1 mg/dL, alkaline phosphatase 91 IU/L, AST 91 IU/L (normal 15–46), ALT 87 IU/L (normal 7–56), and gamma-glutamyltranspeptidase (GGT) 23 IU/L (normal 8–78). Calcium 9.6 mg/dL, phosphorus 4.1 mg/dL. Uric acid 6.3 mg/dL. Cholesterol 402 mg/dL. T_4 less than 1.17 pmol/L (normal 4–12), TSH greater than 50 μU/mL. An abdominal CT scan was normal.

The laboratory studies are helpful. The normal white cell count is not surprising to me. The patient does not have an anemia of chronic disease. The normal sedimentation rate indicates the patient is unlikely to have a significant inflammatory disease. The slightly low sodium level may be due to a mild degree of volume depletion, although the physical examination did not document that. Diabetes seems to be ruled out. The slightly elevated creatinine with the markedly elevated cholesterol makes me wonder about an underlying nephrotic syndrome. A mixed nephritic/nephrotic syndrome is more likely to present with an elevated creatinine. Of course, the cholesterol could be due to an unrelated process. The patient now has developed definite hypothyroidism. He may

have had an elevated TSH earlier, but it had not been checked. The patient likely has a predisposition to autoimmune disorders. I do not think that hypothyroidism explains the whole picture. It is not usually associated with weight loss but rather weight gain. Abdominal pain is not usually present. Could the patient have a pituitary process contributing to multiple endocrine disorders by way of compression? If so, then he would have to have a TSH-producing pituitary tumor with associated adrenal insufficiency from the mass effect of the tumor. I would be interested in seeing whether or not the patient had any hyperpigmentation that would help us to distinguish between primary and secondary adrenal insufficiency.

A diagnosis of severe hypothyroidism was made, and the patient was started on levothyroxine. Over the next 6 weeks as his TSH was falling, the patient felt progressively tired and anorectic. His abdominal discomfort increased, and his weight loss accelerated (to a total of 40 pounds over the course of his illness, from 210 to 170 pounds). In the week before admission, he developed frequent nausea, vomiting, and poor oral intake. When he was first seen he appeared chronically ill, and his systolic blood pressure was 70 mm Hg. He was given intravenous saline and admitted to the hospital.

The treatment of the hypothyroidism was generally appropriate, but in this patient, in whom we are considering adrenal insufficiency, the thyroid replacement could have caused more harm to the patient. Increasing his metabolic demands with thyroid replacement can exacerbate the adrenal insufficiency and cause a crisis. The increasing fatigue, weight loss acceleration, and increase in his abdominal discomfort are compatible with adrenal insufficiency. This patient may have a poly autoimmune endocrine disorder, which needs further testing, especially with a cortisol level and an adrenocorticotropic hormone (ACTH) stimulation test. I am concerned that he is presenting with an adrenal crisis. I want to know if his glucose is low, if his potassium is high, or if his sodium is lower.

He had a sallow complexion. His blood pressure was 90/60 mm Hg supine and 85/60 mm Hg standing. Pulse was 85 per minute supine, rising to 100 per minute on standing. He was afebrile. Other than evidence of chronic weight loss, his physical examination was unremarkable. No skin lesions were noted. There was no lymphadenopathy. The abdomen was benign, with no tenderness or organomegaly. Rectal examination was normal.

His blood pressure does not meet the strict criteria for orthostatic hypotension, which is usually associated with a greater drop in blood pressure and rise in pulse rate. Nonetheless, I would give him fluid replacement. The physical findings are compatible with an endocrine disorder. Crohn disease has fallen down on my list.

Laboratory studies: white cell count 4,500 with 50 polys, 42 lymphs, 6 monos, 2 eos. Hematocrit 47%. Platelet count normal. Sodium 133 mEq/L, potassium 5.6 mEq/L, chloride 100 mEq/L, and total CO_2 23 mEq/L. BUN 25 mg/dL and creatinine 1.4 mg/dL; glucose 53 mg/dL. Serum albumin 4.3 gm/dL. Bilirubin 1.5 mg/dL, alkaline phosphatase 55 IU/L, AST 44 IU/L, ALT 50 IU/L. Free thyroxine index 8.0 (normal) and TSH 17.0 μU/mL. Chest x-ray and electrocardiogram were normal.

The laboratory findings of hyponatremia, hyperkalemia, and the low sugar are all compatible with adrenal insufficiency, probably on a primary basis. The abnormal enzymes bring to mind the possibility of an underlying myopathy from the endocrine dysfunction. We cannot say for sure whether the enzyme elevations are due to liver or muscle pathology. The TSH is improving, suggesting that his hypothyroidism is being treated and the patient is closer to being euthyroid.

Morning cortisol levels before and after administration of synthetic ACTH were undetectable. Adrenal insufficiency was finally diagnosed (in addition to his hypothyroidism), probably on an autoimmune basis. Replacement steroid therapy was added to his levothyroxine. He improved and was discharged.

Analysis

What is so different about this discussant's transcript from almost all the others in this book? If the

reader has not identified its uniqueness, it is worth explaining in some detail. First, in contrast to the nearly disastrous diagnostic strategy of the physicians caring for the patient, in whom they nearly missed the diagnosis of Addison disease entirely, the discussant not only jumped on the diagnosis immediately, but also mentioned it repeatedly until tests proved him right. We should give the physicians caring for the patient the benefit of the doubt: Although the patient's clinical manifestations were quite characteristic for Addison disease, the disease is rare and difficult to diagnose.

However, there is a second, even more convincing explanation for the seemingly "eagle eye" approach of the discussant. In contrast to the physicians caring for the patient, who extracted one element of the history, one element of the physical examination, and one laboratory test at a time, our discussant was given a compiled summary of the patient's clinical course. In one fell swoop, he learned that the patient had an extended history of abdominal discomfort, fatigue, and extensive weight loss. This combination of findings led him to suspect the disease from the beginning.

There are important lessons in this exercise. The first is that when patients present difficult diagnostic dilemmas, it is useful to summarize the observations to date: Such summaries often trigger diagnostic possibilities hitherto unconsidered. Indeed, in such cases, other common conditions have often been "ruled out," thereby increasing the likelihood of other, often rarer causes. Second, we should appreciate that how case material is constructed for purposes of teaching clinical reasoning can profoundly influence the reasoning processes. Multiple compiled cues, as in this instance, provide a far richer context than extracting information piecemeal from a patient.[39] The former is much more analogous to the approach applied when one physician "presents a case" to another physician, the latter is more analogous to an Emergency Department, private office, or clinic first encounter with a patient. In the latter instance, because uncertainty is maximized, the task is simply more difficult.

From a teaching standpoint, neither approach is better, just different. However, when we construct didactic cases, we should do so with awareness of the pedagogic goal.

CASE 61. A COLLECTION OF COGNITIVE DIAGNOSTIC ERRORS

Twenty years ago, we published a classification of cognitive diagnostic errors based on the aspects of the diagnostic process in which the error occurred. As we selected cases for the second edition of this book, we often included cases with cognitive errors, in the belief that demonstrating such errors and pointing out how they occurred would offer special insights into their identification and possibly to their prevention. Of the 41 cases with cognitive errors in the second edition, 17 are holdovers from the former analysis.[77]

As we repeated the task with the cases in this edition, we found again that most cases contained more than one cognitive error, but experience has shown that the decisions about where in the process of diagnosis the errors occurred are not clear-cut. Although all three of the authors agreed on the classification (Table 20.1), we concede that others might have a different interpretation than ours, and we welcome such interpretations. We have made similar, somewhat arbitrary judgments about the consequences of the errors. There is yet no scientific basis for these decisions, but that does not mean that errors should go unclassified.

We also make no claim about the frequency of such errors or about the overall importance of cognitive errors in diagnosis among all diagnostic errors in doctors' offices and in hospitals. Although this issue is important, our goal is pedagogic, not administrative.

The rationale for using the clinical cases to analyze errors is described elsewhere,[77] and we will not repeat it here. However, based on the errors identified in these cases, it is possible to provide striking examples of errors and their influence on individual patients. None of the following examples are taken from previous work.[77]

Triggering Error

A 40-year-old woman (see case 12) who had never smoked had a 2-day history of dyspnea and was admitted to the hospital gasping for breath and breathing at a rate of 40 per minute. Examination of her lungs and chest x-ray disclosed no abnormalities, and despite high concentrations of inspired oxygen, she remained severely hypoxic and required intubation. After a period of slight improvement, the ventilation tube was removed, but within an hour, she had to be reintubated. The correct diagnosis—myasthenia gravis—was triggered subsequently, only after the patient developed bilateral ptosis. Multiple clinical clues to the correct diagnosis had been missed.

Context Error

A 35-year-old man (see case 60) presented with an 8-month history of vague abdominal discomfort and weight loss. His examination and routine tests were unremarkable. Initially he was treated for gastrointestinal reflux. After studies showed that he was hypothyroid, he was given thyroid replacement, but he continued to have abdominal discomfort and lost more weight (the cumulative deficit was 40 pounds). On readmission he was hypotensive, hyponatremic, hyperkalemic, and hypoglycemic, and finally a diagnosis of adrenal insufficiency was made. In retrospect, he probably had adrenal insufficiency from the beginning, but the diagnostic contexts were gastrointestinal disease and thyroid disease.

Error in Data Interpretation

A 59-year-old man (see case 23) with longstanding hypertension was evaluated by his physician for a possible diagnosis of pheochromocytoma when the patient's blood pressure reached a sustained level of 180/120 mm Hg. A measurement of vanillylmandelic acid (VMA) excretion was twice the upper limit of normal, and despite subsequent normal values for excretion of metanephrines and catecholamines, he was started on phenoxybenzamine. Additional diagnostic studies, including measurements of epinephrine, norepinephrine, and dopamine and an abdominal CT scan, were carried out and were normal. The final conclusion was that the first measurement of VMA was a false positive. In this instance, overinterpretation of a diagnostic test led to excessive and unnecessary testing and inappropriate treatment. Fortunately, the treatment caused no harm.

Error in Estimation of Prevalence

A 5 1/2-year-old boy (see case 19) developed malaise, headache, abdominal pain, and shortness of breath after returning from a vacation in the Smoky

TABLE 20.1

Summary of Cognitive Errors in the Cases

| Case | Hypothesis Generation | | Refinement | | | Testing: Test Interpretation | Causal Model |
	Trigger	Context	Data Interpretation	Estimated Prevalence	Faulty Threshold		
3	✓	✓					✓
5	✓						
6	✓		✓				
7		✓					
8		✓			✓		
9		✓				✓	
12	✓	✓					
13			✓				
16							
17							
18	✓	✓					
19				✓			
21						✓	
22	✓						
23				✓		✓	
24		✓	✓				
26			✓			✓	
27		✓	✓	✓			
29			✓				
31			✓				✓
35							✓
36			✓				✓
39							
43			✓				
44	✓						
48			✓				
51						✓	
52							
53							
54	✓	✓	✓				
55	✓						
56			✓				✓
57		✓		✓			
58	✓		✓				✓
59	✓	✓	✓				✓
60		✓	✓				
63	✓						
64	✓	✓					✓
65	✓						
66							

(continued)

TABLE 20.1

(Continued)

Case	Verification	Axiom	No Fault	Diagnostic Delay	Unnecessary/Excessive Testing	Delay in Treatment	Inappropriate Treatment	Risky Consequences
3				✓	✓			
5	✓		✓	✓				✓
6				✓			✓	
7				✓				✓
8				✓		✓		
9				✓	✓			
12				✓			✓	✓
13						✓		
16		✓						
17	✓			✓				
18				✓				✓
19			✓					
21			✓					
22			✓	✓	✓			
23					✓			
24					✓			
26								
27								✓
29					✓			
31				✓				
35				✓			✓	
36								
39	✓					✓		
43	✓						✓	✓
44				✓	✓			
48								
51							✓	
52	✓							
53	✓				✓		✓	
54	✓							
55			✓					
56	✓			✓		✓	✓	
57					✓	✓		
58	✓						✓	
59				✓	✓		✓	
60				✓				
63				✓				
64								
65			✓					
66	✓					✓		

Mountains in Tennessee. His parents, both physicians, recalled removing a tick from his scalp during their vacation, and given their experience with Rocky Mountain spotted fever in an endemic area during their house staff training, were concerned that the child might have this disease. Discussions were held about giving the child a risky antibiotic, but fortunately it was discovered that no cases of the disease had been seen in the Smoky Mountains for years. No antibiotic was given, and the child recovered uneventfully.

Error in Causal Attribution

A 59-year-old woman (see case 59) with severe abdominal pain and weight loss was treated for sprue, which she did not have, and fundoplication for gastroesophageal reflux before the correct diagnosis was made, namely mesenteric ischemia. There were two errors in causal attribution. Both were the assumptions that her symptoms could be explained by two conditions despite deficiencies in evidence for either as the cause of her symptoms. Ignoring findings of overt vascular disease was another error.

Error in Verification (Premature Closure)

A 31-year-old man (see case 56) admitted to the hospital for a liver transplant had a previous extensive medical evaluation. He had been previously been jaundiced and had been diagnosed with hepatitis A and B and subsequently developed ascites and peripheral edema. A liver biopsy was consistent with macro-micronodular cirrhosis. For 2 years the ascites, edema, and weakness persisted, but he had no varices, and when admitted for transplantation his liver function was only mildly abnormal. Echocardiogram on that admission disclosed an enlarged right atrium and findings consistent with elevated right-sided pressure. Although jugular venous pressure was normal, cardiac catheterization disclosed findings consistent with constrictive pericarditis, and the patient improved after pericardiectomy. A primary diagnosis of liver disease was incorrect. This conclusion was reached prematurely without considering that various features did not fit this diagnosis.

No-Fault Errors

We classified several cases as no-fault errors under the supposition that the physicians responsible for the patient's care, no matter how expert in their diagnostic capabilities, would not have arrived at the correct diagnosis. Examples include one patient (see case 5) with complete heart block whose symptoms were vague and whose tests failed to identify the cause for years, one patient (see case 21) who was thought to have a lung tumor but ended up having only a blood clot in the lung, one patient (see case 22) who had vitamin B_{12} deficiency with neurological manifestations but with no anemia, and one patient (see case 55) who had an atrial myxoma—a rare cardiac tumor.

Analysis

Inspection of the table shows that cognitive errors can have diverse and serious consequences. Delays in making the correct diagnosis and unnecessary or excessive testing were the most common consequences, but delays in beginning treatment or inappropriate treatment were quite frequent. Some cognitive errors led only to unnecessary anxiety, but in other instances, they led to grave outcomes, including premature extubation, unnecessary surgery, and loss of a normal kidney.

Avoiding the cognitive errors illustrated here is not easy, and there is no tried-and-true method for doing so.[290,291] As we have argued, exposure to salient examples such as those in this book might heighten the student or physician's sensitivity to the kinds of errors. Providing extensive tables of possible errors and biases has a similar basis.[79] Other procedures have been proposed. Some suggestions are to use a strategy of stepping back from the problem of the moment and only making an action-oriented decision after careful reflection on the problem; providing training to identify specific reasoning flaws; decreasing the reliance on memory by substituting cognitive aids; and providing rapid and reliable feedback at the time that the error is made.[1,79,292]

Although some of these techniques may be helpful, none has stood the test of scientific evaluation.

CHAPTER 21

Some Cognitive Concepts

CASE 62. A MESSAGE ABOUT METHODS

An 18-year-old woman with a history of acute lymphocytic leukemia (ALL) was admitted to the hospital with fever, chills, sweating, myalgias, and headache.

With these symptoms, it sounds to me as if she is infected. It could also be her underlying disease, but that usually does not present in this way. She could have a disseminated bacterial infection or certainly could have a viral infection, given the myalgias and the headache. If it was in the springtime, it could be an adenovirus infection. If it was in the summertime, it could be a Coxsackie virus infection with aseptic meningitis. But it could be other things as well.

The patient's leukemia was diagnosed 3 years earlier and was treated effectively with chemotherapy, including intrathecal methotrexate. Bone marrow morphology remained normal every 3 months thereafter until 4 months before admission, when she had a relapse. Peripheral counts at that time were hematocrit 25%, platelets 81,000, and white cell count 4,600. At that time, malignant cells were again present. Chemotherapy induced another remission. One month before admission, the following values were obtained: hematocrit 39%, platelets 249,000, and white cell count 4,200. Bone marrow was hypocellular with decreased myeloid precursors. During the week before admission, the patient had been taking thioridazine in doses as high as 600 mg per day.

This fever is not thioridazine induced. I am not sure why you are telling me that.

On the day before admission, she had abrupt onset of fever, chills, sweating, myalgias, and headache. She had no neck stiffness, sleepiness, change in mental status, or joint pain and no cardiovascular, pulmonary, or gastrointestinal symptoms. Her temperature was 39°C, pulse 130 per minute, and blood pressure 130/90 mm Hg. Examination disclosed a grade 2/6 systolic ejection murmur but no other abnormalities.

Neither liver nor spleen was palpable. Rectal and pelvic examinations were normal.

The abrupt onset sounds more bacterial than viral, but maybe not. A fever with chills and sweating also sounds more bacterial than viral, but myalgias are more commonly viral. It sounds like a viral infection, but because she has leukemia, she could have a number of different opportunistic infections. The fact that she does not have a stiff neck does not mean that she does not have meningitis either.

Laboratory studies showed hemoglobin 10.1 g/dL, hematocrit 29%, white cell count 13,700 with 70 polys, 15 bands, 7 lymphs, 5 monos, 1 eosinophil, 1 metamyelocyte, and 1 myelocyte. Platelets 173,000. On the blood smear, teardrop forms and a few nucleated red cells were seen. Electrolytes, blood urea nitrogen (BUN), creatinine, coagulation studies, and liver function studies were normal. Lactate dehydrogenase (LDH) was 383 IU/L; Creatine kinase (CK) was 90 IU/L. Chest x-ray and lumbar puncture were normal.

Her hematocrit is 29%, which, with her fever, is probably why she has a systolic ejection murmur. The white count of 13,700 with 70 segs is important. It pushes me immediately in the bacterial direction, away from this being a virus, although the flu sometimes will give you a left shift. But 7 lymphs, 5 monos, 1 eosinophil, 1 metamyelocyte, and 1 myelocyte are a little much for that. The nucleated red cells could mean that she is activating her bone marrow to put out a lot of white cells, or it could mean that she has a myelophthisic process. Or it could be just a result of the bone marrow's recovery from the chemotherapy. LDH was elevated, which would go along with her hyperactive marrow production.

I would get cultures. So far, there is no obvious focus of infection. If she has just come off chemotherapy, she certainly could have small gastrointestinal ulcerations, with easy access to the bloodstream of the gram-negative rods and other things in the gastrointestinal tract. With the left shift, this really concerns me. With that fever and that shift, I probably would treat her broadly with antimicrobial therapy to cover gastrointestinal pathogens, and also cover for Pseudomonas, although she is not neutropenic. What about fungi in a patient with ALL? There is nothing in the chest. Where would the fungus be? Where would it be coming from? I do not see a urinalysis report. There was no diarrhea. This could be candidiasis.

One infection to consider when the bone marrow is active as in this patient is tuberculosis. We have seen disseminated TB (tuberculosis) frequently in our AIDS patients. She could be at high risk for disseminated TB. We do not know her PPD (purified protein derivative) status. So tuberculosis, fungal infection, and gram-negative sepsis without hypotension are all on my list. I would not treat for a fungus or tuberculosis yet, but I might go ahead fairly soon and look at her bone marrow. The fact that she has nucleated reds on her smear could mean that there is something invading the marrow. It could be *Histoplasma* or any organism such as that.

> Thioridazine was discontinued immediately, and cefepime was started on the day after admission. Subsequently, four blood cultures and one urine culture were sterile. Spinal fluid also was sterile. Antibiotic therapy was discontinued. Fever (39°C) persisted for the next 5 days. The white count was 13,800 with 83 polys, 6 bands, 8 lymphs, 2 monos, and 1 basophil. No new symptoms appeared, and physical examination did not change.

The four negative blood cultures and one negative urine culture reduce the likelihood of gram-negative sepsis in this patient. I would have been more concerned about it if she was neutropenic, but she is not. She has lymphocytic leukemia, which pushes you more toward the infections seen in AIDS patients. She has persistent fever. She really does not have any evidence here of reactivation of her leukemia to explain the fever. I think she is going to have something in her bone marrow, and I think it is going to be a fungus, or it might be an acid-fast organism.

> On the fifth hospital day, a bone marrow aspirate showed that the marrow was packed with lymphoblasts that again were similar to her original malignant cells. A new course of chemotherapy was started. Three days later, her fever disappeared, and 7 days later, her blood counts reverted toward normal. A bone marrow study done after 2 weeks showed that the bone marrow also had reverted toward normal. Her fever and constitutional symptoms were attributed to relapse of acute leukemia, but drug fever or an intercurrent viral infection could not be excluded with certainty.

She did have a myelophthisic picture. Rather than having an organism in the marrow, however, she had lymphoblasts in there; I agree that the fever was caused by a relapse of the leukemia. What is surprising to me is the abruptness of the onset of the symptoms. That pushed me much more toward hypothesizing some infectious cause, and the shift to the left pushed me toward a bacterial cause. I would have felt obligated to do what her physicians did, namely to culture and to treat expectantly. It looks to me as if the lymphocytes were acting like an organism in terms of the production of the fever.

Analysis

We put a premium on efficient and accurate diagnostic problem solving. Thus, we must place an even higher premium on understanding the mental processes that we use to solve such problems. The question is how to learn about these mental processes and states. Traditionally, we have trusted the how-to opinions of expert clinicians, who have relied on their introspective accounts of how the process operates.[138,139] Yet we have reason to believe that such accounts are not what they are cracked up to be. Several lines of evidence suggest that people have limited access to the workings of their minds and that they have no privileged knowledge of the factors that influence their cognitive behavior, yet they readily offer extensive explanations of how to proceed in making diagnoses. Such explanations, one assumes, are inferred from personal concepts of their internal processes and state of mind.[88,89,91]

For several decades, psychologists have viewed introspection on the state of one's mind as suspect, or at least seriously deficient.[293] Any study designed to detect and interpret mental states must rely on the integrated response of an individual to a particular stimulus, that is, the implementation of the content of a mental process. Missing in such responses, presumably, are the mental processes and the mental states themselves.

How can we define the nature of these processes and states as they relate to the diagnostic process? Verbal protocols have been used in medicine, as in other domains, to understand the structure of sequential cognitive processes.[18,19,47,61,89] The general procedure is to present a clinician with authentic clinical material in a chronological fashion that mimics a patient's workup. As the clinician responds to the material, he or she thinks out loud, and the monologue is recorded and transcribed verbatim. The protocol, or transcript, is then analyzed by a person who is trained in transcript analysis and familiar with the medical domain.

This commentary provides a running series of responses that, in theory, can be used to infer the sequence of mental states and the processes used to solve a problem.[90] An assumption of the method is that thinking while speaking probably is not unlike thinking without speaking. The analysis of protocols proceeds as follows: First, we observe what data a person pays attention to and assume that this information exists in working memory; then, from this information, the analyst infers a sequence of states; finally, from these sequential descriptions the analyst attempts to understand the general rules that the person used to solve problems. Note that in this approach the analyst, not the subject, makes the inferences about the mental processes involved.

These experimental procedures probably are best at generating hypotheses, that is, plausible analyses of the subject's problem-solving processes. Such procedures are weak in their capacity to develop, test, and reject competing hypotheses; other methods must be used for hypothesis testing. In a few instances, individual subjects have been studied repeatedly, and their problem-solving abilities in narrow domains (recalling sequences of digits) have been characterized extensively. The generalizability of this characterization across subjects and domains, however, is yet to be determined.[92]

The most optimistic view of protocols is that they can provide selective glimpses of intermediate points in clinical reasoning, thereby illuminating the states that people pass through in the performance of a certain task.[93,94] Indeed, there are many reservations about the validity of protocol analysis. The technique diverges from traditional scientific approaches that rely heavily on statistical studies, and thus the analyses lack a certain objectivity. No generally accepted conventions for reporting the data have been developed; thus, the ability to report and compare data from more than one study has been hampered.[94] Collecting and analyzing protocols is a tedious, time- and effort-consuming task. Analysis requires the participation of a person who is professionally familiar with the subject material.[36,61]

There are other reservations about the content of transcripts. Often there is no record of a subject's planning process; usually there is no way of observing a subject's unstated confusion or expressions of difficulty.[94] Another concern is that the findings can be misleading if a subject gives a "canned," or precompiled, version of problem solving instead of an ongoing problem-solving strategy.[61] One also must recognize that because subjects cannot be expected to report all their reasoning as they are thinking aloud, at least some intermediate steps in their reasoning processes will be omitted.[36] Moreover, cognitive biases such as availability, representativeness, anchoring, omission, or framing all occur unconsciously and hence are unlikely to be articulated and captured.[88,91] Finally, in analyzing a protocol, the analyst must pay particular attention to those aspects in which the subject is using his or her medical knowledge and concentrating on explanations rather than on those aspects in which the subject is opining about his or her mental processes.[89]

Despite these reservations, transcript analysis has provided not only interesting hypotheses about the reasoning of physicians, but also valuable insights that have been the basis of didactic approaches and computer programs that model clinical reasoning.[1,162] Studies of the diagnostic process have identified many of its features and the complex interactions among hypothesis generation, hypothesis testing, and hypothesis verification.[18,19] The cause-and-effect relationships between clinical variables, so critical to medical diagnosis and therapeutics, also have been studied by transcript analysis.[47,89] The result is a deeper understanding of how physicians apply causal reasoning in diagnosis and how they revert to "first principles" when precompiled reasoning processes are insufficient to explain peculiarities in clinical data. Indeed, the implementation of the causal model from these analyses as a working computer program demonstrates that the data obtained from the transcripts are sufficient to model the detailed causal reasoning used by the physician subjects.[36]

Finally, even the reasoning that physicians use to make complicated tradeoffs between the choices of tests and treatments under conditions of uncertainty have been subjected to transcript analysis. Such studies suggest that in making decisions about the benefits and risks of tests and treatments, physicians use an incremental planning approach that sometimes ignores the "big picture," and that they sometimes disregard appropriate therapeutic approaches in favor of invasive diagnostic approaches that are no more valuable than other therapeutic measures. These studies also suggest

explanations for some of the cognitive biases inherent in the physician problem solver.[61]

No analysis can be expected to identify all the reasoning processes or all the data used in the process. The best we can hope for is to achieve some insights. The transcript just given contains many such insights about how an expert clinician assembles a diagnosis. We identified all the verb phrases in the transcript and then assembled those that related to any diagnostic hypotheses. By selecting such phrases, we gain assurance that the subject is using her medical knowledge to explain the clinical findings. The results are displayed in Table 21.1.

Note that a large number of the verb phrases are used for generating diagnostic hypotheses (*could be*, *might be*) and that many others make assertions about existing hypotheses (*pushes me*

TABLE 21.1

Verb Phrases Describing Hypotheses

SIMPLE HYPOTHESIS GENERATION	**ASSERTIONS ABOUT HYPOTHESES**
It **could also be** her underlying disease	it **sounds to me** as if she is infected
She **could have** a disseminated bacterial infection	**sounds like** a viral infection
certainly **could have** a viral infection	It **pushes me immediately** in the bacterial direction, away from this being a virus
it **could be** an adenovirus infection	which **would go along with** her hyperactive marrow production
it **could be** other things	She **does not really have any evidence here of**
she **could have** a whole host of opportunistic infections	I **would be very concerned about** that
doesn't mean that she doesn't have meningitis	She **would be at high risk for** disseminated TB
It **could be** a number of those things	**pushes you more toward** the infections seen in AIDS patients
reds **could mean** that she is shifting	I **think she is going to have** something in her bone marrow
it **could mean** a myelophthisic process	I **think it is going to be** a fungus
it **could be** just a result of	That **pushed me much more toward** some infectious cause
she **certainly could have** small ulcerations	**would have pushed me toward** a bacterial cause
What about fungi in a patient with ALL?	
This **could be** candidiasis	**EXCLUSIONARY STATEMENTS**
thing **that you think about** when you talk about the bone marrow	fever **is not** thioridazine-induced
are all on my list	there **is no** focus for infection
could mean that there is something in the marrow	**really rule out** gram-negative sepsis
It **could be** histoplasmosis	**ORDINAL DESCRIPTORS**
it **might be** an acid-fast organism	abrupt onset **sounds more** bacterial **than** viral
	maybe not (**more** bacterial **than** viral)
	also **sounds more** bacterial **than** viral

toward, *sounds like*, *think she is going to have*). Some of these assertions are quite strong (*I think she is going to have*), whereas some are considerably less strong (*sounds to me as if*). Still stronger are assertions that a certain hypothesis has been excluded (*really rules out*). Finally, some assertions are in the form of ordinal descriptors, that is, comparisons between clinical disorders (*sounds more . . . than . . .*).

Of course, the monologue by the discussant contained verb phrases other than those that described hypotheses. We identified (but excluded from the table) phrases that described conditional probabilities, selection of diagnostic tests, causal attributions, and comments conditional on findings that might be present. The assemblage of verb phrases describing hypotheses provides glimpses into how one clinician generates a variety of hypotheses. She juggles many hypotheses, occasionally assesses one type of disease against another, and rejects some hypotheses unequivocally. Eventually, she accepts the weight of evidence as favoring a single hypothesis. These aspects of diagnosis are similar to those identified in earlier studies of the process.[18,19]

CASE 63. MEMORY: HOW WE OVERCOME ITS LIMITATIONS

A 54-year-old man was admitted to the hospital with persistent crushing chest pain. An electrocardiogram (ECG) showed an acute inferior myocardial infarction and 5-mm depression of ST segments in V_1 to V_4. Intravenous nitroglycerin, 5 μg/kg per minute, did not relieve the pain, but insertion of an intraaortic balloon 1 hour after admission led to reduction in the pain and less extreme depression of the precordial ST segments. Three hours later, severe chest pain recurred and the ST segments returned to their original configuration. Pain was not relieved by intravenous nitroglycerin (30 μg/kg per minute), intravenous propranolol, and large doses of morphine. The patient was hemodynamically stable and had no rhythm disturbances.

The patient apparently has an acute inferior myocardial infarction. The ischemia seems to have been relieved after an intraaortic balloon was inserted, leading to pain reduction and improvement in the precordial ST-segment depressions. The patient then has another episode of chest pain that is not responsive to nitroglycerin, beta-blockers, and morphine. It seems to me that he has a fairly established lesion, and my guess is that this is not due to simple vasospasm. I would be suspicious that the patient has a localized lesion due to thrombosis.

Cardiac catheterization disclosed complete or nearly complete occlusion of the left anterior descending, the right coronary, and the circumflex arteries. The ejection fraction was 50%, and the inferior wall of the left ventricle was akinetic. Nitroglycerin, morphine, and propranolol were continued. Although the patient remained hemodynamically stable, he appeared plethoric and somewhat cyanotic despite administration of oxygen by nasal prongs at a rate of 4 L/min. The arterial partial pressure of oxygen (PaO_2) never fell below 69 mm Hg.

His PaO_2 is 69, and yet he is starting to appear cyanotic and plethoric. With this slightly cyanotic appearance, I would be concerned that he is getting high doses of nitroglycerin, which produces a dilation of his capacitance vessels and causes a certain degree of venous pooling. The extraction of oxygen is probably increased, but I would be worried that with all the intravenous nitroglycerin he is getting, methemoglobinemia might be developing. With cyanosis in the face of a normal PaO_2 (or at least an acceptable PaO_2, one that should not give him cyanosis) and with a reasonable blood pressure, I would be concerned that we are overdoing the nitroglycerin. I would order a methemoglobin level at this point.

The patient was taken to the operating room. The surgeon had painted a dark picture of the patient's prognosis to the family, but he was astounded when the blood flowing from the initial incision was neither red nor blue. It was black.

That suggests to me that indeed the patient had methemoglobinemia.

The cardiothoracic surgeon made a diagnosis of methemoglobinemia, stopped the nitroglycerin, infused methylene blue, gave several pints of blood, and bypassed all three occluded coronary arteries. Review of the record disclosed that the patient had been receiving as much as 50 μg/kg per minute of nitroglycerin. The patient recovered uneventfully. He had no evidence of brain damage postoperatively, and chest pain did not recur.

Well done. I cannot remember what the appropriate dose is, but I think that dose was much too high.

Analysis

Here is an interesting paradox: On the one hand, our recall of various items (the name of a person we have just met or a new telephone number) is rather poor, whereas facts about a new patient seem indelibly etched in our minds. If we contemplate the clinical problem-solving process, we appreciate that as we solve diagnostic problems, we must be manipulating an enormous number of details about a patient garnered from the history, physical examination, and laboratory tests. Even more impressive sometimes is how we recall most of the patient's present illness with unerring accuracy and the results of electrolytes to the nearest milliequivalent. What do we know about this paradox? Why should we care about it? What relation does memory have to our ability to solve clinical problems?

Studies in cognitive science have yielded considerable information about memory and have led to the notion that the mind is a powerful information processor but that its processors have sharply limited capacity.[108] This notion becomes less ambiguous when it is understood that memory can be subdivided into two distinctive parts: short term and long term. Short-term, or working, memory is the part that holds only information currently being processed, and long-term memory is the storehouse of all our factual knowledge.[294] Those distinctions, which have become somewhat blurred, are useful in understanding our information-processing capabilities.

Working memory is where we store the items (or "chunks") of information we are manipulating as we are trying to understand or decode them. Working memory is both evanescent and limited in capacity, but retrieval from it is rapid. A new piece of information is maintained in an activated state in working memory as long as attention is devoted to it, and then it fades rapidly thereafter (e.g., a new phone number).[108,115] For reasons that have not yet been identified, working memory is thought to hold only 5 to 10 items; this capacity has been validated repeatedly by memory experiments and is now a widely accepted value.[23,24]

Long-term memory, on the other hand, is thought to be both long lasting and unlimited in capacity.[294] Information appears to be stored in long-term memory as a network of associations among concepts and is retrieved by a spreading activation from working memory through that network.[295] Retrieval from long-term memory is slow.

This description of memory fails to account for the remarkable capacity of clinicians to manipulate the large amounts of information obtained when attempting to solve a clinical problem—for example, trying to come up with a diagnosis for a patient with a set of complaints. The apparent shortcoming probably is explained by what is defined as a chunk of information and by methods for organizing knowledge in long-term memory.[108,296]

Studies show that persons who memorize a string of random digits by attaching a semantic meaning or label to short sequences of the digits are far more efficient at recalling the digits accurately than others who try to memorize the digits without developing a meaningful framework.[108,296] The chunk is defined as a particular amount of information that has semantic meaning.[23,24,296] According to these concepts, working memory and long-term memory can act symbiotically to accomplish effective problem solving while handling a large mass of information. They do so, it is thought, by an approach known as skilled memory. Skilled memory is a process by which experts develop elaborate cognitive structures in long-term memory where information with semantic meaning is stored.[108,137] By "chunking" information into meaningful semantic units and by the use of these cognitive structures, long-term memory becomes an efficient extension of short-term memory.

To what mental tasks do these rather esoteric concepts relate in the clinical arena? Detailed, comparable studies in medical problem solving have not been done, but some relationships seem apparent. First, we do tend to chunk information into meaningful or semantically significant units. Chronological accounts of patients' illnesses and groupings of test results under the function of a particular organ fit this description. Furthermore, medical experts, like chess masters, recognize certain patterns of findings because presumably they (like the masters) have stored in long-term memory patterns of findings that are meaningful and readily retrieved when new information demands their attention.[118,137] Patterns of liver function tests and electrolytes come to mind as examples. Quite likely, the chunking of data and their storage in semantically significant units accounts for the ability of the expert clinician to recall unaided and with near precision the laboratory results for several patients, whereas the student must resort to his or her clipboard for the data.

The transcript of the discussant's immediate responses illustrates some of the features we have considered. We get a few glimpses of the content of his long-term memory, although we can learn little about the structure that houses the knowledge stored there. In addition, although we can glean few insights into the structure of his working memory, we can dissect out of the transcript what appear to be some, and perhaps even most, of the semantic items—the chunks that he manipulates as he solves the diagnostic problem of the patient who turned blue from excessive doses of nitroglycerin. After he is given the initial clinical information, he describes the following semantic units:

- Acute inferior myocardial infarction
- Balloon-related pain relief
- Recurrent pain unresponsive to drugs
- Irreversible myocardial lesion
- Coronary thrombosis

Later, when he is given the follow-up data, he describes the following semantic units:

- PaO_2 of 69
- Plethoric appearance
- Large doses of nitroglycerin
- Venous pooling
- Cyanosis with normal PaO_2
- Methemoglobinemia

How many of these chunks he retains in working memory at any given time we do not know, of course, but it appears that the number is small.

Indeed, it is quite likely that some chunks supplant and replace ones created earlier.[294] For example, "irreversible myocardial lesion" probably supplants "acute myocardial infarction," and "methemoglobinemia" probably supplants "cyanosis with normal PaO_2." It is interesting to appreciate how easy it is to contemplate those sets of chunks and how they illustrate the discussant's problem-solving approach.

We should try to learn something about clinical problem solving from this information on memory. These experiments seem to indicate that what is important is not what you remember, but how you remember it. We should try to design experiments to learn which cognitive structures are useful enhancers of working memory, and we should try to find out how best to organize information so that it has semantic meaning. By doing so, we might improve the performance even of our experts.

CASE 64. DIAGNOSIS AND THE STRUCTURE OF MEMORY; DISEASE POLYMORPHISM AND MENTAL MODELS

A medical consultant was called to evaluate a 69-year-old woman on the Gynecology Service for syncope.

The differential diagnosis of syncope is extremely long. I am not sure what the connection is with a patient on the Gynecology Service. The only thing I think about in somebody this age is a large abdominal mass, either from an ovarian carcinoma or a large fibroid uterus, pressing on the inferior vena cava and causing orthostatic hypotension with subsequent syncope. Otherwise, I would say it is the usual long differential diagnosis of syncope.

The patient had had a total abdominal hysterectomy 6 days previously for endometrial cancer. Since then her course had been uncomplicated. She was preparing to go home (standing, washing herself in the bathroom) when she was overcome by a "wave of weakness" followed by "blackness"; she then lost consciousness for several minutes.

These symptoms are consistent with an orthostatic picture, in that she subsequently just stood up, felt a premonitory syndrome with a wave of weakness, blackness, and then subsequent loss of consciousness. This episode sounds very much like it was caused by depressed cardiac output. Losing consciousness for several minutes is significant, and is not the usual orthostatic picture, but the time course can sometimes be confusing. I would try to eliminate possibilities such as seizures, especially if no one witnessed a seizure or other central nervous system events and assume that this is a cardiovascular cause of syncope.

> Her blood pressure was 80/60 mm Hg, her pulse rate was 90 per minute, and her respiratory rate was 20 per minute. Her blood pressure increased after infusion of saline. She was afebrile. After she regained consciousness, the physical examination was unremarkable except for an occasional extrasystole.

The hypotension is a little bit disturbing. The heart rate is slightly up, and the respiratory rate appears normal. Another thing I was thinking of was whether she had an atypical presentation for a pulmonary embolus after having undergone surgery, being at bed rest, and then subsequently standing up. I do not think that we can exclude a pulmonary embolus based on the data at hand. I know that in terms of the differential diagnosis of syncope, pulmonary embolus is a cause, but it is a rare cause. This diagnosis is still possible, but her normal respiratory rate points against it a little bit. The occasional extrasystole really is of no help diagnostically.

> The patient had no shortness of breath, chest pain, palpitations, perioral paresthesias, bleeding, or symptoms suggestive of a seizure.

As I mentioned, seizures are an uncommon cause of syncope, and it is hard to make this diagnosis unless there is a witness who identifies tonic–clonic activity. Usually patients with seizures also have a postictal picture. The fact that she had no shortness of breath or chest pain is against a diagnosis of myocardial infarction or pulmonary embolus. The lack of palpitations is fairly unreliable from a diagnostic standpoint, but the lack of perioral paresthesias does argue against hyperventila-

tion. Bleeding is still a possibility, and I would like to see a hematocrit, although the sudden onset of symptoms points against that.

> Review of her past history disclosed that she had experienced two to three episodes of lightheadedness and one episode of syncope 1 year previously; each of these episodes were related to defecation. She had a history of atypical chest pain with a positive dipyridamole thallium scan, but a recent cardiac catheterization was normal. She had a history of mild hypertension treated with metoprolol. She had received subcutaneous heparin since surgery and was on no other medications.

She did have some symptoms in the past that could be consistent with orthostatic hypotension or vasovagal episodes. Her atypical chest pain appears to have been worked up. Even though she had a positive dipyridamole thallium scan, the normal cardiac catheterization makes it very unlikely that she has significant coronary artery disease. Another possibility would be valvular disease, but we have no information yet about that. Aortic stenosis is certainly a possibility because chest pain, syncope, and congestive failure are the classic triad of its presentation. I would imagine that during the cardiac catheterization they carried out a left ventriculogram, and thus we should know whether or not she had significant aortic stenosis. Metoprolol certainly could be a cause of orthostatic hypotension. She was not taking any other medications that could contribute. The fact that she received subcutaneous heparin lessens the likelihood that she had a pulmonary embolus, although I am not really aware of the data on subcutaneous heparin as prophylaxis against deep venous thrombosis after total hysterectomy.

> Laboratory data: white blood cells (WBCs) 8,900, hematocrit 30%. Sodium 138 mEq/L, potassium 3.8 mEq/L, chloride 103 mEq/L, total CO_2 25 mEq/L. BUN 11 mg/dL, creatinine 0.8 mg/dL, calcium 8.7 mg/dL. Chest x-ray normal. ECG: normal sinus rhythm with frequent premature ventricular contractions (PVCs). Anterior ST-T wave changes, consistent with ischemia. There is a new $S_1 Q_3$ pattern.

The laboratory studies are normal, except for the slightly low hematocrit, which probably is consistent with the postoperative state. It is not low enough to cause syncope. The normal chest x-ray is not very helpful. Frequent PVCs are not very predictive of anything. The anterior ST-T wave changes are consistent with ischemia, but likewise are not very specific. The $S_1 Q_3$ pattern can be seen with pulmonary emboli, especially when there is right ventricular strain, and that may be what the ST-T wave changes refer to. That may be a strain pattern from acute right ventricular overload, which might be seen with a pulmonary embolus. So that is a little bit worrisome to me. The possibility that she had a myocardial infarct, I suppose, is still there, although I discounted it earlier on the basis of the normal cardiac catheterization, and I still think it is unlikely.

> The patient was transferred to the intensive care unit. Blood gas analysis showed pH 7.42, PaO_2 55 mm Hg, and arterial partial pressure of carbon dioxide ($PaCO_2$) 38 mm Hg (on room air). The patient was started on intravenous heparin, and a stat computed tomography (CT) pulmonary angiogram was ordered.

All of this is consistent with a pulmonary embolus. There is a large alveolar–arterial gradient, and I think it is appropriate that the patient be treated with heparin immediately.

> The medical consultant was less certain of the cause of syncope and his note was more contemplative. He wrote, "probably hypovolemic etiology. . . . I suspect venous pooling upon standing, with known falling hematocrit, accounting for her syncopal event. However, this does not explain the hypoxemia though I suspect postop atelectasis and hypoventilation in an obese person lying supine . . . is the most likely explanation. Yet, the $S_1 Q_3$ pattern on the ECG is new and there is left calf tenderness in a patient obviously at risk for DVT though on prophylactic heparin. As such, P.E. cannot be confidently ruled out without further data."

There are some features in this patient's course that do not fit together particularly well. The duration of the loss of consciousness for several minutes is difficult to explain. The fact that she needed intravenous fluids to raise her blood pressure points to a significant suppression of her cardiac output. I agree that the new $S_1 Q_3$ pattern on the ECG in a patient with a normal coronary arteriogram suggests a pulmonary embolus. Left calf tenderness is often nonspecific, but if it is truly new, it could be significant. I do not think that there are convincing data on the value of prophylactic heparin in patients after total hysterectomies. We know that it fails for other forms of pelvic surgery, and it would not surprise me if it failed in this setting as well. So I certainly agree that the patient should be evaluated further for a pulmonary embolus.

> The consultant recommended aggressive hydration, oxygen, stool softeners, transfusions as necessary to keep hematocrit at 27% or higher, and the following additional tests: three CKs and ECGs at 12-hour intervals, repeat hematocrit, and 24-hour Holter monitor. He also agreed that a CT pulmonary angiogram was indicated.

We need to look at the things that we need to work up aggressively and urgently. The hematocrit was greater than 30% at this point and we have no indication that there is any bleeding, but I agree that a repeat hematocrit after rehydration is indicated. The CKs and ECGs at 12-hour intervals are going to take a long time, and given the story, I think a myocardial infarct is unlikely. I would just put the patient on a cardiac monitor and skip the Holter. The CT scan is indicated, and I think it should be done urgently because of the serious implications of a pulmonary embolus.

> The CT pulmonary angiogram showed multiple bilateral filling defects. It was considered to be "very high probability for pulmonary embolus." The patient was treated with anticoagulants. The remainder of her hospital course was uncomplicated.

Given the previous surgery and her clinical course, I would feel comfortable treating her for a pulmonary embolus based on the noted defects. I would not perform further studies at this point and just maintain her anticoagulation.

Analysis

Both in the clinical material presented here and in the transcript of the discussant's reactions to this material, we see evidence of "waffling" over the diagnosis. After all the information is known, few clinicians would doubt the diagnosis of pulmonary embolism in this patient: she acutely developed hypotension on the sixth postoperative day, and she was found to have a large alveolar–arterial gradient, an S_1 Q_3 pattern on the ECG, and a strongly positive CT scan. Through the "retro-spectroscope," arriving at this diagnosis is easy, but prospectively it was not. Why not? In part, the difficulty stems from the fact that among patients with pulmonary emboli, syncope is an unusual presenting complaint, occurring in just 8% of patients with acute pulmonary embolism.[297] In this instance, the complaint was sufficiently unusual to cast doubt on the correct diagnosis long after many of the typical findings were already known. What do we do when patients fail to fit our preconceived notions of a given disease? What exactly are these preconceived notions? How do we classify unusual instances of disease into existing categories? How are these categories represented in memory?

A loose end in the process of diagnosis is how we store our knowledge about disease entities and how we use this stored information when we encounter a new patient. Why should the process of comparing a new patient's findings to our mental model of various diseases be so difficult at times? The number of diseases is finite, and because long-term memory is thought to be infinite, we should be able to remember all patterns of all diseases and to readily assess a new patient against these patterns. As we contemplate these heady diagnostic issues, a series of questions surface: (1) Why is it that we encounter "classical" cases so infrequently? (2) What are the characteristics of diseases (such as syphilis and vasculitis) that induce us to call them the "great imitators"? (3) What is the conceptual difference between an acute inferior myocardial infarction and syphilis? Between an acute inferior myocardial infarction and a new U.S. $20 bill? (4) What is the basis for the "We see this" assertion by senior clinicians when explaining that a putatively atypical patient actually fits within a well-defined diagnostic category, implying that the patient is simply an outlier within that particular diagnostic category? (5) Why do many discussants in clinico-pathologic conferences (CPCs) in the *New England Journal of Medicine* ignore textbook descriptions of disease entities and dig out individual cases comparable to the one they are discussing? Though some of these questions sound frivolous, we believe they are interrelated and important in understanding the connections between memory and the diagnostic process.

In large part, diagnosis is a classification task. It is the task of recognizing a newly encountered instance of illness as an example of a known disease class or entity. Classifying a patient not only avoids the need to create a new diagnostic category, but also allows one to bring to bear whatever knowledge we have of the existing category. Whatever it is that we retain in memory against which we measure or weigh a new case must capture the variations in all clinical manifestations within a single category. Such variations include the recognized variations in the factors that promote the development of the disease, variations in patients' symptoms (syncope, e.g., as a sign of pulmonary embolism), variations in the appearance of manifestations over time, variations in physical and laboratory findings, and variations in the course of disease and its response to treatment. Whenever we see a patient, an essential aspect of our task is to decide whether he or she fits into a stored diagnostic category (such as pulmonary embolism). We have to decide whether a given patient's manifestations are sufficiently atypical to exclude the patient from the diagnostic category or whether the patient is simply an outlier yet still must be considered to fall within the bounds of the category. Whatever we store in memory must permit us to make these distinctions.

We do not know precisely how we store disease models against which we compare new cases. As we discuss elsewhere, memory is considered by some to be composed of symbols and by others to be represented in the connections between sets of neurons. No matter which concept (or some other) is correct, we can explore some of the ways we might store disease categories for use in identifying and classifying a new patient. How do we reason from what we have learned? The most common concept of the structure of memory holds that in the process of learning medicine we compile and compress "training" cases into some abstract description; then, by comparing a new case to the abstract description, we infer whether the new case can be subsumed under the abstract description. Indeed, if one asks a physician to describe a clinical entity, he or she can readily invent such an abstract description. Such a "typical case" would be replete with all the predisposing factors, clinical features, physical findings, laboratory abnormalities, and responses to therapy.

The problem in understanding memory as a set of monolithic, abstract descriptions is that (as the patient with pulmonary emboli exemplifies) substantial variability exists among well-accepted instances of disease entities; in turn this variability makes it difficult to learn a fixed, uniform set of conditions that are both necessary and sufficient to classify a new instance as an example of a known disease. How are these variations represented in memory? As noted before, a widely accepted view is that we store an abstract model that is sufficiently complex to contain all possible clinical variations of disease entities. This model presumably also contains rules that allow us to exclude a patient from that disease category when certain criteria are not met (if a patient has all the criteria for nephrotic syndrome, e.g., except heavy proteinuria, the diagnosis of nephrotic syndrome is excluded). A second view is that variations in disease categories are stored according to some probabilistic scheme—not necessarily represented by actual numbers, but perhaps by semiquantitative categorical expressions of probability such as "frequently," "common," and "rare."[61] The problem with a probabilistic representation is that although it does express how often certain findings occur in various diseases, it does not describe satisfactorily how disease attributes vary together.

Neither of these notions—namely abstract descriptions and probabilistic associations—fully satisfies the complexities required to store a representation of disease. Another concept of memory is directly relevant to how we store diagnostic categories and how we use these categories to classify the illness of a new patient. To explain this hypothesis we will introduce a concept we alluded to earlier but did not name, that is, disease polymorphism.[98] Polymorphism refers to the large number of variations in the form a disease takes. Although textbooks describe "typical" or "classic"

cases, expert clinicians recognize that these textbook descriptions (and those we obtain by asking a physician to describe a disease category) are excessively simplified. These experts know not only the typical case, but also about anomalous cases and exceptions to the rules.[298] By long experience with disease polymorphism, they develop sophisticated and flexible category definitions, and their accumulated experience allows them to formulate an extremely detailed model of various diseases.

The polymorphism of certain diseases is simply too complex to describe in a textbook or in an oral description of the disease. Yet, in reality, substantial variations exist by which diseases manifest. Some disease entities are probably more polymorphic than others. One can assume that acute inferior myocardial infarctions are less polymorphic than syphilis (the "great imitator"), as also we can assume that new $20 bills are less polymorphic (virtually no discernible variation from one to another) than Dalmatian dogs (which vary in size, age, and pattern of spots) and that Dalmatian dogs are less polymorphic than humans. Among disease conditions, many manifestations vary to produce this polymorphism, including factors that promote the development of the disease, symptoms, appearance of manifestations over time, physical findings, laboratory findings, the course of disease, and its response to treatment. A clear description of disease polymorphism was written almost 250 years ago about a disease we rarely see today, namely scurvy. The description of polymorphism is so apt that we reproduce it verbatim here:

> The disease so frequently attending all long voyages, and, so particularly destructive to us, is surely the most singular and unaccountable of any that affects the human body. For its symptoms are inconstant and irregular; for scarcely any two persons have the same complaints, and where there hath been found some conformity in the symptoms, the order of their appearance has been totally different. However, though it frequently puts on the form of many other diseases, and is therefore, not to be described by any exclusive and infallible criterions; yet there are some symptoms which, more general than the rest, and therefore, occurring the oftenest, deserve a more particular enumeration.[299]

Although we know such polymorphism to occur, we have only a gross qualitative view of the polymorphism of certain diseases. Although we suppose that some diseases (syphilis, vasculitis, lupus) are more polymorphic than others, we have no well-defined measures of the degree of polymorphism by disease.

The concept of disease polymorphism explains several questions we posed earlier. We encounter "classic" cases so infrequently simply because the textbook descriptions of disease are idealized, and patients with only the manifestations described in the books are rare. Students first learning clinical medicine come to believe that diseases follow the monomorphic textbook descriptions. Indeed, studies show that those first learning medicine readily dismiss correct diagnoses that experienced clinicians do not miss because the experienced clinician whose disease category definitions are richer and more flexible knows when a given patient is simply an outlier within a diagnostic category rather than truly outside the category.[77,300] Thus we understand the occasional assertion by an experienced clinician, "We see this," a comment that confirms that some apparently atypical finding is still consistent with a diagnosis. The answer to the question of why many discussants in CPCs in the *New England Journal of Medicine* ignore textbook descriptions of diseases and dig out individual cases comparable to the one they are discussing should also be apparent: In many instances even expert clinicians who encounter uncommon diseases do not have sufficient personal experience with the polymorphism of these diseases and, rather than rely on their own knowledge or on textbook descriptions, they turn to individual case descriptions to get a more complete picture of the disease's varied manifestations.[301] All of these features simply point to the complexity of the storage mechanisms of disease entities.

CASE 65. INTUITIVE AND INSPIRATIONAL, OR INDUCTIVE AND INCREMENTAL?

A 60-year-old woman presented to the hospital with a 4-day history of lethargy, nausea, vomiting, and swelling of the right jaw. On admission, she was markedly confused. She was known to have had non–insulin-dependent diabetes mellitus for 30 years, complicated by mild renal insufficiency and gastroparesis. She had been hospitalized 1 month earlier for a right ureteral calculus complicated by *Escherichia coli* pyelonephritis and urosepsis, and she had been on an antibiotic since discharge. Other medications included glipizide, metoclopramide, and a stool softener.

The most important piece of information is her 30-year history of diabetes. Diabetics are prone to a number of different complications, and the scant information we have about her right jaw swelling is at least consistent with some problem related to the diabetes. We need more information about that. In the diabetic patient who comes in with lethargy, nausea, and vomiting, I would think about problems related to the metabolic consequences of the diabetes and then to its nonmetabolic complications, such as urosepsis. Lethargy, nausea, and vomiting are nonspecific and could be consistent with anything from hypoglycemia to ketoacidosis to sepsis, so I would be interested in knowing her blood sugar, serum electrolytes, BUN, and creatinine.

An infectious complication would be my major concern for several reasons. First, she was hospitalized just a month earlier for a renal calculus and *E. coli* pyelonephritis, and she has been treated with antibiotics. We do not know what her urine culture showed, and we do not know whether that calculus passed. I assume that it either passed spontaneously or was extracted, but we do not have that information. So one complication I would worry about is recurrent urosepsis. Urosepsis in a 60-year-old, non–insulin-dependent diabetic certainly could present with lethargy, nausea, and vomiting. We would expect some other abnormalities, including fever and tachycardia, which I would want to know about.

The other reason that I would be concerned about an infectious problem is her right jaw swelling. I do not know whether it is in the jaw, the parotid gland, or a submandibular gland. There are parotid complications in diabetes, but I do not recall them now and would have to check on them.

The medications that she is taking do not provide many leads. The fact that she has been taking an antibiotic raises the possibility of overgrowth, such as *Candida* infection, and would also raise the possibility of other infectious complications of diabetes.

The patient was obese, in mild respiratory distress, oriented only to person, and rambling incoherently but was able to follow commands. Her temperature was 37°C orally, blood pressure was 158/72 mm Hg, pulse 125 per minute and regular, and respirations 20 per minute. She had a 6-cm mass at the angle of the right mandible, which was tender, fluctuant, and warm. Carotid pulses were symmetrically reduced. The remainder of the physical examination was normal; except for the mental status changes, no focal deficits were present.

So she seems to have an infectious process. She has a 6-cm tender, fluctuant, warm mass at the angle of the right mandible. Interestingly, her temperature is not elevated. The fact that it is an oral temperature might explain a normal value, or it could be an early-morning measurement. We have to keep in mind that diabetics sometimes do not do what nondiabetics do; for example, they may not be as febrile as nondiabetics.

Nonetheless, the mass in the neck would be the focus of my concern. In addition to the things that usually are near the mandible, we would also have to think of parotid duct obstruction, although the size of the mass is extraordinarily large for that kind of problem. I would also like to know whether one could see anything on the inside of her mouth, whether there is any abnormality of the ducts coming from the parotid glands. The mass still could be an enlarged parotid gland, an enlarged node, a cricopharyngeal abscess, or a cyst that had become obstructed and infected.

Results of a complete blood count were WBCs 13,500 with a normal differential, hemoglobin 9.4 g/dL, hematocrit 30%, platelets 89,000. Serum electrolytes were sodium 132 mEq/L, potassium 5.1 mEq/L, chloride 98 mEq/L, total CO_2 11 mEq/L. Blood pH 7.26, arterial PCO_2 21 mm Hg. Blood glucose 763 mg/dL, serum acetone positive at 1:16 dilution. BUN 60 mg/dL, creatinine 3.4 mg/dL. Urinalysis: specific gravity 1.020, protein 3+, glucose 3+, ketones 3+, pH 5. Urine sediment showed no bacteria (on Gram stain) and no white cells. Chest x-ray was normal. ECG showed sinus tachycardia but was otherwise normal. Lumbar puncture and CT scan of brain were normal. Blood, spinal fluid, and urine cultures were obtained.

Those data are helpful because they tell us not only that there is a nonmetabolic complication of diabetes (i.e., whatever is going on under her right mandible), but also that she has diabetic ketoacidosis: Her blood sugar is 763, bicarbonate is 11, anion gap is elevated, and serum acetone is positive. The blood pH is acidic, and the arterial PCO_2 is appropriately reduced for that degree of hypobicarbonatemia. BUN and creatinine are elevated and are consistent with prerenal azotemia from the glucosuria that one would expect, first by history and now demonstrated on urinalysis. Sepsis is one of the classic predisposing causes of ketoacidosis in a diabetic. The common causes of sepsis are pneumonia and urosepsis, but any type of sepsis could cause the same problem. My current thinking is that the lethargy, nausea, and vomiting are the result of severe diabetic ketoacidosis. The questions are, what is the predisposing cause of the ketoacidosis, and what is the cause of the right jaw swelling? As an aside, I do not understand why a CT scan of the brain was done in a diabetic with ketoacidosis.

The patient was treated with intravenous fluids, insulin, and ceftazidime. The right mass was found to be an abscess, and it was incised and drained; cultures of the purulent material were positive for *E. coli.* Antibiotics were continued.

The fact that the organism is *E. coli* is important. *E. coli* is a uropathogen, not an oral pathogen or a "head and neck" pathogen. This finding suggests that during the episode of *E. coli* infection 1 month earlier, the patient had septicemia and *E. coli* localized in some abnormal site, such as a pharyngeal tumor or a cricopharyngeal cyst. I would also be interested to know whether *E. coli* grew out of her blood. All we are told so far is that blood cultures were taken. We also do not have the results of the urine culture. My guess is that the urine is sterile because neither bacteria nor white cells were seen. I would not be surprised if the blood cultures are negative, because the septicemia may have cleared and left us with only a residual abscess.

How much further I would go would depend on what happened to her clinically in the next 24 hours.

> **Ultrasound studies of the gallbladder and kidneys were normal. A 4- to 5-cm aortic aneurysm above the level of the renal arteries was observed. The patient improved for 3 days after neck exploration, but then hypotension suddenly developed (50 mm Hg, systolic), and she sustained acute respiratory arrest. Her hemoglobin had fallen from 9.4 g/dL on admission to 5.5 g/dL. Nasogastric tube drainage was negative for blood.**

During the first 3 or 4 days I would have followed the same plan, namely to try to find out the source of the *E. coli* abscess. The places that were looked at were the kidneys (which makes sense because she previously had had urosepsis) and the biliary tract. In fact, biliary tract disease in a diabetic is a common cause of *E. coli* sepsis.

The aortic aneurysm is potentially important because if she did seed a lesion in the neck with *E. coli,* she also could have seeded an aortic aneurysm. As long as the aneurysm is small enough, I do not think we need to worry about rupture. But something disastrous has happened. Presumably, the patient was getting better, and then she suddenly became acutely hypotensive and had a respiratory arrest. It could be from an overdose of psychotropic agents, but that seems unlikely. It could also be in conjunction with a stroke.

I am trying to put together the neck mass with the respiratory arrest, but I am having a problem doing that. The only way that I could even speculate on that event is that a communication developed with the carotid artery and she bled from an extension of the abscess into the carotid artery or possibly that the mass lesion obstructed her trachea. I think either one of these possibilities is remote. Nonetheless, it would be important to know whether pulsations could be identified over the mass. I suppose I should have asked that early on. Also, we should be able to tell if the artery is visible at the base of the abscess. Finally, if she was easily intubated, it is unlikely that a lesion could account for the respiratory arrest.

There is another striking finding: In 3 days, her hemoglobin fell from 9.4 to 5.5 g/dL. She has mild renal insufficiency, but such severe and rapid development of anemia is too much for the mild renal insufficiency, and it suggests that she bled. Bleeding could occur in three sites. First, she could have bled into the gastrointestinal tract; second, the aortic aneurysm could have ruptured, even though 4- to 5-cm aneurysms typically do not rupture; third, bleeding could be occurring locally, with the abscess involving the carotid artery.

> **Gastroscopy revealed a blood clot in the cardia of the stomach but no ulceration in either the stomach or duodenum. CT scan of the abdomen demonstrated that the aneurysm was in close proximity to the third portion of the duodenum.**

Interesting. The patient has blood in the gastrointestinal tract, with no obvious source of bleeding found in the stomach or duodenum. I am not told if there was gastritis. Most patients who bleed from the stomach have gastritis. I will assume that no lesion was seen that could account for the blood clot in the stomach.

The CT finding of an aneurysm in close proximity to the third portion of the duodenum raises the possibility of an aortoduodenal fistula. Such a perforation would fit with our earlier hypothesis that the patient had *E. coli* sepsis a month ago and that she seeded not only the mass in her neck but also the aneurysm, and now a mycotic aneurysm has eroded into the duodenum. That is a tough diagnosis to make, but it can be made by arteriography. At this time, the emphasis should be on first making sure that she is appropriately intubated and that there is nothing in her neck that is interfering with ventilation, stabilizing her as much as possible, supporting her blood pressure, and then either doing an arteriogram or, if one felt strongly enough that she had an aortoduodenal fistula, taking her directly to the Operating Room.

> **The patient was taken to surgery, where she was found to have an aortoduodenal fistula. The aneurysm was resected, and the specimen was thought to be consistent with a mycotic aneurysm. Postoperatively, her course was complicated by acute renal failure and pulmonary**

embolism. The neck abscess eroded into the right carotid artery, and the patient died.

Analysis

In this clinical exercise, an acute life-threatening problem, namely an aortoduodenal fistula, manifested several days into the patient's hospital course. The clinician, a general internist, initially focused quite appropriately on other features, including the neck lesion, the previous urinary tract infection, and the patient's metabolic state. When the patient became hypotensive and the aortic aneurysm was identified, however, the clinician quickly raised the possibility that a mycotic aneurysm had eroded into the duodenum. How did this possibility occur to him? Was it an intuitive flash of insight, an inspiration? Or was it by an ordinary process of plodding induction, built on a solid foundation of clinical findings and hypotheses? These two metatheories reflect the extremes of the "cognitive continuum" or dual-processing approach ranging from purely analytic to intuitive.[2,3,302]

This problem-solving session provides a fine opportunity to explore clinical insights. The startling revelation that came to Archimedes in the public bath about how to measure the volume of an irregular object is familiar to every schoolchild. Archimedes' discovery and his famous cry of *"Eureka"* ("I have found") as he ran through the streets of Syracuse in the third century B.C. have become synonymous with the "flash of insight" that characterizes some forms of human problem solving. In medicine, too, intuition and creativity have received credit for the almost magical performance of certain physicians who seem to come up with a particularly important insight that others have missed.

The notion that the practice of medicine is as much art as science is probably as old as Archimedes' insight, but even in recent times the exceptional prowess of some physicians—in coming up with the right diagnosis or selecting the right treatment—is still perceived by some as an undecipherable art.[40] In these cases, we have shown several examples of flashes of clinical insight, and probably because we lean toward explicit analyses of clinical problems, we have tended to consider them special cases of well-defined problem-solving tactics, not unique qualities of the individual clinician. We have argued that we should be trying to understand those insights so as to better use and teach them (see cases 2 and 3).

In imaginative experiments, cognitive scientists, neuroscientists, and computer scientists have explored the nature of classical scientific discoveries.[111] We describe their studies in some detail here because it is our conviction that if some of the critical historical "insights" in the hard sciences (physics and chemistry) can be shown to represent examples of already defined problem-solving techniques, it will be even harder to argue that clinical insights are intuitive and undiscoverable aspects of the art of medicine.

Using the computer as a laboratory for studies of cognition is now a well-recognized and accepted technique that produces interesting insights into human behavior.[293] Elsewhere, we refer to parallel processing and connectionism as a model for human reasoning; here we discuss the application of computers in processing symbols. Because behavior can be simulated in the computer by manipulation of symbols, such a simulation can be used effectively to simulate cognition.[36,111] In one study, the investigators reasoned that if they could embody extensively studied and well-accepted problem-solving tactics as computer programs and could then derive some of the classical discoveries of hard science by presenting experimental data to the computer program, the problem-solving tactics they encoded would be considered sufficient to account for the discoveries of the laws of science.

The principal problem-solving tactics on which these investigators focused their attention were heuristics and induction. Heuristics, as we discussed earlier, are short-cuts that drastically reduce the number of steps needed in a search for solutions to a problem (see case 57), and induction is the process of making a generalization from a finite body of data.

The two problem-solving tactics—heuristics and induction—that scientists use to guide their search for regularities in data were modeled in a list-processing computer program as a set of "production rules" in the following general form: *if* (a certain pattern) is found or is present, *then* (identify a goal, or establish a law, or define new terms).

These "if-then" rules gather and record data, detect regularities in the data, assess relationships between sets of data, and compute the values of those relationships. For example, these rules assess whether clusters of data exist, whether a given set of values is either increasing or decreasing, and whether two sets of values are linearly related.

Using a series of computer programs that contained many "if-then" rules, considered by some to be analogous to concepts used by human problem solvers, the investigators tested either physical or chemical data; the data in some instances were identical to those available to the scientists who originally discovered a particular law. Most of the data presented to these computer programs were quantitative, but some were only symbolic.

The results of the experiment were intriguing: The computer programs presented with raw data "discovered" several historically important physical laws, including Boyle's law, which relates the pressure of a gas to its volume; Ohm's law, which relates current, resistance, and voltage; Galileo's law of uniform acceleration under the force of gravity; and Kepler's laws of planetary motion. Even when early knowledge about the nonquantitative relations between acids, bases, and salts were modeled as a computer program, the program defined abstract classes of chemical compounds and formulated reasonable laws stated in terms of these classes. Thus, the programs were applicable not just to a single aspect of scientific discovery, but also in several contexts: finding quantitative laws, generating qualitative laws, inferring the components of substances, and formulating structural models.

Those results imply that the basic processes underlying scientific discovery do not have to be explained as intuition, inspiration, creativity, or genius but can be explained as examples of "normal" problem solving adapted to a particular scientific domain. In other words, no special process needs to be invoked to explain such discoveries other than the plausible heuristic search strategies and inductive approaches used by intelligent humans. These studies might lead one to conclude that that the mental phenomena to which the terms "intuition" and "inspiration" are applied can be explained in terms of information processing, either by the brain or by the computer.

What are we to infer from this experiment about expert problem solving in medicine? First,

we must keep in mind that medical problem solving and the scientific discoveries described here may or may not be analogous. Indeed, the computer studies were almost all data driven. In other words, a set of data points formed the material presented to the programs; no hypotheses predated exposure to the data. It seems quite likely that some problem solving in medicine fits this data-driven format, but that a substantial element is hypothesis driven.[18,19] We have little insight, of course, into what fraction of our diagnostic competence is based on inspiration and how much is based on common induction; there is reason to believe that both elements are at work.[5,34]

However, what of the clinical problem-solving exercise that began this discussion? Was the clinician's "discovery" of the correct diagnosis the consequence of a flash of insight (an inspiration), or did it result only from progressive induction? Based on the transcript, we might conclude that it was that latter, that is, a stepwise, cumulative, and workman-like inductive process. The clinician, we believe, was fully prepared to accept relevant data when the life-threatening problem—namely rupture of a mycotic aneurysm into the duodenum—developed. When considering the jaw mass, he raised the possibility of infection. When considering the *E. coli* cultured from the abscess, he posited a previous urinary tract infection and transmittal of organisms via the bloodstream to the abscess. When the aneurysm was first identified, he hypothesized that it too could have been "seeded" by *E. coli*. Finally, after the CT scan showed the aneurysm in close proximity to the duodenum, he concluded that a mycotic aneurysm probably had ruptured into the duodenum.

The foregoing analysis, however, ignores an evolving body of information on human intuition.[2,3,7] Based on a series of ingenious experiments, some cognitive scientists have posited that much of our intelligence and problem-solving capacities are not conscious but are based on heuristics, namely hunches, gut feelings, and intuition. They argue that our ability to recognize subtle information from the environment (e.g., visual, auditory, or tactile cues such as body positioning, tone of voice, or response to physical examination) has been undervalued, and that a "recognition heuristic" plays an important part in how we process information. A recognition heuristic is analogous to appreciating the "if" concept of condition–action pairs (or production rules) that we described before (see case 48). According to the hypothesis, once a person appreciates a clue from the environment, the brain fills in details and makes predictions based on rather limited information.[6] In contrast to quantitative approaches to solving clinical problems, such intuitive methods are faster and might even be more accurate.[303] The inferences are in the form: I know the meaning, I act on it, but I do not know how I know it.[7] How much of our clinical reasoning is intuitive, how much explicit, and how much driven by accumulated data is not known. How accurate are our diagnostic hunches? In cases throughout the book are examples of striking accuracy and striking mistakes. How to use our clinical intuitions and their value are subjects for further study.

CASE 66. KNOWLEDGE AND CLINICAL EXPERTISE

A 44-year-old engineer was evaluated by his local physician for right flank pain of 3 months' duration. Ultrasound evaluation and CT scan of the abdomen revealed a solid 11-cm right adrenal mass.

At this point, I certainly want to focus on the solid 11-cm right adrenal mass. I think the differential diagnosis would include a large tumor of the adrenal cortex, which could be producing excessive cortical hormones. It also could be a tumor of the adrenal medulla, possibly a pheochromocytoma. I think that if it were an adrenocortical tumor, it would be producing aldosterone, and the patient would have electrolyte and fluid abnormalities and would be hypertensive. If it were a pheochromocytoma, I would also expect the patient to have symptoms indicative of that.

The flank pain could certainly be caused by this mass. A tumor could cause pain solely because of its size and pressure on adjacent tissues, but it could also cause obstruction of the kidney or other distortion of the urinary tract. At this point, I do not know if it is benign or malignant.

The patient had a remote history of episodic paroxysmal atrial fibrillation but no personal or family history of hypertension or endocrine disorders. Plasma cortisol levels were normal, as were 24-hour urinary excretions of vanillylmandelic acid (VMA), metanephrines, and catecholamines on two occasions. The patient was normotensive, and physical examination revealed no abnormalities.

The normal plasma cortisol probably excludes a cortisol-producing tumor. Similarly, the normal VMA, metanephrines, and catecholamines would exclude a pheochromocytoma. There still is a possibility that a tumor of the adrenal cortex that produces aldosterone or an androgen-like substance could be present. I think it is less likely that such a tumor would produce aldosterone without any history of hypertension, but I have not yet learned whether the patient is hypokalemic.

It would be exceedingly unusual for a tumor of this size to be either an aldosterone-producing tumor or a pheochromocytoma. It would also be unusual for either of those tumors not to have revealed itself via a hypertensive syndrome. It is true that in some studies, 50% of cases of pheochromocytoma are diagnosed at autopsy, but most of those patients have a history of hypertension. I believe there are cases of spontaneous bleeding into a pheochromocytoma that could explain this patient's flank pain, but I think that explanation is unlikely.

As for other possible causes of solid adrenal masses, tuberculosis and histoplasmosis are two infections that involve the adrenal gland and usually produce adrenal insufficiency. However, I have never heard of an 11-cm adrenal mass being caused by either of them. I find it hard to explain the mass on the basis of any infectious agent. Another common cause of adrenal masses is metastatic disease. Again, the size of the mass argues against a metastatic lesion, although metastasis should be in the differential.

At surgery, the adrenal mass was adherent to the liver and retroperitoneum, but it was removed uneventfully. Pathology revealed a pheochromocytoma.

I guess this is one of those unusual cases of pheochromocytoma, but I am a little confused.

Most patients with a pheochromocytoma that is not diagnosed during life are nonetheless hypertensive. It is possible to have a pheochromocytoma and still have 24-hour urine collections that are within the normal range; the tumor might not be active or only episodically so. Nevertheless, 90% to 95% of patients with a pheochromocytoma have elevated metanephrine secretion. Recent studies, however, suggest that plasma catecholamines are a more sensitive test.

On the basis of the laboratory studies, I would think this is not a catecholamine-secreting tumor. I wonder whether there are differences between hormone-secreting pheochromocytomas and those that do not secrete excessive catecholamines. I wonder whether the nonsecreting ones are more likely to be malignant—although with these particular tumors, malignancy is defined by the presence or absence of distant metastases.

Six weeks postoperatively, the patient's abdomen was reexplored because of an intraabdominal hemorrhage, but no obvious bleeding site was found. Cells identical to those seen in the original specimen—again, considered characteristic of pheochromocytoma—were identified in tissue taken from a clot near the liver. Postoperative studies revealed no evidence of disseminated intravascular coagulation, clotting factor deficiency, or platelet dysfunction. Intraabdominal bleeding recurred, and the patient was transferred to the Tufts Medical Center.

We now have two problems: First, in view of the fact that more pheochromocytoma cells were identified in the tissue, it appears that the initial tumor was inadequately resected. Second, what is causing the hemorrhage? It is important that the patient did not appear to be bleeding at sites other than the operative one. The blood studies do not reveal any evidence of a coagulation disorder. That does not rule it out, but again I think the overall picture makes a systemic clotting disturbance unlikely. The bleeding most likely is due to the tumor or to an actively bleeding vessel. At this point, therefore, I would ask whether the original diagnosis was correct and, more urgently, how we go about stabilizing the patient so that further bleeding does not occur.

Bleeding continued. Cytologic studies performed on a cell block from the abdominal fluid were consistent with pheochromocytoma. The following laboratory results were obtained shortly after surgery: 24-hour Urine VMA 8 mg (normal, up to 6), metanephrine 189 μg (normal 65–300), normetanephrine 4,908 μg (normal 120–400). Plasma norepinephrine 890 pg/mL (normal 167–515), plasma epinephrine 35 pg/mL (normal 20–109). The findings were attributed to a metastatic pheochromocytoma. An oncologist was consulted to assess whether chemotherapy was feasible.

While the urinary metanephrine is within the normal range, the VMA is slightly elevated, and the normetanephrine excretion is vastly elevated. The plasma levels show that norepinephrine is elevated, while epinephrine is not.

I need to know some facts before I try to interpret these data. For instance, were the blood samples simply obtained at the time of random blood drawing rather than according to a specific protocol? It has been well demonstrated that for one to measure catecholamines in the blood, the patient must be supine in a dark room with a needle placed in the antecubital vein 30 minutes ahead of time. If this protocol is followed, one can more easily interpret the data in terms of the sensitivity and specificity of the elevated levels as either indicative of a tumor or not.

This patient was in a postoperative state and had ongoing hemorrhage; I doubt that such a protocol would have been followed in those circumstances. Therefore, I am not sure how to interpret these elevations. Nonetheless, the elevation of normetanephrine is striking, and I would have to say that the findings are consistent with metastatic pheochromocytoma. I do not know whether metastatic pheochromocytomas have a propensity for hemorrhage.

The oncologist was skeptical of the working diagnosis because recurrent bleeding is rare with pheochromocytomas and more common with other tumors. Slides of the original tumor were obtained. Stains for chromogranin, keratin, and S-100 protein were negative, and cytoplasmic staining for factor VIII–related antigens was

> positive. Those findings, the histology, and the clinical pattern were considered consistent with angiosarcoma.

Well, that is interesting, I guess this case is a good example of accepting somebody else's conclusion and findings. Obviously, however, many aspects of the case were unusual. I commented before on the normal studies of catecholamines in the preoperative evaluation, and certainly the patient's clinical course was unusual in that he appeared to be bleeding from the tumor, which is unusual for a pheochromocytoma.

> Outcome: A trial of chemotherapy was instituted, but the patient did not respond. Bleeding into the abdomen continued, and he became increasingly lethargic. He died 3 weeks after admission. An autopsy was not performed.

Analysis

The physicians responsible for the care of this patient before the oncologist was consulted probably will never forget that bleeding into the abdomen is not characteristic of pheochromocytoma but is a feature of some abdominal sarcomas. Despite the lack of any clinical manifestations of pheochromocytoma, these physicians accepted the pathologist's diagnosis as correct and sought no further confirmation or refutation. Our discussant performed somewhat better but was not sufficiently suspicious of the findings to offer a better diagnosis.

The oncologist who saw the patient immediately "smelled a rat," asked for additional histologic studies, and confirmed his suspicion that the tumor was not a pheochromocytoma but instead was an abdominal sarcoma. Here we illustrate unequivocal dominance of an expert in diagnostic problem solving, a phenomenon identified in some formal studies.[19,116] In this case, the expert quickly recognized that there was a discrepancy between the accepted diagnostic hypothesis (pheochromocytoma) and a single clinical finding (abdominal bleeding). Indeed, the nononcologists appreciated that their working hypothesis was rather weak, yet they had no other reasonable hypothesis to take its place.

Clearly, an important difference in problem-solving ability between the expert and the nonex-

pert is knowledge, and we can presume that the oncologist was a more accurate problem solver than the others because he simply knew more. Unfortunately, we know little about what is almost certainly an exceedingly complex relationship between the extent of an individual's medical knowledge and his or her capacity to solve clinical problems, but we can gain substantial insights into this relationship from attempts to model diagnostic problem solving in the computer.

This branch of computer science is subsumed under the rubric "artificial intelligence" (AI). A computer program that behaves in a fashion such that its output would be considered intelligent if it had emerged from a human brain generally qualifies as an AI program. In medicine, although many prototype AI programs have been written and tested, few are in active use. Rather than elaborate on the accomplishments of those programs, we will describe the organization of knowledge in the memory of some AI programs. If the representation of knowledge in human memory is similar or even analogous, we might deduce a better understanding of the efficiency and accuracy of the expert human problem solver.

In several AI programs, knowledge is stored in the form of symbolic rules.[304,305] An example of such a rule relevant to the patient under discussion might be, "If a patient has an abdominal tumor resembling a pheochromocytoma but has no hypertension or increase in blood or urinary catecholamines, the chance of his having a pheochromocytoma is 0.01." Another rule might be, "If a patient has an abdominal tumor that produces intraabdominal hemorrhage, angiosarcoma is likely, with a probability of 0.4." Some combination of those rules, either by a computer program or by a clinician, might lead to the inference that pheochromocytoma in unlikely and sarcoma is likely.

Another symbolic knowledge representation in AI computer programs is a so-called "frame."[306] A frame is a detailed description of the attributes one would expect to find in a given disease or clinical entity, as well as the attributes one would expect to be absent. A pheochromocytoma frame might include hypertension and increased VMA excretion as findings that typically are present; findings that should be absent are persistently normal blood pressure and intraabdominal hemorrhage. Each finding, either present or absent, may be assigned a weight to be used to compute a score.

To solve a diagnostic problem, the computer program assembles the characteristics of an individual patient and then matches those characteristics to one or more disease frames.[162] It is easy to imagine how such a program—assuming that its frames for pheochromocytoma, sarcoma, and other tumors contained the requisite accurate data—would go about solving the problem in the patient presented here. The pheochromocytoma frame would be a poor match. Even if the histology resembled a pheochromocytoma, the clinical and laboratory features would not, and the combined score of the findings in the pheochromocytoma frame would be quite low. By contrast, sarcoma would be a better fit: Both the clinical and the laboratory characteristics would exist in the sarcoma frame, and the score would be high.

Drawing analogies between AI computer programs and clinical reasoning is not merely an arcane exercise. If a theory of clinical problem solving can be modeled as a computer program, the performance of the program can be considered a test of the validity of the theory.[36] For the program to work, the clinical knowledge and the techniques to manipulate that knowledge must be specified completely and unambiguously. Efforts to test theories of clinical cognition with this approach already have been described.[36] Although writing such programs sounds straightforward, the complexities of clinical medicine make a complete representation of even a single disease formidable, and as a consequence, diagnostic computer programs based on symbolic representations still perform only marginally effectively.

As noted elsewhere, research on knowledge and pattern recognition in chess provides some additional insight into the process we observed in this transcript. When chess grand masters and novices study a chessboard on which the pieces are arranged in a random fashion, there is no difference between the recall of the position of the pieces by the experts and the recall by the novices. When the pieces are arranged in a pattern that could exist in a real game, the grand masters outperform the novices overwhelmingly in recalling the positions of the pieces.[118] The chessboard pattern consisting of the clinical manifestations of the patient presented here was immediately recognized by the oncologist but not by others.

Finally, we note that an ordinarily reliable "gold standard" failed the clinicians who were taking care of this patient. As we assess various results of our clinical inquiries, we do so against some standard: A lung scan may have as its gold standard a pulmonary arteriogram, and a pulmonary arteriogram may have as its standard an autopsied lung. In many circumstances, the histology of tissue is the ultimate gold standard, and we thus rely heavily on its interpretation to confirm or deny our clinical suspicions. In this case, the gold standard was tarnished: The real gold standard in this patient was not the routine histology but one that was highly specialized. Inappropriate reliance on the routine histology submerged the uncharacteristic clinical picture and led to a long-sustained incorrect working diagnosis. But the oncologist was not tricked by "fool's gold": Recognizing the discrepancy between the clinical findings and the histology, he dug deeper until he struck the real thing.

CHAPTER 22

Learning Clinical Problem Solving

CASE 67. LEARNING CLINICAL REASONING FROM EXAMPLES

> A 48-year-old man presented with a 2-day history of headaches and neck stiffness. He also had a mild sore throat, a dry mouth, and a temperature as high as 39°C associated with chills. He had no confusion, nausea, vomiting, or changes in mental status. There was no history of homosexuality, intravenous drug abuse, recent travel, head trauma, tuberculosis, or exposure to tuberculosis.

With the symptoms of fever, headache, and a stiff neck, my first concern is about a central nervous system infection and possible meningitis. I would perform a physical examination first, followed quickly by lumbar puncture. In the emergency room, I would examine the fundi, looking for venous pulsations. If I did not see papilledema, I would do a lumbar puncture. I am concerned that this patient has an infection of the central nervous system; if he has bacterial meningitis, it is a bona fide medical emergency. The history of a mild sore throat suggests a variety of pathogens, specifically meningococcus or pneumococcus, the most common causes of adult acute bacterial meningitis. A sore throat can be the presenting sign of meningococcal disease before central nervous system symptoms appear. The numerous negative symptoms and history reduce the likelihood of opportunistic pathogens associated with acquired immune deficiency syndrome. I would not expect this to be tuberculous meningitis because its manifestations are not so acute. Encephalitis is less likely because the patient's mental status is normal. I would take some more history and prepare to do a lumbar puncture after I ascertained that his vital signs were stable. If papilledema were absent, I would not perform a head CT (computed tomography) scan before the lumbar puncture. If there is concern regarding increased intracranial pressure, introducing the risk of herniation in the course of lumbar puncture, a CT should be performed, but this should not delay empiric administration of antibiotics.

> On physical examination, the patient's blood pressure was 120/70 mm Hg without orthostatic changes. His temperature was 39.5°C. Examination of the head, eyes, ears, nose, and throat was unremarkable. Papilledema was not present. There were scattered nontender cervical and axillary lymph nodes. Nuchal rigidity was present. Lungs, heart, and abdomen were normal. The neurologic exam indicated that the patient was oriented. Cranial nerves were intact. Muscle strength and deep-tendon reflexes were normal.

The scattered lymph nodes could be important. If we are talking about shotty nodes of 0.5 cm or larger, we may be talking about diffuse lymphadenopathy, which would change the list of possible pathogens but not the need to do the lumbar puncture.

> The following initial laboratory data were obtained: White blood cell count was 4,300 with 71 polys, 22 lymphocytes, and 7 monos. Atypical lymphocytes were noted. Hemoglobin was 12.8 g/dL, hematocrit 38.2%, and mean corpuscular volume (MCV) 85. Serum electrolytes, blood urea nitrogen (BUN) and creatinine levels were normal. Serum glucose was 68 mg/dL, calcium 8.8 mg/dL, phosphorus 3.7 mg/dL, and magnesium 2.1 mg/dL. Liver function test results were normal, with the exception of a lactate dehydrogenase (LDH) of 467 IU/L. Total protein was 7.4 gm/dL, and serum albumin was 3.6 g/dL. International Normalized Ratio (INR) and partial thromboplastin time (PTT) were normal. The chest x-ray was normal.

The normal chest x-ray is useful information. In pneumococcal meningitis, a pulmonary infiltrate or pneumonia is frequently a primary event, with hematogenous spread. The CBC (complete blood count) is troublesome. There is no marked leukocytosis. There are an adequate number of lymphocytes—that is, about 1,000 total lymphocytes, if we are concerned about AIDS. In view of the atypical lymphocytes on smear and the sore throat, we certainly cannot ignore the possibility of mononucleosis and Epstein-Barr virus infection. Thus, the possibility of a viral, or aseptic, meningitis certainly has to enter the differential diagnosis. The serum glucose is normal or on the low side, and that will be important in interpreting the spinal fluid glucose concentration.

Is there a chronic infection? Are we looking at some chronic inflammatory process? A hemoglobin of 12.8 in a man is a little low, again suggesting a chronic illness. Results of the liver function studies and coagulation studies are normal. The white cell count may be indicative of overwhelming sepsis, but we have no picture of that. It may be indicative of viral infection but also might make us think a bit about HIV infection. If we believe the history, I would not get an HIV test because this man appears to be in a low-risk group.

> The results of the lumbar puncture were as follows: white blood cell count 187/mL with 19% polys, 65% lymphs, and 7% monos; red blood cell count 111/mL; glucose 40 mg/dL, protein 42 mg/dL. Acid-fast bacilli (AFB) stain, Gram stain, and bacterial antigen studies were negative. Blood culture and urine culture revealed no growth. A throat culture was negative. A rapid plasma regain (RPR) test was positive at 1:1 dilution. Fluorescent treponemal antibody (FTA) was negative.

The patient certainly has a pleocytosis in his spinal fluid with 187 white cells, which is abnormal. The CSF (cerebrospinal fluid) glucose is 40, which is just less than two thirds of the serum concentration of 68. There is no report of a cryptococcal antigen being drawn. We cannot take much comfort from the fact that the AFB stain is negative. I would want to obtain a skin test for tuberculosis in this patient, although if the patient is immunosuppressed, it might be nonreactive despite infection with *Mycobacterium tuberculosis*. The chest x-ray is normal, but tuberculous meningitis can present with a picture like this. In addition, in HIV-infected patients, it is not unusual for tuberculosis to present as extrapulmonary disease, espe-

cially in the lymphatic system. There is nothing atypical about tuberculosis here except the acute nature of the illness. The diagnosis of viral meningitis is one of exclusion, so we have to be careful not to miss a pathogen. I would worry about *Cryptococcus*, and we also have to worry some about AIDS, although now it is low on the list. My approach would be to look for *Cryptococcus* first and, if I found it, then to order the HIV test.

I am comfortable that the patient does not have a bacterial meningitis that must be treated immediately. The Gram stain of the spinal fluid is an important test; in the bacterial meningitides that are likely to affect people in their 40s (including some unusual organisms such as *Listeria*), we might expect to see the organism on smear. We might even see the organism before we saw the cells in the spinal fluid, especially in pneumococcal meningitis, where, early on, there may be an overwhelming proliferation of pneumococci and only a modest inflammatory response. We should also see meningococcus. *Haemophilus* is a rare pathogen in this age group, and other bacterial possibilities in someone without either an immunocompromised state or head trauma become small. I am worried about tuberculous meningitis. I am worried about the chronic meningitides. The diagnosis of exclusion is viral meningitis. A PPD (purified protein derivative) test and a cryptococcal antigen test would be next on my list.

> The patient improved slightly with intravenous fluids and was allowed to go home with a presumptive diagnosis of viral meningitis. His condition deteriorated, however, and he returned to the hospital within hours. His temperature had fallen to 38°C. He had a persistent headache and a stiff neck. The physician noticed some increased lethargy and difficulty in concentrating. The patient's laboratory data were essentially unchanged, with the exception of mild hyponatremia. A repeat chest x-ray was normal. A head CT scan revealed normal brain parenchyma. There was no midline shift. A mass was noted in the right maxillary sinus. A repeat lumbar puncture revealed mild lymphocytosis. Protein was 215 mg/dL, and glucose was 28 mg/dL. The AFB stain, Gram stain, and bacterial antigen testing were negative.

He probably has the syndrome of inappropriate antidiuretic hormone secretion (SIADH), which is seen in all sorts of central nervous system (CNS) processes. The highest prevalence of this syndrome associated with CNS infections was seen in an epidemic of equine encephalitis in Dallas, Texas, where 60% of the patients had at least transient evidence of SIADH. Tuberculous meningitis is another well-recognized cause of SIADH.

The chest x-ray remains normal. A CT scan of the head was now done—appropriately, I think. A mass was noted in the right maxillary sinus. In view of the CSF findings, I have to be very concerned about tuberculous meningitis, but what is this mass in his maxillary sinus? That becomes an important question.

> Antibiotic coverage was started with ceftriaxone and vancomycin. The maxillary sinus was drained, and cultures revealed *Staphylococcus aureus* sensitive to nafcillin. The hyponatremia was controlled with fluid restriction. A PPD was negative. An HIV test was positive both by enzyme-linked immunosorbent assay (ELISA) and Western blot. An HIV viral load and CD4 count were pending.

This combination of antibiotics seems to have a broad enough spectrum. He does turn out to have *S. aureus* in his maxillary sinus, which might dictate the use of an antistaphylococcal agent. It also raises the possibility of a parameningeal focus, namely sinusitis, as the cause of his headache and fever. The positive HIV test is confirmed by Western blot, which makes it almost certainly a true positive; I would treat it as a real finding. As I recall, the patient denied that he was homosexual and denied IV drug abuse. I do not recall a history of transfusions, but he probably did not have any. We either have to discount aspects of the history or wonder whether we are looking at a patient who acquired HIV infection through heterosexual spread. In view of the positive HIV test, I am concerned about what organism is infecting the central nervous system and whether it will be sensitive to traditional medications.

> Over the next 24 hours, the patient became incontinent of urine. A repeat head CT scan revealed no hydrocephalus or mass lesion. There

> was no evidence of right maxillary sinusitis. The patient was transferred to the intensive care unit, and treatment with isoniazid, rifampin, ethambutol, pyrazinamide, pyridoxine, and dexamethasone was begun. A repeat lumbar puncture revealed increased pressure. Lymphocytosis was noted. Protein concentration was increased, and glucose was decreased. An AFB stain, Gram stain, bacterial antigen study, and cryptococcal antigen tests were negative.

At this point, what could we be missing that we could treat? I do not think we would have missed a bacterial meningitis on three lumbar punctures. How about fungal meningitis? We have looked for the important one, cryptococcosis. The cryptococcal antigen, which is a sensitive test, is negative.

What about herpes simplex encephalitis with a meningeal reaction? It usually presents with focal nervous system lesions, specifically in the temporal lobe, but there have not been any such lesions in this patient. This is now looking like a meningoencephalitis. The urinary incontinence troubles me. We are told there is no hydrocephalus and no evidence of cerebral edema. I cannot think of any other infections that I could treat.

I do not think I would treat for toxoplasmosis without a positive radiographic study but feel that an MRI (magnetic resonance imaging) of the brain with gadolinium is indicated. Primary HIV infection of the central nervous system as the cause of this syndrome is possible but unlikely.

> Over the next 24 hours, the patient became increasingly confused. An MRI of the head revealed an area of demyelination involving the right frontal lobe adjacent to the Sylvian fissure. The patient's serum sodium fell to 119 mEq/L but subsequently rose to 126 mEq/L with fluid restriction.

I am beginning to worry and wonder whether we are looking not at tuberculous meningitis but rather at HIV meningoencephalitis, for which—as far as I know—there is no effective treatment. I would continue the antituberculosis therapy, however. I would go back and try to get more history. It is difficult to turn to the patient's family and friends under these circumstances, but I would want to know what the patient's hepatitis B serology was because that is a kind of marker for both intravenous drug abuse and sexual promiscuity. I would like to find an explanation for this patient's HIV infection. Given the uncertainty of the diagnosis and the progressive nature of this illness, a brain biopsy should be performed.

> **On the fifth hospital day, generalized tonic–clonic seizures developed. The neurologic exam revealed bilateral clonus and positive Babinski reflexes. A repeat head CT scan revealed a nonenhancing lucent area involving the left head of the caudate nucleus and anterior limb of the left internal capsule (not seen in the two previous studies). The lateral and third ventricles were dilated.**

The characteristic lesions of toxoplasmosis are enhancing; so are tuberculomas of the central nervous system. Nonenhancing lesions might suggest nonvascular tumors, infarcts, or a series of other things that I do not think I can list on the basis of the data here.

> **On the sixth hospital day, the patient underwent placement of an intracranial bolt for obstructive hydrocephalus. Ganciclovir was added to the medical regimen to empirically cover both herpes encephalitis and cytomegalovirus encephalitis. The results of cerebrospinal fluid studies were unchanged. The patient was considered too unstable to undergo a brain biopsy.**

Patients being considered for brain biopsy often look well for a long time and then rapidly become "too unstable." I do not think I can quarrel with the antiviral drug, but I think it is not going to make much difference. The laboratory findings continue to point to a viral, or possibly malignant, cause of meningitis. I do not have further suggestions for therapy.

> **By the seventh hospital day, the patient was responsive only to deep pain. Apneustic breathing developed, necessitating mechanical ventilation. The patient continued to deteriorate and died on the ninth hospital day. At autopsy, he was found to have extensive tuberculosis involving the brain. The organism was found to be *Mycobacterium tuberculosis,* which was sensitive to all of the antituberculosis drugs that the patient had received.**

What we are looking at here is the fact that immunocompetence is important in treating this infection since the appropriate medications were unable to cure it.

Analysis

One could hardly argue against the virtues of teaching clinical reasoning—how to do it right and how not to do it wrong. Yet major impediments deter even outstanding clinician-teachers from imparting those skills. First, a comprehensive theory of clinical cognition is not available (indeed, a comprehensive theory of human cognition is yet to be formulated); only bits and pieces exist. Second, the clinical reasoning process is sufficiently complex to virtually preclude a step-by-step analysis and a complete description of the process. What is the alternative? Textbook learning is only the initial step in developing the requisite clinical cognitive skills. In fact, the bulk of the learning process consists of refinement of the cognitive skills by practice. None of these concepts should be particularly surprising. Anyone who recalls learning to drive an automobile with the goal of passing a licensure examination appreciates that one really learns to drive solo after passing the test.

How can students refine their cognitive skills if we cannot give them something to memorize and cannot impart it in our lectures? In carrying out this task, medical education departs little from undergraduate education. We teach such refinement by example. In geometry and calculus, we solve one problem after another until we "catch on" to the generalities of problem solving; in medicine, we "work up" one patient after another until the process becomes "second nature."

The principal problem with learning by example is the examples. We may select the examples on the basis of the case types they represent (gastrointestinal bleeding, acute appendicitis, hepatorenal syndrome), but we rarely select them for the cognitive processes—good or bad—that they illustrate. As a consequence, our teaching of clinical cognition with the most powerful tool available—the clinical example—is often incomplete and, at best, spotty. Perhaps we have paid too little attention to this valuable didactic modality. Perhaps it is time to take a page from other educational disciplines and carefully scrutinize this teaching tool.

What value, for example, is the case presented here in terms of understanding the diagnostic process? The discussant is a seasoned infectious disease specialist, and her reasoning processes seem transparent. Once she narrowed her hypothesis down to a central nervous system infection, she began to identify the organisms that produce clinical syndromes similar to the findings in the patient at hand. In the course of her analysis, she mentioned about a dozen different infections, and, notably, she mentioned the correct diagnosis no less than six times, indicating that it remained, or kept popping up, in her working memory. On top of specific pathogens, she also considered purulent meningitis (a summary hypothesis that includes many others) and chronic meningitis. The transcript discloses a typical diagnostic approach used by specialists in this field, and it is one that a student could begin to learn to emulate.

How is it best to learn this aspect of medicine? The ability to learn is one of the most fundamental human attributes. Learning by rote or learning from direct instruction requires little inference on the part of the learner, whereas learning from analogy or learning from examples, when done actively and intentionally, requires considerable inference.[21,307] Learning from example is simply a special form of inductive learning, one that generates plausible general descriptions, concepts, or hypotheses—which, in turn, become useful in a predictive mode.[308,309]

To provide the optimal learning experience, examples should not be produced randomly. If they are, there is no guarantee that a comprehensive set of concepts or hypotheses will emerge. Instead, a teacher should select the examples that fully instantiate the inferences to be made—that is, are sufficiently broad to evoke by inference the appropriate and relevant principles.

With respect to the cognitive aspects of medicine, the examples should instantiate an accepted, tested, excellent problem-solving strategy. However, inclusion of only such positive examples is probably not sufficiently instructive because

a student might well overgeneralize the inferred concept from such examples. To avoid such overgeneralization, the teacher should also provide negative examples, namely instances of faulty clinical reasoning. Such counterexamples are helpful in circumscribing the concepts we want to teach. In fact, some have argued that even more helpful counterexamples in avoiding inductive overgeneralizations are "near hits"—namely, negative examples that just miss being positive by a single significant attribute.[309,310]

Let us proceed from the theoretical to the practical. The cases described in this book are all examples of medical problems, each with a built-in lesson. We believe that there is no better approach to teaching clinical problem solving than teaching by example. The teaching need not be confined to published examples, as in this series, but can be adapted for small group sessions, grand rounds, and demonstrations for as many as 1,000 physicians.[1]

In these cases, however, it has been possible to pick and choose examples that explicate many different aspects of the clinical problem-solving process. Many such cases have been "positive" examples (see cases 4, 34, and 40), and many have been negative examples or counterexamples (see cases 27 and 58). Indeed, several have been near hits (see cases 11, 17, and 44). From these cases, the student can infer, by induction, many problem-solving principles. When the principle is particularly opaque, we have provided some illumination in the form of editors' comments. We do not claim that this series of cases provides a complete picture of the concept of clinical problem solving, only that alert readers can acquire many of the cognitive concepts they need as physicians.

CASE 68. MAKING A SILK PURSE OUT OF A SOW'S EAR

A 55-year-old physician asked his primary care physician, whom he had been seeing for 10 years, if he should have an electrocardiographic (ECG) stress test.

This is an example of caring for the "worried well." If I were his physician, I would say no, unless he was having symptoms. I think the data are fairly convincing that exercise testing for coronary disease in asymptomatic individuals is not cost-effective. In a patient with a low prior probability of coronary disease, false-positive results are frequent, and in such patients, the costs of testing far exceed the benefits of early detection. In addition, the evidence that intervention early on in the asymptomatic state alters the natural history of coronary artery disease is also scanty at best. Generally, I would argue that if you uncover disease in this early stage, it is not at a state in which intervention would make a difference. So, unless this patient is having some symptoms, I would recommend no test. But whether he is really symptom-free is one of the important things to be sure of. If someone had been followed for a long time and all of a sudden asks if he should have a test but denies symptoms, be suspicious. Go hunting for the symptoms. There is something that may be making that patient worry now that he was not worried about before.

It is important to uncover whether in fact the patient thinks he may have angina and he's denying symptoms. But maybe he is asking for the test and thinking that he will find out first whether there is anything to worry about before he tells you what is really going on. Maybe his father died at 55 of a myocardial infarction and that is why he is worried. Then that is an important thing to talk about, but even if this history were obtained, the test is still not necessarily justified.

> The patient had no chest pain or dyspnea. He was riding a bicycle 25 miles per week and walking as well. On a recent trip, he had jogged for several miles along a beach without difficulty. He had long-standing hypertension that was under excellent control with enalapril.

I am reassured at least up to this point that he is not symptomatic and is really physically active. So my first inclination is reinforced, namely that a screening exercise test is not indicated at this particular time.

> Ten years earlier, during an evaluation for mild mitral valve prolapse and atrial premature contractions, an ECG stress test was performed and was negative.

Again, I worry about doing a stress test in this patient because of the high likelihood of nonspecific findings and false-positive results commonly seen in the presence of mitral prolapse. It is reassuring that the test was negative then, but of course that does not tell us for sure that he does not have coronary disease now. He could have had insignificant disease that progressed. This history does not change my estimate of the probability of significant coronary disease at this point in time. and it does not change my view about his need for a stress test now. If I can use this opinion as reassurance for the patient, that is fine.

> Ten years earlier, the patient was deemed overweight and was advised to lose weight. The following values have been obtained since (HDL, high-density-lipoprotein cholesterol; LDL, low-density-lipoprotein cholesterol; all measurement except weight in mg/dL; weight in pounds):

Years Ago	Cholesterol	Triglycerides	HDL	EST LDL	Weight
10	267	168	39	173	
3	266	309		178	
2	287	293	37	191	174
1	235	290	31	146	
Current	231	290	31	146	182

> During this time, he received only antihypertensive agents.

His weight has gone up, his HDL cholesterol has fallen, his triglycerides have risen, and his total cholesterol still is around 230. So, this patient clearly needs some counseling. He is worried, and he has some good reasons to be worried. But rather than do a stress test, I would emphasize dietary management. He is exercising, and maybe he needs to exercise more. Clearly, however, he needs to deal with the issues of diet for weight loss and cholesterol control.

> Family history: His father developed angina at age 50 years but lived to age 89 years. Uncles on both his maternal and paternal sides had suffered from myocardial infarctions. His older brother had a coronary bypass graft for angina at age 51 years.

So he has another reason to be worried, and because he is a physician this is probably something that he is very aware of. Men in his family had symptomatic manifestations of coronary disease in the 50s, and he is 55 now. Again, rather than pursue the exercise test at this point, I would try to use this information to provide the incentive to him for lifestyle modifications and behavioral changes that stand the best chance of improving his long-term outcome.

> The primary care physician was not certain what to do. He was reluctant to recommend the test, given the absence of any symptoms. He wondered about the implication of testing based on risk factors alone. He wondered about what to do if the test were positive, given that most of the data in the literature on such tests were derived from patients with chest pain. He wondered about the obligation to carry out repeated tests if the test was negative.

Well, these were all issues that I alluded to at the beginning and show why I think the screening stress test is not an effective strategy. There certainly are times when, in order to take care of a particular patient, we do something that we would not recommend as a universal strategy for health care. I think that is an important issue to acknowledge. Assuming that I knew the patient well, I would first spend a lot of time talking to him. I would explain to him all the implications of doing the test. Only then would I do something that I would not generally do in everybody else. I have been in situations in which I have decided to go ahead and do a test I usually would not do, but in such instances, I have done it because I think it is an effective strategy for managing a particular patient. But I would also spend a lot of time with such a patient before I gave in. I would encourage him to exercise more and give him incentives to modify his lifestyle.

> The primary care physician referred the patient to a cardiologist.

Now, that is like choosing your confessor! We know in our own institutions which cardiologists are aggressive and invasive and which ones are conservative and have a preventive medicine approach. So again, as an internist, referrals become

self-fulfilling prophecies. But at least if you refer someone, you then can throw up your hands and say, "I didn't make the decision; someone else did."

> A nuclear stress test was carried out. It showed an inferior defect with partial redistribution; there were no Q waves in corresponding leads in the ECG. There also was evidence of lung uptake of the isotope, signifying left ventricular dysfunction.

Well, now we got what we asked for. Are we happy or not? The patient underwent a nuclear exercise test with greater specificity and sensitivity than the standard stress test. If his baseline ECG was entirely normal, I would still argue that if one were going to do a stress test, that the appropriate one would be just an ECG stress test. Since we were told that he had mitral prolapse, he may have some baseline repolarization abnormalities and, if so, if you were inclined to do a stress test, then choosing the test with higher sensitivity and specificity might be warranted as your first test, even acknowledging the greater expense.

Given the result of this test, the probability of coronary disease is probably 90% or 95% certain. It appears to be limited to one vessel, at least by the perfusion abnormality. The inferior wall is often the hardest one to interpret, particularly at the apex. Movement changes can make the interpretation of the nuclear scan in the apical region difficult. The increased lung uptake often reflects evidence of more extensive coronary disease and significant left ventricular dysfunction. It has been shown at least in postinfarction patients to be a powerful prognosticator for future events because of its high correlation with significant three-vessel disease. We have a dissociation between the extent of the perfusion abnormality and this increased lung uptake. We have to decide what we are going to emphasize. To some extent, the interpretation of these findings depends on personal bias. If you tend to be aggressive, you might synthesize the findings thus: "Here's a 55-year-old man with several risk factors who has a positive stress test with lung uptake. He must have extensive coronary disease, and we'd better carry out cardiac catheterization." Or, if you tend to be conservative, you might frame the problem another way: "Here's an asymptomatic 55-year-old man with a limited perfusion abnormality. He may have coronary disease, but if he has, it's limited. Because he's asymptomatic, a conservative management is in order." I would choose the latter approach because he is asymptomatic and has a limited perfusion defect. Yet he probably has coronary disease, but it's probably limited. What he needs is dietary counseling, lifestyle modification, and medications.

> The coronary arteriogram revealed the following stenoses: 75% left main, 75% proximal left anterior descending (LAD), 40% mid-LAD, 80% left circumflex artery, 75% proximal right coronary artery (RCA), and 80% distal RCA.

So he went to an aggressive cardiologist, and we have evidence of three-vessel disease. I am surprised at the extent of disease. Clearly, the increased lung uptake on the nuclear study meant something. In patients with diffuse coronary artery disease, the scan may underestimate the severity of disease because it is dependent on comparisons of perfusion. In retrospect, the scan underestimated the extent of coronary disease because the myocardium was more symmetrically hypoperfused. The increased lung uptake was indeed a marker of the extent of the coronary disease.

This example indicates the messiness of clinical medicine. What lesson should we take home from this experience? One possible lesson goes like this: "You never know who has disease and you better exercise everybody, and perform catheterizations and operations on more people." I would be reluctant to provide that as the message from this patient.

What we have is an asymptomatic patient in whom we have almost accidentally discovered severe and potentially life-threatening coronary disease. We know that we can prolong life with surgery in symptomatic patients with left main and three-vessel disease, but whether this result is the same in asymptomatic patients is simply unknown. Nonetheless, the survival data in symptomatic patients are so impressive in that group that even a conservative cardiologist like me would recommend surgical intervention in this patient with the expectation that bypass surgery would prolong life.

> The patient had five coronary artery bypass grafts 3 days after cardiac catheterization. The

> internal mammary arteries were grafted to the distal circumflex and the left anterior descending arteries; vein grafts were used to bypass the right coronary, obtuse marginal, and diagonal arteries. The patient recovered from surgery uneventfully and left the hospital on the fourth postoperative day.

Well, the patient and his doctors were lucky. In this particular instance, the exercise test and the catheterization yielded a favorable outcome. But there is a danger in using the outcome of a decision as the measure for the validity of the decision-making process. Even after seeing the outcome, I believe that by and large a conservative approach to a patient like this is the right approach. Given a population of similar patients with his family history and laboratory findings, the number in whom you are going to find unexpected left main disease is very, very small. Nevertheless, the experience with this patient illustrates why it is so difficult to make hard and fast rules that govern how you are going to approach all patients.

Analysis

With respect to the varied aspects of the clinical problem-solving process, there are few, if any, issues raised in the discussant's remarks that we have not covered before. Familiar items that quickly surface include interpretation of test results, efficacy of therapeutic approaches, patient involvement in decision making, extrapolation of data from existing studies to patients who do not fit precisely the study group, and the occasional discrepancy between outcomes and choices in medical decision making. What is special about this case is the controversy it produces when used to teach clinical problem solving. Some observers are laudatory about its use in the didactic mode, but others have been strongly critical. The argument of the critics is simple. They argue that it broadcasts the wrong message, namely, that the exercise test was an appropriate choice in this asymptomatic patient and that students or physicians who pay attention to the testing approach in this patient would extrapolate the same approach to other patients. The ultimate outcome of this lesson would be excessive and inappropriate testing, presumably resulting, overall, in more harm than good. Because the only purpose of presenting this particular patient was to teach, this criticism deserves serious assessment.

In another instance (see case 67), we point out the value of teaching clinical reasoning by example. We emphasized that, because a comprehensive theory of clinical problem solving is yet to be formulated, it is difficult to teach all the elements of reasoning, but because many aspects are well recognized, that using specific examples to teach clinical reasoning was an alternate approach that can be used today. We also made three other points: (1) When using specific examples to teach clinical reasoning, the examples must be selected with care because not all cases are paradigms of specific reasoning strategies. (2) When selecting examples, the choice should include not only samples of optimal reasoning, but also samples of poor reasoning and "near hits," namely examples that miss by some small attribute. Such counterexamples limit overgeneralization and falsify incorrect ideas. (3) Teaching reasoning by instantiation (use of specific examples) is not different from, and simply an extrapolation of, the way we teach the facts of clinical medicine, namely by selecting a series of cases of, say, jaundice or acute renal failure for

students to "work up" until they become comfortable with the clinical entities. In another instance (see case 64), we discussed one additional possible rationale for this pedagogic approach, namely the nature of storage of information in memory. If memory of reasoning concepts consists of a polyglot of images of the concept rather than a single model (or a single generalization) (as proposed for memory of facts—see case 64),[311] then presenting concepts using multiple examples (good or bad) or presenting concepts from multiple vantage points should be beneficial to the learner.

Before trying to decide whether the decision making by this particular patient's physicians was optimal or suboptimal, let us first examine the concepts generated in this particular instantiation, as generated by the discussant. Table 22.1 contains a brief description of many of the concepts illustrated by the discussion. The reader can identify at which point in the discussion these issues were considered by reference to the "chunk" of information that preceded the discussion of the concept. Note that each concept is different, that the total set embraces a large and important group of clinical problem-solving principles, and that, in all, at least

TABLE 22.1

Examples of Problem-Solving Concepts in Response to Information Chunks

Chunk	Concept
1	Cost-effectiveness of exercise testing in coronary artery disease
1	High likelihood of false-positive results in patients with a low prior probability of disease
1	Efficacy of coronary bypass grafting in asymptomatic patients
1	When to be suspicious of a patient's history
3	Interpretation of repetitive tests over time
4, 5, 7	Conservative vs. aggressive approach of certain physicians
6	Departure from common practice in individual patient
6	Importance of sharing information on risks with the patient
8	Sensitivity and specificity of one test vs. another
8	Posterior probability after a positive test result
8	Test results that predict the severity of disease
8	Alternative interpretations of compiled clinical data
9	Using established clinical data as an anchor point for a patient whose clinical features differ from established data in some essential respect
10	Just because an outcome is favorable does not ensure that the decision was optimal

14 items were considered. Considering the "down side" of presenting this patient that we alluded to before (putatively it teaches the wrong message), are the benefits listed in the table sufficiently large to outweigh the negatives? Clearly, this choice is a matter of judgment. We believed that the benefits substantially outweigh the risks or we would not have used the example. Others may not agree.

Finally, we admit we may have invoked a "straw man." We have declared the case to be an example of inappropriate patient management, and by the title, we have implied that we have used a case of poor (or at least debatable or controversial) medical practice to do good clinical teaching. But was the practice of medicine in this patient flawed? Clearly, our discussant would have opted for a far less aggressive approach involving exercise, diet, and weight loss. Yet, even she acknowledges that clinical medicine is messy and that, from time to time, it is appropriate to violate general rules for individual patients. Clearly, the decision to test was a borderline one, yet the cardiologist felt strongly that testing was in order. Our discussant sensed that there might be more than meets the eye when she warned us that when a patient "all of a sudden asks if he should have a test, but denies symptoms, be suspicious." The discussant was aware that the patient is a physician. Physicians, other health care workers, and well-informed individuals from the lay public probably qualify for special attention. When these individuals raise concerns about testing, one should be aware that some clinical information may be hidden, either consciously or not. The cardiologist who saw the patient in consultation actually wondered if he had obtained the "whole story," and this suspicion pushed him over the testing threshold.[59] Quite likely the patient's life expectancy was extended as the consequence of this decision. Bad medicine? Good medicine? Judge for yourself. Good teaching material? We think so.

CASE 69. OPTIMIZING CASE DISCUSSIONS

Whereas teachers of clinical medicine recognize the importance of careful case selection and advance preparation in teaching aspects of physiology and pathophysiology, we should expend the same thoughtfulness and energy in preparing cases to teach clinical problem solving. Although grand rounds formerly was a venue for such didactic sessions, it no longer is. Over the years, many hospitals have given up patient-oriented grand rounds.[312] Sometimes a patient's history is still the focal point for discussion, but often no live patient is presented. The patient has often been replaced by an isolated lecture on a new research approach, a disease entity, a new treatment, or a new diagnostic procedure. Many factors are responsible for this evolution: shorter hospital stays, concern for patients' privacy, clinicians' uneasiness with impromptu case discussions, and reduced availability of house officers to present cases. The ease of giving "canned" talks, the time-consuming preparation of a detailed discussion oriented exclusively around a single patient, and discomfort with a free-wheeling, unstructured discussion may have contributed. Nonetheless, conferences devoted to discussions of individual patients still survive but are now usually in intimate settings with small groups. Morning report conferences in departments of medicine are prototypes of such discussions, and in many institutions, such conferences have more or less supplanted grand rounds. Such conferences are ideal for teaching not only the nuts and bolts of clinical medicine (pathology, mechanisms of disease, pathophysiology, drug doses), but also aspects of clinical reasoning. To do so, however, case selection and sequence of case material are critical. An approach that has been widely adopted across the country incorporates the following attributes:

- An exclusive discussion of the clinical and cognitive aspects of a single case
- Careful selection and preparation of patient problems for presentation
- Presentation of clinical material prospectively
- Impromptu problem solving by participants, holding any "canned" discussions until the end
- Active involvement of participants

One such format is completely unstructured. The patient selected for presentation is intentionally known only to a restricted number of people in attendance. Information is made available corresponding to the chronological sequence in which the data accumulated. No advance information is given to anyone who will be discussing the problem. Participants are invited to "think out loud" as they interpret the available data; they are encouraged to ask for information, but in doing so explain why they asked it when the rationale for their question is not immediately apparent. Then, once they have been given the new information, they are asked to interpret the data in light of the current diagnostic strategy. All members (except those who know the details or outcome of the case) are asked to participate: to offer opinions, ask questions, challenge interpretations, comment on pathophysiology, and make predictions about the patient's outcome.

All elements of diagnostic and therapeutic problem solving, including the knowledge required to solve the patient's problem, can be explored in a session of this kind. If the session is conducted properly, the participants feel little pressure, and the problem-solving session proceeds with good humor in a congenial climate.

The most important aspect of selecting a case for discussion is the lesson it teaches. Cases should be selected if their exposition and solution explicate something special about medical knowledge, diagnostic reasoning, or therapeutic decision making. These "paradigm cases" should not be canonical examples—that is, they should be selected not merely on the basis of their similarity to a "classic case" but because they exemplify some special aspect of problem solving.[298] For example, a patient with hemochromatosis should be selected not on the basis of the prevalence of the disease but because of the interesting way a clinician happened to think of the diagnosis or because of the particular way in which the clinician made a decision about the risks and benefits of various therapeutic approaches. Presentation of rare diseases with no intrinsic lesson (e.g., tularemia meningitis) is likely to fall flat; a routine case of a disease presented only because of its rarity may not contain an important lesson about clinical reasoning.

This book provides numerous examples of paradigm cases. Table 22.2 lists those cases and the problem-solving goals that they were designed to illustrate. The goal need not necessarily fall into one of these formal categories. Cases can be selected because a serious outcome was narrowly averted (see case 16) or because a finding was startling and unexpected (see case 67). Even the most mundane case can evoke exciting discussions if a special aspect of the problem is highlighted.

Another major criterion for case selection is veridicality. All cases should be real, and all relevant clinical material should be included. Deliberate omission of critical data (a classic ECG in a patient with pericarditis, a remarkably elevated creatine kinase in a patient with rhabdomyolysis) converts the exercise into a guessing game. Indeed, the roads of the real world of medicine are cluttered with enough red herrings without creating new ones. The goal is not to trick the participants but merely to provide powerful examples of the real day-to-day inductive and inferential process of solving clinical problems. The ability to correctly interpret and overcome these natural hurdles is precisely what we wish to convey in teaching exercises.

Another format also works exceptionally well and has been used for more than 20 years at the annual meeting of the American College of Physicians. As characteristic of most of the cases in the book, material is presented in chunks that simulate the chronological sequence of data that became available. In installments the initial or early clues consist only of laboratory data (see cases 2, 14, and 34), but often the presentation is initiated by a slide containing only the patient's age, sex, race, and presenting complaints. In the exposition of the sequential information, special care must be given to the real mystery and drama involved in explaining discrepancies, discovering the diagnosis, and elaborating on testing and treatment options. Preparing material in this fashion generates interest, creates anticipation, and engages participants in trying to unravel the dilemma. This case construction capitalizes on one of the fundamental motivations of physicians to practice medicine: its intellectual challenges.

When possible, material presented in this fashion should disclose the nearly subliminal clues that led a clinician to generate a hypothesis that no one else had considered, the reason why a clinician avoided using a test that might have been disastrous, or how a clinician weighed the benefits and risks of two or more therapeutic approaches in arriving at a difficult decision. Our cases were infrequently constructed according to the traditional package containing a chief complaint, a history of the current illness, a review of systems, a family history, a social history, a physical examination, and the full battery of laboratory tests. Constructions

TABLE 22.2

Paradigm Cases and Associated Problem-Solving Acquisition Goals

Goal	Case	Goal	Case
Diagnostic Issues			
Generation of diagnostic hypotheses	45	Physiologic reasoning in hypothesis assessment	32, 34, 36
Single cues or clusters of cues that yield new hypotheses	1, 11, 63	False-positive cues in the history	17
Variations in clinical attributes of a disease	13, 64	Persistent diagnostic uncertainty	9, 41
Influence of prior probability on data interpretation	21, 26, 29	Discrimination between hypotheses	18, 38
Laboratory results as clinical data	14	Interpretation of discrepant data	40
Cognitive Errors			
Defective hypothesis generation	5, 55	Error attributable to the availability heuristic	57
Faulty context formulation	7, 9		
Faulty assessment of prior and conditional probabilities	27	Error attributable to faulty causal reasoning	58
Failure to appreciate the significance of a single clinical cue	39, 54	Faulty application of a clinical axiom	16
Error attributable to the representativeness heuristic	23	Faulty hypothesis verification ("premature closure")	43, 52, 56, 66
Testing Issues			
Screening for rare diseases	22	Influence of therapeutic efficacy on testing decisions	25
Concept of test or treatment threshold	24, 45	Interpretation of false test results	20, 27, 36, 51
Therapeutic Issues			
Tradeoff between immediate and long-term risk of two therapeutic approaches	46	Tradeoff between risks and benefits of surgical vs. medical treatments	44, 50
Tradeoff between quality of life and immediate risk of death	47		

conforming to this approach often miss the drama and, more important, the critical problem-solving aspects of data presented in a chronological mode.

The "CPC mode," a valuable teaching venue itself, is not ideally suited to teaching clinical reasoning. In the typical clinicopathologic conference, all of the patient's data are predigested, and the problem solving begins after consideration of all, or almost all, of the patient's findings. For teaching clinical problem solving, the CPC mode has several disadvantages. First, retrospective bias has a powerful influence on the problem-solving practices of participants. Merely knowing which tests and treatments were selected and which laboratory tests were positive or negative gives major clues to the thinking of the clinicians caring for the patient. Second, the availability of all the data inhibits a clinician from discussing his or her rationale for collecting such data. In addition, a CPC discussant is always looking for "zebras" and often fails to consider the actual prevalence of diseases likely to be encountered.[313]

Finally, the sequence of materials should be clinically logical. If an expert clinician might immediately order a CT scan of the head for an alcoholic or AIDS patient with new neurologic findings, there is no need to insert a lot of extraneous clinical material before giving the results of the CT scan. If a good clinician chose to order a serum potassium and thyroid function studies in a young Asian man who presented with muscle weakness, it would be appropriate to present the data in that sequence. Failing to follow the logical sequence of the diagnostic (or therapeutic) process may stifle the discussion.

In this format, it is useful to have someone act as a discussion facilitator. If the participants are unable to explicate their reasoning tactics or are unable to explain the findings, the facilitator can quickly advance the slides and disclose more information. The facilitator can also keep the discussion on course by minimizing blind alleys and discussions that miss the mark. The facilitator can also enliven the exercise by challenging or questioning interpretations of data and even by gently puncturing irrelevant comments (e.g., a participant who regularly posits a diagnosis of amyloidosis).

Properly conducted, such problem-solving sessions can be informative, exciting, and enjoyable. Clear expositions of diagnostic and therapeutic reasoning, examples of faulty reasoning, and communication of knowledge can be conveyed. Judging by the attendance at conferences of this kind and by the comments after each session, the exercise is a popular one. The value of educational innovations is extremely difficult to assess, however, and we have no data to substantiate our assumption that people acquire knowledge and problem-solving skills from these exercises. Furthermore, we have no evidence that they learn more facts or different skills (problem solving) with this format. Some notable educators have described this approach as more show biz than education. Perhaps so, but since "80% of success is showing up" (Woody Allen), the audience response encourages us to recommend the method. Lack of an evaluative mechanism has not deterred curricular reform in the past, and we believe it should not.[1] Thus, we make cautious claims about the benefits of this didactic approach. New features of this refined format include suggestions for case selection and case construction, a series of published examples of case types and constructs, a facilitator to direct the discussion, and a framework of cognitive research as the basis for the diagnostic and therapeutic aspects to be explicated.

Try it; you will like it.

GLOSSARY

Adequacy: Diagnostic sufficiency. An adequate diagnostic hypothesis is one that encompasses all elementary hypotheses under consideration and accounts for all of the patient's findings, whether abnormal or normal.

Ambiguity: The degree of uncertainty in a probability assessment. The degree of confidence in a probability assessment. A second-order probability; the probability of a probability.

Anchoring heuristic; anchor point: The likelihood of an event or an outcome is assessed based on some starting point or initial value.

Artificial intelligence: The branch of computer science that programs computers to carry out tasks that would require intelligence if done by humans. Principal themes of artificial intelligence include the organization of knowledge, search strategies, the control of the order of processes, and learning.

Availability heuristic: The likelihood of an outcome is assessed on the basis of the ease with which readily recallable, striking, or impressive similar outcomes come to mind.

Bayes' rule (Bayes' theorem; Bayesian analysis): An algebraic expression for calculating posterior probabilities of a set of disorders (diseases, conditions, or syndromes) from data on the prior probabilities of each of the disorders and the conditional probabilities of various findings in these disorders.

Bayesian revision: The process by which diagnostic hypotheses are revised and refined using Bayes' rule.

Bias: A process at any stage of inference tending to produce results that vary systematically from the true values.

Case-based reasoning: A problem-solving method that involves recall of a previous similar situation and application of the results of that situation to the current problem. Individual experiences act as exemplars on which to base later decisions.

Case building: The process of revision and refinement of diagnostic hypotheses in response to accumulation of clinical data. See hypothesis refinement.

Catchall hypothesis: A diagnostic category consisting of a group of closely related, undiscovered hypotheses.

Categorical reasoning: Compiled knowledge from any source in the form of unambiguous rules; see rule-based reasoning and deterministic reasoning.

Causal model: A chain of related features consisting of stimuli and their responses. Frequently applied to physiologic systems.

Causal reasoning: Forming inferences, judgments, and conclusions that depend on the cause-and-effect relations between variables. The cause is a condition whose presence makes a critical difference to the occurrence of the outcome.

Chunk: A configuration or package of information, typically organized in a semantically meaningful form.

Close call: Toss-up.

Cognition: The process of perceiving and knowing.

Cognitive Science: The discipline that views the human mind as an information processing system and studies how the mind receives, stores, retrieves, transforms, and transmits information.

Coherency: A coherent diagnosis is one in which a patient's findings, risk factors, and complications are consistent with the altered pathophysiology and causality of the hypothesized disease state.

Compiled knowledge: Already synthesized, packaged information. Accepted rules of procedure.

Condition–action pairs: The statements in production rules that define the feature or features to be identified and the consequences invoked by these features. See production rules.

Conditional probability: The probability of a finding among patients with a known disorder.

Confirmation strategy: A tactic in the process of hypothesis refinement in which questions are used to seek data that are expected to enhance the likelihood of a diagnostic hypothesis.

Connectionism: A theory of information, storage, and retrieval based on the anatomic structure of the brain. Such models process information through the parallel activation of simple processing units (neurons in the case of the brain) through excitatory and inhibitory connections. Concepts and entities are represented by a pattern of activity distributed across many units.

Context: The cognitive representation of a problem, which frames or constrains the solution to the problem. In medicine, typically some diagnostic category such as a disease entity or syndrome.

Data-driven strategy: A problem-solving reasoning approach that begins with data and works toward a hypothesis.

Decision analysis: The formulation in quantitative terms of the principles of reaching optimal decisions in the face of uncertainty. An explicit prescriptive approach in which the problem is broken into its components and typically represented as a decision tree. Chance events are represented as probabilities and the values of outcomes as numerical utilities.

Decision theory: The set of axioms and logical relations (probability theory and utility theory) that form the basis for decision analysis.

Decision tree: A structure used to display the logical and temporal relations in a decision problem; in this structure, all relevant choices and their outcomes are represented and the expected outcomes of the choices are calculated and analyzed.

Descriptive approach: The method of study of clinical reasoning in which theories are generated about clinical problem-solving strategies from experimental studies of individuals actually engaged in problem solving.

Deterministic reasoning: Inferences about clinical problems that are already compiled and are in the form of rules of procedure. See compiled knowledge and rule-based reasoning.

Diagnosis: An iterative, inferential process of determining by examination the nature and circumstances of a diseased condition.

Diagnostic hypothesis: One or more disease entities, conditions, or syndromes that could be responsible for causing a patient's clinical features.

Diagnostic uncertainty: Lack of distinction or differentiation; diagnostic entropy.

Diagnostic verification: The final step in the diagnostic process in which one or more hypotheses are accepted as sufficiently valid to permit further (invasive or risky) testing, therapeutic decision making, or prognostic judgments.

Differential diagnosis: A set of surviving, competing diagnostic hypotheses.

Discrimination strategy: A tactic in the process of hypothesis refinement in which questions and diagnostic tests are used to distinguish between two or more competing diagnostic hypotheses.

Domain expert: An individual with special skill or knowledge in a specific field of thought; a specialist.

Elimination strategy: A tactic in the process of hypothesis refinement in which information is sought to reduce the likelihood of an unlikely hypothesis.

Exemplar: A specific instance or example.

Expected utility: Averaged outcome value resulting from a choice in formal decision analysis.

Expert: An individual with special skill or knowledge in some particular field.

False-negative result: Negative test result in a patient known to have a given disease.

False-positive result: Positive test result in a patient known not to have a given disease.

Falsification: The process during hypothesis revision or verification by which certain features, clearly identified as inconsistent with a hypothesis, discredit the currently favored hypothesis and thus call for revision of competing hypotheses.

Frame: A list of declarative (factual) and procedural (processing) aspects that describe a given entity. A frame for a disease entity would consist of some hierarchical structure into which the entity fits, findings necessary and sufficient to define the entity, factors that cause the disorder, complications of the disorder, approaches to distinguish it from other entities, and some mechanism to score the relative importance of expected findings.

Framework: The context within which a problem is likely to be solved.

Generate-and-test strategy: A problem-solving tactic that involves unmotivatedly selecting possible actions, carrying each out until progress is apparent, and then reevaluating the problem situation. One of the "weak" problem-solving methods.

Goal-directed strategy: See top-down processing.

Gold standard: A relatively irrefutable standard that constitutes recognized and accepted evidence that a certain disease exists.

Heuristic: Rule of thumb, or short-cut, used to make inferences about data; a judgment that appeals to an intuitive sense of plausibility. See representativeness heuristic and availability heuristic.

Hypothesis: A proposition or set of propositions set forth as an explanation for the occurrence of some specified group of phenomena.

Hypothesis confirmation strategy: See confirmation strategy.

Hypothesis elimination strategy: See elimination strategy.

Hypothesis generation: Evocation or introduction of diagnostic hypotheses. Triggering.

Hypothesis modification (hypothesis refinement): Sequential revision of diagnostic hypotheses in response to accumulated clinical data. See case building.

Hypothesis revision: See hypothesis modification.

Hypothesis verification: See diagnostic verification.

Inductive reasoning: Inferential reasoning processes that extend an individual's knowledge in the face of uncertainty.

Inference: Reasoning process by which conviction in one set of beliefs comes to affect conviction in another.

Instance script: A script that captures information about a specific event or phenomenon. In medicine, a script might contain information about a single patient.

Instantiate: Exemplify; provide a specific example or exemplar.

Learning: Any process whereby people increase their knowledge or improve their skill.

Long-term memory: Information that remains out of the immediate sphere of consciousness for minutes to years and then is retrieved or brought back into conscious attention when it is relevant to some ongoing thought process. A store of large capacity and relatively permanent storage but slow access time.

Markov process: A mechanism in decision analysis for making choices between strategies in which future events that occur at various intervals from some reference time are modeled. Patients are considered to be in one of a set of discrete health states; the rules that govern the movement from one state to another are defined as a matrix of transition probabilities, and calculations of the expected utility of all possible outcomes determine the optimal strategy.

Means–end analysis: A problem-solving method by which the individual selects operators (means) that will achieve the solution (end) to the problem. The principle of operator selection is to reduce the difference between the current state of the problem and the desired end, or goal. One of the "weak" problem-solving methods.

Monte Carlo simulation: A form of sensitivity analysis in which dependent variables (probabilities and utilities) are varied randomly and simultaneously.

Normative models: Prescriptions for ideal performance.

Ockham's razor: The law of parsimony; the simplest diagnosis that explains the patient's findings.

Parallel distributed processing: Simultaneous activation of units without the control of a central mechanism. The units are neurons in the brain, and microprocessors in computers. See connectionism.

Parsimonious: Economical; the simplest possible explanation.

Physical symbol system hypothesis: The concept that mental activity and intelligence can be explained in terms of symbols (objects, events, relations between objects, relations between events) manipulated by an information processing system.

Polymorphism: The quality of natural concepts of being variable in observable features.

Posterior (posttest) probability: The likelihood of a given disease after test results are known.

Premature closure: Accepting a diagnosis before it is fully verified.

Prescriptive approach: A normative approach to diagnosis and therapy based on probability and utility theory. Bayesian analysis and decision analysis are two examples.

Prevalence: The frequency of a given disease in the population of interest at a given point in time.

Prior (pretest) probability: The likelihood of disease before a given test result is available.

Probabilistic model: A representation of clinical data in terms of the probabilistic relations between variables.

Probability distribution: An exhaustive set of diagnostic possibilities and the probabilities associated with each.

Problem space: The subject's representation of the task environment that permits the consideration of different problem solutions and sets limitations on possible operations that can be applied to the problem; a sort of maze of mental activity through which individuals wander when searching for a solution to a problem.

Production rule: Compiled knowledge in the form of an "*if-then*" statement, with the *if* part of the statement representing some semantically meaningful condition and the *then* part of the statement representing some action to be implemented whenever the *if* condition is satisfied.

Productions: The statements of production rules.

Protocol analysis: See transcript analysis.

Random search: A strategy of discovery based exclusively on chance.

Reasoning: Forming inferences, judgments, and conclusions from facts or premises.

Regret: A bias introduced into clinical decision making when the decision maker (usually the physician) is uncomfortable about the possibility of an adverse patient outcome.

Representativeness heuristic: The likelihood of an outcome is assessed on the basis of the close resemblance to other well-defined outcomes.

Retrospective bias: After-the-fact reasoning; considering or critiquing a process after the outcome has been revealed.

Rule-based reasoning: Categorical or deterministic strategies based on compiled information.

Rules of procedure: See deterministic reasoning and compiled knowledge.

Script: An organized knowledge structure that captures general information about a routine series of events or recurrent type of event. In medicine, a script might contain information about the course of a particular illness.

Search strategies: Methods of finding solutions to problems.

Sensitivity: The likelihood of a positive test result in a patient known to have a disease.

Sensitivity analysis: The process in decision analysis of assessing the effect of variations in problem structure or data (probabilities and utilities) on the choices in a decision; a method of assessing the stability of the conclusions of a decision analysis.

Short-term memory: The site in which we store the items of information we are manipulating as we are trying to understand or decode them; a sensory store of short duration and limited capacity.

Skilled memory (working memory): An efficient extension of short-term memory created by "chunking" together semantically meaningful units in long-term memory.

Specificity: The likelihood of a negative test result in a patient known not to have a given disease.

Strong problem-solving methods: Purposive, highly directed, and domain-specific approaches to problem solutions.

Sutton's law: A clinical axiom of uncertain validity, which asserts that a decision to focus a diagnostic test should be based on the "obvious" location of a pathologic process. Based on the supposed reply of the infamous bank robber Willie Sutton, who, when asked why he robbed banks, answered, "That's where the money is."

Systematic search: A strategy of discovery based on investigation of all possible solutions to a problem.

Testing threshold: The probability or utility value at which the expected utility of performing a given test is the same as not performing the test. The alternative choice often is either to give a certain treatment or not give the treatment.

Therapeutic threshold; treatment threshold: The probability or utility value at which the expected utility of one choice (giving a certain treatment) is equivalent to another choice (giving another treatment or giving no treatment).

Threshold: A reference value for clinical decision making and sensitivity analysis. A probability or a utility that, when exceeded, calls for one choice and, when short of the value, calls for a different choice. At the threshold (the break-even value), the choices are of equivalent value.

Top-down processing: Search strategy driven by hypotheses, expectations, or inferences.

Toss-up: A circumstance in decision making in which the expected utility of one choice is not substantially different from the expected utility of a competing choice.

Transcript analysis: The detailed examination and interpretation of transcribed material from recorded "thinking aloud" sessions of individuals engaged in problem solving.

Triggering: See hypothesis generation.

True-negative result: A negative test result in a patient known not to have a given disease.

True-positive result: A positive test result in a patient known to have a given disease.

Utility: A numerical expression of the value of an outcome used in decision analyses.

Weak problem-solving methods: General problem-solving tactics used for attacking problems. They impose order on the process of using what one knows when it is not clear how to proceed. See means–end analysis and generate-and-test strategy.

Working diagnosis: A diagnostic hypothesis sufficiently accepted to form the basis for planning the next step in patient management—to order additional tests, to arrive at a certain forecast about the patient's subsequent clinical course, to observe the patient without further tests or studies, or to embark on a course of treatment.

Working memory (skilled memory): An expansion of short-term memory made possible by the chunking together of semantically meaningful information.

BIBLIOGRAPHY

1. Kassirer JP. Teaching clinical medicine by iterative hypothesis testing. Let's preach what we practice. *N Engl J Med.* 1983;309:921–923.
2. Hamm RM. Clinical intuition and clinical analysis: Expertise and the cognitive continuum. In: Dowie J, Elstein AS, eds. *Professional Judgment: A Reader in Clinical Decision Making.* New York: Cambridge University Press; 1988:78–105.
3. Hammond KR. Coherence and correspondence theories in judgment and decision making. In: Connolly T, Arkes HR, Hammond KR, eds. *Judgment and Decision Making: An Interdisciplinary Reader.* 2nd ed. New York: Cambridge University Press; 2000:53–65.
4. Norman G. Research in clinical reasoning: Past history and current trends. *Med Educ.* 2005;39:418–427.
5. Eva KW. What every teacher needs to know about clinical reasoning. *Med Educ.* 2005;39:98–106.
6. Schwartz A, Elstein AS. Clinical reasoning in medicine. In: Higgs J, Jones MA, Loftus S, et al., eds. *Clinical Reasoning in the Health Professions.* 3rd ed. Boston: Elsevier; 2008:223–234.
7. Gigerenzer G. *Gut Feelings: The Intelligence of the Unconscious.* New York: Viking Penguin; 2007.
8. Bowen JL. Educational strategies to promote clinical diagnostic reasoning. *N Engl J Med.* 2006;355:2217–2225.
9. Dhaliwal G. Clinical decision-making: Understanding how clinicians make a diagnosis. In: Saint S, Drazen JM, Solomon CG, eds. *New England Journal of Medicine: Clinical Problem Solving.* New York: McGraw-Hill; 2006:19–29.
10. Hunink MGM, Glasziou PP, Siegel JE, et al. *Decision Making in Health and Medicine: Integrating Evidence and Values.* New York: Cambridge University Press; 2001.
11. Sox HC, Blatt MA, Higgins MC, et al. *Medical Decision Making.* Philadelphia: ACP Press; 2007.
12. Elstein AS, Schwartz A. Clinical problem solving and diagnostic decision making: Selective review of the cognitive literature. *BMJ.* 2002;324:729–732.
13. Schmidt HG, Norman GR, Boshuizen HP. A cognitive perspective on medical expertise: theory and implication. *Acad Med.* 1990;65:611–621.
14. Schmidt HG, Rikers RMJP. How expertise develops in medicine: Knowledge encapsulation and illness script formation. *Med Educ.* 2007;41:1133–1139.
15. Norman G. Building on experience—-The development of clinical reasoning. *N Engl J Med.* 2006;355:2251–2252.
16. Grossman PD, Rodriguez MA. Clinical diagnostic reasoning. *N Engl J Med.* 2007;356:1273; author reply, 1273–1274.
17. McColl GJ, Groves MA. Clinical diagnostic reasoning. *N Engl J Med.* 2007;356:1272; author reply, 1273–1274.
18. Elstein AS, Shulman LS, Sprafka SA. *Medical Problem Solving: An Analysis of Clinical Reasoning* Cambridge, MA: Harvard University Press; 1978.
19. Kassirer JP, Gorry GA. Clinical problem solving: A behavioral analysis. *Ann Intern Med.* 1978;89:245–255.
20. Szolovits P, Pauker SG. Categorical and probabilistic reasoning in medical diagnosis. *Artificial Intelligence.* 1978;11:115–144.
21. Holland JH, Holyoak KJ, Nisbett RE, et al. *Induction: Processes of Inference, Learning, and Discovery* Cambridge, MA: MIT Press; 1989.
22. Szolovits P, Pauker SG. Categorical and probabilistic reasoning in medicine revisited. *Artificial Intelligence.* 1993;59:167–180.
23. Miller GA. The magical number seven plus or minus two: Some limits on our capacity for processing information. *Psychol Rev.* 1956;63:81–97.
24. Miller GA. The magical number seven, plus or minus two: Some limits on our capacity for processing information. 1956. *Psychol Rev.* 1994;101:343–352.
25. Fisher SD, Gettys CF, Manning C, et al. Consistency checking in hypothesis generation. *Organ Behav Hum Perform.* 1983;31:233–254.
26. Gettys CF, Fisher S. Hypothesis plausibility and hypothesis generation. *Organ Behav Human Decision Processes.* 1979;24, 93–110.

27. Kahneman D, Slovic P, Tversky A. *Judgment under Uncertainty: Heuristics and Biases.* New York: Cambridge University Press; 1982.

28. Tversky A, Kahneman D. Judgment under uncertainty: Heuristics and biases. *Science.* 1974;185:1124–1131.

29. Schiffmann A, Cohen S, Nowik R, et al. Initial diagnostic hypotheses: Factors which may distort physicians' judgment. *Organ Behav Hum Perform.* 1978;21:305–315.

30. Newell A, Simon HA. *Human Problem Solving.* Englewood Cliffs. NJ: Prentice-Hall; 1972.

31. Einhorn HJ, Hogarth RM. Behavioral decision theory: Processes of judgment and choice. *Annu Rev Psychol.* 1981;32:53–88.

32. Keren G. On the importance of identifying the correct "problem space." *Cognition.* 1984;16:121–128.

33. Bordage G. Prototypes and semantic qualifiers: From past to present. *Med Educ.* 2007;41:1117–1121.

34. Norman G, Young M, Brooks L. Non-analytical models of clinical reasoning: The role of experience. *Med Educ.* 2007;41:1140–1145.

35. Bassok M, Trope Y. People's strategies for testing hypotheses about another's personality: Confirmatory or diagnostic? *Social Cognition.* 1983;2:199–216.

36. Kassirer JP, Kuipers BJ, Gorry GA. Toward a theory of clinical expertise. *Am J Med.* 1982;73:251–259.

37. Skov RB, Sherman SJ. Information-gathering processes: Diagnosticity, hypothesis-confirmatory strategies, and perceived hypothesis confirmation. *J Exp Soc Psychol.* 1986;22:93–121.

38. Trope Y, Bassok M. Confirmatory and diagnosing strategies in social information gathering. *J Pers Soc Psychol.* 1982;43:22–34.

39. Hall KH. Reviewing intuitive decision-making and uncertainty: The implications for medical education. *Med Educ.* 2002;36:216–224.

40. McCormick JS. Diagnosis: The need for demystification. *Lancet.* 1986;2:1434–1435.

41. Cutler P. *Problem Solving in Medicine: From Data to Diagnosis.* 3rd ed. Baltimore: Lippincott Williams & Wilkins; 1998.

42. Harvey AM, Bordley JI. *Differential Diagnosis: The Interpretation of Clinical Evidence.* 3rd ed. Philadelphia: WB Saunders; 1979.

43. Sershon PD, Barry MJ, Oesterling JE. Serum prostate-specific antigen discriminates weakly between men with benign prostatic hyperplasia and patients with organ-confined prostate cancer. *Eur Urol.* 1994;25:281–287.

44. Einhorn HJ, Hogarth RM. Judging probable cause. *Psychol Bull.* 1986;99:3–19.

45. Susser MW. *Causal Thinking in the Health Sciences: Concepts and Strategies of Epidemiology.* New York: Oxford University Press; 1973.

46. Kuipers B. Commonsense reasoning about causality—Deriving behavior from structure. *Artific Intell.* 1984;24:169–203.

47. Kuipers B, Kassirer JP. Causal reasoning in medicine: Analysis of a protocol. *Cognitive Science.* 1984;8:363–385.

48. Patel VL, Arocha JF, Zhang J. Thinking and reasoning in medicine. In: Holyoak KJ, Morrison RG, eds. *The Cambridge Handbook of Thinking and Reasoning.* New York: Cambridge University Press; 2005:727–750.

49. Cheng PW. Causal reasoning. In: Wilson RA, Keil F, eds. *The MIT Encyclopedia of the Cognitive Sciences.* Cambridge, MA: MIT Press; 2001:106–108.

50. Jonassen DH, Ionas IG. Designing effective supports for causal reasoning. *Educ Technol Res Dev.* 2008;56:1042–1629.

51. Hume D. *A Treatise of Human Nature.* 2nd ed. Oxford: Clarendon Press; 1978.

52. Graber ML, Franklin N, Gordon R. Diagnostic error in internal medicine. *Arch Intern Med.* 2005;165:1493–1499.

53. McSherry D. Avoiding premature closure in sequential diagnosis. *Artific Intell Med.* 1997;10:269–283.

54. Eva KW, Cunnington JPW. The difficulty with experience: does practice increase susceptibility to premature closure? *J Contin Educ Health Prof.* 2006;26:192–198.

55. Berner ES, Graber ML. Overconfidence as a cause of diagnostic error in medicine. *Am J Med.* 2008;121:S2–23.

56. Eva KW, Norman GR. Heuristics and biases—A biased perspective on clinical reasoning. *Med Educ.* 2005;39:870–872.

57. Eisenberg JM, Hershey JC. Derived thresholds. Determining the diagnostic probabilities at which clinicians initiate testing and treatment. *Med Decis Making.* 1983;3:155–168.

58. Pauker SG, Kassirer JP. Therapeutic decision making: A cost–benefit analysis. *N Engl J Med.* 1975;293:229–234.

59. Pauker SG, Kassirer JP. The threshold approach to clinical decision making. *N Engl J Med.* 1980;302:1109–1117.

60. Kassirer JP, Pauker SG. The toss-up. *N Engl J Med.* 1981;305:1467–1469.

61. Moskowitz AJ, Kuipers BJ, Kassirer JP. Dealing with uncertainty, risks, and tradeoffs in clinical decisions. A cognitive science approach. *Ann Intern Med.* 1988;108:435–449.

62. Evidence-Based Medicine Working Group. Evidence-based medicine. A new approach to teaching the practice of medicine. *JAMA.* 1992;268: 2420–2425.

63. Sackett DL, Rosenberg WM, Gray JA, et al. Evidence based medicine: What it is and what it isn't. *BMJ.* 1996;312:71–72.

64. Guyatt G, Rennie D, Meade M, et al. *Users' Guides to the Medical Literature: A Manual for Evidence-Based Clinical Practice.* 2nd ed. New York: McGraw-Hill; 2008.

65. Guyatt G, Sackett D, Taylor DW, et al. Determining optimal therapy—Randomized trials in individual patients. *N Engl J Med.* 1986;314:889–892.

66. Montori VM, Wilczynski NL, Morgan D, et al. Optimal search strategies for retrieving systematic reviews from Medline: Analytical survey. *BMJ.* 2005;330:68.

67. Haynes RB, Wilczynski NL. Optimal search strategies for retrieving scientifically strong studies of diagnosis from Medline: Analytical survey. *BMJ.* 2004;328:1040.

68. Greenhalgh T. *How to Read a Paper: The Basics of Evidence-Based Medicine.* 3rd ed. Malden, MA: Blackwell; 2006.

69. Guyatt GH, Rennie D. Users' guides to the medical literature. *JAMA.* 1993;270:2096–2097.

70. Grimes DA, Schulz KF. An overview of clinical research: The lay of the land. *Lancet.* 2002;359: 57–61.

71. Straus SE, Richardson WS, Glasziou P, et al. *Evidence Based Medicine: How to Practice and Teach EBM.* 3rd ed. Philadelphia: Elsevier; 2005.

72. Yusuf S, Wittes J, Probstfield J, et al. Analysis and interpretation of treatment effects in subgroups of patients in randomized clinical trials. *JAMA.* 1991; 266:93–98.

73. Committee on Quality of Health Care in America. *To Err Is Human: Building a Safer Health System.* Washington DC: National Academy Press; 2000.

74. Zhang J, Patel VL, Johnson TR. Medical error: Is the solution medical or cognitive? *J Am Med Inform Assoc.* 2002;9:S75–S77.

75. Bordage G. Why did I miss the diagnosis? Some cognitive explanations and educational implications. *Acad Med.* 1999;74:S138–S143.

76. Graber M, Gordon R, Franklin N. Reducing diagnostic errors in medicine: What's the goal? *Acad Med.* 2002;77:981–992.

77. Kassirer JP, Kopelman RI. Cognitive errors in diagnosis: Instantiation, classification, and consequences. *Am J Med.* 1989;86:433–441.

78. Croskerry P. Achieving quality in clinical decision making: Cognitive strategies and detection of bias. *Acad Emerg Med.* 2002;9:1184–1204.

79. Croskerry P. The importance of cognitive errors in diagnosis and strategies to minimize them. *Acad Med.* 2003;78:775–780.

80. Redelmeier DA, Cialdini RB. Problems for clinical judgement: 5. Principles of influence in medical practice. *CMAJ Can Med Assoc J.* 2002;166:1680–1684.

81. Dawson NV, Arkes HR. Systematic errors in medical decision making: Judgment limitations. *J Gen Intern Med.* 1987;2:183–187.

82. Kuhn GJ. Diagnostic errors. *Acad Emerg Med.* 2002;9:740–750.

83. Redelmeier DA. Improving patient care. The cognitive psychology of missed diagnoses. *Ann Intern Med.* 2005;142:115–120.

84. Ioannidis JP, Lau J. Evidence on interventions to reduce medical errors: An overview and recommendations for future research. *J Gen Intern Med.* 2001;16:325–334.

85. Fischhoff B. Debiasing. In: Kahneman D, Slovic P, Tversky A, eds. *Judgment under Uncertainty: Heuristics and Biases.* New York: Cambridge University Press; 1982:422–444.

86. Yates J, Veinott ES, Patalano AL. Hard decisions, bad decisions: On decision quality and decision aiding. In: Schneider SL, Shanteau J, eds. *Emerging Perspectives on Judgment and Decision Research.* New York: Cambridge University Press; 2003:1–63.

87. Graber M. Metacognitive training to reduce diagnostic errors: Ready for prime time? *Acad Med.* 2003;78:781.

88. Nisbett RE, Wilson TD. Telling more than we can know: Verbal reports on mental processes. *Psychol Rev.* 1977;84:231–259.

89. Kuipers BJ, Kassirer JP. Knowledge acquisition by analysis of verbatim protocols. In: Kidd AL, ed. *Knowledge Acquisition for Expert Systems: A Practical Handbook.* New York: Plenum Press; 1987:45–71.

90. Anderson JR. Methodologies for studying human knowledge. *Behav Brain Sci.* 1987;10:467–477.

91. Baron J. *Thinking and Deciding.* 4th ed. New York: Cambridge University Press; 2008.

92. Ericsson KA. The scientific induction problem: A case for case studies. *Behav Brain Sci.* 1987;10:480–481.

93. Reed AV. Ways and means. *Behav Brain Sci.* 1987; 10:488–489.

94. Seifert C, Norman DA. Levels of research. *Behav Brain Sci.* 1987;10:490–492.

95. Brooks LR. Non-analytic concept formation and the memory for instances. In: Rosch E, Lloyd BL, eds. *Cognition and Categorization.* Hillsdale, NJ: Lawrence Erlbaum; 1978:169–211.

96. Medin DL, Dewey GI, Murphy TD. Relationships between item and category learning: Evidence that abstraction is not automatic. *J Exp Psychol Learn Mem Cogn.* 1983;9:607–625.

97. Feltovich PJ, Barrows HS. Issues of generality in medical problem solving. In: Schmidt HG, de Volder ML, eds. *Tutorials in Problem-Based Learning: A New Direction in Teaching the Health Professions.* Assen, Netherlands: Van Gorcum; 1984:128–142.

98. Bareiss R. *Exemplar-Based Knowledge Acquisition: A Unified Approach to Concept Representation Classification, and Learning.* Boston: Academic Press; 1989.

99. Kolodner JL. Maintaining organization in a dynamic long-term memory. *Cogn Sci.* 1983;7:243–280.

100. Kolodner JL. Reconstructive memory: A computer model. *Cogn Sci.* 1983;7:281–328.

101. Koton P. A medical reasoning program that improves with experience. *Comput Methods Programs Biomed.* 1989;30:177–184.

102. Shank RC. *Dynamic Memory Revisited.* 2nd ed. New York: Cambridge University Press; 1999.

103. Kassirer JP. Diagnostic reasoning. *Ann Intern Med.* 1989;110:893–900.

104. Crick F. The recent excitement about neural networks. *Nature.* 1989;337:129–132.

105. Pessoa L, Ungerleider LG. Top-down mechanisms for working memory and attentional processes. In: Gazzaniga MS, ed. *The Cognitive Neurosciences.* 3rd ed. Cambridge, MA: MIT Press; 2004:919–930.

106. Grossberg S. *Neural Networks and Natural Intelligence.* Cambridge, MA: MIT Press; 1988.

107. Anderson JR. *The Architecture of Cognition.* Mahwah, NJ: Lawrence Erlbaum; 1983, reprinted 1996.

108. Waldrop MM. The workings of working memory. *Science.* 1987;237:1564–1567.

109. Search In: Barr A, Feigenbaum EA, eds. *Handbook of Artificial Intelligence.* Vol. 1. Los Altos, CA: William Kaufmann; 1981:19–140.

110. Lesgold A. *Problem solving.* New York: Cambridge University Press; 1988.

111. Langley P, Simon HA, Bradshaw GL, et al. *Scientific Discovery: Computational Explorations of the Creative Processes* Cambridge, MA: MIT Press; 1987.

112. Patel VL, Groen GJ, Frederiksen CH. Differences between medical students and doctors in memory for clinical cases. *Med Educ.* 1986;20:3–9.

113. Bobrow DG, Norman DA. Some principles of memory schemata. In: Bobrow DG, Collins A, eds. *Representation and Understanding: Studies in Cognitive Science.* San Diego, CA: Academic Press; 1975: 131–149.

114. Anderson JR. Skill acquisition: Compilation of weak-method problem situations. *Psychol Rev.* 1987;94:192–210.

115. Stillings NA, Feinstein MH, Garfield JL, et al. Topics in cognitive psychology. In: *Cognitive Science: An Introduction.* Cambridge, MA: MIT Press; 1987:73–86.

116. Patel VL, Groen GJ. Knowledge based solution strategies in medical reasoning. *Cogn Sci.* 1986; 10:91–116.

117. Goldman AI. Perception. *Epistemology and Cognition.* Cambridge, MA: Harvard University Press; 1986:181–198.

118. de Groot AD. *Thought and Choice in Chess.* 2nd ed. Cambridge: Cambridge University Press; 1978.

119. Chi MTH, Feltovich PJ, Glaser R. Categorization and representation of physics problems by experts and novices. *Cogn Sci.* 1981;5:121–152.

120. Reyna VF, Lloyd FJ. Physician decision making and cardiac risk: Effects of knowledge, risk perception, risk tolerance, and fuzzy processing. *J Exp Psychol Appl.* 2006;12:179–195.

121. Weber EU, Bockenholt U, Hilton DJ, et al. Determinants of diagnostic hypothesis generation: Effects of information, base rates, and experience. *J Exp Psychol Learn Mem Cogn.* 1993;19:1151–1164.

122. Bordage G, Zacks R. The structure of medical knowledge in the memories of medical students and general practitioners: Categories and prototypes. *Med Educ.* 1984;18:406–416.

123. Charlin B, Boshuizen HPA, Custers EJ, et al. Scripts and clinical reasoning. *Med Educ.* 2007; 41:1178–1184.

124. Chang RW, Bordage G, Connell KJ. The importance of early problem representation during case presentations. *Acad Med.* 1998;73:S109–111.

125. Nendaz MR, Bordage G. Promoting diagnostic problem representation. *Med Educ.* 2002;36:760–766.

126. Mandin H, Jones A, Woloschuk W, et al. Helping students learn to think like experts when solving clinical problems. *Acad Med.* 1997;72:173–179.

127. Barrows HS, Norman GR, Neufeld VR, et al. The clinical reasoning of randomly selected

physicians in general medical practice. *Clin Invest Med.* 1982;5:49–55.

128. Clancy W, Letsinger R. NEOMYCIN: Reconfiguring a rule–based expert system for application to teaching. In: Clancy WJ, Shortliffe EH, eds. *Readings in Medical Artificial Intelligence: The First Decade.* Reading, MA: Addison-Wesley; 1984:361–381.

129. Feltovich PJ, Johnson PE, Moller JH, et al. LCS: The role and development of medical knowledge in diagnostic expertise. In: Clancy WJ, Shortliffe EH, eds. *Readings in Medical Artificial Intelligence: The First Decade.* Reading, MA: Addison-Wesley; 1984:275–319.

130. Kulikowski CA. Artificial intelligence methods and systems for medical consultation. In: Clancy WJ, Shortliffe EH, eds. *Readings in Medical Artificial Intelligence: The First Decade.* Reading, MA: Addison-Wesley; 1984:72–97.

131. Gruppen LD, Woolliscroft JO, Wolf FM. The contribution of different components of the clinical encounter in generating and eliminating diagnostic hypotheses. *Res Med Educ.* 1988;27:242–247.

132. Neufeld VR, Norman GR, Feightner JW, et al. Clinical problem-solving by medical students: A cross-sectional and longitudinal analysis. *Med Educ.* 1981;15:315–322.

133. Fisher SD. Cue selection in hypothesis generation: Reading habits, consistency checking, and diagnostic scanning. *Organ Behav Hum Decis Process.* 1987;40:170–192.

134. Gettys CF, Mehle T, Fisher S. Plausibility assessments in hypothesis generation. *Organ Behav Hum Decis Process.* 1986;37:14–33.

135. Kahneman D, Tversky A. Subjective probability: A judgment of representativeness. *Cogn Psychol.* 1972;3:430–454.

136. Coderre S, Mandin H, Harasym PH, et al. Diagnostic reasoning strategies and diagnostic success. *Med Educ.* 2003;37:695–703.

137. Larkin J, McDermott J, Simon DP, et al. Expert and novice performance in solving physics problems. *Science.* 1980;208:1335–1342.

138. Feinstein AR. An analysis of diagnostic reasoning. I. The domains and disorders of clinical macrobiology. *Yale J Biol Med.* 1973;46:212–232.

139. Feinstein AR. The 'chagrin factor' and qualitative decision analysis. *Arch Intern Med.* 1985;145:1257–1259.

140. Dennett D, Miller J. Artificial intelligence and the strategies of psychological investigation. In: Miller J, ed. *States of Mind.* New York: Pantheon; 1983:66–81.

141. Barrows HS, Bennett K. The diagnostic (problem solving) skill of the neurologist. Experimental studies and their implications for neurological training. *Arch Neurol.* 1972;26:273–277.

142. Kwoh CK, Beck JR, Pauker SG. Repeated syncope with negative diagnostic evaluation. To pace or not to pace? *Med Decis Making.* 1984;4:351–377.

143. Fischhoff B. Hindsight not equal to foresight: The effect of outcome knowledge on judgment under uncertainty. 1975. *Quality Safety Health Care.* 2003;12:304–311; discussion, 311–302.

144. Wood G. The knew-it-all-along effect. *J Exp Psychol Hum Percept Perform.* 1978;4:345–353.

145. Fischhoff B. Hindsight is not equal to foresight: The effect of outcome knowledge on judgment under uncertainty. *J Exp Psychol Hum Percept Perform.* 1975;1:288–299.

146. Tversky A, Kahneman D. The framing of decisions and the psychology of choice. *Science.* 1981;211:453–458.

147. Bordage G, Lemieux M. Some cognitive characteristics of medical students with and without diagnostic reasoning difficulties. *Res Med Educ.* 1986;25:185–190.

148. Kaplan MM. Personal Communication.

149. Seller RH. *Differential Diagnosis of Common Complaints.* 5th ed. Philadelphia: WB Saunders; 2007.

150. Greenberger NJ, Berntsen MS, Jones DK, et al. *Handbook of Differential Diagnosis in Internal Medicine: Medical Book of Lists.* 5th ed. St. Louis, MO: Mosby; 1998.

151. Price RB, Vlahcevic ZR. Logical principles in differential diagnosis. *Ann Intern Med.* 1971;75:89–95.

152. Hoc J-M. *Cognitive Psychology of Planning.* San Diego, CA: Academic Press; 1988.

153. Chase WG, Simon HA. The mind's eye in chess. In: Chase WG, ed. *Visual Information Processing.* New York: Academic Press; 1973:215–281.

154. Fitzgibbons JP. Teaching clinical medicine by iterative hypothesis testing. *N Engl J Med.* 1984;310:600–601.

155. Griner PF, Mayewski RJ, Mushlin AI, et al. Selection and interpretation of diagnostic tests and procedures. Principles and applications. *Ann Intern Med.* 1981;94:557–592.

156. Sox HC Jr. Probability theory in the use of diagnostic tests. An introduction to critical study of the literature. *Ann Intern Med.* 1986;104:60–66.

157. Sonnenberg FA, Kassirer JP, Kopelman RI. An autopsy of the clinical reasoning process. *Hosp Pract (Off Ed).* 21:45–49.

158. Kassirer JP, Kopelman RI. Leaving no stone unturned. *Hosp Pract (Off Ed).* 1987;22:18–21.

159. Gorry GA, Kassirer JP, Essig A, et al. Decision analysis as the basis for computer-aided management of acute renal failure. *Am J Med.* 1973;55:473–484.

160. Barrows HS, Bennett K. Experimental studies on the diagnostic (problem solving) skills of the neurologist and their implications for neurological training. *Trans Am Neurol Assoc.* 1971;96:51–54.

161. Popper KR. *The Logic of Scientific Discovery.* Oxford: Basic Books; 1959.

162. Pauker SG, Gorry GA, Kassirer JP, et al. Towards the simulation of clinical cognition. Taking a present illness by computer. *Am J Med.* 1976;60:981–996.

163. Centers for Disease Control and Prevention. Rocky Mountain spotted fever. Epidemiology. Available at: http://www.cdc.gov/ncidod/dvrd/rmsf/Epidemiology.htm. Accessed March 27, 2009.

164. Lindenbaum J, Healton EB, Savage DG, et al. Neuropsychiatric disorders caused by cobalamin deficiency in the absence of anemia or macrocytosis. *N Engl J Med.* 1988;318:1720–1728.

165. Weinberger MH. Systemic hypertension. In: Kelley WN, ed. *Textbook of Internal Medicine.* 2nd ed. Philadelphia: JB Lippincott; 1992:236–247.

166. Kaplan NM. Hypertension in the population at large. In: Kaplan NM, ed. *Clinical Hypertension.* 5th ed. Baltimore: Williams & Wilkins; 1990:1–25.

167. Kaplan NM. Hypertension in the individual patient. In: Kaplan NM, ed. *Clinical Hypertension.* 5th ed. Baltimore: Williams & Wilkins; 1990:26–53.

168. Bravo EL. Pheochromocytoma: New concepts and future trends. *Kidney Int.* 1991;40:544–556.

169. Ingelfinger JA, Mosteller F, Thibodeau LA, et al. *Biostatistics in Clinical Medicine.* New York: Macmillan; 1983.

170. Kaplan NM. Pheochromocytoma. In: Kaplan NM, ed. *Clinical Hypertension.* 5th ed. Baltimore: Williams & Wilkins; 1990:350–367.

171. Feldman JM. Diagnosis and management of pheochromocytoma. *Hosp Pract (Off Ed).* 1989;24:175–179, 187–179.

172. Stewart BH, Bravo EL, Haaga J, et al. Localization of pheochromocytoma by computed tomography. *N Engl J Med.* 1978;299:460–461.

173. Young MJ, Dmuchowski C, Wallis JW, et al. Biochemical tests for pheochromocytoma: Strategies in hypertensive patients. *J Gen Intern Med.* 1989;4:273–276.

174. Likelihood and odds. In: Lusted LB, ed. *Introduction to Medical Decision Making.* Springfield, Il: Charles C Thomas; 1968:20–23.

175. Feinstein AR. Clinical biostatistics. XXXIX. The haze of Bayes, the aerial palaces of decision analysis, and the computerized Ouija board. *Clin Pharmacol Ther.* 1977;21:482–496.

176. Pauker SG, Kassirer JP. Decision analysis. *N Engl J Med.* 1987;316:250–258.

177. Politser P. Reliability, decision rules, and the value of repeated tests. *Med Decis Making.* 1982;2:47–69.

178. Bravo EL, Tarazi RC, Gifford RW, et al. Circulating and urinary catecholamines in pheochromocytoma. Diagnostic and pathophysiologic implications. *N Engl J Med.* 1979;301:682–686.

179. Henry JB. *Clinical Diagnosis and Management by Laboratory Methods.* 17th ed. Philadelphia: WB Saunders; 1984.

180. Shapiro B, Copp JE, Sisson JC, et al. Iodine-131 metaiodobenzylguanidine for the locating of suspected pheochromocytoma: Experience in 400 cases. *J Nucl Med.* 1985;26:576–585.

181. Yusuf S, Fallen E, Harrington RA, et al. Clinical decisions. Management of stable coronary disease. *N Engl J Med.* 2007;357:1762–1766.

182. Bravata DM, Gienger AL, McDonald KM, et al. Systematic review: The comparative effectiveness of percutaneous coronary interventions and coronary artery bypass graft surgery. *Ann Intern Med.* 2007;147:703–716.

183. Smith PK, Califf RM, Tuttle RH, et al. Selection of surgical or percutaneous coronary intervention provides differential longevity benefit. *Ann Thorac Surg.* 2006;82:1420–1428; discussion, 1428–1429.

184. Cheng S, Jarcho J. Clinical decisions. Management of stable coronary disease—Polling results. *N Engl J Med.* 2007;357:e28.

185. Poses RM, Krueger JI, Sloman S, et al. Physicians' judgments of survival after medical management and mortality risk reduction due to revascularization procedures for patients with coronary artery disease. *Chest.* 2002;122:122–133.

186. Poses RM, De Saintonge DM, McClish DK, et al. An international comparison of physicians' judgments of outcome rates of cardiac procedures and attitudes toward risk, uncertainty, justifiability, and regret. *Med Decis Making.* 1998;18:131–140.

187. Diamond GA, Forrester JS. Analysis of probability as an aid in the clinical diagnosis of coronary-artery disease. *N Engl J Med.* 1979;300:1350–1358.

188. Gorry GA, Pauker SG, Schwartz WB. The diagnostic importance of the normal finding. *N Engl J Med.* 1978;298:486–489.

189. Bayes T. An essay towards solving a problem in the doctrine of chances. *Phil Trans R Soc Lond.* 1763;53:269–271.

190. Bayes T. An essay towards solving a problem in the doctrine of chances. 1763. *MD Comput.* 1991;8:157–171.

191. Kassirer JP. The wild goose chase and the elephant's relevance. *JAMA.* 1986;256:256–257.

192. Lederle FA, Walker JM, Reinke DB. Selective screening for abdominal aortic aneurysms with physical examination and ultrasound. *Arch Intern Med.* 1988;148:1753–1756.

193. Kassirer JP. Adding insult to injury. Usurping patients' prerogatives. *N Engl J Med.* 1983;308:898–901.

194. Sox HC, Jr., Liang MH. The erythrocyte sedimentation rate. Guidelines for rational use. *Ann Intern Med.* 1986;104:515–523.

195. Beck JR, Pauker SG. The Markov process in medical prognosis. *Med Decis Making.* 1983;3:419–458.

196. Sindelar WF, Kinsella TJ, Mayer RJ. Cancer of the pancreas. In: DeVita VTJ, Hellman S, Rosenberg SA, eds. *Cancer: Principles & Practice of Oncology.* 2nd ed. Philadelphia, PA: JB Lippincott; 1985:691–739.

197. Freeny PC, Marks WM, Ball TJ. Impact of high-resolution computed tomography of the pancreas on utilization of endoscopic retrograde cholangiopancreatography and angiography. *Radiology.* 1982;142:35–39.

198. Van Dyke JA, Stanley RJ, Berland LL. Pancreatic imaging. *Ann Intern Med.* 1985;102:212–217.

199. Hessel SJ, Siegelman SS, McNeil BJ, et al. A prospective evaluation of computed tomography and ultrasound of the pancreas. *Radiology.* 1982;143:129–133.

200. Redman HC. Standard radiologic diagnosis and CT scanning in pancreatic cancer. *Cancer.* 1981;47:1656–1661.

201. Freeny PC. Computed tomography of the pancreas. *Clin Gastroenterol.* 1984;13:791–818.

202. Manabe T, Miyashita T, Ohshio G, et al. Small carcinoma of the pancreas. Clinical and pathologic evaluation of 17 patients. *Cancer.* 1988;62:135–141.

203. Cello JP. Carcinoma of the pancreas. In: Wyngaarden JB, Smith LHJ, eds. *Cecil Textbook of Medicine.* 18th ed. Philadelphia: WB Saunders; 1988:781–784.

204. Freeny PC, Ball TJ. Endoscopic retrograde cholangiopancreatography (ERCP) and percutaneous transhepatic cholangiography (PTC) in the evaluation of suspected pancreatic carcinoma: diagnostic limitations and contemporary roles. *Cancer.* 1981;47:1666–1678.

205. Moskowitz AJ, Kassirer JP, Pauker SG. Empiric therapy [Abstract]. *Med Decis Making.* 1986;6:267.

206. Einhorn HJ, Hogarth RM. Ambiguity and uncertainty in probabilistic inference. *Psychol Rev.* 1985;92:433–461.

207. Welch WP, Miller ME, Welch HG, et al. Geographic variation in expenditures for physicians' services in the United States. *N Engl J Med.* 1993;328:621–627.

208. Curley SP, Young MJ, Yates JF. Characterizing physicians' perceptions of ambiguity. *Med Decis Making.* 1989;9:116–124.

209. Marschak J, Degroot MH, Marschak J, et al. Personal probabilities of probabilities. *Theory Decision.* 1975;6:121–153.

210. Curley SP, Yates J, Abrams RA. Psychological sources of ambiguity avoidance. *Organ Behav Hum Decis Process.* 1986;38:230–256.

211. Kassirer JP. Our stubborn quest for diagnostic certainty. A cause of excessive testing. *N Engl J Med.* 1989;320:1489–1491.

212. Doubilet P, Begg CB, Weinstein MC, et al. Probabilistic sensitivity analysis using Monte Carlo simulation. A practical approach. *Med Decis Making.* 1985;5:157–177.

213. Doyle AC. The five orange pips. In: *The Complete Sherlock Holmes.* New York: Doubleday; 1930:224–225.

214. Waldrop MM. The necessity of knowledge. *Science.* 1984;223:1279–1282.

215. Tolstoy L. *War and Peace.* New York: Knopf; 2007.

216. Miller DJ, Miller C. On evidence, medical and legal. *J Am Physicians Surgeons.* 2005;10:70–75.

217. Voytovich AE, Rippey RM, Suffredini A. Premature conclusions in diagnostic reasoning. *J Med Educ.* 1985;60:302–307.

218. Carnap R. *The Continuum of Inductive Methods.* Chicago: University of Chicago Press; 1952.

219. Weed LL. *Medical Records, Medical Education, and Patient Care: The Problem-Oriented Record as a Basic Tool.* Cleveland, OH: Case Western Reserve University Press; 1969.

220. Levi P. *The Periodic Table.* New York: Schocken Books; 1984.

221. Schwartz WB, Gorry GA, Kassirer JP, et al. Decision analysis and clinical judgment. *Am J Med.* 1973;55:459–472.

222. Matz R. More principles of medicine. *N Y State J Med.* 1977;77:1984–1985.

223. Feinstein AR. Clinical biostatistics. XLVI. What are the criteria for criteria? *Clin Pharmacol Ther.* 1979;25:108–116.

224. Feinstein AR. Clinical biostatistics. XLV. The purposes and functions of criteria. *Clin Pharmacol Ther.* 1978;24:779–792.

225. Jones criteria (revised) for guidance in the diagnosis of rheumatic fever. *Circulation.* 1965;32:664–668.

226. Rosenberg M, Patterson R, Mintzer R, et al. Clinical and immunologic criteria for the diagnosis of allergic bronchopulmonary aspergillosis. *Ann Intern Med.* 1977;86:405–414.

227. International Study Group for Behcet's Disease. Criteria for diagnosis of Behcet's disease. *Lancet.* 1990;335:1078–1080.

228. Arnett FC, Edworthy SM, Bloch DA, et al. The American Rheumatism Association 1987 revised criteria for the classification of rheumatoid arthritis. *Arthritis Rheumatism.* 1988;31:315–324.

229. Hochberg MC. Updating the American College of Rheumatology revised criteria for the classification of systemic lupus erythematosus. *Arthritis Rheumatism.* 1997;40:1725.

230. Iezzoni LI, Burnside S, Sickles L, et al. Coding of acute myocardial infarction. Clinical and policy implications. *Ann Intern Med.* 1988;109:745–751.

231. Moroff SV, Pauker SG. What to do when the patient outlives the literature, or DEALE-ing with a full deck. *Med Decis Making.* 1983;3:313–338.

232. The PIOPED Investigators. Value of the ventilation/perfusion scan in acute pulmonary embolism. Results of the Prospective Investigation of Pulmonary Embolism Diagnosis (PIOPED). *JAMA.* 1990;263:2753–2759.

233. Bilezikian JP, Potts JT, Fuleihan GEH, et al. Summary statement from a workshop on asymptomatic primary hyperparathyroidism: A perspective for the 21st century. *J Clin Endocrinol Metab.* 2002;87:5353–5361.

234. Ambrogini E, Cetani F, Cianferotti L, et al. Surgery or surveillance for mild asymptomatic primary hyperparathyroidism: a prospective, randomized clinical trial. *J Clin Endocrinol Metab.* 2007;92:3114–3121.

235. Beck JR, Pauker SG, Gottlieb JE, et al. A convenient approximation of life expectancy (the "DEALE"). II. Use in medical decision-making. *Am J Med.* 1982;73:889–897.

236. Geerts WH, Pineo GF, Heit JA, et al. Prevention of venous thromboembolism: The Seventh ACCP Conference on Antithrombotic and Thrombolytic Therapy. *Chest.* 2004;126:338S–400S.

237. World Health Organization. WHO Research into global hazards of travel (WRIGHT) project. Available at: http://www.who.int/cardiovascular_diseases/wright_project/phase1_report/WRIGHT%20REPORT.pdf. Accessed July 28, 2008.

238. Philbrick JT, Shumate R, Siadaty MS, et al. Air travel and venous thromboembolism: A systematic review. *J Gen Intern Med.* 2007;22:107–114.

239. Buller HR, Agnelli G, Hull RD, et al. Antithrombotic therapy for venous thromboembolic disease: The Seventh ACCP Conference on Antithrombotic and Thrombolytic Therapy. *Chest.* 2004;126:401S–428S; Erratum, *Chest.* 2005;127(1):416.

240. Hirsh J, Guyatt G, Albers GW, et al. Executive summary: *American College of Chest Physicians Evidence-Based Clinical Practice Guidelines* (8th Edition). *Chest.* 2008;133:71S–109S.

241. Kearon C, Gent M, Hirsh J, et al. A comparison of three months of anticoagulation with extended anticoagulation for a first episode of idiopathic venous thromboembolism. *N Engl J Med.* 1999;340:901–907; Erratum, *N Engl J Med.* 1999;341(4):298.

242. Agnelli G, Prandoni P, Becattini C, et al. Extended oral anticoagulant therapy after a first episode of pulmonary embolism. *Ann Intern Med.* 2003;139:19–25.

243. Ridker PM, Goldhaber SZ, Danielson E, et al. Long-term, low-intensity warfarin therapy for the prevention of recurrent venous thromboembolism. *N Engl J Med.* 2003;348:1425–1434.

244. Barritt DW, Jordan SC. Anticoagulant drugs in the treatment of pulmonary embolism. A controlled trial. *Lancet.* 1960;1:1309–1312.

245. Eckman MH, Levine HJ, Salem DN, et al. Making decisions about antithrombotic therapy in heart disease: Decision analytic and cost-effectiveness issues. *Chest.* 1998;114:699S–714S.

246. Linkins L-A, Choi PT, Douketis JD. Clinical impact of bleeding in patients taking oral anticoagulant therapy for venous thromboembolism: A meta-analysis. *Ann Intern Med.* 2003;139:893–900.

247. Rosand J, Eckman MH, Knudsen KA, et al. The effect of warfarin and intensity of anticoagulation on outcome of intracerebral hemorrhage. *Arch Intern Med.* 2004;164:880–884.

248. Committee on Quality of Health Care in America. *Crossing the Quality Chasm: A New Health System for the 21st Century.* Washington, DC: National Academy Press; 2001.

249. O'Connor AM, Wennberg JE, Legare F, et al. Toward the 'tipping point': Decision aids and informed patient choice. *Health Aff (Millwood).* 2007;26:716–725.

250. Barry MJ. Health decision aids to facilitate shared decision making in office practice. *Ann Intern Med.* 2002;136:127–135.

251. Elwyn G, Edwards A, Kinnersley P. Shared decision-making in primary care: The neglected second half of the consultation. *Br J Gen Pract.* 1999;49:477–482.

252. Edwards A, Elwyn G. *Evidence-Based Patient Choice.* Oxford University Press; 2001.

253. Briss P, Rimer B, Reilley B, et al. Promoting informed decisions about cancer screening in communities and healthcare systems. *Am J Prev Med.* 2004;26:67–80.

254. Barry MJ. Commentary: How serious is getting a diagnosis of prostate cancer? *Oncologist.* 2008;13: 306–308.

255. McNaughton Collins M, Ransohoff DF, Barry MJ. Early detection of prostate cancer. Serendipity strikes again. *JAMA.* 1997;278:1516–1519.

256. Benson MC, Whang IS, Pantuck A, et al. Prostate specific antigen density: A means of distinguishing benign prostatic hypertrophy and prostate cancer. *J Urol.* 1992;147:815–816.

257. Thompson I, Thrasher JB, Aus G, et al. Guideline for the management of clinically localized prostate cancer: 2007 update. *J Urol.* 2007;177:2106–2131.

258. Walsh PC, DeWeese TL, Eisenberger MA. Clinical practice. Localized prostate cancer. *N Engl J Med.* 2007;357:2696–2705.

259. Pinthus JH, Witkos M, Fleshner NE, et al. Prostate cancers scored as Gleason 6 on prostate biopsy are frequently Gleason 7 tumors at radical prostatectomy: Implication on outcome. *J Urol.* 2006;176: 979–984; discussion, 984.

260. Albertsen PC, Hanley JA, Fine J. 20-year outcomes following conservative management of clinically localized prostate cancer. *JAMA.* 2005;293:2095–2101.

261. Albertsen PC, Hanley JA, Barrows GH, et al. Prostate cancer and the Will Rogers phenomenon. *J Natl Cancer Inst.* 2005;97:1248–1253.

262. Draisma G, Boer R, Otto SJ, et al. Lead times and overdetection due to prostate-specific antigen screening: Estimates from the European Randomized Study of Screening for Prostate Cancer. *J Natl Cancer Inst.* 2003;95:868–878.

263. Parker C, Muston D, Melia J, et al. A model of the natural history of screen-detected prostate cancer, and the effect of radical treatment on overall survival. *Br J Cancer.* 2006;94:1361–1368.

264. Martin RM, Gunnell D, Hamdy F, et al. Continuing controversy over monitoring men with localized prostate cancer: A systematic review of programs in the prostate specific antigen era. *J Urol.* 2006;176:439–449.

265. Klotz L. Active surveillance for prostate cancer: For whom? *J Clin Oncol.* 2005;23:8165–8169.

266. Moneta GL, Edwards JM, Papanicolaou G, et al. Screening for asymptomatic internal carotid artery stenosis: Duplex criteria for discriminating 60% to 99% stenosis. *J Vasc Surg.* 1995;21:989–994.

267. Moneta GL, Edwards JM, Chitwood RW, et al. Correlation of North American Symptomatic Carotid Endarterectomy Trial (NASCET) angiographic definition of 70% to 99% internal carotid artery stenosis with duplex scanning. *J Vasc Surg.* 1993;17:152–157; discussion, 157–159.

268. Halliday A, Mansfield A, Marro J, et al. Prevention of disabling and fatal strokes by successful carotid endarterectomy in patients without recent neurological symptoms: Randomised controlled trial. *Lancet.* 2004;363:1491–1502; Erratum, *Lancet.* 2004;364(9432):416.

269. Executive Committee for the Asymptomatic Carotid Atherosclerosis Study. Endarterectomy for asymptomatic carotid artery stenosis. *JAMA.* 1995;273:1421–1428.

270. Yadav JS, Wholey MH, Kuntz RE, et al. Protected carotid-artery stenting versus endarterectomy in high-risk patients. *N Engl J Med.* 2004;351:1493–1501.

271. Iafrati MD, Salamipour H, Young C, et al. Who needs surveillance of the contralateral carotid artery? *Am J Surg.* 1996;172:136–139.

272. Roederer GO, Langlois YE, Lusiani L, et al. Natural history of carotid artery disease on the side contralateral to endarterectomy. *J Vasc Surg.* 1984;1:62–72.

273. Couser WG. Glomerular disorders. In: Wyngaarden JB, Smith LH, Bennett JC, eds. *Cecil Textbook of Medicine.* 19th ed. Philadelphia: WB Saunders; 1992:551–568.

274. Glassock RJ, Adler SG, Ward HJ, et al. Primary glomerular diseases. In: Brenner BM, Rector FCJ, eds. *The Kidney.* 4th ed. Philadelphia: WB Saunders; 1991:1182–1279.

275. Lee HA, Stirling G, Sharpstone P. Acute glomerulonephritis in middle-aged and elderly patients. *Br Med J.* 1966;2:1361–1363.

276. Glassock RJ, Cohen AH, Adler SG, et al. Secondary glomerular diseases. In: Brenner BM, Rector FCJ, eds. *The Kidney.* 4th ed. Philadelphia: WB Saunders; 1991:1280–1368.

277. Holdsworth S, Boyce N, Thomson NM, et al. The clinical spectrum of acute glomerulonephritis and lung haemorrhage (Goodpasture's syndrome). *Q J Med.* 1985;55:75–86.

278. Johnson JP, Whitman W, Briggs WA, et al. Plasmapheresis and immunosuppressive agents in anti–basement membrane antibody–induced Goodpasture's syndrome. *Am J Med.* 1978;64:354–359.

279. Wiggins RC. Renal biopsy and therapy in glomerular diseases. In: Kelley WN, ed. *Textbook of Internal Medicine.* 2nd ed. Philadelphia: JB Lippincott; 1992:774–787.

280. Keane WF, Michael AL. Renal diseases. In: Samter M, ed. *Immunological Diseases.* Vol. 2. 4th ed. Boston: Little Brown; 1988:1809–1850.

281. Madaio MP, Harrington JT. Current concepts. The diagnosis of acute glomerulonephritis. *N Engl J Med.* 1983;309:1299–1302.

282. Doyle AC. A study in scarlet. In: *The Complete Sherlock Holmes.* New York: Doubleday; 1930:49–50.

283. Doyle AC. The crooked man. In: *The Complete Sherlock Holmes.* New York: Doubleday; 1930:412.

284. Doyle AC. The sign of four. In: *The Complete Sherlock Holmes.* New York: Doubleday; 1930:91.

285. Reagan R. *Farewell address to the nation.* Washington DC: Oval Office; 1989.

286. Elstein AS. Heuristics and biases: Selected errors in clinical reasoning. *Acad Med.* 1999;74:791–794.

287. Pollard P. Human reasoning: Some possible effects of availability. *Cognition.* 1982;12:65–96.

288. Arkes HR. Impediments to accurate clinical judgment and possible ways to minimize their impact. *J Consult Clin Psychol.* 1981;49:323–330.

289. Steel K, Gertman PM, Crescenzi C, et al. Iatrogenic illness on a general medical service at a university hospital. *N Engl J Med.* 1981;304:638–642.

290. Graber ML. Taking steps towards a safer future: Measures to promote timely and accurate medical diagnosis. *Am J Med.* 2008;121:S43–46.

291. Schiff GD. Minimizing diagnostic error: The importance of follow-up and feedback. *Am J Med.* 2008;121:S38–42.

292. Bradley CP. Can we avoid bias? *BMJ.* 2005;330:784.

293. Erneling CE, Johnson DM. *The Mind as a Scientific Object: Between Brain and Culture.* New York: Oxford University Press; 2005.

294. Schachter DL. Memory VI. Introduction. In: Gazzaniga MS, ed. *The Cognitive Neurosciences III.* 3rd ed. Cambridge, MA: MIT Press; 2004:643–645.

295. Anderson JR. Retrieval of information from long-term memory. *Science.* 1983;220:25–30.

296. Simon HA. How big is a chunk? *Science.* 1974;183:482–488.

297. Stein PD, Beemath A, Matta F, et al. Clinical characteristics of patients with acute pulmonary embolism: Data from PIOPED II. *Am J Med.* 2007;120:871–879.

298. Hunter L. Knowledge acquisition planning—Using multiple sources of knowledge to answer questions in biomedicine. *Math Comput Modelling.* 1992;16:79–91.

299. Walker R [1748]. George Anson, A Voyage Round the World in the Years 1740–44. In: Carey J, ed. *Eyewitness to History.* New York: Avon Books; 1987:221.

300. Johnson PE, Duran AS, Hassebrock F, et al. Expertise and error in diagnostic reasoning. *Cogn Sci.* 1981;5:235–283.

301. Case records of the Massachusetts General Hospital. Weekly clinicopathological exercises. Case 26–1987. A 67-year-old man with progressive renal failure. *N Engl J Med.* 1987;316:1642–1651.

302. Croskerry P, Norman G. Overconfidence in clinical decision making. *Am J Med.* 2008;121:S24–S29.

303. Hammond KR, Hamm RM, Grassia J, et al. Direct comparison of the efficacy of intuitive and analytical cognition in expert judgment. *IEEE Trans Syst Man Cybernet.* 1987;17:753–770.

304. Davis R, Buchanan B, Shortliffe E. Production rules as a representation for a knowledge-based consultation program. *Artific Intell.* 1977;8:15–45.

305. Kulikowski CA. Artificial-intelligence methods and systems for medical consultation. *IEEE Trans Pattern Analysis Machine Intelligence.* 1980;2:464–476.

306. Minsky M. A framework for representing knowledge. In: Winston PH, ed. *The Psychology of Computer Vision.* New York: McGraw-Hill; 1975:211–277.

307. Carbonell JG, Michalski RS, Mitchell TM. An overview of machine learning. In: Carbonell JG, Michalski RS, Mitchell TM, eds. *Machine Learning: An Artificial Intelligence Approach.* Los Altos, CA: Morgan Kaufman; 1983:3–23.

308. Michalski RS. A theory and methodology of inductive learning. In: Carbonell JG, Michalski RS, Mitchell TM, eds. *Machine Learning: An Artificial Intelligence Approach.* Los Altos, CA: Morgan Kaufman; 1983:83–134.

309. Dietterich TG, Michalski RS. A comparative review of selected methods for learning from examples. In: Carbonell JG, Michalski RS, Mitchell TM, eds. *Machine Learning: An Artificial Intelligence*

Approach. Los Altos, CA: Morgan Kaufman; 1983: 41–81.

310. Winston PH. Learning structural descriptions from examples. In: Winston PH, ed. *The Psychology of Computer Vision.* New York: McGraw-Hill; 1975:157–209.

311. Schank RC, Collins GC, Hunter LE. Transcend- ing inductive category formation in learning. *Behav Brain Sci.* 1986;9:639–651.

312. Bogdonoff MD. A brief look at medical grand rounds. *Pharos.* 1982;45:16–18.

313. Eddy DM, Clanton CH. The art of diagnosis: solv- ing the clinicopathological exercise. *N Engl J Med.* 1982;306:1263–1268.

INDEX

Page numbers followed by f denote figures, and those followed by t denote tables.

Adequacy of diagnostic hypothesis, 191
Ambiguity, in diagnosis, 15
Anchoring heuristic, 41
Artificial intelligence, 4, 6, 45, 57, 75, 124, 259, 293
Availability heuristic, 104, 255–262

Bayes' rule, 17–18
   advantages, 22–23
   caveats, 23
   in diagnostic tests, 141–143, 141t
   in hypothesis refinement, 14, 22
Benefit-risk ratio (see also Threshold)
   diagnostic tests, 25f
   treatment, 36
Bias, 32

Case-based reasoning, in hypothesis refinement, 12
Case building (see Diagnostic hypothesis, refinement)
Catchall hypothesis, 23
Categorical rules, in reasoning, 75
Causal field, 171, 183
Causal reasoning/model
   definition, (cases 32, 34, 35)
   explaining relations between variables, (cases 11, 33, 34, 36)
   in hypothesis refinement, 11
   in hypothesis verification, language used in, 31
   physiological mechanisms in, 31
   using a causal model, (cases 11, 32, 33, 35, 36)
   where in the diagnostic model does causal reasoning fit?, (cases 11, 33, 34)
Causality, cues to, 183
Cause-effect link, strength, 183
Chunks of information, 55, 280
Clinical reasoning, definition, 3
Clinicopathological conference, as teaching method, 218, 284, 306
Close call decision, 147
Cognition
   definition, 42, (case 65)
   expertise in, 43, 46, (cases 2, 3, 11, 66)
   in problem solving, 5
   search strategies and, 44–46
   structure of memory, (cases 63, 64, 66)
   studying mental processes, (cases 62, 65)
   theories on, 8–9
Cognitive errors (see under Errors)
Cognitive science
   definition, 42
   information chunks in (see Chunks of information)
Coherency
   diagnostic hypothesis
      language used in, 32
Compiled knowledge, in reasoning, 30
Computer programs (see also Artificial intelligence)
   for study of problem-solving processes, 277
   vs. brain function, 44
Condition-action pairs (see also If-Then statements: production rules)
   in memory, 65
Conditional probability, 14, 19f, 23
Confidence, in diagnostic tests, 167–168
Confirmation strategy, in hypothesis refinement, 13
Connectionism, in memory, 44
Context
   causal field as, 171
   for information gathering
      diagnostic classification and, 11–12
      hypothesis generation and, 9
      language used in, 48
Costs, diagnostic tests, 15, 25f
Criteria, for hypothesis verification, 31

Data-driven reasoning, in information processing, 45–46, 45t
Decision analysis
   in treatment, 221, 225
   threshold calculation, 26, 34–35, 160
Decision making (see also Information processing Problem solving)
   close-call, 34, 147
   in test ordering, 134
   in treatment, 4
   in uncertain conditions, 22, 23
   quantitative, 34–35
   toss-up, 34
   trade-offs in, 34
Decision theory, 4, 34, 112

Decision threshold (*see* Threshold)

Decision tree, 35, 161–162, 162f

Descriptive approach
  to information gathering, 112–113
  to reasoning study, 42

Deterministic reasoning, in hypothesis refinement, 11

Diagnosing strategy, in hypothesis refinement, 112–113

Diagnosis
  as probability distribution, 22
  differential, in hypothesis refinement, 102, 119, 124
  inference in, 247

Diagnostic classification
  context for information gathering and, 39, 111–112

Diagnostic entropy reduction, 111

Diagnostic hypothesis, 111
  adequacy, 76, 87
  alternatives to, 112–113
  as framework, 183
  basis for, 66, 68, 73, 74, 83
  coherency, 76
  discarding, 8
  evolution, 12
  falsification, 31
  forms for, 8
  function, 31
  generation, 56–88
    causal reasoning in, 29–30
    classification, (cases 16, 27, 54, 55, 57, 58)
    cognitive basis, 8–9, (cases 1, 3, 6, 23, 57, 63)
    context for information gathering, 111–112
    cues for, 100
    errors in, 9–10, (cases 3, 9, 54, 58, 66)
    expertise for, 9–10, 60–63, (cases 3, 9, 54, 58, 66)
    false starts in, 73
    hypotheses and cues, (cases 1, 2, 3, 4, 16)
    hypotheses as a context, (cases 7, 8)
    in atypical disease, 83
    in life-threatening situations, 9
    in rare disease, 63
    information gathering for, 93
    language used in, 57, 66
    models for, 202
    short cuts in, 8–9
  intermediate, 86
  parsimonious, 76
  premature closure, 31–32
  priority assignment, language used in, 209, 237
  reappearance during evolution, 12
  refinement
    boundaries, 101
    causal reasoning in, 11, 93
    context and diagnostic classification, (cases 7, 9, 63, 64)
    context for information gathering, 111–112
    data collection sequence in, 12–13
    diagnostic entropy reduction in, 13–14, 111
    differential diagnosis, (cases 10, 18, 38)
    discrimination in, language used in, 121–125
    discrimination strategy in, 13, 14
    disease variations and, 11

  errors in, 13, 124
  evolution in, 12
  hypotheses active in, 93
  hypothesis evolution, (cases 1, 10, 12, 16, 33)
  language used in, 99
  priority assignment, 14
  probabilistic approach in, 14
  reducing diagnostic uncertainty, (cases 9, 12, 15, 18, 38)
  relation to formal probabilistic approach, (cases 23, 27, 42)
  sequence of data collection, (cases 14, 24, 45)
  testing in, 12–13
  where refinement begins and ends, (cases 1, 12, 13, 16, 17, 37, 38)
  triggering, 60–63
  verification, (*see also* working diagnosis)
    after refinement, 11
    definition, 11, (cases 37, 38, 39, 56)
    errors in, 32
    final, 31, 191
    language used in, 155
    premature closure in, 31–32, (cases 5, 8, 12, 33, 39, 53, 56)
    unclear diagnosis in, 236
    validity criteria in, 31, (cases 12, 17, 38, 39, 40, 43)
    working diagnosis, (cases 9, 39, 41)

Diagnostic tests
  ambiguity in, 15, 147, 167
  Bayes' rule and, 17–18, 142–143, (cases 20, 23, 30, 51)
  Bayesian revision for multiple disease with multiple attributes, (cases 23, 27)
  benefit-risk ratio, 25f
  confirmatory, 18, 23, 136
  cost, 136
  decisions to perform, 4
  disease prevalence in, 5
  errors in, 13
  expected utility, 112, 160, 164
  false negative/positive results, 16f, 17, 18f
  for multiple disease with multiple attributes, 21–22
  function, 15
  gold standard in (*see* gold standard)
  interpretation
    causal reasoning in, 12
    disease stage and, 23
    language used in, 48
    probabilistic, 15–16
  interpreting results, (cases 20, 23, 26, 29)
  negative results, 16f, 20f
  positive results, 20f, 25
  pragmatic considerations in probabilistic approach, 22–23, (cases 23, 31, 42, 43)
  prevalence of disease and, 127
  principles, 18–19
  quantifying testing decisions, 15–16, (cases 20, 23, 26, 27, 29, 30, 31)
  sensitivity, 16–17, (cases 20, 23, 26)
  specificity, 16–17, (cases 20, 23, 26)
  testing principles, (cases 20, 22, 23, 29)
  testing thresholds, (cases 25, 29, 30, 51)
  therapeutic threshold and, 24–25, 25f, (cases 22, 45, 51)

threshold concept and, 24, (cases 24, 29, 30, 45, 51, 52)
true negative/positive results, 16, 16f
when to test, (cases 23, 25, 28, 29, 30, 45)
Diagnostic uncertainty, 13–14, 33, 73, 111–112, 202
Differential diagnosis, in hypothesis refinement
language used in, 99
Discrimination strategy, in hypothesis refinement, 191
Disease stages, test interpretation and, 23
Domain expert, transcript analysis by, 42

Elimination strategy, in hypothesis refinement, 112
Entropy, diagnostic reduction, 111
Errors
cognitive, 39–41
classification, 39, 40t, (cases 16, 27, 54, 55, 57, 58)
consequences, 40–41, (cases 16, 43, 52, 56, 57, 58)
in hypothesis generation, 39, 272t
in hypothesis refinement, 272t
in hypothesis verification, 277
in laboratory, 40, (case 57)
nature of, 39–40, (cases 31, 36, 39, 54, 55, 56, 57, 58)
psychological factors in, 39, (case 5)
no fault, 39, 40t, 274
types, 39
Evolution, diagnostic hypothesis, 12
Examining evidence
Evidence-based medicine, (cases 23, 48, 49, 50)
Examples, in learning problem solving, 49–50
Exemplar, information storage in, 43
Expected utility
diagnostic tests, 19, 160
treatment, 164, 165
Expertise
characteristics, 46–47
in hypothesis generation, 63
problem solving, 48

False negative/positive results, diagnostic tests, 16–17, 16f
Falsification, diagnostic hypothesis, 31
Frame
in artificial intelligence, 293–294
in memory, 42–43

Generate and test strategy, in information processing, 45
Generation, hypothesis (see under Diagnostic hypothesis)
Goal-driven reasoning, in information processing, 45–46
Gold standard, diagnostic tests
unreliability, 294
Grand rounds, as teaching method, 49, 299, 304

Heuristic(s)
anchoring
cognitive errors and, 40
availability, 40–41, 66
expert use of, 46
in diagnostic hypothesis generation, 59
representativeness, 60
Hypothesis, diagnostic (see Diagnostic hypothesis)
Hypothesis confirming strategy (see Confirmation strategy)

Hypothesis elimination strategy (see Confirmation strategy)
Hypothesis generation, 9–10, 39, 40t, 56–88
Hypothesis modification, 5
Hypothesis verification, 31, 277
Hypothetico-deductive reasoning, 45

If-Then statements
in computer program, 289–290
in memory, 42
Inductive reasoning, 5
Inference, in diagnosis, 5
Information, interpretation (see also Diagnostic tests, interpretation)
Information gathering (see also Diagnostic tests)
context for
diagnostic classification and, 11–12
hypothesis generation and, 185
in abnormal situation, 11
language used in, 34, 48
errors in, 39
for decision analysis, 34
for diagnostic classification, 11–12
for hypothesis refinement
descriptive approach, 112–113
prescriptive approach, 112
sequence, 12–13
in medical education, 298
strategies for, 290
Information processing (see also decision making: problem solving)
cognitive science view, 42
errors in, 274
expertise in, 291–294
memory in (see Memory)
search strategies in, 44–46
top-down, 45t
Information storage (see also Chunks of information: Memory)
in scripts, 12
Instance scripts, information storage in, 43
Instantiate (instantiation), in learning problem solving, 51
Interpretation, diagnostic test (see under Diagnostic tests)
Intuition, in problem solving, 13

Language used in diagnosis, 34
Learning clinical problem solving
facts versus process, (cases 46, 60, 67, 69)
learning by instantiation, (cases 67, 68, 69)
pedagogic principles, (cases 60, 69)
specific example, (case 69)
Long-term memory, 280–281

Markov process, in decision analysis, 161
Means-end analysis, in information processing, 45
Memory
connectionism in, 44
in hypothesis refinement, 11–12
limitations, 12
long-term, 280, 284
neuronal function in, 249–250

Memory (*Continued*)
    parallel distributed processing in, 44
    short-term, 44
    skilled (working), 12, 44, 46, 75, 83, 100, 120, 185, 277, 280–281, 299
    structure, 279–281
    working (skilled) , 12, 44, 46, 75, 83, 100, 120, 185, 277, 280–281, 299
Mental processes, in reasoning (*see also* Information processing: memory; search strategies)
Models, causal (*see* Causal reasoning/model)
Monte Carlo simulation, 168
Multiple diseases, test interpretation in, 21–22

Negative results, diagnostic tests, 130–131
No fault errors, 40t, 274

Ockham's razor, 6

Parallel distributed processing, in memory, 44
Parsimony, diagnostic hypothesis, 31
Physical symbol system hypothesis of memory, 42–44
Physiological mechanisms, in causal reasoning, 28, 29, 30, 31, 37
Polymorphism, in disease
    memory storage and, 281–286
Positive results, diagnostic tests
    levels, 25, 25f
Posterior probability, 15–16, 19f, 20f, 21f, 22f, 22, 23, 232
Premature closure, diagnostic hypothesis, 31–32
Prescriptive approach, to information gathering, 112
Prescriptive process, in hypothesis refinement, 14
Prevalence of disease
    diagnostic tests and, 127
    in hypothesis generation, 142
    in hypothesis refinement, 15, 17, 18, 29
    language used in, 48, 57, 66, 155
Prior probability, 15–16, 17t, 18f, 19f, 20f, 21f, 22f, 22–23, 123, 130, 142, 145, 155, 162, 215, 228
Probabilistic approach
    ambiguity in, 15, 168
    disease polymorphism and, 281–286
    in diagnostic testing, 15–16
    in hypothesis refinement, 13, 14
    vs. causal reasoning, 28, 29–30
Probability
    conditional, 14, 16, 19f, 22, 22f, 23, 113, 155, 202, 279
    posterior, 15–16, 19–21f, 22–23, 112, 155, 163, 197, 232
    prior, 15–16, 17t, 18f, 19f, 20f, 21f, 22f, 22–23, 123, 130, 142, 145, 155, 162, 215, 228
    threshold (therapeutic threshold), 24, 25f, 26f, 131, 215, 238
Probability distribution, 22
Problem-based learning, 51
Problem solving (*see also* Decision making; information processing)
    expertise in, 46–47
    intuition in, 13
    learning, 51

    brain function in, 44
    case selection for, 304–305
    clinicopathological conference in, 48
    examples for clinical rotation group, 49
    facilitator role in, 51, 307
    facts vs. process in, 48–49
    format preparation for, 299
    grand rounds methods in, 49
    instantiation in, 50–51
    language used in, 48
    pedagogic principles in, 49
    techniques for, 47
    vs. problem—based learning, 51
    mental processes in, 42
    strategies for, 5
    strong methods for, 45–46
    weak methods for, 44–45
Problem space, in hypothesis refinement, 13, 80
Production rules (*see also* If-Then statements)
    in memory, 291
Protocol analysis, 42, 277
Psychological factors, in errors, 39

Quantitative decision making, 22

Reasoning
    case-based, in hypothesis refinement, 12
    causal (*see* Causal reasoning/model)
    data-driven, in information processing, 45–46
    definition, 179
    deterministic, in hypothesis refinement, 75
    expertise in, 46–47
    goal-driven, in information processing, 45–46, 45t
    inductive, 286–291
    mental processes in, 42
    search strategies in, 44–46
Refinement, diagnostic hypothesis (*see under* Diagnostic hypothesis)
Regret, as error factor, 160
Reminding (*see also* Triggering)
    in information processing, 43–44
Representativeness heuristic
    cognitive errors and, 40, 41
Retrospective bias, in reasoning, 40, 118, 211
Rule-based reasoning, 75
Rules (*see also* Production rules)
    in artificial intelligence, 124, 259, 293
    procedural, in treatment, 42

Script, information storage in
    instance, 43
Search strategies, in information processing, 44–46
Sensitivity of diagnostic tests, 16–17
Sensitivity analysis
    in test interpretation, 151–152
    in test ordering, 134
    in treatment, 151
Short-term memory
    in diagnostic hypothesis generation, 75

Skilled (working) memory, 44, 280
Specificity, diagnostic tests, 16–17
Strategy
    confirmation, 13, 112
    diagnosing, 112–113
    discrimination, 13, 191
    elimination, 13, 32, 112–113
    search, 44–46
Strong problem-solving methods, 45–46
Sutton's law, in diagnosis, 113–118
Systematic search, in information processing, 44–46

Testing threshold, 25–27, 26f, 160, 163–164, 164f
Therapeutic decision making
    incommensurate options, (cases 46, 47)
    quantitative decision making, (cases 23, 30, 45, 47, 51)
    treatment under conditions of uncertainty, (cases 41, 44, 48, 50, 53)
    when value of therapeutic choices is close, (cases 25, 26, 46, 50, 51)
Therapeutic principles, 6–7
Therapeutic threshold, 24–25, 25f, 233–234
Threshold
    definition, 7
    function, 7
    in diagnostic testing, 24
    testing, 25–27, 26f, 160, 163–164, 164f
    therapeutic, 24–25
Top-down processing, 45
Toss-up decision, 34, 218
Trade-offs, in decision making, 34
Transcript analysis, 42, 124, 277–278
Treatment
    benefit-risk ratio in, 25

    causal reasoning in, 28–30
    close choices for, 34
    decision analysis in, 7
    decision making in, 23
    diagnosis linked to, 7
    expected utility, 164
    in uncertain conditions, 33
    incommensurate options for, 34
    patient preferences in, 226
    reliance on randomized controlled trials, 33
    sensitivity analysis in, 35, 164–165, 165f
    threshold concept and, 24
    withholding, 24–27
Triggering, diagnostic hypothesis, 60–63
True negative/positive results, diagnostic tests, 16–17, 16–17f, 18f

Uncertainty (*see also* Entropy)
    language expressing, 34, 57
    treatment under, 33
Utility, expected
    diagnostic tests, 164
    treatment, 164

Variables, relations between, causal reasoning and, 28, 30, 178–179
Verification, hypothesis (*see under* Diagnostic hypothesis)

Weak problem solving methods, 44–45
Working diagnosis, 5, 32, 195, 208
    causal reasoning in, 30
    coherency, 28, 30, 31–32
    criteria, 31
Working (skilled) memory, 44, 280